Practical Atlas of Breast Pathology

Simona Stolnicu • Isabel Alvarado-Cabrero
Editors

Practical Atlas of Breast Pathology

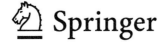 Springer

Editors
Simona Stolnicu
Department of Pathology
University of Medicine and Pharmacy
Tîrgu Mureş
Romania

Isabel Alvarado-Cabrero
Department of Pathology
Hospital de Oncologia
Centro Medico Nacional Siglo XXI
Instituto Mexicano del Seguro Social
Mexico City
Mexico

ISBN 978-3-319-93256-9   ISBN 978-3-319-93257-6   (eBook)
https://doi.org/10.1007/978-3-319-93257-6

Library of Congress Control Number: 2018949947

This Springer imprint is published by Springer Nature, under the registered company Springer International
Publishing AG
The registered company address is: Gewerbestrasse 11, 6330 Cham, Switzerland

To my family, for their endless love and support to achieve an academic career.

Simona Stolnicu

To my mother, who taught me the love for reading.
To my siblings for the shared adventures.
To you.... the wind beneath my wings.

Isabel Alvarado-Cabrero

Foreword

As the title indicates, this breast pathology atlas is focused on providing the reader with a practical approach to breast pathology. The editors have assembled an international group of breast pathology experts who present up-to-date criteria for diagnosis and differential diagnosis of breast lesions. Succinct text is accompanied by numerous illustrations. The focus of the atlas is, as it should be, on diagnosis of breast lesions using hematoxylin- and eosin-stained sections, but the role of adjunctive studies to aid in diagnosis is emphasized and illustrated where appropriate. Important contemporary issues such as core needle biopsy (with an emphasis on the importance of radiologic–pathologic correlation), sentinel lymph node biopsy, and treatment-related changes are each addressed in their own chapters, as are the role of immunohistochemistry in breast pathology, prognostic and predictive factors, and molecular pathology basics. This atlas should serve as a useful, easy-to-use resource for pathology trainees and practicing pathologists alike.

Stuart J. Schnitt, MD
Dana-Farber Cancer Institute/Brigham and Women's
Hospital Breast Oncology Program
Dana-Farber/Brigham and Women's Cancer Center
Harvard Medical School,
Boston, MA, USA

Preface

In recent decades, there has been remarkable progress due to many changes and discoveries that have been published in the breast pathology field. Diagnosis of breast lesions has become challenging for pathologists, but also very important concerning the impact on the patient's treatment and, consequently, on survival.

There are many breast pathology textbooks available on the market that often present exhaustive information. Our book is an atlas, designed as a practical approach for understanding and practicing breast pathology through pictures.

This atlas is mainly dedicated to trainees and practicing pathologists in surgical pathology with an interest in breast pathology and tackling the daily sign-out. This easy-to-use practical guidebook explains how to tackle the diagnosis, emphasizing diagnostic clues for each entity as well as pitfalls and mimickers. This is the reason why each chapter includes short and concise text mostly illustrated with numerous high-quality pictures with explanatory legends highlighting the pearls and pitfalls in the diagnosis of breast lesions. This manner of presentation will help readers quickly assimilate the essential information about all breast lesions.

We have included the most important and frequent benign and malignant lesions of the breast. We have also included a separate chapter dedicated to normal breast anatomy and histology, which is very important for understanding breast pathology, and a separate chapter for breast radiology–pathology correlations, which is essential in understanding and diagnosing the breast lesions especially in a multidisciplinary team. We dedicated a special chapter to the core needle biopsy with radiological–pathological correlations since breast lesions are diagnosed using this method in most medical centers all over the world. Additionally, because cytology is still used in many breast units to diagnose breast lesions, we have added a chapter dedicated to this technique, which is easy to apply and cheaper compared to others, although sometimes it has its limitations. Sampling is essential in breast pathology and for this reason we have demonstrated the grossing method in a separate chapter. The molecular classification and its surrogate immunohistochemical evaluation have completely changed the diagnosis and treatment for breast carcinoma, which is why we have dedicated special chapters to these topics.

We hope that both pathologists and clinicians with a particular interest in this area will find this book interesting.

Tîrgu Mureş, Romania   Simona Stolnicu, MD, PhD
Mexico City, Mexico   Isabel Alvarado-Cabrero, MD, PhD

Acknowledgments

We would like to thank Adrian Naznean from the Foreign Language Department, University of Medicine and Pharmacy of Tirgu Mures, for translating and correcting several chapters of this book. We would also like to thank Dr. Susan DeWyngaert for providing the radiologic images and Dr. Esteban Gnass for his help with the images in Chapter 9. We thank our colleagues who provided interesting and challenging cases in consultation over the years. Also, we would like to thank our residents who helped us in our daily practice but also for raising interesting questions that helped us to better understand breast pathology.

Simona Stolnicu, Tîrgu Mureş, Romania
Isabel Alvarado-Cabrero, Mexico City, Mexico

Contents

1 **Histology of the Normal Breast, Normal Changes, and Abnormalities of Breast Development** 1
Simona Stolnicu

2 **Radiology of the Normal Breast and Overview of Breast Imaging Reporting and Data System** 27
Eloisa Asia Sanchez-Vivar and Isabel Alvarado-Cabrero

3 **Core-Needle Biopsy: Radiologic-Pathologic Correlation** 43
Isabel Alvarado-Cabrero and Eloisa Asia Sanchez-Vivar

4 **Fine Needle Aspiration of Breast Cytology** 63
Rana S. Hoda and Rema A. Rao

5 **Inflammatory and Reactive Lesions of the Breast** 91
Simona Stolnicu

6 **Papillary Tumors of the Breast** 109
Helenice Gobbi and Marina De Brot

7 **Benign Lesions (Proliferations) and Tumors of the Breast** 125
Simona Stolnicu

8 **Myoepithelial Lesions and Tumors of the Breast** 173
Michael Z. Gilcrease

9 **Fibroepithelial Lesions of the Breast** 183
Danielle Fortuna, Adam Toll, and Juan P. Palazzo

10 **Diagnostic Evaluation of Usual Ductal Hyperplasia and Atypical Ductal Hyperplasia** 205
Anna Biernacka and Melinda F. Lerwill

11 **Ductal Carcinoma In Situ** 227
Isabel Alvarado-Cabrero

12 **Microinvasive Carcinoma** 239
Simona Stolnicu

13 **Atypical Lobular Hyperplasia and Lobular Carcinoma In Situ** 243
Isabel Alvarado-Cabrero

14 **Infiltrating Carcinoma of No Special Type** 251
Simona Stolnicu

15 **Special Types of Invasive Breast Carcinoma** 263
Javier A. Arias-Stella III, Isabel Alvarado-Cabrero, and Fresia Pareja

16 **Hematopoietic Lesions of the Breast** 293
Isabel Alvarado-Cabrero

17 **The Role of Immunohistochemistry in Breast Pathology** 305
    Syed A. Hoda

18 **Prognostic and Predictive Factors in Breast Carcinoma** 327
    Simona Stolnicu

19 **Basic Molecular Pathology in Breast Carcinoma** 357
    Maria Comanescu

20 **Morphologic Changes Induced by the Oncologic Treatment for
    Breast Carcinoma (Chemotherapy, Radiotherapy, Hormonal Therapy)** 373
    Aziza Nassar

21 **Evaluation of Residual Tumor After Neoadjuvant Treatment** 383
    Aziza Nassar

22 **Sentinel Lymph Node: Clinicopathologic Features** 391
    Isabel Alvarado-Cabrero and Sergio A. Rodríguez-Cuevas

23 **Mesenchymal Tumors of the Breast** 403
    Helenice Gobbi and Cristiana Buzelin Nunes

24 **Breast Lesions/Neoplasms in Men** 423
    Filippo Borri and Alessandro Bombonati

25 **Lesions of the Nipple** 445
    Simona Stolnicu

26 **Metastatic Tumors to the Breast** 459
    Isabel Alvarado-Cabrero

27 **Sampling and Evaluation of the Breast Surgical Specimens** 475
    Raquel Valencia-Cedillo

28 **Dermatologic Diseases of the Breast and Nipple** 491
    Anca Chiriac

Index 509

Contributors

Isabel Alvarado-Cabrero, MD, PhD Department of Pathology, Hospital de Oncologia, Centro Medico Nacional Siglo XXI, Instituto Mexicano del Seguro Social, Mexico City, Mexico

Javier A. Arias-Stella III, MD Department of Pathology, Memorial Sloan Kettering Cancer Center, New York, NY, USA

Anna Biernacka, MD, PhD Department of Pathology, The University of Chicago Medicine and Biological Sciences, Chicago, IL, USA

Alessandro Bombonati, MD Pathology and Laboratory Medicine Department, Einstein Medical Center, Philadelphia, PA, USA

Filippo Borri, MD Pathology and Laboratory Medicine Department, Einstein Medical Center, Philadelphia, PA, USA

Pathology Department, University of Rome, Tor Vergata, Rome, Italy

Marina De Brot, MD, PhD Department of Anatomic Pathology, A. C. Camargo Cancer Center, Sao Paulo, Brazil

Anca Chiriac, MD, PhD Department of Dermatology, Nicolina Medical Center, Iaşi, Romania

Department of Dermato-Physiology, Apollonia University, Iaşi, Romania

P. Poni Institute of Macromolecular Chemistry, Iaşi, Romania

Maria Comanescu, MD, PhD Department of Pathology, University of Medicine and Pharmacy "Carol Davila", Bucharest, Romania

Danielle Fortuna, MD Department of Pathology, Thomas Jefferson University, Philadelphia, PA, USA

Michael Z. Gilcrease, MD, PhD Pathology and Laboratory Medicine, Department of Pathology, The University of Texas M. D. Anderson Cancer Center, Houston, TX, USA

Helenice Gobbi, MD, PhD Department of Surgery, Institute of Health Sciences, Federal University of Triangulo Mineiro, Uberaba, MG, Brazil

Rana S. Hoda, MD CBLPath, Rye Brook, NY, USA

Syed A. Hoda, MD New York Presbyterian Hospital-Weill Cornell Medical College, New York, NY, USA

Melinda F. Lerwill, MD Department of Pathology, Massachusetts General Hospital and Harvard Medical School, Boston, MA, USA

Aziza Nassar, MD, MPH Pathology and Laboratory Medicine, Mayo Clinic, Jacksonville, FL, USA

Cristiana Buzelin Nunes, PhD Department of Anatomic Pathology, Faculty of Medicine, Federal University of Minas Gerais, Belo Horizonte, MG, Brazil

Juan P. Palazzo, MD Department of Pathology, Thomas Jefferson University Hospital, Philadelphia, PA, USA

Fresia Pareja, MD, PhD Department of Pathology, Memorial Sloan Kettering Cancer Center, New York, NY, USA

Rema A. Rao, MD Papanicolaou Cytology Laboratory, Weill Cornell Medicine/New York Presbyterian Hospital, New York, NY, USA

Sergio A. Rodríguez-Cuevas, MD Breast Institute, FUCAM, Mexico, Mexico

Eloisa Asia Sanchez-Vivar, MD Radiology Department, Hospital de Oncologia, Centro Medico Nacional Siglo XXI, Instituto Mexicano del Seguro Social, Mexico City, Mexico

Simona Stolnicu, MD, PhD Department of Pathology, University of Medicine and Pharmacy, Tîrgu Mureş, Romania

Adam Toll, MD Department of Pathology, St. Luke's University Health Network, Bethlehem, PA, USA

Raquel Valencia-Cedillo, MD Department of Pathology, Hospital de Oncologia, Centro Medico Nacional Siglo XXI, Instituto Mexicano del Seguro Social, Mexico City, Mexico

Histology of the Normal Breast, Normal Changes, and Abnormalities of Breast Development

Simona Stolnicu

The breast, a modified sweat gland and target for different hormones, lies on the anterior chest wall over the pectoralis major muscle and has the specialized function of feeding the newborn infant. The breast displays various morphologic alteration throughout the reproductive life cycle (menarche, pregnancy, lactation, and menopause, in addition to maternal hormonal effects in utero). By understanding its normal morphology, normal changes, and immunohistochemical profile, breast pathologists are better able to identify and diagnose breast lesions, also by using ancillary examinations. A variety of abnormalities can occur during the development of the breast, most of which can be easily corrected with the help of cosmetic surgery.

1.1 Histology of the Normal Breast and Normal Changes

The mammary gland is a modified sweat gland, influenced by the hormones prolactin, estrogen, and progesterone, which have active or passive roles in its physiology. This gland is located on the anterior thoracic wall, corresponding to the space between ribs 2 and 6 in the vertical axis and between the sternal edge and the midaxillary line in the horizontal axis, wrapped by the superficial pectoral major muscle fascia, which is the posterior/deep margin, and the underlying deep pectoral fascia (which covers the pectoralis major muscle). The two fasciae are connected by fibrous strips (Cooper's ligament attachment), which is a natural support for the breast tissue.

The shape, weight, size, density, and spread of breast tissue into the adjacent tissue (for example, within pectoralis muscle fibers) differ from one person to another and are influenced by the individual's body habitus. This has a very practical impact on cosmetic surgery, but also results in the fact that even a total mastectomy does not achieve the removal of all breast glandular tissue, meaning that prophylactic mastectomy substantially, but not entirely, reduces the risk of developing breast cancer [1].

Primitive mammary crests (or milk lines) develop in the human embryo in the fifth week of gestation and consist of two epidermal thickenings, which stretch from the armpit to the groin. Immediately after their formation, the greatest part regresses, except for a small portion of the pectoral region. In weeks 12–16 of gestation, the nipple and areola develop. Sequentially, the underlying epithelial buds appear. All these changes are independent of hormonal influences. The first differences between the sexes occur at the end of the first

S. Stolnicu, MD, PhD
Department of Pathology, University of Medicine and Pharmacy, Tîrgu Mureș, Romania

© Springer International Publishing AG, part of Springer Nature 2018
S. Stolnicu, I. Alvarado-Cabrero (eds.), *Practical Atlas of Breast Pathology*, https://doi.org/10.1007/978-3-319-93257-6_1

trimester of pregnancy, under the action of estrogen and testosterone. Throughout the third trimester (weeks 20–32), under the influence of placental hormones, a channeling system develops from the epithelial buds, initially in the form of full cords in which ducts form in time, which will give rise to lactiferous ducts. The myoepithelial cells are differentiated in weeks 24–28 of intrauterine life, and will undergo subsequent quantitative or morphological changes only in pathological lesions. Between weeks 32 and 40, nipple and areola pigmentation occur.

Immediately after birth, a transient breast hyperplasia may occur, due to the transplacental action of maternal hormones. Breast tissue appears as dilated ducts filled with secretory material, which is also observed as a liquid in the nipple in both sexes. This typically continues until weeks 3–4 postpartum, but can sometimes extend to several months or even up to puberty. This type of breast hyperplasia should not be confused with a pathological process because its surgical excision leads to amastia.

Until puberty, the primary duct system branches, but remains at a rudimentary stage in both sexes (Figs. 1.1 and 1.2).

At puberty, the mammary gland in females develops under the action of hormones secreted by the pituitary gland and ovaries. This occurs by the continuous branching of the ducts simultaneously with the proliferation of periductal stroma (under the effect of ovarian estrogen) and by the development of lobules (under the effect of estrogen and progesterone). Regarding the lobules, at the end of elongated and branched ducts, an initial thickening of the channeling epithelium will occur, forming the so-called "waiting buds." They consist of small spheroid masses composed of polygonal epithelial cells, which do not define a lumen. These spherules, along with intralobular channels, will form Type 1 lobules, features of nulliparous women (Fig. 1.3). In younger patients (during puberty), as compared to adults, the intralobular stroma is dense and appears to have a similar appearance to the extralobular one (Fig. 1.4). This increase in the amount of connective tissue at this age can produce pseudo-nodular areas on palpation (by the clinicians) but also on macroscopic and microscopic examination (especially by inexperienced pathologists), and should not be confused with the pathologic process of fibrosis because it may lead to unnecessary surgery.

Sometimes, before puberty, an increase in the size of the mammary gland may occur under the action of endogen hormones. This anomaly is called premature thelarche and, on microscopy, it is characterized by a proliferation of the ducts and acini, arranged in a denser collagenous stroma. Simultaneously, an increase in the volume of adipose tissue occurs. These patients may be at early puberty, but studies have also shown frequent association of this condition with the subsequently development of breast carcinoma.

The mammary gland presents complete pigmentation of the areola and nipple in adults. The nipple is located in the central area of the breast and is surrounded by areola. It consists of bundles of smooth muscle fibers and elastic tissue, passed through by lactiferous ducts (14–24 ducts may be seen within each nipple), which end in an opening. Smooth muscle fibers are arranged radially and longitudinally (Figs. 1.5, 1.6, and 1.7). In some cases, in the region of the nipple the smooth muscle bundles show hyperplasia, which may lead to the increase of the nipple volume (Fig. 1.8). This process must be differentiated from leiomyoma (a benign nodule with well-defined margins) or leiomyosarcoma (a malignant tumor with infiltrative margins, atypia, presence of atypical mitoses and areas of necrosis) of the nipple. In up to 20% of cases, careful examination of the nipple will also reveal mammary lobules (this is the reason that some special subtypes of breast carcinoma also occur initially within the nipple and not only in the terminal duct-acini unit) (Figs. 1.9 and 1.10) [2, 3]. The epidermis covering the nipple and areola is composed of stratified squamous epithelium in the thickness of which clear cells can be identified in some patients (considered Paget precursor cells, also known as Toker cells) (Figs. 1.10 and 1.11). These cells are larger than the adjacent keratinocytes, with a round or oval nucleus and pale cytoplasm, but no intracytoplasmic mucin is present, and they are negative for carcinoembryonic antigen (CEA). Some authors have highlighted pre-Paget dysplastic changes within these cells. As such, they should not be confused with Paget cells. The dermis may present sebaceous and eccrine sweat glands, and hair follicles may sometimes appear on the margin of the areola (Fig. 1.12). Some large sebaceous glands open to the surface through a duct, corresponding to 10–15 small rounded uniform formations called Montgomery tubercles (present in both women and men) (Fig. 1.13). These structures can proliferate after puberty and become prominent during pregnancy, but they undergo atrophy with age and have little importance in the routine practice because pathological lesions develop very rarely at this site. However, sebaceous gland hyperplasia was described for the first time in the areolar area in an adult patient, as a bilateral lesion developed after the patient gave birth [4]. Few other communications of this lesion have been published in either women or men; most of those that have been reported were of a bilateral presentation, whereas in others the presentation was unilateral [5]. Macroscopically, nipple sebaceous gland hyperplasia consists of multiple, soft, normal-colored or yellowish papules or nodules, with central umbilication (Fig. 1.14). When the lesions involve large areas of the nipple and areola, and when they develop in postmenopausal patients, Paget's nipple disease associated with malignant breast lesions should be ruled out from a clinical point of view. Microscopically, the lesion is represented by hyperplastic and hypertrophic mature sebaceous glands aggregated in the dermis, sometimes extending into the epidermis (Fig. 1.15).

The area of the areola increases in size during pregnancy and becomes more pigmented, changes that do not disappear subsequently. Inverted nipple is a congenital anomaly that can sometimes occur, predisposing the female to the development of mammary duct ectasia (Figs. 1.16 and 1.17). It should not be confused with an invasive malignancy on macroscopic or microscopic examination (Fig. 1.18).

The adult mammary gland is composed of 15–20 independent glandular units called mammary lobes, arranged radially around the nipple. Each lobe drains through a single channel, called the lactiferous canal, which opens in the nipple. A lobe is in turn constituted by a ductal-acini structure, surrounded by fibrous connective septa. The septa separate one breast lobe from another and divide each lobe into a variable number of lobules. Highlighting the septa is difficult in terms of both surgical and anatomical pathology. For this reason it is almost impossible to define the boundaries between lobes from a surgical point of view and to perform a "segmentectomy" in some of the breast lesions. The connective tissue, which forms the septa, is not hormone-dependent. Histologically, the ductal (canalicular) system is divided into several segments. The deep segment of the ductal system is called terminal duct and comprises an intralobular portion and an extra-lobular one. Several terminal ducts unite and constitute subsegmental ducts, which in turn drain into segmental ducts. Segmental ducts unite and form lactiferous ducts, which open in the nipple (Fig. 1.19).

The superficial portion of the duct orifice is covered by squamous epithelium, which may extend for a short distance into the most distal portion of the duct (Fig. 1.20). The squamous-columnar junction, where the squamous epithelium joins the columnar epithelium, is normally distal to a dilated segment of the duct called the lactiferous sinus. The extension of the squamous epithelium beyond the lactiferous sinus is called squamous metaplasia, a condition that may lead to the obstruction of the lactiferous duct and the development of a subareolar abscess.

Except for a small portion adjacent to the nipple, in which the system of ducts is covered by squamous epithelium, the whole ductal system is lined by two layers of cells: the inner continuous layer formed by epithelial cells (which can be flattened, cuboidal, or columnar, and have pale eosinophilic cytoplasm and uniform oval nuclei), and the outer layer consisting of myoepithelial cells (often showing a bipolar elongated dense nuclei and small cytoplasm; however, the cytoplasm contains glycogen, which gives a cleared appearance in the Hematoxylin-Eosin stained slides) (Fig. 1.21). Sometimes, the myoepithelial cells have a myoid appearance with a spindle shape and dense eosinophilic cytoplasm (Fig. 1.22). Of interest, the myoepithelial layer may be discontinuous, or, in very rare instances, it may be absent, even in normal breast tissue (Fig. 1.23) [6]. At the periphery, the two layers are surrounded by a basement membrane and fibroblasts. Also, elastic tissue fibers are variably present around normal ducts while they are absent at the lobular level. Terminal ducts deepen into mammary acini, called by some authors "terminal ductules." The intralobular segment of the terminal duct, along with the acini, will constitute mammary lobules, also called terminal ductal-lobular units (TDLU) (Figs. 1.24 and 1.25). This is the level where most benign or malignant breast lesions occur. Breast lesions will be further divided and called *ductal* or *lobular* depending on the morphological and immunohistochemical appearance of proliferation, but also because they are, from a clinical and developmental point of view, totally different from one another. The terms "ductal" and "lobular" do not relate to the origin of the lesion within ducts or acini (lobule). Acini are also lined by the two cell layers, and are surrounded by a basement membrane and fibroblasts. Some authors have suggested the presence of a third layer of intermediate cells called basal cells or clear cells in both the acini and in the ducts. Also, some authors describe the existence of stem cells (also called progenitor cells) spread throughout the system of mammary ducts and acini, more numerous in the acini. These cells proliferate during pregnancy, and some studies suggest that they are the origin of the capability of different breast tumor lesions to differentiate into both glandular epithelial cells and myoepithelial cells.

Around the acini and the ducts, the stroma is hormone-dependent and is more cellular (intralobular stroma), while interlobular stroma is less cellular and is not hormone-dependent (Fig. 1.26). Hormone-dependent stroma consists of collagenous connective bundles, abundant fundamental substance, and fibroblast cells. The laxity of intralobular stroma facilitates the distension of acini during pregnancy and lactation. Also, the intralobular stroma often displays a mucoid character (positive for Alcian blue) (Fig. 1.27). Of interest, the intralobular stroma of mammary glands free of pathological changes usually presents a varying number of lymphocytic and/or plasma cells (Fig. 1.28). Additionally, these cells do not normally occur in the epithelium of the ducts or acini. Also, mast cells, histiocytes, and ochrocytes (periductal histiocytes with lipofuscin pigment) are sometimes present around ducts [7]. The interlobular stroma is composed of a dense connective tissue, consisting of thick connective tissue bundles, with a low level of fundamental substance and reduced number of cells. Adipose tissue can be found only between mammary lobes, and it never appears intralobularly (Fig. 1.29). The adipose tissue varies quantitatively according to the age of the patient and among individuals. The interlobular stroma may also present multinucleated giant cells or bizarre cells (Fig. 1.30). Their significance is unknown, and they should not be misinterpreted as malignant cells. This interlobular tissue may also host encapsulated lymph nodes, usually with less than 5 mm, which may appear as densities on mammography and can be detected when grossing a surgical specimen (Fig. 1.31). The presence of these nodes (most often incidentally identified in surgical specimens) is important because they may play a fundamental role in the metastasis of breast carcinoma. If present, the metastases of a breast carcinoma must be recorded in the histopathological report along with axillary lymph nodes metastases, and must be taken into account when staging the breast carcinoma.

During the early follicular phase, the acini show poorly defined lumina surrounded by epithelial cells with dark, centrally located nuclei and very rare mitoses and eosinophilic cytoplasm. During the luteal phase, it shows vacuolization and swallowing of the myoepithelial cells due to the increase in the amount of glycogen cytoplasmic contents, while the epithelial cells have prominent apical snouting (Figs. 1.32 and 1.33). Also, during the luteal phase, the lumen of the acini is enlarged and contains eosinophilic secretory material, while the intralobular stroma is loose edematous with congested blood vessels (Fig. 1.34). In contrast, the intralobular stroma is dense cellular with plump fibroblasts in the follicular phase. Sometimes, the epithelial cells in the TDLU show prominent clear cell changes in the cytoplasm at any age, and unrelated to pregnancy or exogenous hormonal administration (Fig. 1.35). A potential pitfall is mistaking benign clear cell change for involvement of lobules by clear cell variants of *in situ* carcinoma. Very rarely, it may represent metastatic clear cell carcinoma from other sites.

In contrast with females, the breast of adult males is primarily composed of ductal structures within collagenized stroma, with lobular elements absent or rare as compared to the female breast. The lobular elements in males develop under hormonal stimulation (Fig. 1.36). The nipple, however, has a similar appearance to that of females (Fig. 1.37).

Epithelial and myoepithelial cells present distinct immunohistochemical features and this information is of great importance for the breast pathologist when dealing with differential diagnosis of a breast lesion. Epithelial cells are strongly positive for low molecular weight cytokeratin (CK) such as CK 7, 8, 18, and 19. Also, epithelial cells express a heterogeneous reaction for high molecular weight cytokeratin such as CK34betaE12, and CK 5/6, and are variably positive for S-100 protein and negative for Cytokeratin 20 [8]. The epithelial cells are also sporadically positive for estrogen receptor (ER), progesterone receptor (PR), and androgen receptor (AR) (Fig. 1.38). This positivity is variable with age, location (ducts versus acini or within different lobules), and menstrual phase. The epithelial cells also express E-cadherin, Mammaglobin, GCDFP-15, and GATA 3. In contrast, the myoepithelial cells are positive for Actin (smooth muscle actin or muscle-specific actin), smooth muscle myosin heavy chain, calponin, p63, CD10, 14-3-3 sigma,

and sometimes for S-100 protein. For a practical perspective, the markers highlighting the myoepithelial cells vary in both specificity and sensitivity. Myoepithelial cells are almost always negative for ER, PR, and AR [8, 9]. The vast majority of myoepithelial cells are negative for low molecular weight CK or may show focally and have weak positivity. Also, the myoepithelial cells may show a heterogeneous positivity for high molecular weight CK such as CK34betaE12, and CK 5/6 [8]. It has been shown that there is an endocrine cell population in a normal mammary gland positive for Chromogranin, discontinuously located between the epithelial cells. Intralobular stroma is negative for RE, RP, and AR. Basement membrane is positive for Laminin, and Collagen IV.

During pregnancy, significant hormonal changes occur. The placenta and the pregnancy corpus luteum produce large amounts of estrogen and progesterone, leading to higher levels of prolactin. Increased hormone secretion causes mammary gland secretion. The most significant changes occur in the lobules. As the pregnancy progresses, the number of acini increases, along with progressive accumulation of secretory material and, consequently, the lobules become bigger. The waiting buds turn into glandular acini and thus type 2 lobule develops (Figs. 1.39 and 1.40). Myoepithelial cells become obscured by the epithelial cells, but are still present (the positivity for myoepithelial markers confirms this, using ancillary examinations). Proliferative activity, reflected in the number of mitoses, is greatest in the 20th week of pregnancy and declines afterwards. The appearance of epithelial cells is different in the acini as opposed to the ones that line the ducts, due to the fact that the secretory material accumulates particularly in the cytoplasm of the epithelial cells of the acini, which becomes vacuolated.

During pregnancy, especially during the third semester, localized adenomatous lactational hyperplasia may lead to the development of one or more nodules, called lactational adenomas (Figs. 1.41 and 1.42). Also, pronounced areolar pigmentation and dilation of superficial cutaneous veins become apparent.

During lactation, the amount of estrogen and progesterone decreases, whereas that of prolactin increases. Because of the secretory activity, their lumen accumulates lactation and the acini expand, developing mammary alveoli (type 3 lobules). Myoepithelial cells continue to have a weakened appearance.

The act of sucking stimulates the nipple and leads to the release of oxytocin, which stimulates the myoepithelial cells to contract and release milk from the mammary alveoli. The process of lactation ceases 7–10 days after the cessation of nipple stimulation. The process of breast tissue involution, called post-gestational involution, lasts 3–4 months and is not uniform. In its first stage, the lobules regress, and become irregular in shape due to the uneven distribution of acini and ducts and due to their angular shape of these structures, especially of the ducts. The epithelium is flattened and the basement membrane is castellated, while the intralobular stroma shows an inflammatory lymphoplasmacytic infiltrate. In time, the lobules become fibrotic and hyalinized, decrease in size and number, and the amount of fibrous tissue and fat around them increases (Figs. 1.43 and 1.44). In some mammary alveoli, in which milk secretion persists, the expansion of the lumen (called galactocele) and the rupture of the wall can occur (Figs. 1.45 and 1.46). The involution process is controlled by hormonal changes and reduction in the level of prolactin, but other vascular or cellular factors (the presence of macrophages with phagocytic action) are also involved.

In general, the florid changes and areas of infarction seen during pregnancy and lactation can be alarming for an inexperienced pathologist. However, pseudolactational changes may occur in patients under treatment with medication. These patients can present with changes that are usually incidentally diagnosed; in some cases, however, they can produce a nodule. Microscopic examination reveals partial involvement of some of the terminal ductal-lobular units, which are composed of dilated acini lined by vacuolated epithelial cells, while the myoepithelial cells are attenuated. Some of the cases may also show hobnail cells (hobnail type of pseudolactational changes) (Figs. 1.47 and 1.48).

After menopause, due to the decrease in estrogen and progesterone levels, breast tissue atrophy occurs by a reduction in the number of acini, epithelial and myoepithelial cells mitigation, luminal obliteration, and basement membrane thickening. The hormone-dependent stroma turns into a dense hyaline tissue. Over time, the ducts and acini atrophy and become completely hyalinized, forming hyaline nodules (Figs. 1.49, 1.50, 1.51, and 1.52). Sometimes, the acini expand and become cystic, a change termed cystic atrophy, which needs to be differentiated on microscopic examination from fibro-cystic changes (Fig. 1.53). Of interest, cystic atrophy is never associated with ductal or lobular hyperplasia (Fig. 1.54). Myoepithelial cells can sometimes become prominent due to hypertrophy or hyperplasia. This transformation was termed *myoepithelial atrophy*, a misnomer considering that myoepithelial cells become more prominent. The stroma undergoes involution changes, with alterations of elastic and collagen fibers and fat-tissue growth. The process of atrophy may occur in a heterogeneous way, in which some lobules are changed while others are not. The process of post-menopausal mammary involution is not uniform throughout the gland; on palpation, therefore, more consistent areas in the vicinity of flaccid ones are often detected. Occasionally, microcalcifications can occur in atrophic acini

and ducts, being diagnosed on mammography and identified during microscopic examination (Fig. 1.55). Vascular calcifications become more prominent, especially in those with coronary artery disease and diabetes. Elastosis (excess elastic fibers) is found in 50% of women aged 50 years and older without breast disease, either diffusely in stroma, around vessels, or around ducts. Also, arteries in the breast undergo sclerotic changes comparable to those seen in other organs with increasing age. Arterial calcifications may be seen in the breast in postmenopausal women, which can be detected on mammography but are different from those associated with glandular parenchyma.

Blood circulation in the breast is ensured by the thoracic branches of the axillary artery, internal thoracic artery (internal mammary artery), and intercostal arteries. The venous vessels are the branches of the axillary vein and internal thorax.

The lymphatic vasculature is particularly important in breast pathology because it is the main route of metastasis of breast carcinoma. Most of the lymph drains into the axillary lymph nodes, a smaller quantity into the internal mammary lymph nodes, and a very small amount drains into the posterior intercostal lymph nodes. The breast tissue is divided into upper outer, upper inner, lower outer, and lower inner quadrants, the subareolar area, and the axillary tail of the upper outer quadrant (of interest, glandular tissue is most abundant in the upper outer quadrant of the breast and as a result, half of all breast cancers occur here). In general, tumors located in upper and external quadrants metastasize to the axillary lymph nodes, whereas tumors located in central or internal quadrants metastasize to the internal mammary lymph nodes. However, this is not a general rule. It is possible to encounter metastases with paradoxical localization due to anatomic variations or blockage of the lymphatic pathways. Sappey's subareolar plexus drains the lymph in subcutaneous channels.

Regional lymph nodes are divided into four categories: axillary, infraclavicular, internal mammary, and supraclavicular. Axillary lymph nodes are the primary lymph nodes likely to metastasize due to a breast carcinoma. They are divided into three levels according to their location along the axillary vein and its branches. Rotter interpectoral lymph node is also included in the category of axillary lymph nodes. With the introduction of the sentinel lymph node method, extensive studies regarding the mammary lymphatic drainage have been reported. The existence of more than one sentinel lymph node in some of the patients implies that a hierarchy exists in the anatomical and functional distribution of the lymph nodes in the axilla as they relate to the breast.

Mammary gland innervation is ensured by the anterior and lateral cutaneous branches of intercostal nerves II–IV.

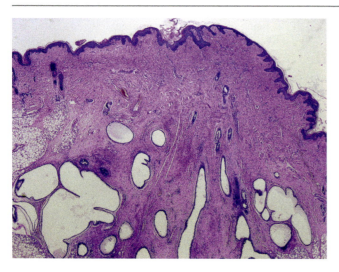

Fig. 1.1 Breast tissue in the newborn: primary duct system branches can be detected on microscopic examination (19 days old)

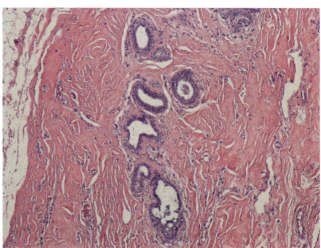

Fig. 1.4 During puberty, the intralobular stroma is dense and has a similar appearance to the extra-lobular stroma (12-year-old patient)

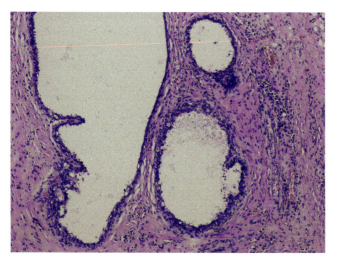

Fig. 1.2 Breast tissue in the newborn: primary ducts are lined by epithelial and myoepithelial cells and some of them are cystically dilated (19 days old)

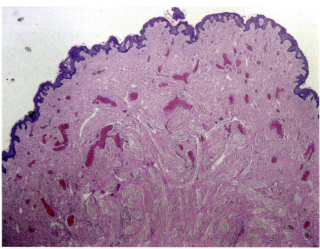

Fig. 1.5 The nipple of an adult female consists of bundles of smooth muscle fibers and elastic tissue

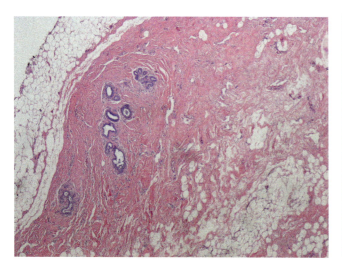

Fig. 1.3 At puberty in females, under the action of hormones, the lobules develop (12-year-old patient)

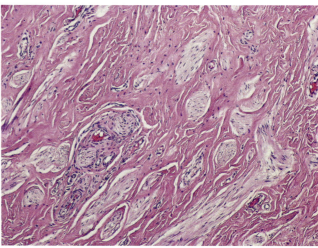

Fig. 1.6 The nipple of an adult female: smooth muscle fibers are arranged radially and longitudinally

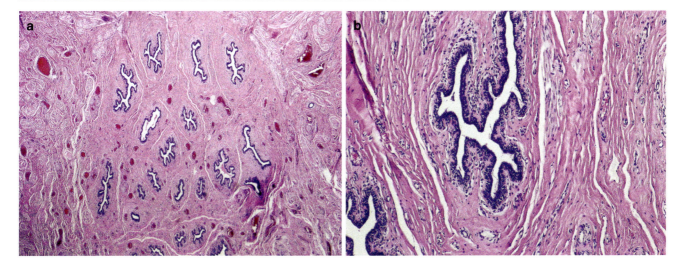

Fig. 1.7 (**a**) Nipple with lactiferous ducts. (**b**) Cross-section reveals that the duct is lined by two layers of cells

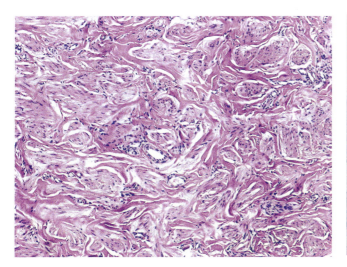

Fig. 1.8 In some cases, in the region of the nipple, smooth muscle bundles may show hyperplasia, which may lead to the increase of the nipple volume

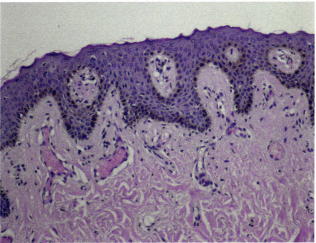

Fig. 1.10 The epidermis covering the nipple and areola is composed of stratified squamous epithelium

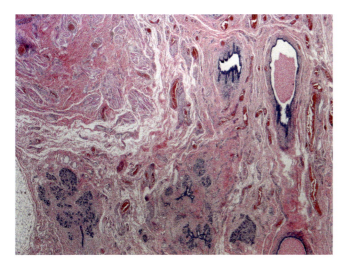

Fig. 1.9 Careful examination of the nipple may also reveal mammary lobules in some cases

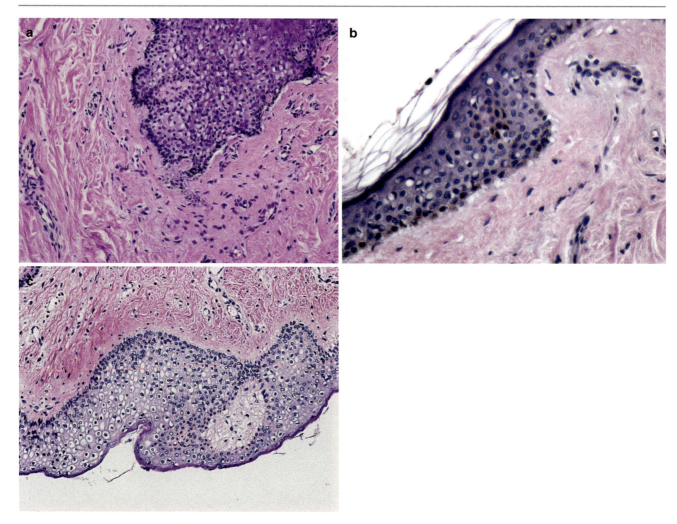

Fig. 1.11 (**a**) In the thickness of the epidermis covering the nipple, clear cells known as Toker cells can be identified in some patients. (**b**) These cells are larger than the adjacent keratinocytes, with a round or oval nucleus and pale cytoplasm, but no intracytoplasmic mucin can be detected using special stains. (**c**) Toker cells can also be appreciated in the epidermis covering the nipple of a newborn patient

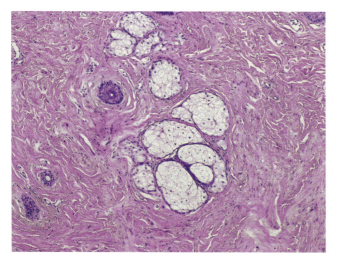

Fig. 1.12 In the nipple, the dermis may present sebaceous glands

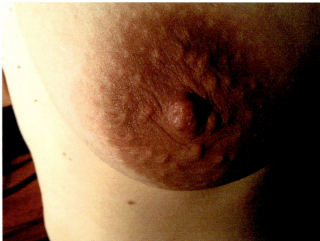

Fig. 1.13 Nipple: some large sebaceous glands open to the surface through a duct, corresponding to small rounded uniform formations called Montgomery tubercles (Courtesy of Dr. Marius Florin Coros)

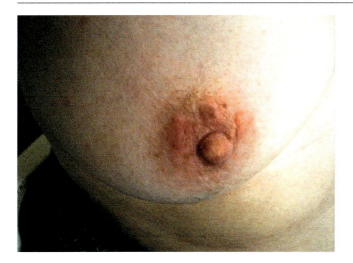

Fig. 1.14 Nipple sebaceous gland hyperplasia: multiple soft, yellowish papules or nodules, with central umbilication (Courtesy of Dr. Anca Chiriac)

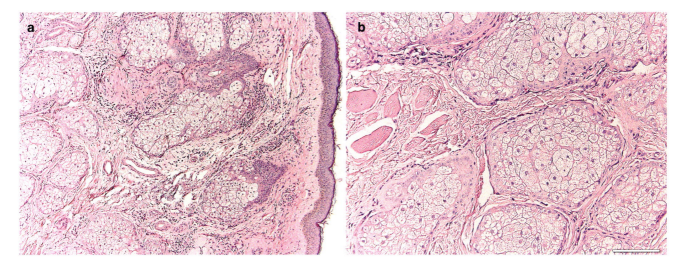

Fig. 1.15 (**a**) Nipple sebaceous gland hyperplasia: the lesion is microscopically represented by hyperplastic and hypertrophic mature sebaceous glands aggregates involving the dermis, (**b**) lacking atypical features (Courtesy of Dr. Sabina Zurac)

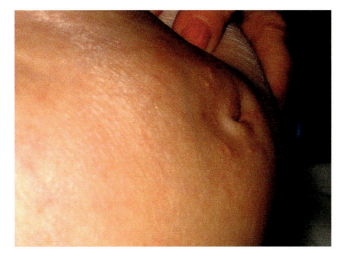

Fig. 1.16 Congenital inverted nipple: macroscopic appearance (Courtesy of Dr. Marius Florin Coros)

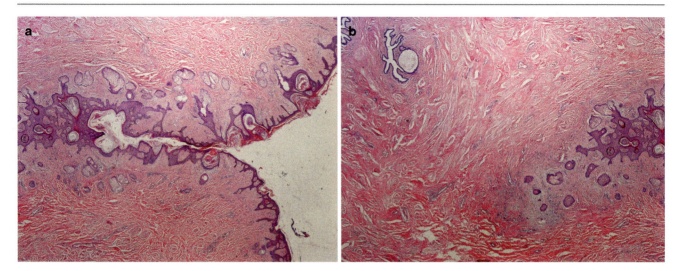

Fig. 1.17 Congenital inverted nipple: (**a**) microscopic examination revealed the squamous epithelium invaginated into the underlying stroma and (**b**) in the vicinity of lactiferous ducts, some of which can become dilated

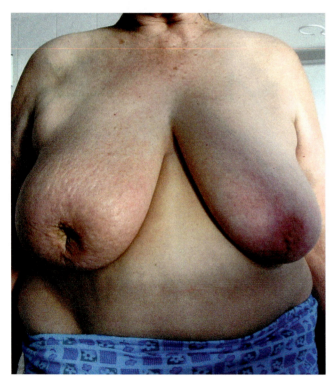

Fig. 1.18 Acquired inverted nipple of the right breast in a patient with invasive carcinoma (Courtesy of Dr. Marius Florin Coros)

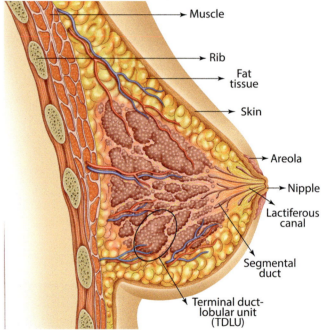

Fig. 1.19 The deep segment of the ductal system is called terminal duct; several terminal ducts unite and constitute subsegmental ducts that drain into segmental ducts; segmental ducts unite and form lactiferous ducts that open in the nipple (*From* Alexilusmedical/Shutterstock; *with permission*)

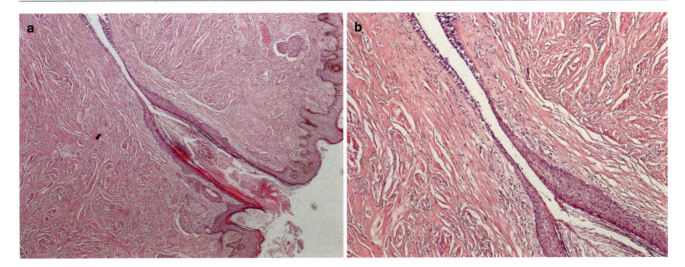

Fig. 1.20 (**a**) The superficial portion of the duct orifice is covered by squamous epithelium, and this epithelium may extend for a short distance into the most distant portion of the duct. (**b**) The area where the squamous epithelium joins the columnar epithelium is called the squamous-columnar junction

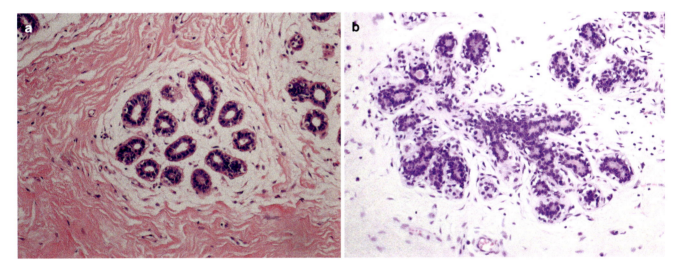

Fig. 1.21 (**a**) The whole ductal system as well as the acini are lined by two layers of cells: the inner layer of epithelial cells (flattened/cuboidal/columnar, with pale eosinophilic cytoplasm and uniform oval nuclei), and the outer layer of myoepithelial cells (the cytoplasm of which contains glycogen, which gives a cleared appearance in the Hematoxylin-Eosin stained slides). (**b**) At the periphery, the two layers are surrounded by a basement membrane and fibroblasts

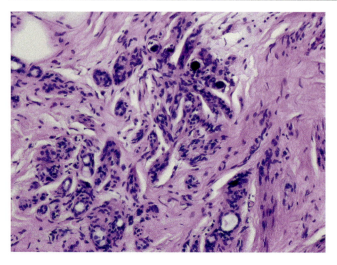

Fig. 1.22 The myoepithelial cells sometimes have a myoid appearance with a spindle shape and dense eosinophilic cytoplasm

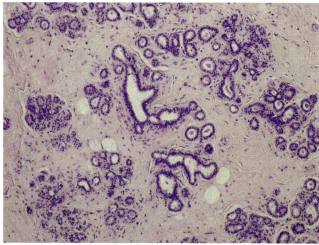

Fig. 1.24 The intralobular segment of the terminal duct along with the acini will constitute mammary lobules, also called terminal ductal-lobular units (TDLU)

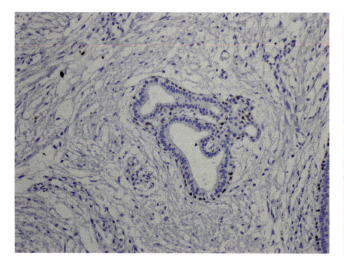

Fig. 1.23 p63 stain highlights the discontinuity of the myoepithelial layer in normal ducts

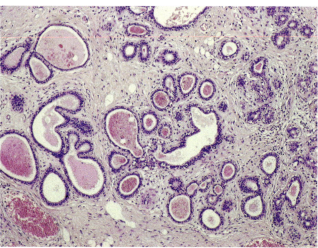

Fig. 1.25 In contrast with normal TDLU, the unfold lobule consists of acini and ducts that become larger and cystically dilated

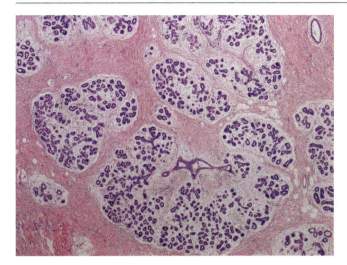

Fig. 1.26 Around the acini and the ducts, the stroma is hormone-dependent and is more cellular (intralobular stroma), while interlobular stroma is less cellular and is not hormone-dependent

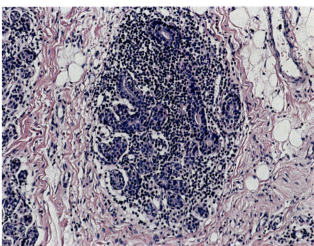

Fig. 1.28 The intralobular stroma of mammary glands free of pathological changes usually presents a varying number of lymphocytic and/or plasma cells

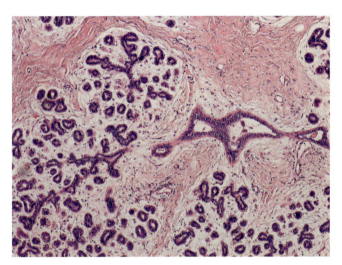

Fig. 1.27 Intralobular stroma consists of collagenous connective bundles, abundant fundamental substance, fibroblast cells, and often displays a mucoid character (positive for Alcian blue—not shown here)

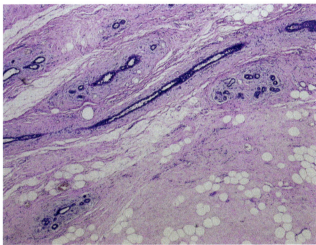

Fig. 1.29 Adipose tissue can be found only between mammary lobes and it never appears intralobularly

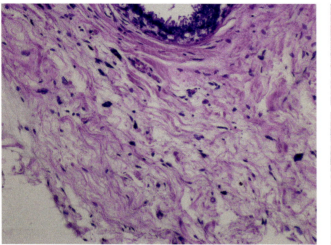

Fig. 1.30 The interlobular stroma may present multinucleated giant cells or bizarre cells

Fig. 1.31 The interlobular tissue may host encapsulated lymph nodes

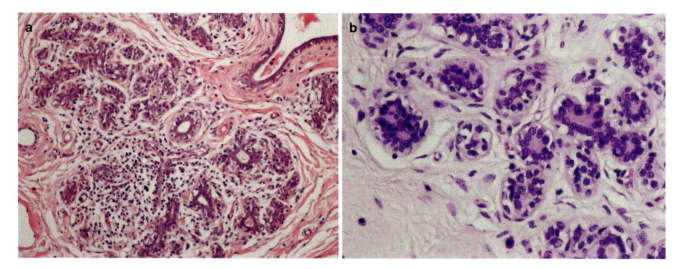

Fig. 1.32 The early follicular phase: (**a**) the acini show poorly defined lumina, (**b**) surrounded by epithelial cells with dark centrally located nuclei, very rare mitoses and eosinophilic cytoplasm

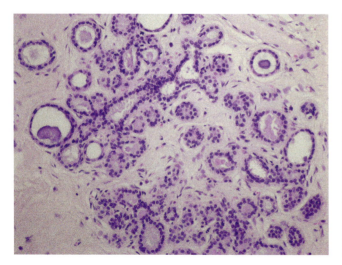

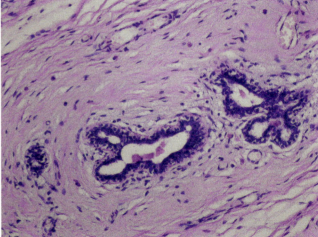

Fig. 1.33 The luteal phase vacuolization and swallowing of the myo-epithelial cells due to the increase in the amount of glycogen cytoplas-matic contents; the epithelial cells have prominent apical snouting

Fig. 1.34 The luteal phase: the lumen of the acini and ducts is enlarged and contains eosinophilic secretory material

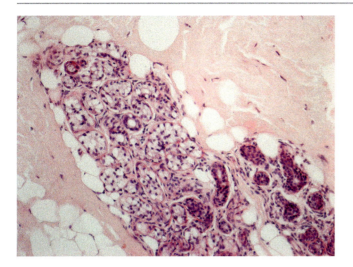

Fig. 1.35 The epithelial cells in the TDLU may show prominent clear cell changes in the cytoplasm (clear cell metaplasia)

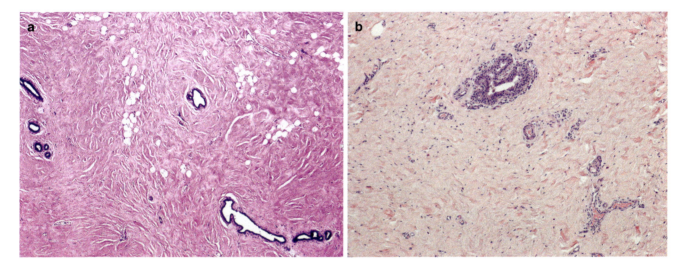

Fig. 1.36 (**a**) In adult males, the breast is primarily composed of ductal structures within collagenized stroma, (**b**) with no lobular elements compared to female breast

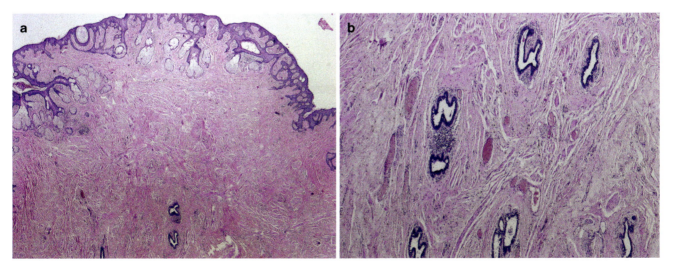

Fig. 1.37 (**a**) The male nipple has a similar appearance to that of females, and (**b**) contains lactiferous ducts

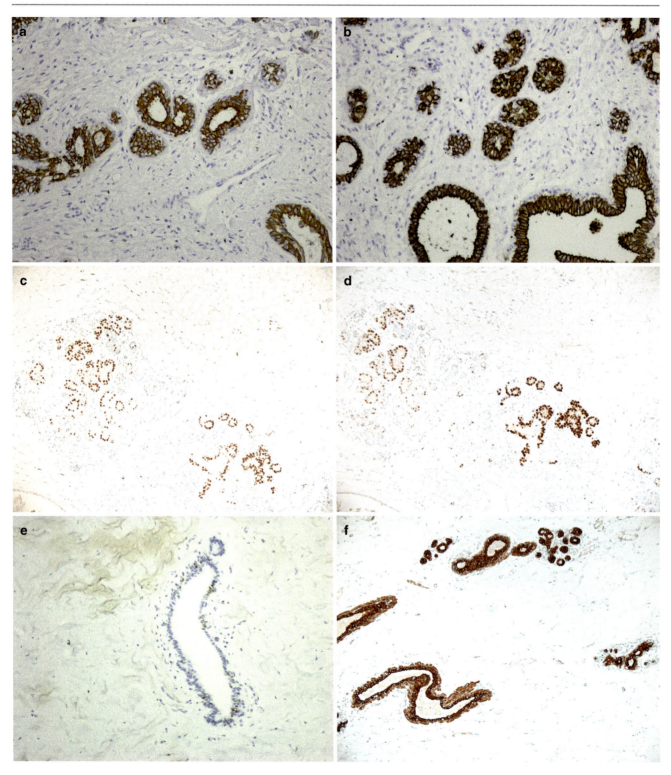

Fig. 1.38 (**a**) The epithelial cells are strongly positive for Cytokeratin 8; (**b**) 18; (**c**) sporadically positive for estrogen receptor; (**d**) progesterone receptor, and (**e**) androgen receptor; (**f**) positive for Cytokeratin 7. (**g**) Both epithelial and myoepithelial cells are heterogeneously positive for Cytokeratin 5; (**h**) myoepithelial cells are positive for Actin and (**i**) CD 10. (**j**) Epithelial cells also express E-cadherin, (**k**) Mammaglobin, and (**l**) GCDFP-15 (Courtesy of Dr. Cristina Terinte)

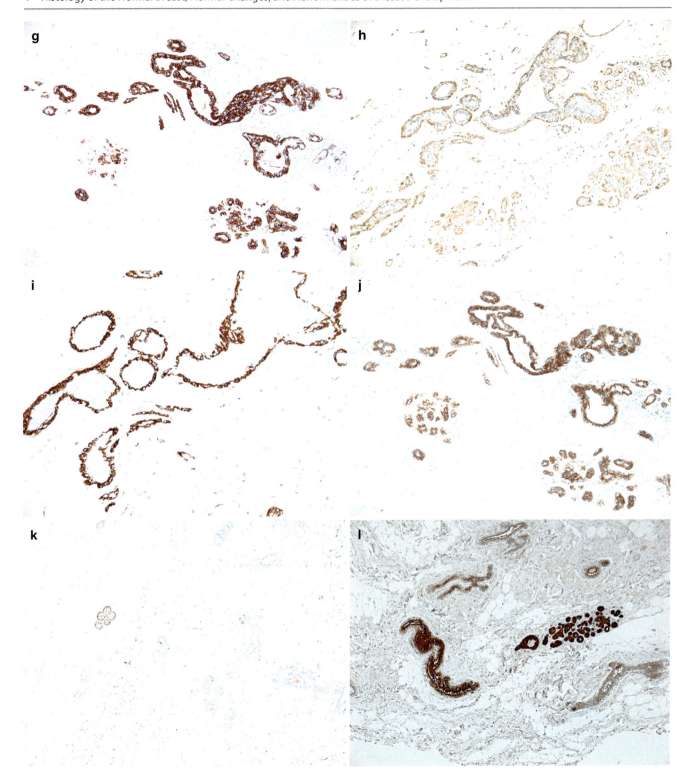

Fig. 1.38 (continued)

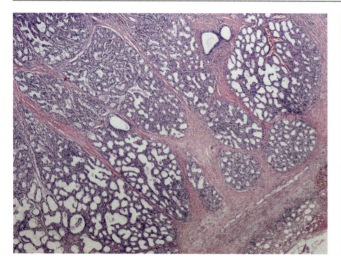

Fig. 1.39 Pregnancy changes: due to the hormonal stimulation, the number of acini increases, along with progressive accumulation of secretory material and, consequently, the lobules become bigger (type 2 lobule)

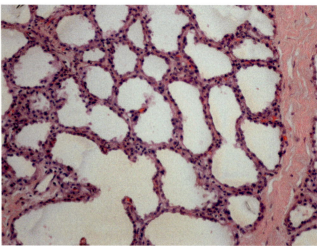

Fig. 1.42 Lactational adenoma: high-power view reveals the dilated acini lined by vacuolated epithelial cells without atypia, while the myoepithelial ones are obscured, but still present

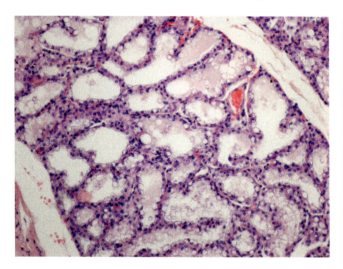

Fig. 1.40 Pregnancy changes: the acini are dilated and contain secretory material; the epithelial cells are prominent, and the myoepithelial cells become obscured by the epithelial cells, but are still present

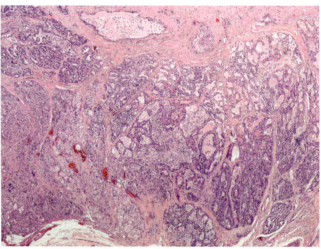

Fig. 1.43 Postgestational involution: regression of the lobules is not uniform

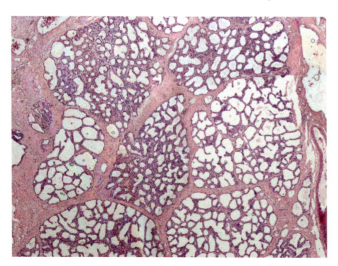

Fig. 1.41 During pregnancy, localized adenomatous lactational hyperplasia may lead to the development of nodules, called lactational adenomas

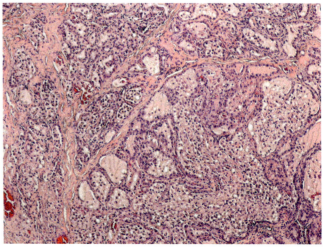

Fig. 1.44 Post-gestational involution: the epithelium is flattened, the basement membrane is castellated, while the intralobular stroma shows an inflammatory lymphoplasmacytic infiltrate

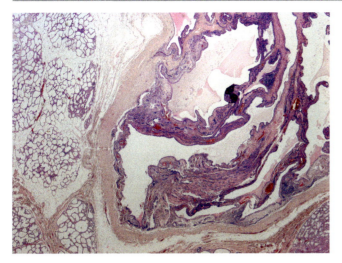

Fig. 1.45 Galactocele: persisting of milk secretion may lead to the expansion of ducts lumina and formation of a cyst

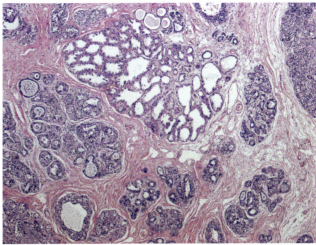

Fig. 1.48 Pseudolactational changes: some of the epithelial cells have hyperchromatic nuclei protruding into the lumina (hobnail cell changes)

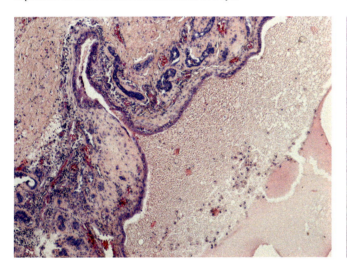

Fig. 1.46 Galactocele: rupture of the cystic wall can occur and is associated with inflammatory infiltrate

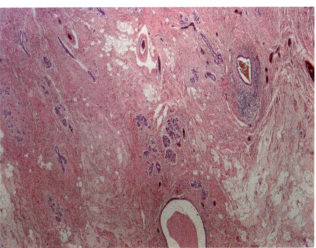

Fig. 1.49 Breast tissue atrophy in menopause: reduction in the number of acini and transformation of the hormone-dependent stroma into a dense hyaline tissue

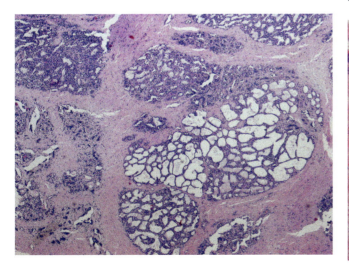

Fig. 1.47 Pseudolactational changes: dilated acini containing secretory material only partially involving some of the terminal ductal-lobular units

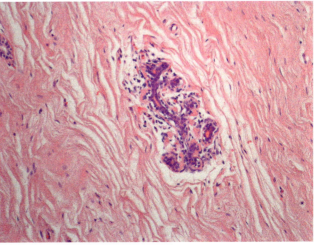

Fig. 1.50 Breast tissue atrophy in menopause: epithelial and myoepithelial cells mitigation, luminal obliteration, and basement membrane thickening

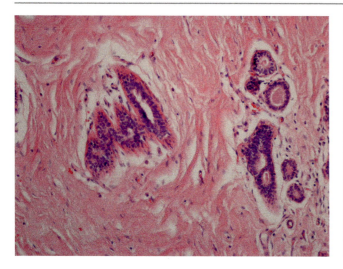

Fig. 1.51 Breast tissue atrophy in menopause: basement membrane has been thickened and transformed into a pink thick line at the periphery of the acini and ducts

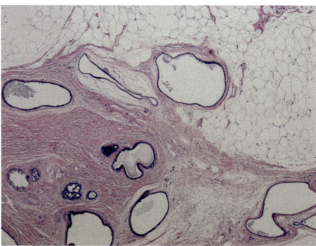

Fig. 1.53 Cystic atrophy of the breast: the acini expand and become cystic

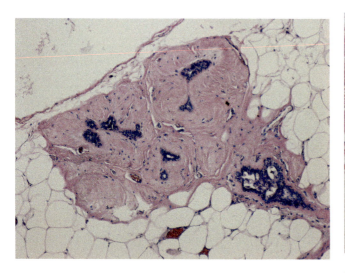

Fig. 1.52 Breast tissue atrophy: over time, the ducts and acini undergo atrophy and become completely hyalinized forming hyaline nodules

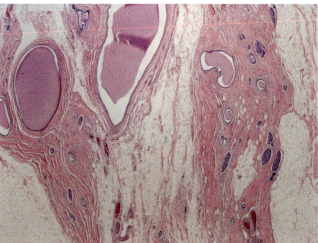

Fig. 1.54 Cystic atrophy of the breast: the stroma undergoes involution changes, with fat tissue growth; the layers lining the cysts are flat, cystic atrophy usually not being associated with ductal or lobular hyperplasia, in contrast to fibro-cystic changes; however, minor usual hyperplasia and/or apocrine metaplasia may occur (as shown in the picture) but these changes are not in favor of fibro-cystic changes

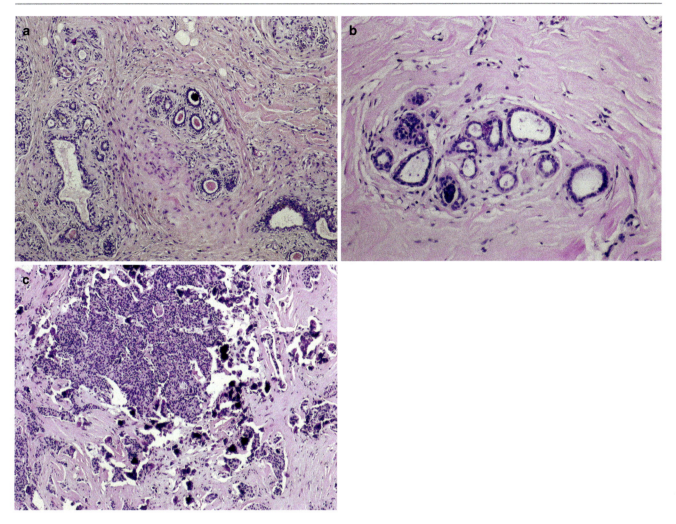

Fig. 1.55 (**a**) Microcalcifications associated with normal breast tissue, (**b**) atrophy, and (**c**) invasive breast carcinoma

1.2 Abnormalities of Breast Development

Amastia, the complete absence of breast and nipple, is a very rare condition that can be unilateral or bilateral. It can also be familial, when it may be accompanied by another developmental defect of the shoulder, chest, arm, or in the complex genetic defect of acrorenal ectodermal dysplasia with lipoatrophic diabetes syndrome (Fig. 1.56) [10–12]. *Athelia* is the complete absence of the nipple and it is the rarest of all congenital anomalies. *Hypoplasia* is the underdevelopment of the breast (usually consisting of only fibrous stroma and ducts without acini). It can also be unilateral or bilateral [13] and is also very rare, while minor variation in the size of the two breasts (asymmetry) is a very common condition (Figs. 1.57, 1.58, and 1.59). Congenital hypoplasia must be differentiated from acquired hypoplasia caused by damage to the mammary bud by previous biopsies, trauma, or radiation of the thoracic wall. *Macromastia* is excessive breast growth and can occur in adolescents (microscopically represented by stromal collagen and fat, rarely by glandular tissue or pseudoangiomatous hyperplasia), but can also occur in the form of gravid macromastia (occurring shortly after the onset of pregnancy, microscopically represented by fibrosis, collagenization, pseudoangiomatous hyperplasia, and, rarely, lactational hyperplasia) or penicillamine-induced macromastia or macromastia in women with HIV treated with indinavir (Fig. 1.60) [14, 15]. Incomplete regression or persistence of different portions of the milk line (from the axilla to the anterior chest wall, to the pubis and upper thighs) results in accessory mammary tissue or accessory mammary gland (polymastia). However, polymastia is most often located in the axilla or vulva (the extreme ends of the mammary ridge) and can be familial (Fig. 1.61). These patients may develop symptoms such as pain and premenstrual tenderness, but also swelling of the lesion and, in time, they can also develop different benign or malignant breast-like lesions [16]. *Polytelia* is an accessory nipple, which can also occur anywhere along the milk line but most occurs frequently on the anterior chest wall above or below the normal breast (Figs. 1.62, 1.63, and 1.64). The accessory nipples consist microscopically of normal nipple components, including lactiferous ducts, smooth muscle, and sometimes breast glandular tissue. Aberrant breast tissue is defined as breast parenchyma found in the region beyond the usual anatomic extent of the breast. In this situation, the breast tissue is not well-organized like normal tissue and it does not form a nipple or areola, but it can develop breast lesions.

This variety of congenital malformations that can occur during the development of the breast can be easily corrected with the aid of cosmetic surgery.

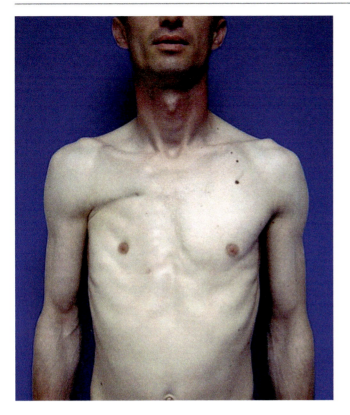

Fig. 1.56 Complete absence of the right pectoral muscle in a male patient (Courtesy of Dr. Calin Dobos)

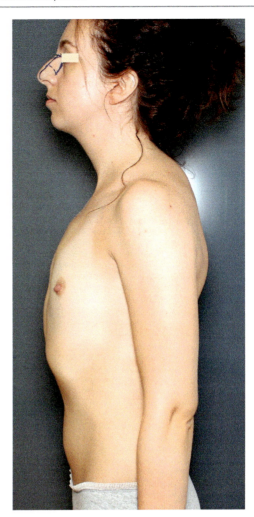

Fig. 1.57 Bilateral congenital breast hypoplasia: underdevelopment of both breasts in a female patient (Courtesy of Dr. Calin Dobos)

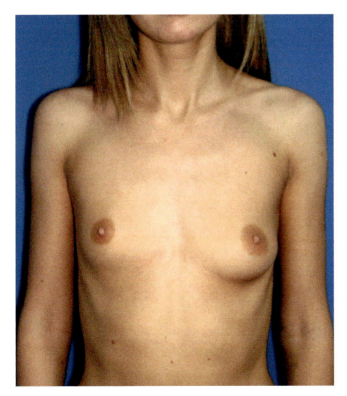

Fig. 1.58 Asymmetry of the breast: minor variation in the size of the two breasts: the right breast is smaller than the left breast (Courtesy of Dr. Calin Dobos)

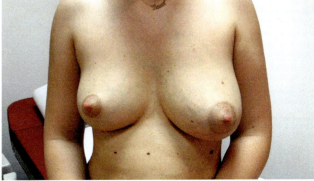

Fig. 1.59 Asymmetry of the breast: a different case with more pronounced asymmetry between the two breasts (the right breast is smaller) (Courtesy of Dr. Marius Florin Coros)

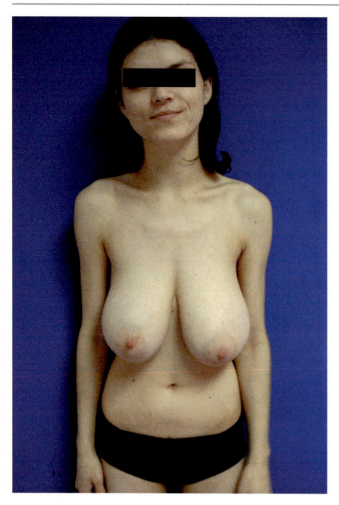

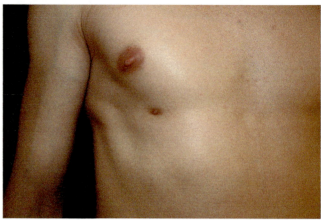

Fig. 1.62 Polytelia in a young male patient located on the right side of the anterior chest wall below the normal breast (Courtesy of Dr. Calin Dobos)

Fig. 1.60 Bilateral macromastia (Courtesy of Dr. Calin Dobos)

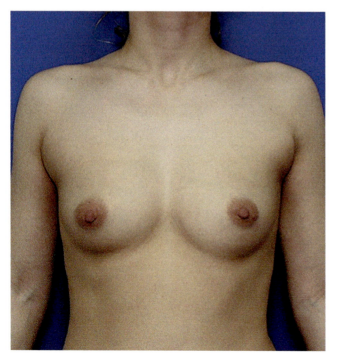

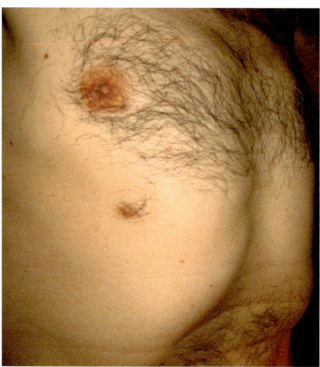

Fig. 1.63 Polytelia in an older patient located on the right side of the anterior chest wall below the normal breast (Courtesy of Dr. Marius Florin Coros)

Fig. 1.61 Accessory mammary tissue in the axillary region, bilateral involvement (Courtesy of Dr. Calin Dobos)

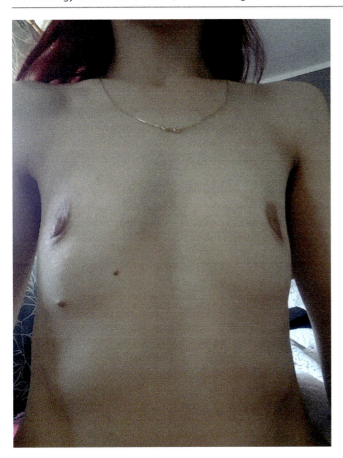

Fig. 1.64 Polytelia located on the right side of the anterior chest wall below the hypoplasic breast associated with bilateral breast hypoplasia in a young female patient (Courtesy of Dr. Calin Dobos)

References

1. Schnitt SJ, Collins L. Biopsy interpretation of the breast. Philadelphia, PA: Lippincott Williams and Wilkins; 2009. p. 1.
2. Giacometti L, Montagna W. The nipple and the areola of the human female breast. Anat Rec. 1962;144:191–7.
3. Stirling JW, Chandler JA. The fine structure of ducts and subareolar ducts in the resting gland of the female breast. Virchow Arch. 1977;373:119–32.
4. Catalano PM, Ioannides G. Areolar sebaceous hyperplasia. J Am Acad Dermatol. 1985;13:867–8.
5. Chiriac A, Moldovan C, Coros MF, Podoleanu C, Moncea D, Stolnicu S. Bilateral areolar sebaceous hyperplasia in a postmenopausal woman. Eur J Dermatol. 2016;26(3):299–300.
6. Cserni G. Benign apocrine papillary lesions of the breast lacking or virtually lacking myoepithelial cells—potential pitfalls in diagnosing malignancy. APMIS. 2012;120(3):249–52.
7. Rosen PP. Rosen's breast pathology. Philadelphia, PA: Lippincott Williams and Wilkins; 2009. p. 8.
8. Moinfar F. Essentials of diagnostic breast pathology. New York, NY: Springer; 2007. p. 236.
9. Tavassoli FA. Pathology of the breast. New York, NY: McGraw-Hill; 1999.
10. Rees TD. Mammary asymmetry. Clin Plast Surg. 1975;2:371–4.
11. Zilli L, Stefani G. Unilateral agenesis of the pectoralis muscle associated with mammary hypoplasia. Friuli Med. 1960;15:1522–30.
12. Breslau-Siderius EJ, Toonstra J, Baart JA, Koppeschar HP, Maassen JA, Beemer FA. Ectodermal dysplasia, lipoatrophy, diabetes mellitus and amastia. A second case of AREDYLD syndrome. Am J Med Genet. 1992;44:374–7.
13. Trier WC. Complete breast absence. Case report and review of the literature. Plast Reconstr Surg. 1965;36:431–9.
14. Wolf Y, Pauzner D, Groutz A, Walman I, David MP. Gigantomastia complicating pregnancy. Case report and review of the literature. Acta Obstet Gynecol Scand. 1995;74:159–63.
15. Lui A, Karter D, Turett G. Another case of breast hypertrophy in a patient treated with indinavir. Clin Infect Dis. 1998;26:1482.
16. Levy RL. Adenocarcinoma of the mammary chain. Breast Dis. 1994;7:383–6.

Radiology of the Normal Breast and Overview of Breast Imaging Reporting and Data System

Eloisa Asia Sanchez-Vivar and Isabel Alvarado-Cabrero

Until breast cancer can be prevented, regular screening programs are widely recommended for asymptomatic women. The goal of breast cancer screening is early detection of disease, to be followed by appropriate treatment. Evaluating any screening program is challenging, and breast cancer screening has been subject to many controversies over the years. The many modalities that have been studied for possible inclusion in screening programs include screening mammography, ultrasound, and magnetic resonance imaging. Awareness of the breast anatomy is essential in order to generate an accurate differential diagnosis and guide patient management. Use of standardized terminology, report organization, and assessment structures allows radiologists to communicate breast imaging findings to referring physicians clearly and succinctly. The Breast Imaging Reporting and Data System (BI-RADS) lexicon was released by the American College of Radiology (ACR) with the goal of standardizing mammography reporting by providing a specific lexicon of imaging features. The purpose of this chapter is to review current knowledge of breast anatomy with a focus on relevant anatomy for diagnosis and intervention, and to provide a general overview of the BI-RADS lexicon.

2.1 Normal Anatomy of the Female Breast

Understanding breast anatomy and its appearance on imaging studies is important for several reasons. First, any interventionist would not want to mistake variations in normal anatomy for a pathologic disorder and possibly harm a patient with an intervention. Second, recognizing the location of abnormality in the breast, within the normal background anatomy, often narrows the list of possible diagnoses for the abnormality. Third, knowledge of breast anatomy enables safe approaches to breast intervention, especially to avoid interventional breast procedures complications (e.g., bleeding or pneumothorax) [1, 2].

The breast is a symmetrical organ located on the front of the chest on both sides of the midline. It occupies an area that stretches from the third to the seventh rib and from the edge of the sternum to the armpit. The volume, shape and degree of development are very variable in relation to various factors such as age, gland development, amount of fat and relative influence of endocrine stimulation [3].

At the center of the breast are the nipple and areola. The areola is a flat hyperpigmented area of skin with a round-to-oval

E. A. Sanchez-Vivar, MD
Radiology Department, Hospital de Oncologia, Centro Medico Nacional Siglo XXI, Instituto Mexicano del Seguro Social, Mexico, Mexico

I. Alvarado-Cabrero, MD, PhD (✉)
Department of Pathology, Hospital de Oncologia, Centro Medico Nacional Siglo XXI, Instituto Mexicano del Seguro Social, Mexico City, Mexico

© Springer International Publishing AG, part of Springer Nature 2018
S. Stolnicu, I. Alvarado-Cabrero (eds.), *Practical Atlas of Breast Pathology*, https://doi.org/10.1007/978-3-319-93257-6_2

shape and of variable diameter, usually between 3.5 and 6 cm. The nipple, at center of areola has a variable size and shape (conical, cylindrical). At its apex there are several small depressions that represent the outlets of the ducts. The areola surface is irregular due to the presence of the 8–12 tubercles of Morgagni, representing sebaceous glands (Fig. 2.1) [4].

The mammary gland is made of three components: glandular, adipose, and fibrous tissue (Fig. 2.2) [4]. The breast parenchyma is contained by a two-layer fold of the subcutaneous superficial fascia, that may be divided in two parts: (1) the superficial layer that covers the gland and contains fibrous septa, called Cooper's ligaments, which penetrate the gland and form the support structure of the parenchyma; and (2) the deep layer, which covers the posterior portion of the gland and separates it from the underlying superficial fascia of the pectoralis major muscle. Cooper's ligaments are the suspensory ligaments of the breast gland, and divide the parenchyma into lobes [3, 5].

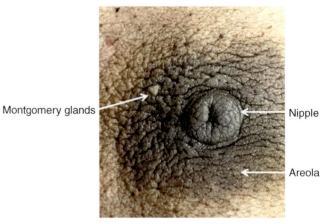

Fig. 2.1 Nipple-areolar complex (NAC). The NAC contains the montgomery glands, large intermediate-stage sebaceous glands that are embryologically transitional between sweat glands and mammary glands

Fig. 2.2 Breast normal anatomy. (**a**, **b**) Mammary gland is made of three components: glandular, adipose, and fibrous tissue

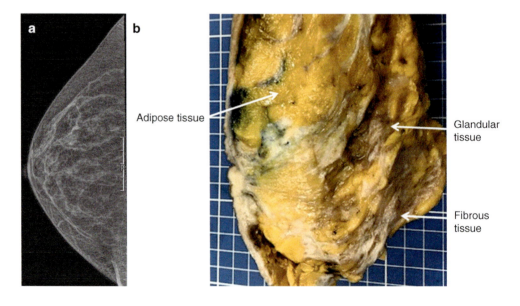

2.2   Normal Mammographic Anatomy

The mammographic appearance of the normal breast depends of the amount of each of the main components: fat tissue appears radiolucent, while the stroma and the gland appear radiopaque. The sensitivity of mammography strongly depends on the density of the breast. A mammogram is usually performed in two projections, the MLO (medio-lateral-oblique) and CC (cranio-caudal) after compression [6].

The skin appears as a thin, continuous, radiopaque rim of homogeneous density of about 1 mm, and is readily distinguishable from the radiolucency of the underlying subcuta-neous fat tissue. The areola usually has a thickness of 3–5 mm, with a central opacity of cylindrical shape corresponding to the nipple. Posteriorly there is the retroareolar region, a triangular-shaped area that is of particular interest because it may hide focal anomalies such as breast tumors (Fig. 2.3) [7].

The subcutaneous fat appears as a thick radiolucent layer, crossed by fibrous linear structures that correspond to the crest of Duret and Cooper's ligaments. Behind the breast gland the fat tissue outlines the retromammary space, which separates the breast from the pre-pectoral fascia overlying the pectoralis major muscle (Fig. 2.4) [8].

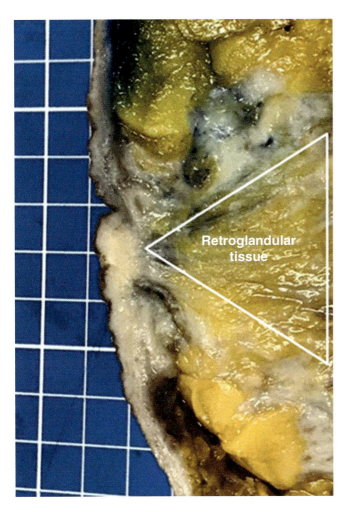

Fig. 2.3 Retroareolar region. Triangular-shaped area that may hide focal anomalies

Fig. 2.4 Normal mammographic anatomy

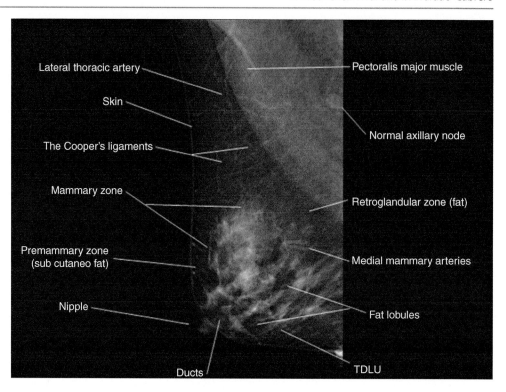

2.3 Normal Ultrasonographic Anatomy

The normal breast as observed with ultrasound presents the skin line, the fibroglandular tissue (also known as the mammary gland), and the pectoralis muscle as hyperechoic (maximum sound reflection and little sound transmission) and the subcutaneous fat and retromammary fat are visualized as hypoechoic, which is to say that they bounce back only a small amount of sound and allow maximum transmission through them (Fig. 2.5) [9].

The course of the ducts imaged by ultrasound from the nipple into the breast is diverse and complicated. The cen-

tral ducts do not extend in a radial fashion from the nipple toward the chest wall, whereas the peripheral ducts drape over the central ducts in a radial fashion. (Fig. 2.6). The breast has alternate hyperechoic and hypoechoic layers as follows [10, 11]:

1. Skin-hyperechoic
2. Subcutaneous fat-hypoechoic
3. Fibroglandular parenchyma-hyperechoic
4. Retromammary fat-hypoechoic
5. Muscle, mainly the pectoralis major-hyperechoic

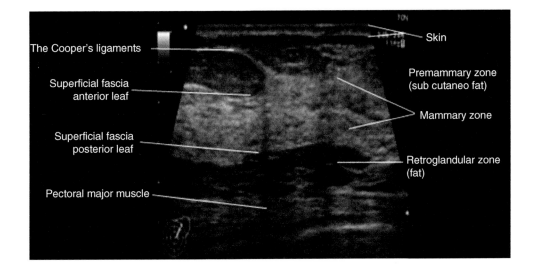

Fig. 2.5 Normal ultrasound anatomy

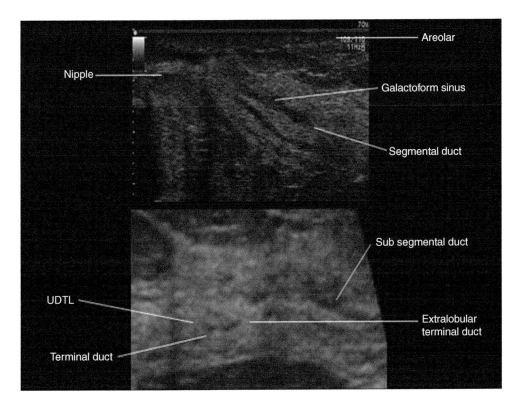

Fig. 2.6 Normal ultrasound anatomy of breast ducts

2.4   Magnetic Resonance (MR), Normal Anatomy

Normal anatomic components of the breast can be visualized and distinguished on MR imaging by assessing signal intensity. On T1-weighted imaging without fat saturation, adipose tissue is of high signal intensity and breast fibroglandular elements appear relatively intermediate-to-dark [12]. The pres-ence of fat can be confirmed by assessing the same region on T1-weighted images with fat saturation, where adipose signal would be expected to be nulled. In T1-weighted images with fat saturation, the relative signal intensity of fibroglandular elements then becomes intermediate-to-bright, given that the fat appears dark. Similarly, on T2-weighted series with fat saturation, fat appears dark while breast parenchyma appears intermediate to bright (Fig. 2.7) [13].

Fig. 2.7 (**a**, **b**) Breast magnetic resonance: normal anatomy

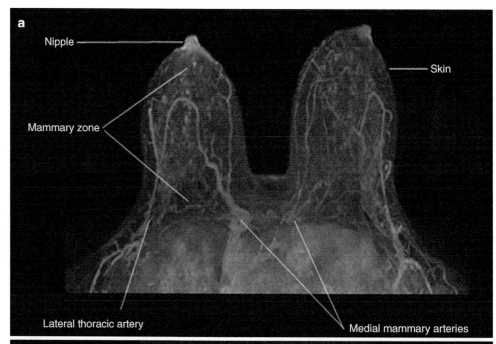

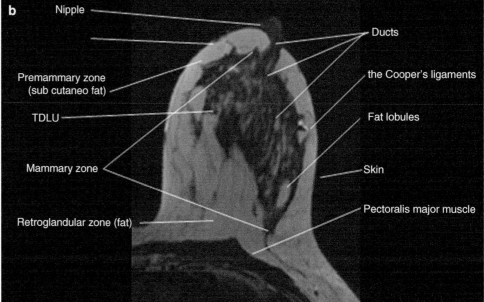

2.5   Breast Imaging Reporting and Data System (BI-RADS) Lexicon Fifth Edition (2013)

Before the development of the BI-RADS lexicon, mammography reports contained ambiguous and often unintelligible descriptions that made clinical management difficult for referring physicians. The first edition of the BI-RADS lexicon was released by the American College of Radiology (ACR) in 1993, with the goal of standardizing mammography reporting by providing a specific lexicon of imaging features. Lexicon descriptors were designed to predict both benign and malignant disease, eliminate ambiguity, allow automated data collection, and facilitate communication with referring physicians. Structured reports were organized into several categories, including breast density, description of findings, and a final decision-oriented assessment. Revisions were made in 1995, 1998 (the addition of an imaging atlas with examples of each descriptor), 2003 (revised terminology, subdivided category 4 findings, and introduction of US and MR imaging standardization) [14], and 2013. Use of the BI-RADS lexicon now facilitates quality assurance, communication, research, and improved care [15].

2.5.1   Density

In the BI-RADS edition of 2003, the assignment of the breast composition was based on the overall density resulting in ACR category 1 (<25% fibroglandular tissue), category 2 (25–50%), category 3 (51–75%), and category 4 (>75%). In the BI-RADS edition of 2013, the use of percentage is discouraged, because in individual cases it is more important to take into greater account the chance that a mass can be obscured by fibroglandular tissue than the percentage of breast density as an indicator for breast cancer risk. The assignment of breast composition is changed into categories a, b, c, and d, each followed by a description:

(a) The breasts are almost entirely fatty (Fig. 2.8)
(b) There are scattered areas of fibroglandular density
(c) The breasts are heterogeneously dense, which may obscure small masses
(d) The breasts are extremely dense, which lowers the sensitivity of mammography (Fig. 2.9)

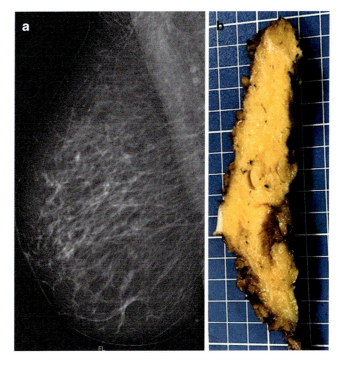

Fig. 2.8 Breast composition (fibroglandular tissue within the breast). ACR category a. (**a**) Mammography. (**b**) Gross aspect of a breast almost entirely fat

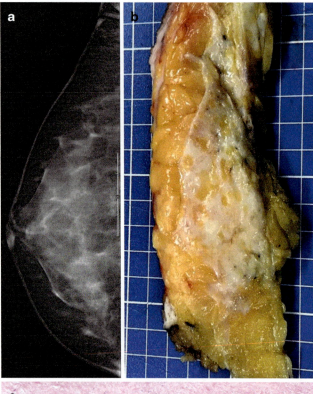

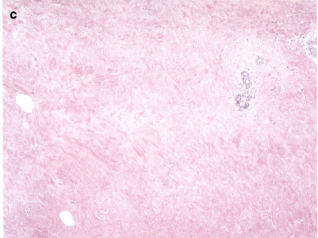

Fig. 2.9 The breast is extremely dense. Breast composition category *d*. (**a**) Mammography, the breast is dense, which may obscure small masses. (**b**, **c**) Gross and microscopic features of a dense fibroglandular tissue

2.5.2 Assessment

All final assessments (BI-RADS categories 1, 2, 3, 4, 5, and 6) should be based on thorough evaluation of the mammographic features of concern or after determination that an examination is negative or benign (Table 2.1).

An incomplete (category 0) assessment is usually given for screening examinations when additional imaging evaluation is recommended before it is appropriate to render a final assessment. There may be rare situations in the screening setting in which a category 4 or 5 assessment is used, but this practice is discouraged because it may compromise some aspects of outcome analysis [15].

A recall (category 0) assessment should include specific suggestions for the next course of action (spot-compression magnifications views, US, etc.) [16].

Table 2.1 BI-RADS assessment categories

Category	Assessment
0	Incomplete-need additional imaging evaluation and/or prior mammograms for comparison
1	Negative
2	Benign
3	Probably benign
4	Suspicious
4A	Low suspicion for malignancy
4B	Moderate suspicion for malignancy
4C	High suspicion for malignancy
5	Highly suggestive of malignancy
6	Known biopsy–proven malignancy

2.5.3   Masses

Mass shapes are reduced to three categories in the fifth edition: oval, round, and irregular (Fig. 2.10). The term lobular has been eliminated and absorbed into the term round or oval or, if there are more than two or three gentle lobulations, the term irregular [17].

Margin categorization is unchanged, with five categories described; circumscribed, obscured, microlobulated, indistinct, and spiculated. The majority of masses with circumscribed margins are benign, such as fibroadenomas (Fig. 2.11), and about 95% of the spiculated masses (Fig. 2.12) or microlobulated masses (Fig. 2.13) are malignant.

It is advisable to perform a targeted breast ultrasonogram (USG) whenever there is a palpable or focal mammographic abnormality in the breast. Although USG is not efficacious as a screening modality, combined mammography and USG pick up more cancer than mammography alone [18]. Fibroadenoma is usually homogeneous, well-circumscribed, hypoechoic, ellipsoid, wider than tall, and may even show posterior enhancement on USG (Fig. 2.14), and intracystic or intraductal papillomas show a complex cyst (Fig. 2.15).

Simple cysts in the breast are completely anechoic, with a thin echogenic capsule, posterior enhancement, and thin edge shadowing (Fig. 2.16).

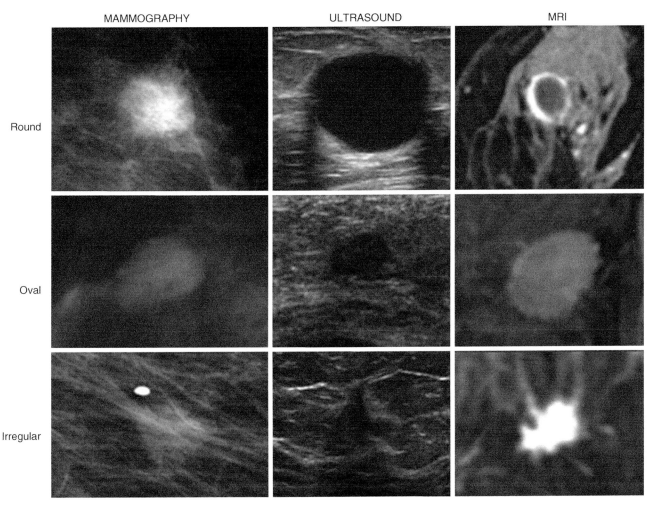

(Top) Shape Masses ACR-BIRADS

Fig. 2.10 BI-RADS margins. Radiologists describe masses according to both overall shape and margins. Digital zoom projection images show round, oval, and irregular masses (left to right: breast mammography, ultrasound, and magnetic resonance imaging)

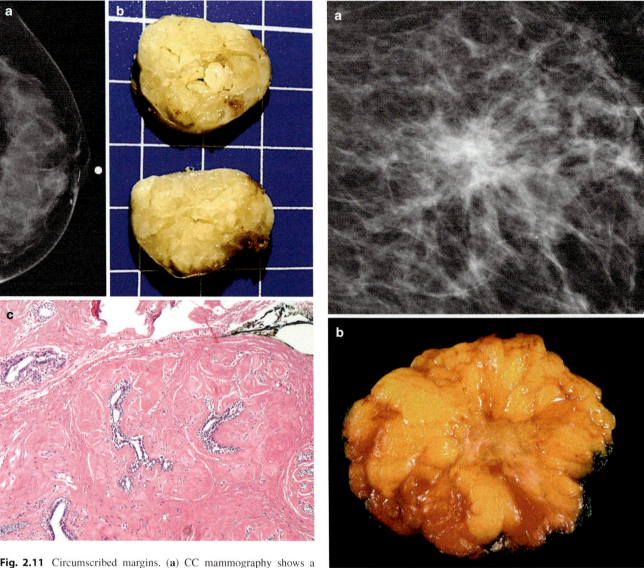

Fig. 2.11 Circumscribed margins. (**a**) CC mammography shows a round mass with well-circumscribed margins. (**b**) Gross: the lesion has a smooth rounded outline with a suggestion of a lobulated structure. (**c**) Fibroadenoma showing demarcation from the surrounding compressed breast tissue

Fig. 2.12 Spiculated margins. (**a**) Mammography shows a mass with spiculated margins. (**b**) Invasive ductal carcinoma not otherwise specified (NOS), gross appearance of breast resection specimen with spiculated lesion

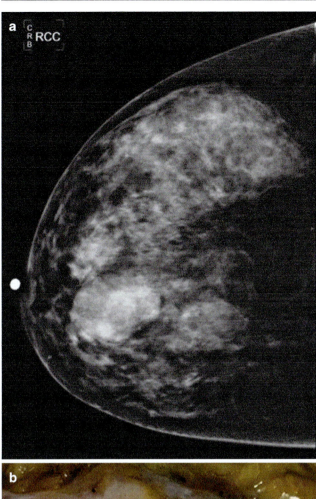

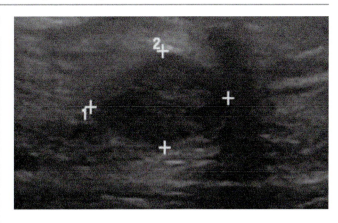

Fig. 2.14 Fibroadenoma. Breast USG shows homogeneous, hypoechoic, gently lobulated lesion suggestive of a fibroadenoma

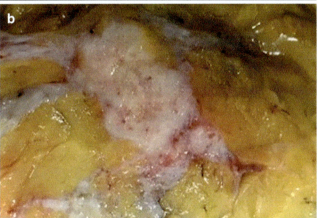

Fig. 2.13 Circumscribed margins. (**a**) Mammography shows circumscribed microlobulated mass. (**b**) Gross aspect of the specimen with a lobulated tumor. US guided biopsy confirmed Invasive Ductal Carcinoma NOS

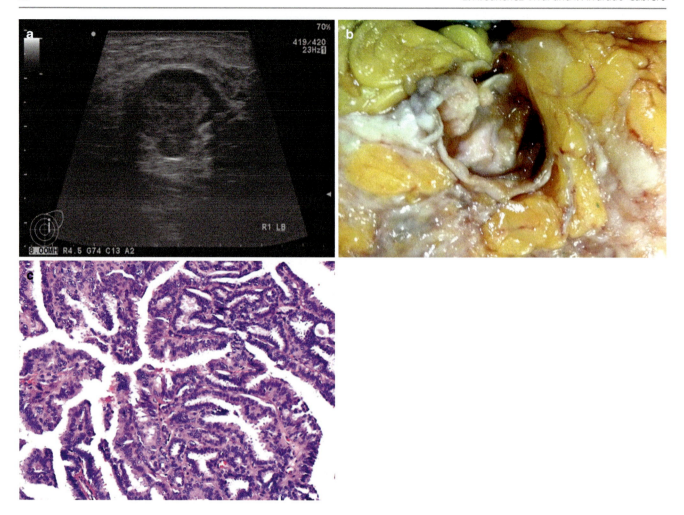

Fig. 2.15 Intraductal papilloma. (**a**) Breast US shows a complex cyst. (**b**) Large duct with an intraductal mass. (**c**) A benign intraductal papilloma with arborescent papillary fronds and well developed fibrovascular cores

Fig. 2.16 Circumscribed margins. (**a**) Ultrasound shows an anechoic imperceptible wall. (**b**) Excisional biopsy shows a simple cyst

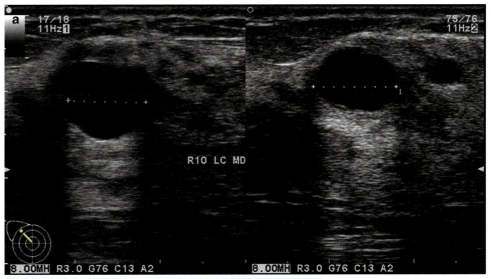

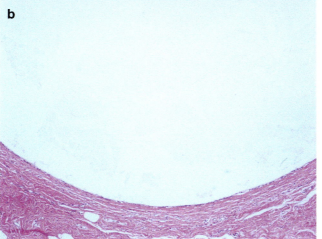

2.5.4 Calcifications

The previous BI-RADS mammography lexicon used the terms "grouped or clustered" for calcifications less than 1 cc in volume, and the term "regional" for calcifications greater than 2 cc. These terms did not address the group of calcifications measuring 1–2 cc in volume. The new edition has resolved this inconsistency by expanding the definition of "grouped" to a volume extending up to 2 cc. In addition, the terms "group or clustered," which could be used interchange- ably with the previous BI-RADS edition, are being phased out and have been changed to the term "grouped" (histori- cally clustered). The ultimate intention is to change it to "grouped" in a later revision [19].

Calcifications are now consolidated into two categories: (1) benign (Fig. 2.17); and (2) suspicious morphology. Amorphous, coarse heterogeneous, and fine linear branching calcifications are now placed in the "suspicious morphol- ogy" category (Fig. 2.18).

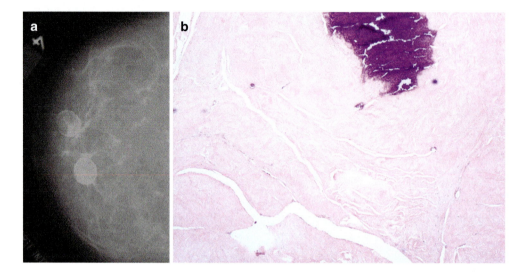

Fig. 2.17 Calcifications. (**a**) Calcifications surrounding a circumscribed lucent mas (Egg-shell). (**b**) Excisional biopsy (same patient) shows a fibroadenoma with macrocalcifications

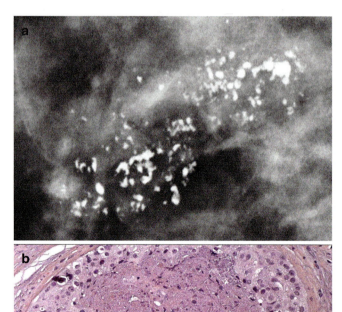

Fig. 2.18 Calcifications. (**a**) Mammography shows coarse heteroge- neous calcifications. (**b**) Biopsy showed a high-grade ductal carcinoma in situ with comedo type necrosis

2.5.5   Architectural Distortion

Architectural distortion is the alteration of the normal breast architecture with thin spiculations radiating from a point without a definitive mass; focal retraction or distortion may be seen at the parenchyma margin. It can be a primary finding associated with a mass, asymmetry, or calcifications [2, 9].

The term architectural distortion (Fig. 2.19) is unchanged in the fifth edition.

2.5.6   Asymmetries

There are some descriptive terms in the updated BI-RADS that have been expanded, such as the terms that describe an "asymmetry," which often represents summation artifacts. In addition, a new term, "developing asymmetry," which describes a focal asymmetry that is new, growing, or more conspicuous, has been added to the existing types of asymmetries in the mammography lexicon [14, 15].

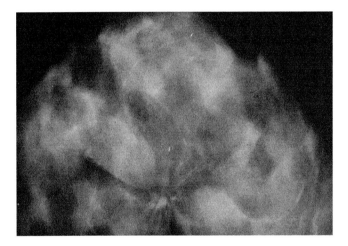

Fig. 2.19 Mammography of a palpable thickening shows an area of architectural distortion

2.5.7   Lesion Location

The new BI-RADS also provides clarification of terms used to describe lesion location on mammography. Previously, in cases where a lesion was located in the central breast or at the 12 o'clock location, a specific quadrant could not be assigned. The new BI-RADS has expanded the terminology for lesion location by adding terms such as "upper/lower/outer/inner central." This terminology allows for direct correlation of lesion location on ultrasound and MRI. Increased clarification has also been provided to describe the use of subcategories for the BI-RADS assessment Category 4. The new BI-RADS provides specific PPV cut-off points for BI-RADS 4A/4B/4C, which match certain specific imaging findings [15].

References

1. Jesinger RA. Breast anatomy for the interventionalist. Tech Vasc Interv Radiol. 2014;17:3–9.
2. Kettler MD. Breast overview. In: Berg WA, Birdwell RL, Gombos EC, editors. Diagnostic imaging: breast. Salt Lake City, UT: Amirsys; 2006. p. 12–130.
3. Hassiotou F, Geddes D. Anatomy of the human mammary gland. Current status of knowledge. Clin Anat. 2013;26:29–48.
4. Geddes DT. Inside the lactating breast: the latest anatomy research. J Midwifery Womens Health. 2007;52:556–63.
5. Going JJ, Moffat DF. Escaping from flatland: clinical and biological aspects of human mammary duct anatomy in three dimensions. J Pathol. 2004;203:538–44.
6. Stines J, Tristant H. The normal breast and its variations in mammography. Eur J Radiol. 2005;54:26–36.
7. Taplin SH, Rutter CM, Finder C, Mandelson MT, Houn F, White E. Screening mammography: clinical image quality and the risk of interval breast cancer. AJR Am J Roentgenol. 2002;178:797–803.
8. Majid AS, de Paredes ES, Doherty RD, Sharma NR, Salvador X. Missed breast carcinoma: pitfalls and pearls. Radiographics. 2003;23:881–95.
9. Agbenorku P, Agbemor Brayn VE, Aitpillah F, Akpaloo J, Aboah K, Agbenorku E. Ultrasonography as a breast imaging modality: a review. Br J Med Med Res. 2015;9:1–8.
10. Gokhale S. Ultrasound characterization of breast masses. Indian J Radiol Imaging. 2009;3:242–7.

11. Crystal P, Strano SD, Shcharynski S, Koretz MJ. Using sonography to screen women with mammographically dense breasts. AJR Am J Roentgenol. 2003;181:177–82.
12. Heywang-Kobrunner SH, Bick U, Bradley WG Jr, Boné B, Casselman J, Coulthard A, et al. International investigation of breast MRI: results of a multicenter study (11 sites) concerning diagnostic parameters for contrast-enhanced MRI based on 519 histopathologically correlated lesions. Eur Radiol. 2001;11:531–46.
13. Gavenonis SC. Breast MR imaging: normal anatomy. Magn Reson Imaging Clin N Am. 2011;19:507–19.
14. D'Orsi CJ, Mendelson EB, Ikeda DM. Breast imaging reporting and data system: breast imaging atlas. 4th ed. American College of Radiology: Reston, VA; 2003.
15. D'Orsi C, Sickles EA, Mendelson EB, Morris EA, ACR BI-RADS Atlas. Breast imaging reporting and data system. Reston VA: American College of Radiology; 2013.
16. Graf O, Helbich TH, Fuchsjaeger MH, Hopf G, Morgun M, Graf C, et al. Follow-up of palpable circumscribed noncalcified solid breast masses at mammography and US: can biopsy be averted? Radiology. 2004;233:850–6.
17. Mainiero MB, Goldkamp A, Lazarus E, Livingston L, Koelliker SL, Schepps B, et al. Characterization of breast masses with sonography. Can biopsy of some solid masses be deferred? J Ultrasound Med. 2005;24:161–7.
18. Berg WA, Blume JD, Cormack JB, Mendelson EB, Lehrer D, Böhm-Vélez M, et al. Combined screening with USG and mammography vs. mammography alone in women at elevated risk of breast cancer. JAMA. 2008;299:2151–63.
19. Henrot P, Leroux A, Barlier C, Génin P. Breast microcalcifications: the lesion in anatomical pathology. Diagn Interv Imaging. 2014;95:141–52.

Core-Needle Biopsy: Radiologic-Pathologic Correlation

Isabel Alvarado-Cabrero and Eloisa Asia Sanchez-Vivar

Percutaneous core-needle biopsies comprise the most common type of breast specimens in current practice. The indications for such biopsies include palpable and nonpalpable breast lesions. In most cases, the result of the procedure provides a definitive diagnosis or at least provides information that is used to plan the further management of the patient. Imaging-pathology correlation is of critical importance in imaging-guided breast biopsies to detect such a possible sampling error and avoid a delay in diagnosis. Pathologists should be familiar with the imaging features of various breast lesions and be able to appropriately correlate imaging findings with pathologic results after a core-needle biopsy. The purpose of this chapter is to review derived categories and corresponding management for an imaging-pathology correlation after performing an imaging-guided biopsy, and to illustrate the selected images for each category.

3.1 Introduction

Accurate preoperative diagnosis of a breast lesion is considered essential for designing an optimal treatment algorithm to achieve a definitive diagnosis without delay and with minimal biopsies. Core-needle biopsy (CNB) is increasingly being used in the investigation of breast disease [1].

The principal aim of core-needle biopsy is to provide a diagnosis of a breast abnormality before, and in many cases avoiding the need for, open surgical biopsy. In addition, CNB generally provides more reliable information compared to fine-needle aspiration biopsy cytology for providing architectural or histological information [2].

However, the cases receiving preoperative systemic therapy have increased in an effort to reduce the tumor volume and eliminate possible micrometastases for patients with locally advanced breast carcinoma. Consequently, clinical demands on pathologists have markedly increased for clinicians in institutions of many parts of the world [3] as they are expected to provide not only histological diagnosis but also prognostic and predictive information for patients, including the determination of estrogen receptor, progesterone receptor, ki67 and human epidermal growth factor receptor 2 (HER2) for treatment planning.

The radiologist breast physician or surgeon chooses which CNB device to use. The choice is determined by a number of interrelated factors with regard to the nature of the breast abnormality (palpable or impalpable): the availability of the various core biopsy instruments (conventional or vacuum-assisted); the imaging modalities (mammography, ultrasound, or MRI); the cost and patient-specific factors such as age and ability to undergo the biopsy procedure [4].

Proper care of patients undergoing breast biopsy requires complete cooperation by the entire breast care team. The team includes a variety of professionals, but centrally involved are radiologist, pathologists, surgeons, and medical oncologists [5].

I. Alvarado-Cabrero, MD, PhD (✉)
Department of Pathology, Hospital de Oncologia, Centro Medico Nacional Siglo XXI, Instituto Mexicano del Seguro Social, Mexico City, Mexico

E. A. Sanchez-Vivar, MD
Radiology Department, Hospital de Oncologia, Centro Medico Nacional Siglo XXI, Instituto Mexicano del Seguro Social, Mexico, Mexico

© Springer International Publishing AG, part of Springer Nature 2018
S. Stolnicu, I. Alvarado-Cabrero (eds.), *Practical Atlas of Breast Pathology*, https://doi.org/10.1007/978-3-319-93257-6_3

3.2 Breast Imaging Modalities

Although a comprehensive knowledge of imaging is not a prerequisite for a pathologist reporting core-needle biopsy, it helps in the interpretation of the pathology findings if the pathologist appreciates the correlation between imaging categories and pathology [1].

The intent is not for the pathologist replace the radiologist as a mammographer or diagnostic ultrasonographer. Instead, it is intended to educate the pathologist to better understand the significance of findings made by the radiologist on mammogram and breast ultrasound, and correlate them with the pathologic findings on ultrasound-guided core-needle biopsies [6].

The three modalities commonly used to evaluate the breast are mammography, ultrasound, and magnetic resonance imaging (MRI).

3.3 Mammography [7]

3.3.1 Mammography-Screening

Mammography-Screening (MS) is a proven system for early breast cancer detection. It is carried out on patients who do not have any symptoms of breast disease. MS has been shown to decrease the death rate from breast cancer.

3.3.2 Mammography-Diagnostic

A diagnostic mammogram is provided when a patient has a clinical abnormality such as: a breast lump, thickening skin, or nipple changes, axillary mass, or unknown primary malignancy. It is also used when a breast irregularity is seen on a screening mammography exam.

3.4 Ultrasound

Breast ultrasound plays a major role in the identification, diagnosis, and staging of breast cancer. Breast lesions that are initially identified on mammography and MRI can be further characterized with ultrasound [8].

3.5 Magnetic Resonance Imaging (MRI)

A breast MRI is mainly used for women who have been diagnosed with breast cancer to evaluate local extent of disease, look for other tumors in the breast, and check for tumors in the opposite breast. It is particularly helpful in young women ≤45 years old and in cases involving dense breast, invasive lobular histology, and extensive intraductal carcinoma [9].

3.6 Core-Needle Biopsy: Radiologic–Pathologic Correlation

A radiologist typically performs the biopsies triggered by an abnormal mammogram. The most important initial step is to get all the necessary information about the clinical examination and imaging studies so that the pathologist can document the information required to perform radiologic–pathologic correlation. It may be useful to aid the physicians to collect and document all the useful clinical information on the pathology requisition.

3.7   Sclerosing Adenosis

In the available literature, the most frequent microcalcifications patterns associated with sclerosing adenosis are: bilateral mammography benign-appearing microcalcifications throughout one or both breasts, punctate, or amorphous calcifications [10]. In one study, 80% of the microcalcifications were in clusters, and the remainder were scattered diffusely (Fig. 3.1) [11].

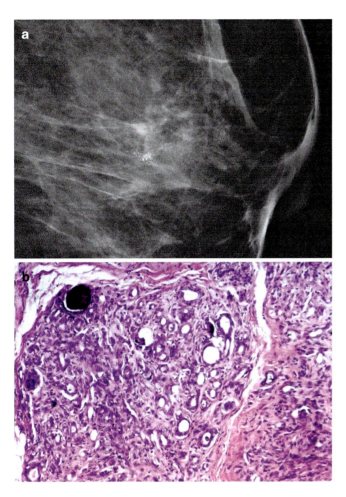

Fig. 3.1 Sclerosing adenosis. (**a**) Mammography magnification shows clusters of powdery, indistinct, calcifications. (**b**) Histopathology showed sclerosing adenosis with psammoma body-like calcifications

3.8   Radial Sclerosing Lesions

Radial Sclerosing Lesions (RSL) refers to both radial scars and larger complex sclerosing lesions (when over 1–2 cm).

The lesions appear as isodense masses, with an oval, lobular, or irregular shape. The margin is obscured, indistinct, or spiculated (Fig. 3.2) [12].

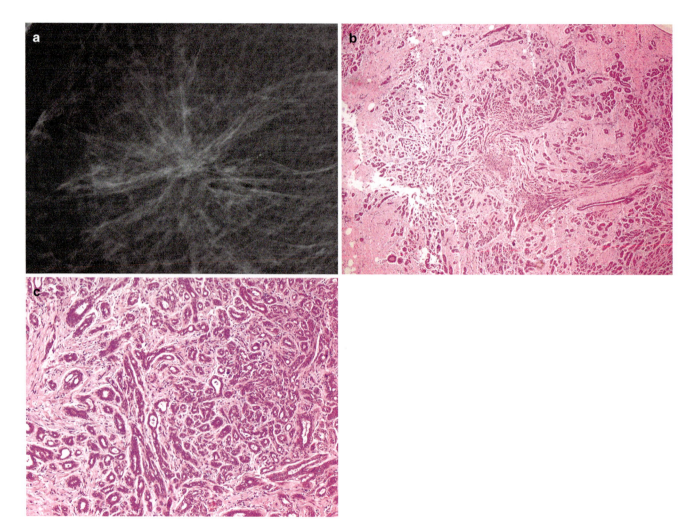

Fig. 3.2 Complex sclerosing lesion. (**a**) Mammography shows radiolucent central core and radiating spicules. (**b**) Ducts become distorted and appear angulated, giving rise to pseudoinfiltrative appearance. (**c**) Entrapped ducts retain myoepithelial layer of cells

3.9   Malignant Lesions

Most mammographic cancers appear as masses, calcifications, asymmetry, distortion, or a combination of the four. Masses and calcifications account for about 90% of all cancer appearances [13]. Masses account for nearly half of all mammographic cancers. Masses refer to space-occupying lesions. Because of the infiltrative biologic nature of most breast cancers, irregular- or lobulated-shaped masses are more likely associated with malignancy than round or oval masses [14].

The margin between a mass and the surrounding breast tissue is the key feature for analysis of masses because it relates to the infiltrating pattern of cancer. Margins are often obscured by breast tissue, rendering this evaluation impossible. Margins that are indistinct or microlobulated suggest infiltration into normal breast tissue and a higher risk of malignancy. Masses with spiculated borders forming a stellate or star-type pattern of radiating lines are associated with the highest risk of malignancy [15].

3.10   Ductal Carcinoma In Situ

The mammographic features of ductal carcinoma in situ (DCIS) have been well described in the literature, with microcalcifications being the dominant feature (Fig. 3.3). Fine linear calcifications in clustered or segmental distribution are almost always due to high-grade DCIS (Fig. 3.4). Other findings, such as masses, architectural distortions, dilated retroareolar ducts, and developing densities, have also been reported [16].

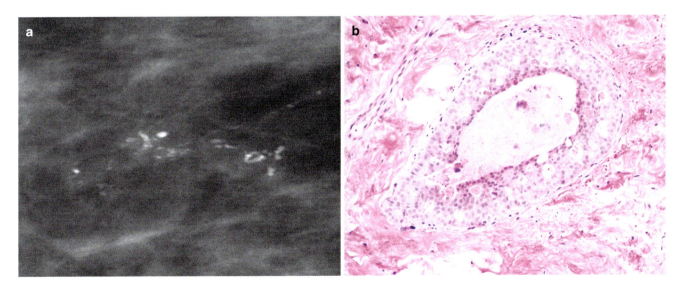

Fig. 3.3 Ductal carcinoma in situ. (**a**) Mammography magnification shows a few punctate and coarse Ca++ in a linear distribution. (**b**) Core-needle biopsy revealed ductal carcinoma in situ, intermediate grade with calcifications

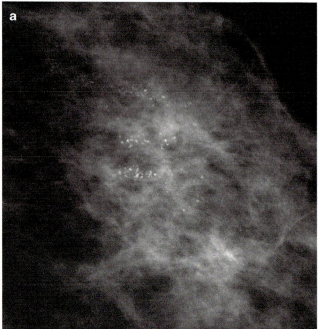

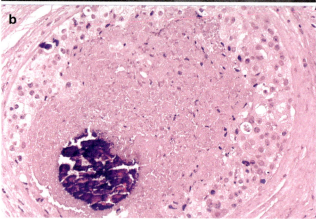

Fig. 3.4 Ductal Carcinoma in situ. (**a**) Mammography magnifications shows fine, pleomorphic calcifications with a segmental distribution. (**b**) Breast biopsy shows a high-grade ductal carcinoma in situ, comedo pattern

3.11 Invasive Carcinomas

- The mammography finding of **infiltrating carcinoma not otherwise specified (NOS)** is typically a dense mass with spiculated margins (Fig. 3.5). Focal asymmetric density ± distortion (Fig. 3.6), enlarging density, or as a mass have also been reported (Fig. 3.7). **Invasive lobular carcinoma** tends to present as a focal asymmetry with distortion, or as a spiculated mass, and calcifications are rare (1–11%) (Fig. 3.8) [17].

- The imaging characteristics of **invasive micropapillary carcinoma** are highly suggestive of malignancy. The lesion is a high-density irregular mass with indistinct margins associated with microcalcifications (Fig. 3.9) [18].

- **Medullary carcinoma** is typically seen as an oval, round, or lobular mass with partially circumscribed margins. There can be varying degrees of lobulation, while calcification is usually not a feature (Fig. 3.10) [19]. **Mucinous carcinoma** tends to present as a round, oval, or lobulated dense mass, and at least a portion of the margin is typically indistinct, particularly in mixed type (Fig. 3.11) [20].

- Mammographic findings of **encapsulated papillary carcinomas** include round or oval, circumscribed solitary or clustered masses, which may be associated with microcalcifications (Fig. 3.12). Spiculations are fairly uncommon, probably due to the lack of fibrosis. On ultrasound, the lesion may appear as an intraductal mass, with or without ductal dilatation, a complex solid cystic mass, or single or multiple solid nodules (Fig. 3.13). These lesions are usually vascular and have a tendency to bleed spontaneously, resulting in intracystic fluid-debris levels [21].

- The mammographic appearance of **metaplastic carcinoma** (MPC) has been described as a high-density mass with either circumscribed, obscured, irregular, or circumscribed with partially spiculated margins. On the other hand, the sonographic appearance of MPCs have been previously described as a heterogeneous or hypoechoic solid mass (Fig. 3.14) [22].

- Mammographically, **adenoid cystic carcinomas** (ACC) have been reported as smooth or irregular masses or asymmetric densities. Sonographically, ACCs have been reported as heterogeneous or hypoechoic, irregular masses (Fig. 3.15) [23].

- **Invasive cribriform carcinoma** (ICC) of the breast is a rare type of invasive carcinoma that shows a favorable prognosis. Few imaging findings related to ICC have been reported. Lee et al. [24] evaluated imaging findings of twenty-eight cases of ICC. The most common mammographic findings were of irregular shape (72.8%), spiculated margin (63.7%) (Fig. 3.16), and a high-density mass (81.8%).

- Calcifications can be associated **with lobular carcinoma in situ** and therefore concordant at core-needle biopsy. The classic form may be incidental and clinically innocuous. The pleomorphic form is morphologically similar to ductal carcinoma in situ, and may have a greater tendency to invasion (Fig. 3.17) [25].

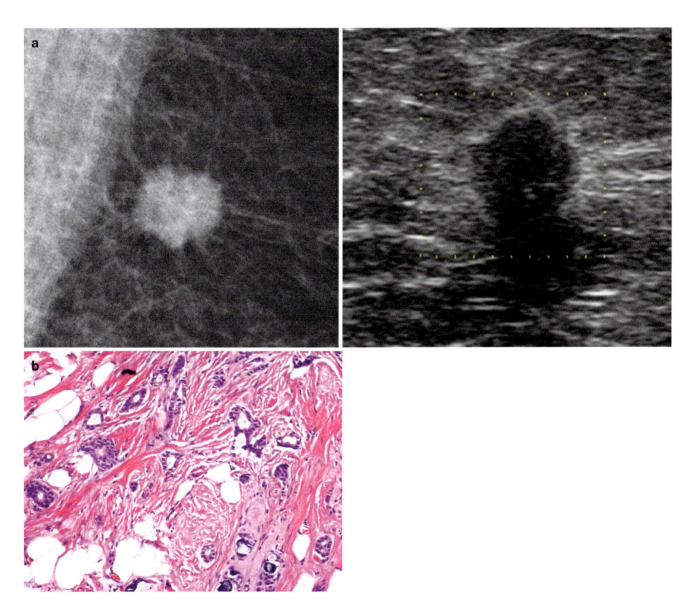

Fig. 3.5 Infiltrating ductal carcinoma not otherwise specified (NOS). (**a**) Mammographic findings, irregular mass, spiculated margins ± calcifications. Ultrasonography (US) shows hypoechoic mass with posterior shadowing. (**b**) US-guided biopsy showed Grade I invasive ductal carcinoma NOS

Fig. 3.6 Invasive ductal carcinoma not otherwise specified (NOS). (**a**) Mammography spot compression demonstrates architectural distortion. (**b**) US-guided biopsy showed Grade II invasive ductal carcinoma NOS

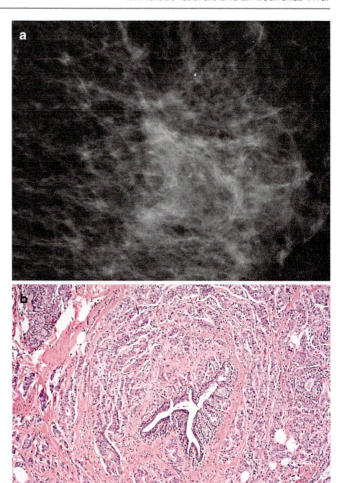

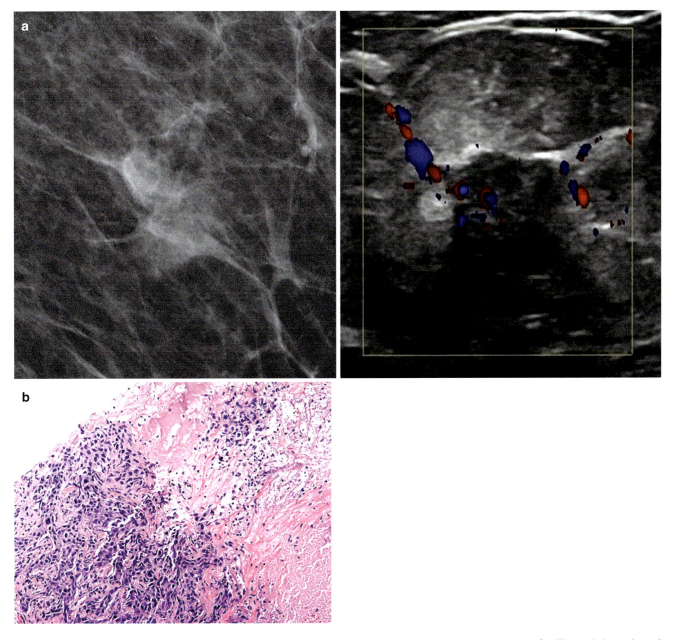

Fig. 3.7 (**a**) Invasive ductal carcinoma not otherwise specified (NOS). Mammography magnification shows a high-density, oval mass. Ultrasound shows hypoechoic, oval mass with angular margins and prominent peripheral vascular structures. (**b**) Histopathology showed Grade III invasive ductal carcinoma NOS

Fig. 3.8 Invasive lobular carcinoma. (**a**) Mammography magnification shows irregular mass with spiculated margins and nipple retraction. (**b**) Biopsy showed the cytological features characteristic of invasive lobular carcinoma

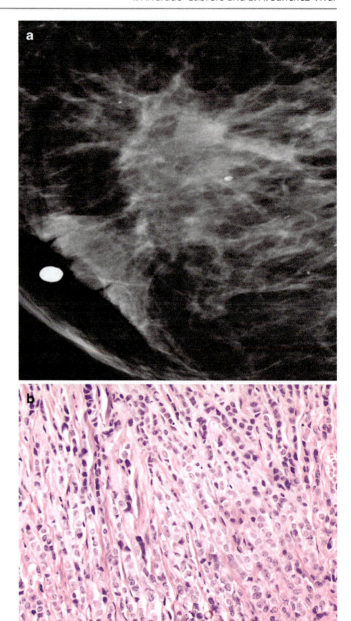

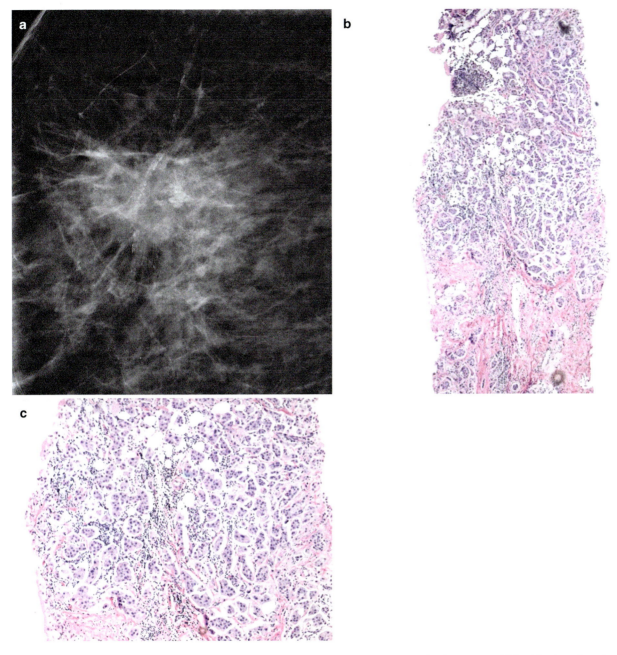

Fig. 3.9 Micropapillary carcinoma. (**a**) Mammography spot compression shows spiculated dense mass with microcalcifications. (**b**) Low-power view illustrates tumor cells in glans and nests, most of which appear to be within clear spaces. (**c**) In this view, the micropapillary clusters lack fibrovascular cores

Fig. 3.10 Medullary
carcinoma. (**a**) Spot
compression view
demonstrates an oval mass
with microlobulated margins.
(**b**) The tumor is composed of
a syncytium of epithelial cells
with an associated
lymphoplasmacytic infiltrate

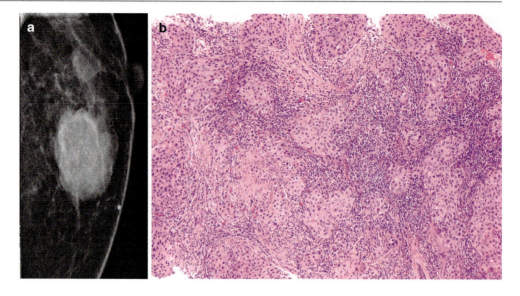

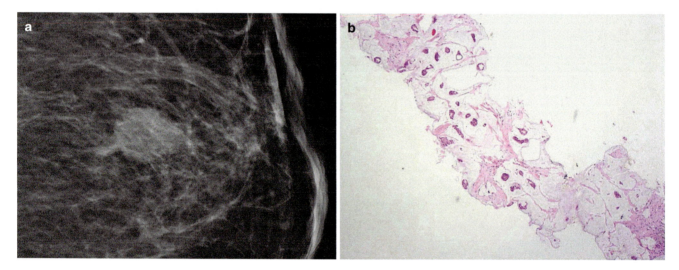

Fig. 3.11 Mucinous carcinoma(MC). (**a**) Mammography shows a dense microlobulated mass. (**b**) MC is characterized by abundant extracellular pools of mucus

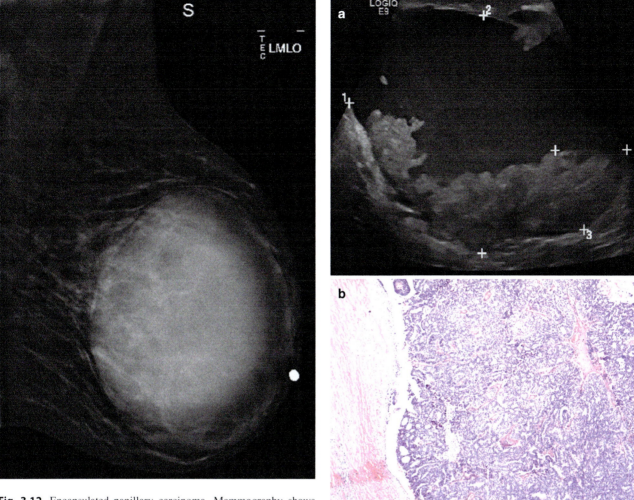

Fig. 3.12 Encapsulated papillary carcinoma. Mammography shows nonspecific, circumscribed mass without microcalcifications

Fig. 3.13 Encapsulated papillary carcinoma. (**a**) Ultrasound shows a complex thick-walled cystic lesion with intracystic masses. (**b**) A diagnosis of encapsulated carcinoma was suggested on core-needle biopsy. Excision confirmed the diagnosis

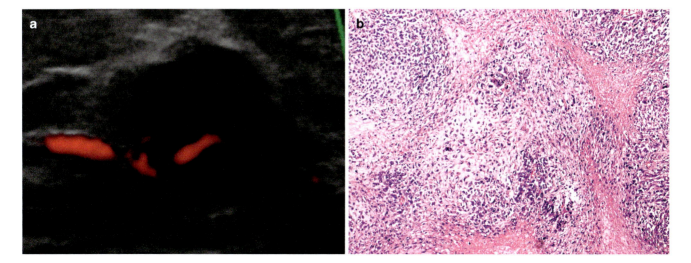

Fig. 3.14 Metaplastic carcinoma. (**a**) Color Doppler ultrasound shows vertically-oriented, hypoechoic, partially circumscribed mass with a feeding artery (or internal vascularity). (**b**) core-needle biopsy showed a metaplastic carcinoma with chondroid matrix

Fig. 3.15 Adenoid cystic carcinoma (ACC). (**a**) Irregular heterogeneous and hypoechoic mass with minimal vascularity on color Doppler imaging. (**b**) Ultrasound-guided biopsy showed an ACC with a cribriform pattern

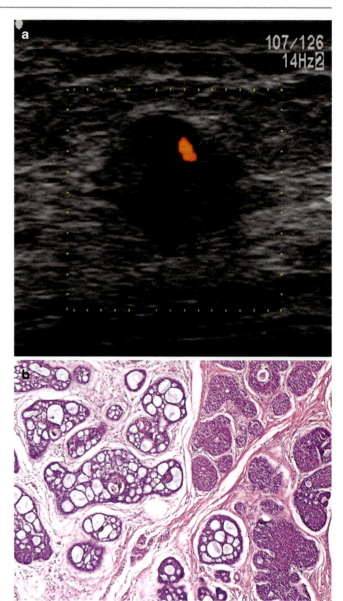

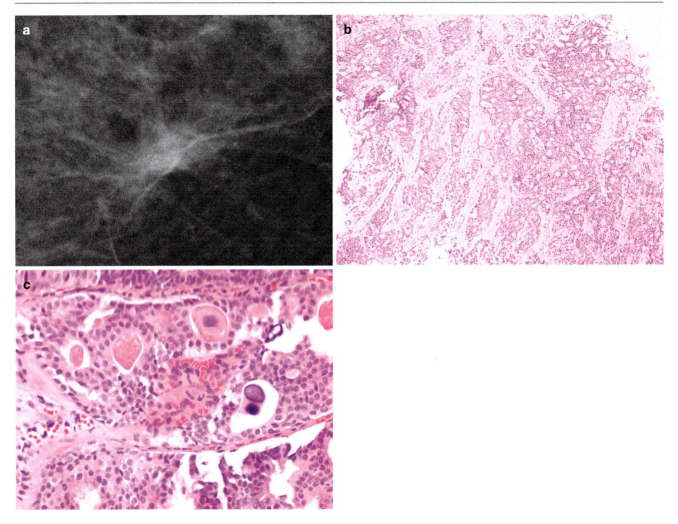

Fig. 3.16 Invasive cribriform carcinoma. (**a**) Mammography shows spiculated dense mass with associated architectural distortion and calcifications. (**b**) The tumor is composed of fenestrated cell nests with contours that vary from smooth to angulated and irregular. (**c**) Tumor cell nests with multiple calcifications

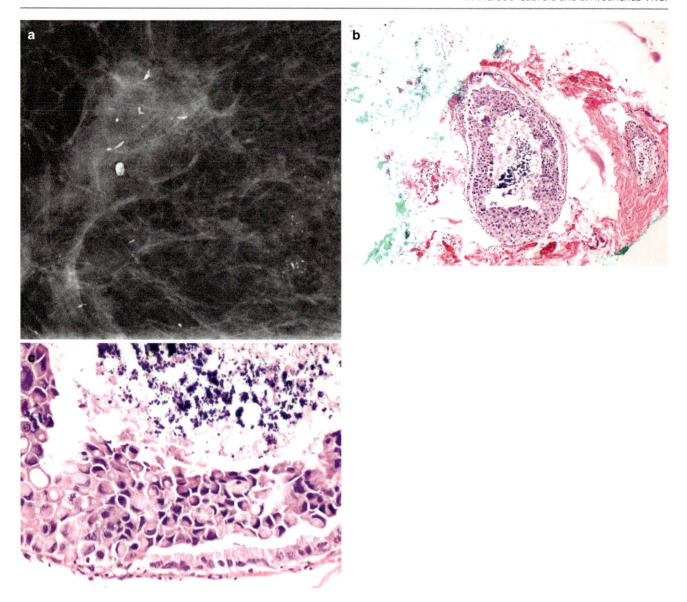

Fig. 3.17 Lobular carcinoma in situ with calcifications. (**a**) Mammography magnification shows coarse heterogeneous calcifications in a segmental distribution. (**b**) Lobular carcinoma in situ with calcifications. (**c**) Lobular carcinoma in situ with signet ring cells, necrosis, and calcifications

3.12   Breast Core-Needle Biopsy: Specimen Processing

The cores should be processed and fixed in formalin immediately after removal. The cold ischemic time (the time from cessation of blood flow to the tissue to exposure of the lesion to formalin) is generally shorter than 5 min, making the preservation of biomolecules optimal in these specimens. Core-needle biopsies are processed in a routine manner to paraffin embedding. The container label is correlated with the patient name and unit number on the requisition form (Fig. 3.18) [26]. The gross evaluation of core-needle biopsies is very simple and similar to other small biopsy speci-

mens. The cores should be counted and measured, and their nature as fatty or fibrous should be noted (Fig. 3.19). It is useful to document the number of cores submitted in each cassette. The tissue cassettes containing the targeted cores should be clearly identified in the gross description of the specimen. The final pathology report on these samples cannot be reliably completed in the current standard of practice without certain pieces of information. The pathology report on these samples requires correlation with findings on imaging studies that triggered the biopsy, in addition to the clinical presentation and clinical breast examination. The physician who performs the biopsy is responsible for the final correlation [27].

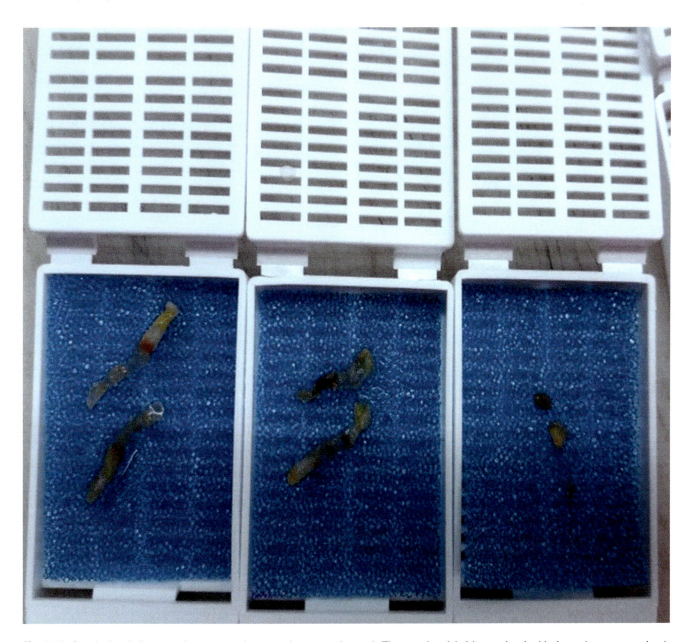

Fig. 3.18 Standard pathology specimen processing procedures must be used. The container label is correlated with the patient name and unit number on the requisition form. The color, number, and labeling of cassettes is verified if this method is used

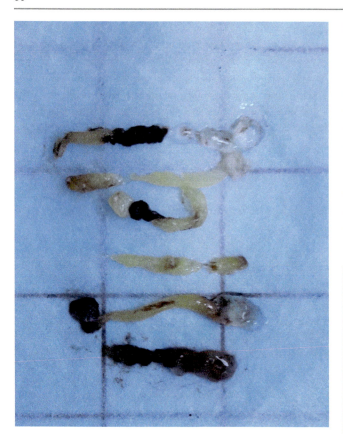

Fig. 3.19 Gross appearance of breast cores. These cores were obtained using ultrasound guidance. Some of them have a soft and gelatinous consistency. Histopathology showed a mucinous carcinoma

3.13 Specimen Radiograph

3.13.1 Core-Needle Biopsy

Biopsies for calcifications are radiographed by the radiologist to demonstrate that the targeted calcifications have been removed (Fig. 3.20). It can be helpful to separate the cores with calcifications, as malignancy is more likely to be found in these cores, compared to the cores without calcifications. Additional levels to find calcifications can be directed toward the blocks with radiologic calcifications. However, significant lesions can also be present in the cores without calcifications [28].

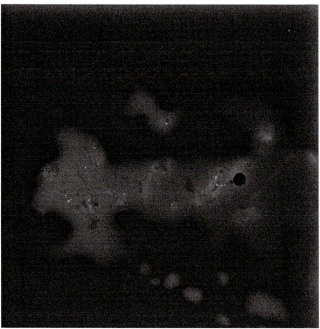

Fig. 3.20 After removing the cores for calcifications on the mammogram, the radiologist images the core

3.14 Evaluation of Breast Specimens Removed by Needle Localization Technique

It is standard practice for excisional specimens performed for lesions identified by imaging to undergo radiographic examination after excision (Fig. 3.21). The breast specimen when received should be measured and grossly inspected for any orientation designated by the surgeon. The specimen, still intact, should be placed on an x-ray plate and a radiograph should be taken. The radiograph should be evaluated with comparison to the patient's prior mammogram that showed the suspicious microcalcifications and/or abnormal soft-tissue densities (ASTD) (this is best evaluated by a radiologist.) If calcification/ASTD are identified which correspond to those observed mammographically, the surgeon should be informed immediately [29].

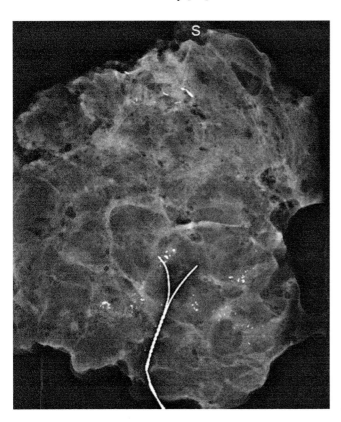

Fig. 3.21 Specimen radiograph. Wire marks cluster of calcifications

References

1. Bilous M. Breast core needle biopsy: issues and controversies. Mod Pathol. 2010;23:S36–45.
2. Tamaki K, Sasano H, Ishida T, Miyashita M, Takeda M, Amari M, et al. Comparison of core needle biopsy (CNB) and surgical specimen for accurate preoperative evaluation of ER, PgR and HER2 status of breast cancer patients. Cancer Sci. 2010;101:2024–79.
3. Uy GB, Laudico AV, Carnate JM, Lim FG, Fernandez AM, Rivera RR, et al. Breast cancer hormone receptor assay results of core needle biopsy and modified radical mastectomy specimens from the same patients. Clin Breast Cancer. 2010;10:154–9.
4. Liberman L. Percutaneous image-guided core breast biopsy. Radiol Clin N Am. 2002;40:483–500.
5. Rogers LW. Breast biopsy: a pathologist's perspective on biopsy acquisition techniques and devices with mammographic-pathologic correlation. Semin Breast Dis. 2006;8:127–37.
6. Lieu D. Breast imaging for interventional pathologists. Arch Pathol Lab Med. 2013;137:100–19.
7. Sickles EA, Miglioretti DL, Ballard-Barbash R, Geller BM, Leung JW, Rosenberg RD, et al. Performance benchmarks for diagnostic mammography. Radiology. 2005;235:775–90.
8. Candelaria RP, Hwang L, Bouchard RR, Whitman GJ. Breast ultrasound: current concepts. Semin Ultrasound CT MR. 2013;34:213–25.
9. Yamaguchi K, Schacht D, Senett CA, Newstead GM, Imaizumi T, Irie H, et al. Decision making for breast lesions initially detected at contrast-enhanced breast MRI. AJR Am J Roentgenol. 2013;201:1376–85.
10. Spruill L. Benign mimickers of malignant breast lesions. Semin Diagn Pathol. 2016;33:2–12.
11. Taskin F, Köseoğlu K, Unsal A, Erkuş M, Ozbaş S, Karaman C. Sclerosing adenosis of the breast: radiologic appearance and efficiency of core needle biopsy. Diagn Interv Radiol. 2011;17:311–6.
12. Inoue S, Inoue M, Kawasaki T, Takahashi H, Inoue A, Maruyama T, et al. Six cases showing radial scar/complex sclerosing lesions of the breast detected by breast cancer screening. Breast Cancer. 2008;15:247–51.
13. Pisano ED, Gatsonis C, Hendrick E, Yaffe M, Baum JK, Acharyya S, et al. Diagnostic performance of digital versus film mammography for breast-cancer screening. N Engl J Med. 2005;353:1773–83.
14. Nelson HD, Tyne K, Naik A, Bougatsos C, Chan BK, Humphrey L, et al. Screening for breast cancer: an update for the U.S. Prevention Services Task Force. Ann Intern Med. 2009;151:727–37.
15. Giess CS, Chikarmane SA, Sippo DA, Birdwell RL. Clinical utility of breast MRI in the diagnosis of malignancy after inconclusive or equivocal mammographic diagnostic evaluation. Am J Roentgenol. 2017;208:1378–85.
16. Van Zee KJ, White J, Morrow M, Harris JR. Ductal carcinoma in situ and microinvasive carcinoma. In: Harris JR, editor. Diseases of the breast. Philadelphia, PA: Lippincott, Williams and Wilkins; 2014. p. 337–59.

17. Evans AJ, Pinder SE, James JJ, Ellis IO, Cornford E. Is mammographic spiculation an independent, good prognostic factor in screening-detected-invasive breast cancer? AJR Am J Roentgenol. 2006;187:1377–80

18. Adrada B, Arribas E, Gilcrease M, Yang WT. Invasive micropapillary carcinoma of the breast: mammographic, sonographic, and MRI features. AJR Am J Roentgenol. 2009;193:58–63.

19. Yilmaz E, Lebe B, Balci P, Sal S, Canda T. Comparison of mammographic and sonographic findings in typical and atypical medullary carcinomas. Clin Radiol. 2002;57:640–5.

20. Matsuda M, Yoshimoto M, Iwase T, Takahashi K, Kasumi F, Akiyama F, et al. Mammographic and clinicopathological features of mucinous carcinoma of the breast. Breast Cancer. 2000;7:65–70.

21. Jagmohan P, Jane Pool F, Choudary Putti T, Wong J. Papillary lesions of the breast: imaging findings and diagnostic challenges. Diagn Interv Radiol. 2013;19:471–8.

22. Leddy R, Irshad A, Rumboldt T, Cluver A, Campbell A, Ackerman S. Review of metaplastic carcinoma of the breast: imaging findings and pathologic features. J Clin Imaging Sci. 2012;2:21.

23. Glazebrook KN, Reynolds C, Smith RL, Gimenez EI, Boughey JC. Adenoid cystic carcinoma of the breast. AJR Am J Roentgenol. 2010;194:1391–6.

24. Lee YJ, Choi BB, Suh KS. Invasive cribriform carcinoma of the breast: mammographic, sonographic, MRI, and 18 F-FDG PET-CT features. Acta Radiol. 2015;56:644–51.

25. Alvarado-Cabrero I, Picón Coronel G, Valencia Cedillo R, Canedo N, Tavassoli FA. Florid lobular intraepithelial neoplasia with signet ring cells, central necrosis and calcifications: a clinicopathological and immunohistochemical analysis of ten cases associated with invasive lobular carcinoma. Arch Med Res. 2010;41:436–41.

26. Hoda SA, Harigopal M, Harris GC, Pinder SE, Lee AH, Ellis IO. Expert opinion: what should be included in reports of needle core biopsies of the breast? Histopathology. 2003;43:84–90.

27. Renshaw AA. Adequate histologic sampling of breast core needle biopsies. Arch Pathol Lab Med. 2001;125:1055–7.

28. Margolin FR, Kaufman L, Jacobs RP, Denny SR, Schrumpf JD. Stereotactic core breast biopsy of malignant calcifications: diagnostic yield of cores with and cores without calcifications on specimen radiographs. Radiology. 2004;233:252–4.

29. Dua SM, Gray RJ, Keshtgar M. Strategies for localization of impalpable breast lesions. Breast. 2011;20:246–53.

Fine Needle Aspiration of Breast Cytology

4

Rana S. Hoda and Rema A. Rao

Breast carcinoma is the most common malignant tumor and the leading cause of carcinoma-related deaths in women worldwide [1]. Fine needle aspiration (FNA) continues to play an integral part in the pre-operative assessment of a breast mass [2, 3] and is the least invasive, fastest, and most cost-effective technique available. Although needle core biopsy (NCB) has largely replaced FNA for diagnosing most solid breast lesions, particularly in the USA, FNA is still used in most countries and displays good clinical performance [1–4].

4.1 FNA and NCB of Breast

The NCB has a better sensitivity than FNA (87% versus 74%) with similar specificity (98% versus 96%) [1, 4]. The indications for FNA include confirmation of the targeted nodule prior to performing NCB, sampling of cystic breast lesions, lesions difficult to access via NCB, and for diagnosis of metastatic disease [1–3]. The diagnostic sensitivity of FNA ranges from 74% to 99%, specificity ranges from 60% to 100%, and accuracy from 72% to 95%. The false-negative and false-positive rates of FNA ranges from 1.7% to 13.3% and from 0.6% to 6.5% respectively [2, 3].

4.2 Advantages and Limitations of FNA of Breast

The "triple test" approach is utilized to accurately analyze a breast mass. The triple test uses the clinical and radiological findings, and cytological features on breast FNA to arrive at a diagnostic interpretation. If all three findings are positive, the diagnostic accuracy for a malignant neoplasm approaches 100% [5].

The advantages of FNA of breast lesions include: (1) the ability to sample cystic lesions; (2) the ability to sample lesions that are difficult to access through NCB, such as lesions in the retroareolar location and chest wall recurrence of breast carcinoma; (3) detecting metastatic breast carcinoma in bone, lungs, and body cavity fluids; and (4) ability to perform prognostic and predictive markers on FNA material from metastatic sites.

Limitations of breast FNA include: (1) Inability to distinguish *in situ* ductal carcinoma (DCIS) from invasive carcinoma of no special type (NST); (2) inability to distinguish low-grade ductal carcinoma from fibroadenoma and atypical epithelial hyperplasia; and (3) inability to perform prognostic and predictive markers, such as Her2-neu in primary breast carcinoma [2, 3, 5].

4.3 Slide Preparation and Staining Techniques

Conventional smears and cellblocks have traditionally been used as the preferred preparations from an FNA of the breast. However, liquid-based preparations (LBP), including ThinPrep (TP; Hologic, Boxborough, MA) and SurePath (SP; BD Diagnostics, Burlington, NC), are increasingly being used as either sole preparations or in conjunction with the traditional preparations for diagnosing breast lesions. Although the LBP produce minor changes in cytomorphology and background features, the diagnostic sensitivity and specificity are similar to conventional preparatory techniques [6].

R. S. Hoda, MD (✉)
CBLPath, Rye Brook, NY, USA
e-mail: rhoda@cblpath.com

R. A. Rao, MD
Papanicolaou Cytology Laboratory, Weill Cornell Medicine/New York Presbyterian Hospital, New York, NY, USA
e-mail: rer9052@med.cornell.edu

© Springer International Publishing AG, part of Springer Nature 2018
S. Stolnicu, I. Alvarado-Cabrero (eds.), *Practical Atlas of Breast Pathology*, https://doi.org/10.1007/978-3-319-93257-6_4

Slide preparations include conventional smears (CS), cytospins, LBP (including TP and SP), and cellblocks (CB). The CS and cytospins can be air-dried and stained with Romanowsky stain or alcohol-fixed and stained with Papanicolaou (Pap) stain. LBP are alcohol-fixed and stained with Pap stain. Hematoxylin and eosin (H&E) stain is used to stain CB sections [2, 6].

The CS can also be stained with ultra-fast (UF) Pap stain. This is a modified Pap stain that hemolyzes the background blood and makes cells flatter and larger due to air-drying and rehydration in saline. In addition, the alcohol fixative used in this process contains formalin. This stain can be performed in 90 seconds and is thus termed ultra-fast. UF-Pap stain has similar background, nuclear staining, and cell morphology as the standard Pap stain [7].

Multiple studies have demonstrated the utility of LBP for breast FNA. Aside from some minor cytomorphological and background differences between LBP and CS, LBP has been shown to be a reliable technique with a diagnostic accuracy equivalent to CS. The advantages include a single standardized and uniform preparation with no obscuring elements, which makes it easier to screen and interpret. Ancillary tests, such as immunocytochemistry, can be formed on additional LBP. Collection technique is uniform and the sample collection vial, containing preservative solution, is easier to transport and store. The main disadvantage of LBP is that on-site adequacy assessment cannot be performed.

Cytological alterations in LBP include: (1) Cells appear smaller; (2) cell groups may become fragmented, and more single cells may be seen; (3) epithelial cells may become dissociated with stromal components, such as in fibroadenoma; (4) due to immediate liquid fixation, nucleoli may become apparent even in benign lesions; and (5) myoepithelial cells may retain their cytoplasm and mimic cells of invasive ductal carcinoma. The main alteration in the background features include reduced or lack of background elements such as mucin or necrosis, and the background material tends to clump instead of being diffuse as seen in CS [6].

4.4   Reporting of Breast FNA

In 1996, the National Cancer Institute (NCI) in the United States proposed the probabilistic approach of breast FNA, based on cytological features, for uniform reporting. The NCI approach has been widely adopted and is comprised of five diagnostic categories: unsatisfactory (C1), benign (C2), atypical (C3), suspicious/favor malignancy (C4), and malignant (C5). The International Academy of Cytology is developing a reporting system similar to the NCI version. A draft of the system will soon be available at the IAC website for review and critique by breast pathologists [8, 9].

4.5   Benign Epithelial Cells

The morphology of ductal and lobular epithelial cells varies with the age of the woman, phase of menstrual cycle, and pregnancy. The majority of ductal epithelial cells are columnar or cuboidal. The cytoplasm contains abundant organelles involved in secretion. Histologically, myoepithelial cells lie between the epithelial cells and basal lamina. Cytologically, they are dark and crescentic, are interspersed between ductal epithelial cells, and appear in different planes of focus. The lobules, both histologically and cytologically, appear as rounded clusters comprising round-to-cuboidal cells with vacuolated cytoplasm (Fig. 4.1) [1–3].

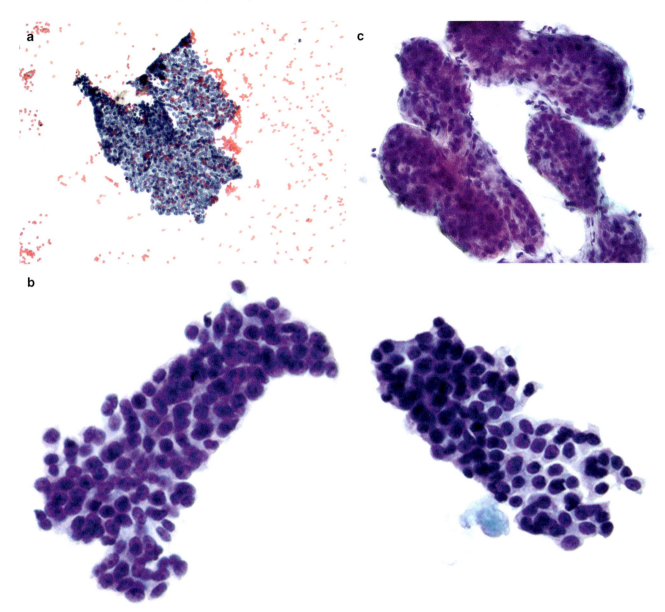

Fig. 4.1 Benign ductal and lobular cells: (**a**) Benign ductal cells in a conventional smear show cohesive sheets and tight clusters of cells with bland nuclei, pale nuclear chromatin, and small inconspicuous nucleoli. Myoepithelial cells appear as darker crescentic cells on a different plane of focus than epithelial cells (Pap stain); (**b**) Benign ductal cells in a ThinPrep shows ductal cell groups with regular thin nuclear membranes, pale chromatin, and small inconspicuous nucleoli. Note the darker myoepithelial cells. Cytological features are similar to those seen in the CS. However, the background is clean (Pap stain); (**c**) Benign lobules are composed of terminal ducts and many small acini. Flattened myoepithelial cells surround the tight cohesive group of benign terminal ductal epithelium (TP, Pap)

4.6   Non-neoplastic Entities

4.6.1   Cystic Apocrine Metaplasia

Apocrine metaplasia can occur in any benign proliferative lesion. Histologically, cystic apocrine metaplasia is composed of flat cuboidal cells, which may form a single layer or as blunt papillae. The cells are evenly spaced with round nuclei with nucleoli and abundant finely granular eosinophilic cytoplasm (Fig. 4.2) [1–3, 6].

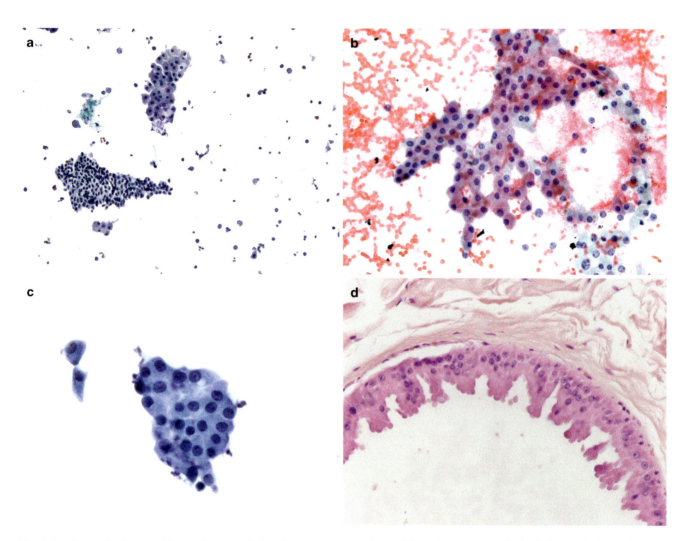

Fig. 4.2 Fibrocystic change with apocrine metaplasia: (**a**) A benign ductal cell group with no cytologic atypia, noted adjacent to a group of apocrine metaplastic cells. The apocrine metaplastic cells contain abundant granular cytoplasm, well-defined cellular outlines, round nuclei, prominent nucleoli, and bland chromatin. The background elements of foamy histiocytes and cystic debris are retained (TP, Pap); (b) Apocrine metaplastic cells in conventional smear: The cells have moderately abundant granular cytoplasm, well-defined cellular outlines, round and regular nuclei, small nucleoli and bland chromatin. Note abundant background blood (Pap stain); (**c**) Apocrine metaplastic cells in ThinPrep: Higher magnification of the apocrine metaplastic cells showing similar features as the conventional smear. Lack of blood in the background allows for better appreciation of cytology (Pap stain); (**d**) Apocrine metaplastic cells in histology: Excisional biopsy shows a cystically enlarged duct lined by apocrine cells, a feature of nonproliferative fibrocystic change or apocrine cyst (H&E)

4.6.2 Fibroadenoma

Fibroadenomas comprise one-fifth of all benign breast masses and usually occur at a mean age of 30 years. It clinically presents as a palpable, painless, firm, and solitary mass. The non-palpable fibroadenoma are detected on imaging. Fibroadenomas arise from the epithelium and stroma of terminal duct-lobular units. Histologically, epithelial and stromal components are noted. Squamous and apocrine metaplasia and duct hyperplasia may be seen within the epithelial component. Fibroadenomas are frequently sampled and diagnosed by FNA. Accurate cytological diagnosis of this common benign lesion is important so that the patient can be treated by conservative surgery or clinically followed. Cytological findings should be correlated with clinical and imaging findings. Cytologically, a confident diagnosis of fibroadenoma shows staghorn epithelial configurations, stromal fragments, and numerous background myoepithelial cells, some of which appear as stripped nuclei (Fig. 4.3). However, fibroadenoma is a well-recognized source of false-positive diagnosis and may be misdiagnosed as a low-grade ductal carcinoma because of shared cytomorphologic features [1–3, 6, 10].

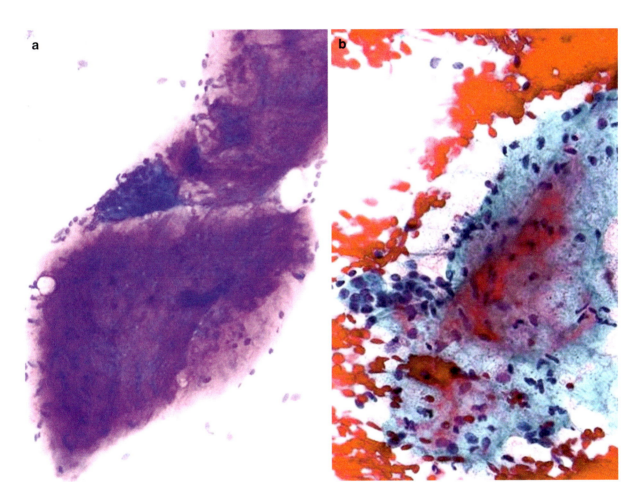

Fig. 4.3 Fibroadenoma: (**a**, **b**) FNA of fibroadenoma are characterized by staghorn arrangements of epithelial cells intermixed with spindled cells embedded in stromal fragments. The nuclei can occasionally show atypia that can be mistaken for malignancy. In these CS, the stromal fragments are intermixed with benign ductal cell groups. The stromal fragments stain magenta on air-dried Romanowsky stain (DQ stain) (left) and greenish-blue on alcohol fixed Pap stain (right); (**c**, **d**) ThinPrep shows clusters of tightly cohesive ductal cells with minimal nuclear atypia and stromal fragments. The background is clean with singly-distributed myoepithelial cells with oval-to-crescentic dark nuclei and scant cytoplasm. In CS, these cells appear as "stripped nuclei." The diagnosis of fibroadenoma may be more difficult on LBP, due to epithelial cells and stromal dissociation. Moreover, in LBP, the myoepithelial cells may retain their cytoplasm and may mimic isolated cells of IDC (TP, Pap); (**e**) Excisional biopsy of fibroadenoma showing the biphasic morphology with elongate staghorn-like benign ductal elements and a background bland appearing hypocellular stromal component with no nuclear atypia, mitoses, or necrosis (H&E)

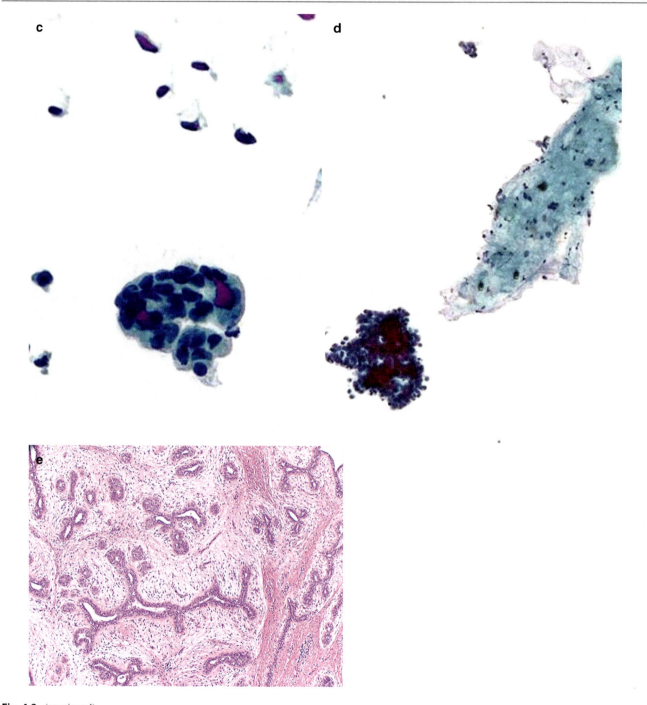

Fig. 4.3 (continued)

4.6.3   Lactational Change

In pregnancy, secretory changes occur evenly throughout the breast. The terminal ducts and the lobules enlarge, with the latter being of different shapes and irregularly distended. Histologically, the cells within the lobules enlarge and proliferate and display vacuolated cytoplasm, hyperchromatic nuclei, and prominent nucleoli. Cytologically, the architec-

tural and cellular features are similar to histology and are also similar in CS and LBP. In addition, the background shows lipid droplets and proteinaceous material with "stripped" nuclei with prominent nucleoli embedded within. FNA of breast masses in pregnant or lactating women is an uncommon procedure, and cytological interpretation is considered problematic due to atypia inherent to secretory change in glandular epithelia (Fig. 4.4) [6, 11].

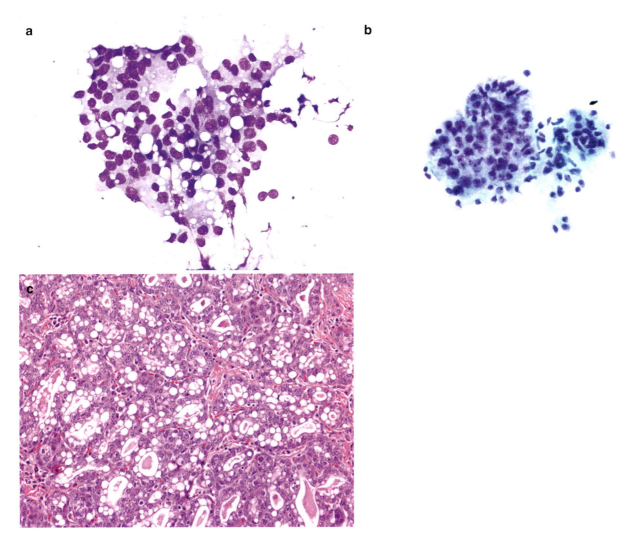

Fig. 4.4 Lactational adenoma/change: (**a**) Lactational adenoma/change presents as a well-circumscribed mass during or immediately after pregnancy. FNA specimens tend to be hypercellular. In this conventional smear, the ductal cell groups are loosely cohesive and show nuclear enlargement without size variation, foamy cytoplasm, and prominent nucleoli. "Bare" nuclei are present in the background. Conventional air-dried smears tend to best show the foamy material in the background, whereas the LBP tend to have a clean background (DQ stain); (**b**) In ThinPrep, the ductal cells are arranged as cohesive groups, appear monotonous, with prominent nucleoli; the cytoplasm is foamy and delicate. All background elements of lactational adenoma/change are retained in LBP, but may be reduced and tend to be more cohesive rather than being diffuse (Pap stain); (**c**) Excisional biopsy of lactational adenoma/change: shows hypersecretory change in mammary glands with closely packed glands and abundant luminal secretions. The lesional cells are similar to those on cytology (H&E)

4.6.4 Fat Necrosis

Fat necrosis may result from trauma, prior surgery, or radiation therapy, and may affect any part of the breast. Patients usually present with a superficially located painless breast mass with retraction of the overlying skin. Fat necrosis may be difficult to distinguish from breast carcinoma, both clinically and radiologically. Histologically, fat necrosis initially shows disruption of fat and hemorrhage, followed by infiltration of histiocytes, some containing hemosiderin, foreign-body giant cells, other inflammatory cells, and occasional foci of calcifications. Fibrosis occurs in late stages. Cytological features are similar to histological features (Fig. 4.5) [1–3, 6].

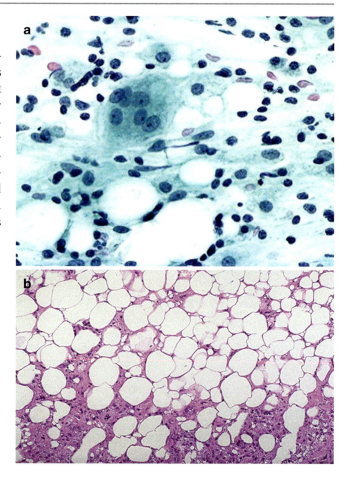

Fig. 4.5 Fat necrosis: (**a**) Aspirates of fat necrosis are usually hypocellular and consist predominantly of histiocytes some forming multinucleate and pigmented giant cells, with coarse vacuolated cytoplasm, on a background of fibroadipose tissue. Occasional foci of calcification may also be seen (CS, Pap); (**b**) Fat necrosis on the corresponding biopsy shows necrotic adipocytes and intermixed histiocytes that are similar to those on cytology (H&E)

4.7   Atypical Breast Lesions

Histologically, ductal hyperplasia without atypia shows orderly epithelial growth with varied structural patterns. The nuclei are smooth, round, oval-to-spindly and may show uneven spacing and overlap. Nucleoli are not conspicuous, chromatin distribution is uniform, cytoplasm is scant and may appear vacuolated. Nuclear-to-cytoplasmic (N:C) ratio is low [1]. In contrast, atypical ductal hyperplasia (ADH) is a proliferative lesion, which fulfills some, but not all criteria for DCIS. ADH may show a solid, cribriform, micropapillary or papillary growth patterns. The nuclei are enlarged, hyperchromatic, with irregular chromatin distribution and nucleoli. N:C ratio is high. Mitoses may be seen [1].

Cytologically, atypical diagnosis poses a management dilemma. The NCI atypical category C3 is characterized by cytological features between clearly malignant or clearly benign, thus making a definitive cytological diagnosis impossible [12]. The rate of C3 is 3–7% of all breast FNA. Causes of atypical diagnoses include sampling and technical reasons such as low cellularity and smear-related artifacts of air-drying, thick cellular areas, and excess blood. Cytopathologists' experience may lead to misinterpretation, such as overcall of atypia that is occasionally seen in a fibroadenoma as atypical. Unfamiliarity with cytomorphologic features on LBP may also cause misinterpretation (Fig. 4.6) [1–3, 6, 12].

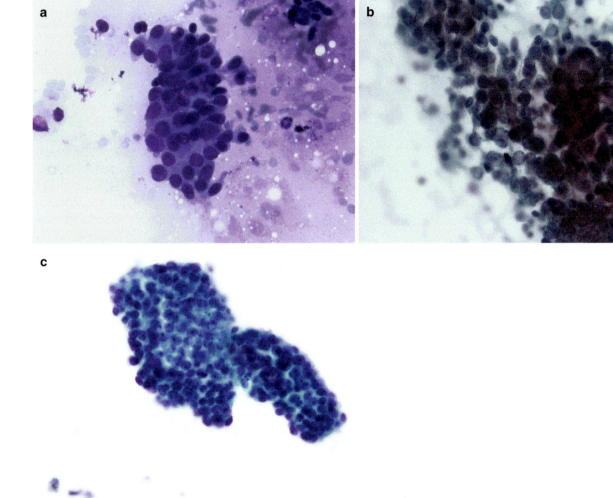

Fig. 4.6 Atypical: (**a**) A loosely cohesive cluster of ductal cells with nuclear enlargement, loss of polarity, and high N:C ratio. Note the single cells with similar cytology in the background. Scant cellularity of these atypical ductal groups precludes a more definitive interpretation and therefore this aspirate is best classified as "atypical" (CS, DQ); (**b**) A cohesive cluster of ductal epithelial cells with nuclear enlargement, overlap, loss of polarity, high N:C ratio, and prominent nucleoli. Scattered in between these atypical ductal cells are dark and crescentic myoepithelial cells. The overall findings raise the possibility of sampling of DCIS or atypical ductal hyperplasia, although these entities are not definitively diagnosed on cytology and therefore best classified as "atypical" (CS, UFPAP); (**c**) A single tight cohesive cluster of ductal cells reminiscent of a "staghorn" cluster in a fibroadenoma, Fibroadenoma (FA) but exhibit cytologic atypia with nuclear enlargement, overlap, and prominent nucleoli, and therefore best classified as "atypical." Note similarity with the conventional smears (TP, Pap)

4.8   Neoplastic Entities

4.8.1   Breast Cancer

Breast carcinoma is the most common malignant tumor in women and the leading cause of carcinoma-related deaths in women worldwide. Breast cancer makes up 25% of all new cancer diagnoses in women globally [1]. Breast carcinoma can be of no special type or lobular type and can be in situ or invasive. Cytology cannot distinguish between in situ or invasive disease due to similar cytomorphology of malignant cells and lack of cytological criteria that can accurately identify invasive carcinoma. This chapter will therefore describe only invasive breast carcinoma.

4.8.2   Invasive Carcinoma of No Special Type (NST)

Invasive carcinoma of no special type (NST), also previously known as invasive ductal carcinoma, not otherwise specified (NOS), is the largest group of malignant tumors in the breast and accounts for 75–80% of all breast carcinomas. Clinical presentation is usually of a solid mass involving any part of the breast, and it can occur at any age. The initial diagnosis can be made on FNA and NCB. Histologically, the tumors can be graded into well, moderately, and poorly-differentiated, based on architectural and nuclear features and mitotic rate. The advantage of FNA in examining NST is that it can be used as an adjunctive diagnostic test to accurately assess the targeted lesion prior to NCB. The limitations of FNA in examining NST include: (1) false-negative diagnoses due to sampling of tumors with abundant fibrosis where malignant cells may not be adequately aspirated; (2) interpretive issues, where well-differentiated carcinoma of NST type may be misinterpreted as fibroadenoma; (3) false-positive diagnosis may be rendered in fibroadenoma and lactational changes, due to cellular atypia of isolated cells; and (4) inability to grade NST because the parameters used in histologic grading cannot be accurately reproduced in cytology (Figs. 4.7 and 4.8) [1–3, 6].

Although FNA is a reliable method for the diagnosis of breast carcinoma, difficulties in the recognition of the various subtypes of NST still exist [1–3, 6, 13]. Haji et al. [13] concluded that NST, as well as other types of infiltrating breast carcinoma such as mucinous, medullary, apocrine, and papillary, have specific cytomorphological features that differentiate them from one another and from IDC, NST (Fig. 4.8). They described the frequency of 20 cytomorphological features, including architectural pattern, forms of neoplastic cells and their nuclear and cytoplasmic characteristics, accompanying cells, and background materials and semi-quantitative analysis of five features including cellularity, pleomorphism, nuclear irregularity, presence of cells in loose cohesive clusters, and singly dispersed cells. Specific features are discussed in the sections on the four variants of infiltrating breast carcinoma described below.

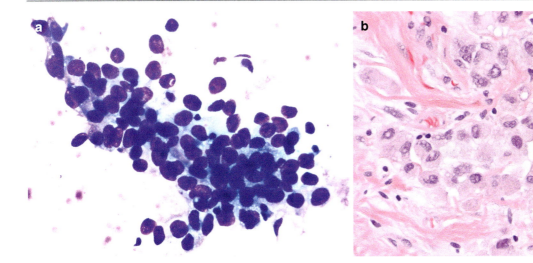

Fig. 4.7 Invasive ductal carcinoma-NST, high-grade: (**a**) The cytomorphologic features are similar to adenocarcinoma seen elsewhere: clusters of three-dimensional (3-D) cells with nuclear pleomorphism, hyperchromasia, and irregular nuclear borders. In this case, the cell clusters are loosely cohesive with nuclear pleomorphism and prominent nucleoli. The cytoplasm is vacuolated. It is not possible to distinguish infiltrating ductal carcinoma (IDC) from ductal carcinoma in situ on cytology alone (CS, DQ); (**b**) Invasive carcinoma-NST, high-grade, on the corresponding histologic section, showing irregular angulated glands composed of cells with similar cytology as previously described (H&E)

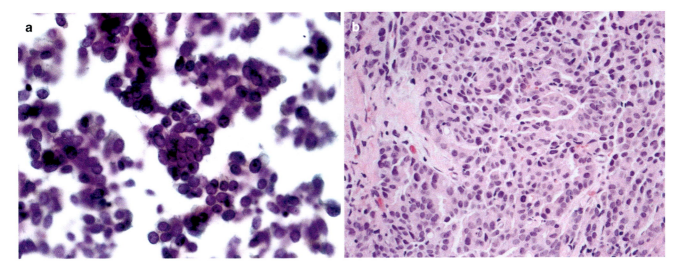

Fig. 4.8 Invasive carcinoma-NST, low-grade: (**a**) Cohesive clusters of malignant cells with low nuclear grade features such as mild-to-moderate nuclear enlargement, mild increase in N:C ratios, fairly regular nuclear membranes and moderately abundant vacuolated cytoplasm seen on Ultra-fast Pap stain (CS, UF Pap); (**b**) Invasive carcinoma-NST, low-grade on concurrent histologic section, showing tumor cells with similar cytomorphology with low nuclear grade and tubule formation (H&E)

4.8.2.1 Tubular Carcinoma

Tubular carcinoma is a highly differentiated infiltrating breast carcinoma accounting for <2% of all female breast carcinomas. Histologically, it is composed of well-defined tubules lined by a single layer of tumor cells and surrounded by abundant fibrous stroma. The tubules are angulated, open, and haphazardly infiltrate the breast parenchyma. The cells are cuboidal or columnar with basally-located round or oval hyperchromatic nuclei, finely granular chromatin, and inconspicuous nucleoli. Cytoplasm is usually amphophilic and apocrine snouts may be seen towards the luminal cell surface. Cytological features are similar to those described for NCB. Most cases of tubular carcinoma are detected by mammography. The sensitivity for the diagnosis of tubular carcinoma is higher with NCB than with FNA. Because of limited sampling, most tubular carcinomas are interpreted as atypical and not outright malignant by FNA. Other histologic types of breast carcinoma may often occur with tubular carcinoma (Fig. 4.9) [1–3, 6].

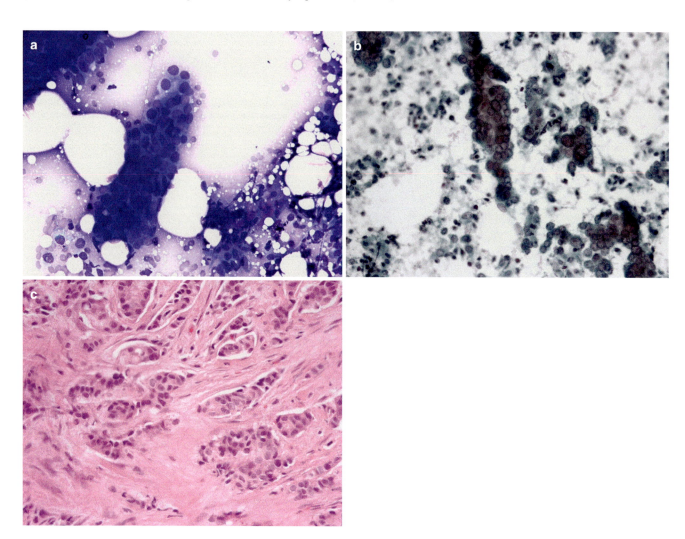

Fig. 4.9 Tubular carcinoma: (**a**) Cohesive clusters of tumor cells in honeycombed sheets and clusters showing tubule formation and low nuclear grade (CS, DQ); (**b**) Cellular aspirate with cohesive clusters of tumor cells with low nuclear grade and prominent tubule like formation (CS, UF Pap); (**c**) Concurrent core biopsy showing the prominent tubule formation and tumor cells with low nuclear grade (H&E)

4.8.2.2 Mucinous (Colloid) Carcinoma

Pure mucinous carcinoma is an uncommon variant of infiltrating breast carcinoma with distinctive histologic and cytologic features, which include loosely cohesive aggregates and acini of bland tumor cells with smooth borders, floating in abundant extracellular mucin. The nuclei may occasionally show moderate pleomorphism. Intracytoplasmic mucin can appear as a large vacuole forming signet-ring cells. Pure or nearly pure mucinous carcinoma diagnosis is restricted to tumors composed of more than (>) 90% of the components described above. Mucinous carcinoma accounts for 2% of all infiltrating breast carcinomas and the usual clinical presentation is of a breast mass. The sensitivity for the diagnosis of pure mucinous carcinoma is significantly higher with NCB than with FNA. Due to limited sampling, cytology cannot distinguish pure mucinous carcinoma from NST type with mucinous features, and should therefore be reported as the latter. Differential diagnosis also includes mucocele of the breast and metastasis of mucinous carcinoma from other sites such as colon, lung, and gynecological tract. In cytology preparations, mucin stains as red-violet to magenta on air-dried Romanowsky-type stains, such as Diff-Quik (DQ) stain and bluish-green on alcohol-fixed Pap-stained slides. Mucinous carcinoma is better diagnosed on DQ-stained CS compared to Pap-stained CS and TP slides (Fig. 4.10) [1–3, 6, 14].

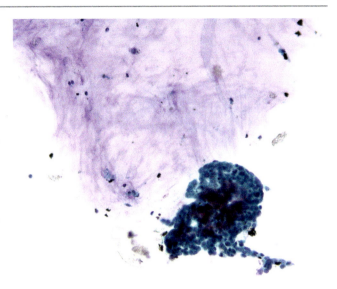

Fig. 4.10 Mucinous carcinoma: the carcinoma cells are present in clusters that float amid abundant extracellular mucin. The malignant cells show moderate to high nuclear grade with vesicular chromatin and prominent nucleoli. Note the rigid borders of both, the dense mucin and the cell cluster. Mucinous carcinoma is better diagnosed on DQ-stained CS compared to Pap-stained CS and TP slides (TP, Pap)

4.8.2.3 Micropapillary Carcinoma

Invasive micropapillary carcinoma is a distinct type of infiltrating breast carcinoma in which the tumor cells are arranged in morule-like clusters. In pure micropapillary carcinoma, at least 75% of the tumor should have this growth pattern. In mixed micropapillary carcinoma, conventional NST type may be the predominant pattern. Due to limited sampling, cytology cannot distinguish the two patterns of micropapillary carcinoma, pure and mixed. Histologically, the carcinoma cells are cuboidal-to-columnar, with granular or dense eosinophilic cytoplasm, with intermediate-to-high-grade nuclei. The clusters of tumor cells have a serrated border and may show a central lumen. Each tumor cell cluster is surrounded by a clear space with intervening stroma. Cytological features are similar to those described on histology. In cytology, this clear space surrounding malignant cell clusters is known as a "lacunar space." Lacunar spaces are commonly seen in almost all malignancies, in the cell block section, CS and LBP (Fig. 4.11) [1–3, 6].

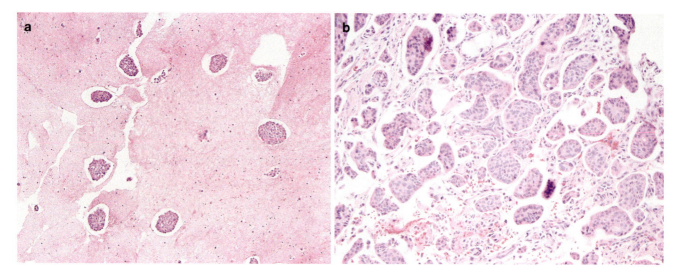

Fig. 4.11 IDC, micropapillary pattern: (**a**) This H&E-stained section of the cell block (CB) made from FNA is characterized by cohesive tufts of cells with nuclear monotony arranged in pseudopapillary structures and surrounded by empty, clear spaces (lacunar space) (H&E); (**b**) H&E-stained sections of the corresponding excisional biopsy showing the tumor composed of morula-like clusters floating in empty, clear spaces lined by delicate strands of stroma. The clusters often have a serrated outer border. They display an inside-out arrangement, with the luminal aspect of the cell present on the outer surface of the cluster (H&E)

4.8.2.4 Apocrine Carcinoma

Apocrine carcinoma is a sub-type of breast carcinoma composed predominantly of malignant apocrine-type cells. It accounts for 1% of all infiltrating breast carcinomas, and the clinical presentation varies from asymptomatic to the presence of a hard, unilateral breast lump with irregular borders. The cells of apocrine carcinoma are reminiscent of apocrine metaplasia and some of these carcinomas probably arise from pre-existing apocrine change. Histologically, the pattern of growth can be similar to NST, although apocrine carcinoma is usually poorly differentiated with more dyscohesion. The tumor cells have abundant eosinophilic, foamy, or granular cytoplasm and large, round, and vesicular nuclei with prominent nucleoli. Nuclear pleomorphism, hyperchromasia, and size of nucleoli vary with the grade of the tumor. Intracytoplasmic lumens with secretions can be seen. Cytology aspirates tend to be moderate to highly cellular with nuclear pleomorphism, overlap, and crowding, irregularity of membranes, macronucleoli, and high N:C ratio. Other cytologic features are similar to those described for histology. Cytological differential diagnoses include apocrine cyst, apocrine metaplasia and apocrine adenosis. Apocrine carcinoma is distinguished from these benign apocrine lesions by the pleomorphic nuclear features (Fig. 4.12) [1–3, 6, 13].

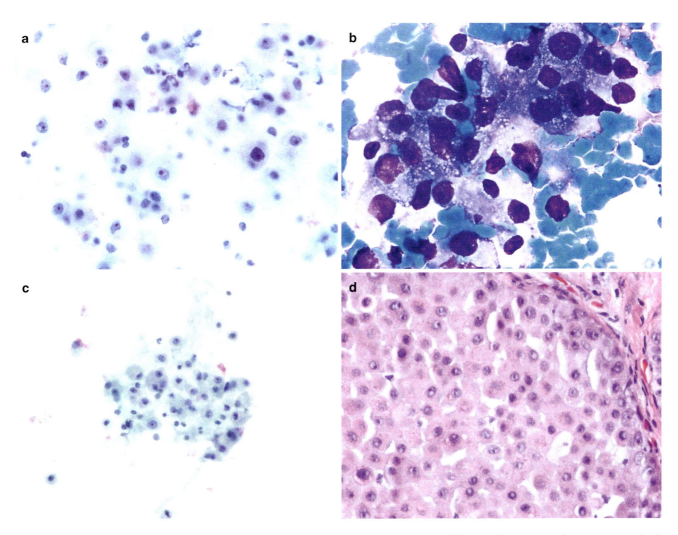

Fig. 4.12 IDC, Apocrine type: (**a**) Loosely cohesive large tumor cells can be seen with a large amount of granular cytoplasm. While the abundant dense and finely vacuolated cytoplasm may give a bland appearance, the enlarged and irregular nuclei with macronucleoli seen in these cells indicate malignancy (CS, Pap); (**b**) The pleomorphic nuclei are more apparent in the DQ stain. The cytoplasm however appears both dense and finely-vacuolated (CS); (**c**) Appearance of apocrine carcinoma on the ThinPrep slide is similar to the Pap-stained conventional smear (Pap); (**d**) The granular eosinophilic cytoplasm can be better appreciated on the resection specimen (H&E)

4.8.2.5 Metaplastic Carcinoma

Metaplastic carcinoma is a high-grade tumor that is considered to represent patterns of gene expression rather than histiogenesis, a conclusion supported by the presence of p53 gene mutation in several components of metaplastic carcinoma [1]. The tumor comprises <1% of infiltrating breast carcinoma, and clinically presents as a large tumor without axillary lymph node involvement. Metaplastic carcinoma can be divided into two categories based on histologic components: squamous and heterologous or pseudosarcomatous. Differential diagnoses include both benign and neoplastic entities. The benign differential diagnoses for metaplastic carcinoma with squamous differentiation include squamous metaplasia in a sub-areolar abscess and squamous metaplasia following lumpectomy and irradiation. Clinical history, radiological features, site of the lesion, and cytologically malignant keratinized squamous cells, aid with the differential diagnoses. For metaplastic carcinoma with mesenchymal (spindle cell) differentiation, the differential diagnoses include primary breast sarcoma and angiosarcoma. Immunohistochemistry is helpful in the detection of metaplastic carcinoma. Metaplastic carcinoma should be considered in the differential diagnosis of any spindle cell tumor in the breast (Fig. 4.13) [1–3, 6, 13, 14].

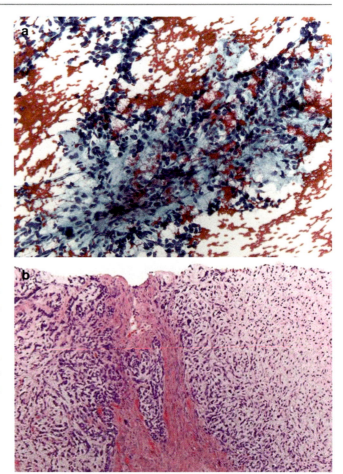

Fig. 4.13 IDC, Metaplastic type. (**a**) Ductal carcinoma of the breast can occasionally be metaplastic and contain sarcomatous elements. In this case, the carcinoma has developed an area resembling chondrosarcoma; the stroma appears light blue, the spindled cells have enlarged, overlapping nuclei, and are disorganized (CS, Pap). (**b**) Corresponding excisional biopsy shows numerous pleomorphic spindle cells present within a chondroid matrix (H&E)

4.8.2.6 Medullary Carcinoma

Medullary carcinoma is a "well-circumscribed" carcinoma composed of large poorly-differentiated cells with scant stroma and prominent lymphoid infiltration [1]. It accounts for <5% of all breast carcinomas. Histologic features include tumor cells in syncytial sheets with high nuclear grade, lymphoplasmacytic infiltration, and high mitotic rate. A definitive diagnosis of medullary carcinoma cannot be rendered on FNA or NCB because of limited sample. However, a possibility of the tumor should be suggested. Clinical differential diagnosis of medullary carcinoma includes a fibroadenoma because of the circumscribed nature of the tumor. Pathologic differential diagnoses include chronic mastitis, intramammary lymph node, and lymphoma of the breast. The benign entities are distinguished from medullary carcinoma by the absence of tumor cells. Lymphoma lacks the syncytial arrangement or loosely-cohesive clusters of tumor cells. Immunohistochemistry can be applied. The distinction between medullary carcinoma and poorly differentiated NST type is also not possible on FNA and NCB. This is an important distinction with prognostic implications, as the former has a better overall prognosis (Fig. 4.14) [1–3, 6, 13].

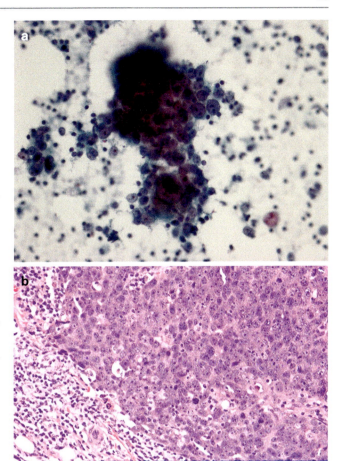

Fig. 4.14 Medullary carcinoma: (**a**) The tumor cells are arranged singly and in clusters of large undifferentiated cells with markedly enlarged and overlapping nuclei, variation in nuclear size, marked nuclear border irregularities, and prominent nucleoli. Small mature lymphocytes can be seen admixed within the tumor cell groups (CS, UF-Pap); (**b**) Markedly pleomorphic tumor cells with similar cytology as described above surrounded by small mature lymphocytes on the resection (H&E)

4.8.3 Invasive Lobular Carcinoma

Invasive lobular carcinoma (ILC), with classic and variant histologic appearance, accounts for approximately 5–14% of all invasive breast carcinomas. These tumors occur at all age ranges, but are more common in older women. Clinical presentation is usually a mass with ill-defined margins. It may also present as a vague thickening or nodularity of the breast. Patients with ILC have a relatively high frequency of bilateral disease when compared with other types of invasive carcinomas. Histologically, ILC shows a linear (cords of cells) and swirling pattern of growth with lack of solid, papillary, and glandular patterns. The tumor cells are fairly monotonous, small, and uniform, and may be mistaken for inflammatory cells. The nuclei are eccentrically placed and uniform with inconspicuous nucleoli. Tumor cells can also exhibit mucin-rich intracytoplasmic vacuoles that impart a signet-ring appearance to the cells. The linear pattern of tumor cells is likened to an "Indian file." Cytological features are similar to those described for histology. In pleomorphic lobular carcinoma, the tumor cells are large with abundant apocrine-type cytoplasm and relatively enlarged hyperchromatic nuclei. Cytologic diagnosis of ILC is one of the most common causes of false-negative FNA due to scant cellularity of tumor cells and small tumor cell size (Fig. 4.15) [1–3, 6, 15, 16].

Fig. 4.15 Invasive lobular carcinoma (ILC), classic type: (**a**) Small carcinoma cells with little cytoplasm can be seen in loosely-cohesive sheets or singly in an otherwise clean background. The linear "Indian-file" pattern of growth is obvious. The nuclear borders are irregular, with moderate variation in shapes and sizes. In clustered cell groups, the nuclei seem to "mold." Appearance of lobular carcinoma is similar to conventional smears (TP, Pap); (**b**) While cytoplasmic vacuoles are not always present, some cells have large vacuoles that give the cells a "signet ring" appearance (the nucleus is compressed to the periphery by the vacuole). In this field, one cell contains condensed mucin which has stained pink on Pap stain (TP, Pap); (**c**) On surgical pathology, the neoplastic cells are loosely cohesive and enlarged when compared to adjacent red blood cells. Some cells have prominent nucleoli and most have an eccentrically placed nucleus. The cytoplasm is foamy, with some cells showing mucin vacuoles (H&E); (**d**) In this surgical pathology section, some cells have prominent nucleoli and most have an eccentri-cally placed nucleus. The cytoplasm is foamy, with some cells showing mucin vacuoles and eccentrically placed compressed nucleus imparting a "signet ring"-like appearance (H&E); (**e**) ILC, pleomorphic type: The TP is cellular and the cells are arranged predominantly in a dyshesive pattern, occasionally forming a few, small aggregates. Note the prominent linear pattern of growth "Indian-file" pattern. Tumor cells display significant nuclear pleomorphism, membrane irregularity, prominent nucleoli, and abnormal chromatin distribution. Cytoplasm is abundant, pale-to-eosinophilic, and can be granular or vacuolated (TP, Pap); (**f**) ILC, pleomorphic type: Cellular aspirate with predominantly dyshesive malignant cells, occasionally forming small aggregates but mostly as single cells. Note the prominent linear pattern of growth ("Indian-file") pattern. The tumor cells as seen here are pleomorphic, enlarged, with relatively-enlarged nuclei, prominent nucleoli. and abundant cytoplasm. Occasional multinucleated malignant cells can be seen and mitoses can be frequent (TP, Pap)

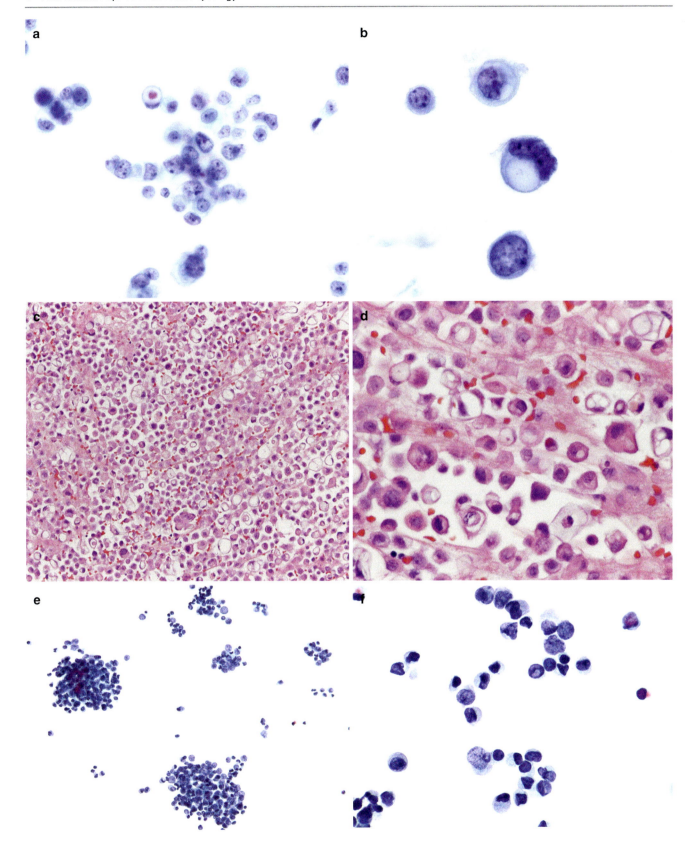

4.9 Papillary Lesions/Neoplasms

Papillary neoplasms of the breast include a wide spectrum of mammary lesions, both benign and malignant, the differential diagnosis of which can be problematic not only in FNA but also in NCB. A diagnosis of an intraductal papilloma or papillary carcinoma on these two modalities warrants surgical excision. Immunostains for smooth muscle actin, calponin, or p63 may be useful in identifying myoepithelial cells, which may favor papilloma [1–3, 6, 13, 17].

4.9.1 Intraductal Papilloma

Central solitary papilloma is a discrete benign papillary tumor that arises from a lactiferous duct usually from the central part of the breast. Clinically, it presents as a palpable subareolar mass. Central solitary papilloma can occur at any age and are usually associated with a nipple discharge that is more commonly non-bloody. Histologically, the papilloma comprises of branching fronds of stroma lined by a layer of cuboidal to columnar epithelium and myoepithelium. The stroma contains thin-walled capillaries and histiocytes. Papilloma can also become complex. Cytologically, pseudo-papillary or papillary structures and cell balls, comprising columnar-to-round ductal cells, can be seen. Background is either proteinaceous or bloody and contains macrophages (Fig. 4.16) [1–3, 6, 14].

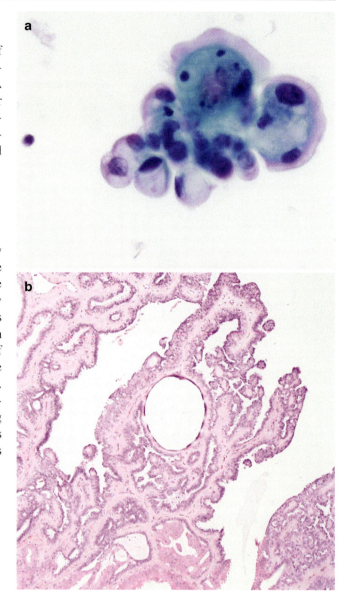

Fig. 4.16 Intraductal papilloma: (**a**) Intraductal papilloma tend to occur as solitary retroareolar tumors but can also occur anywhere in the breast. On FNA, the cells are cuboidal-to-columnar and arranged in a papillary-like cluster or in a cell ball, as shown here. The nuclei are round and regular with fine chromatin and small nucleoli. Note the cytoplasmic vacuolation (TP, Pap); (**b**) The corresponding excisional biopsy shows an intraductal papilloma with multiple papillae containing vascularized fibroconnective tissue. Apocrine metaplasia can be seen (H&E)

Fig. 4.17 Papillary carcinoma: (**a**) This CS shows a very cellular specimen with columnar cells, many of which are loosely attached to thin fibrovascular cores with complex branching. The monotony of these cells and the bland nuclear features may not suggest carcinoma; however, the specimen is hypercellular, and lacks obvious myoepithelial cells. Note the many isolated columnar cells in the background (CS, Pap); (**b**) Papillary carcinoma shows tumor cell clusters with a papillary-like configuration. The columnar cells are well appreciated at the edges of the cell clusters. Differentiating between benign and malignant papillary lesions on FNA and NCB can be challenging (CS, Pap); (**c**) Papillary carcinoma on ThinPrep show complex and cellular papillary-like clusters with columnar cells arranged around the edges. The nuclei demonstrate hyperchromasia, anisonucleosis, and overlapping. The LBP shows few or no single epithelial cells and the background appears clean and less bloody as opposed to the CS (Pap stain). (**d**) Another case of papillary carcinoma on LBP. Note the clean background with few or no single epithelial cells and less blood as opposed to the CS (TP, Pap)

4.9.2   Papillary Carcinoma

Papillary carcinoma comprises 1–2% of all breast carcinomas. It is a term used for carcinomas that histologically show frond formation. The main distinguishing features between a papilloma and papillary carcinoma are: in papillary carcinoma the predominant growth pattern is frond-like papillae with less evenly-distributed and more complex fibrovascular cores compared to papilloma; the epithelial cells are less orderly, nuclei are hyperchromatic with uneven chromatin distribution and have high N:C ratio compared to papilloma; myoepithelial cells are absent in papillary carcinoma but uniformly present in papilloma; and lastly, mitoses are more frequent in papillary carcinoma (Fig. 4.17) [1–3, 6, 13].

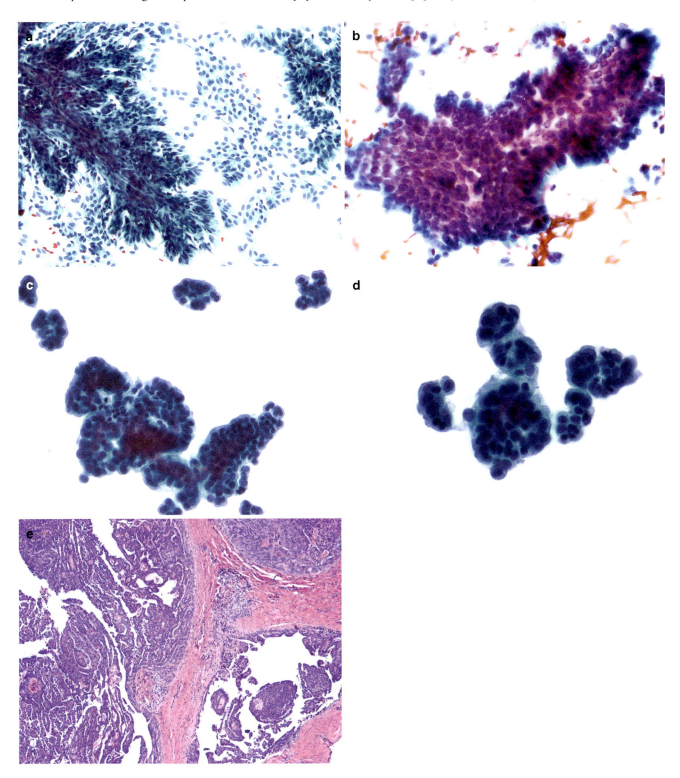

4.10 Role of Immunohistochemistry in Breast Carcinoma

Immunohistochemical staining for breast markers in cytology preparations is usually performed to confirm metastatic breast carcinoma, to evaluate the predictive/prognostic markers in metastatic breast carcinoma, and to distinguish between ductal versus lobular carcinoma.

4.10.1 Metastatic Breast Carcinoma

Metastatic breast carcinoma, both NST and lobular types, is one of the most common metastases analyzed in any cytology laboratory. The common sites for metastatic breast carcinoma are bone, lungs, and liver [1–3]. Immunohistochemistry (IHC), specific to breast carcinoma and to the organ where the metastasis is detected, can be performed on CB sections, conventional smears, or LBP for diagnosis (Figs. 4.18, 4.19, and 4.20) [1–3, 6, 18, 19]. The markers commonly used in practice to confirm a malignancy of breast origin include GATA-3, GCDFP15, and mammaglobin. Of these three markers, GATA-3 offers the most sensitivity, up to 94%, and high specificity, especially for tumors that are ER positive as well. GATA-3 is a zinc binding transcription factor that regulates the differentiation of many human tissue types, including the mammary gland, and shows positive staining of the tumor cell nuclei. Although the sensitivity of GATA-3 in triple negative breast cancers (TNBC) is significantly lower than in non-TNBC, it still has added value in the work up of metastatic TNBC because ER, PR, and HER-2 immunostains ideally cannot serve as markers for detection of these tumors. Approximately 40–70% of breast carcinomas are GCDFP-15 positive, and 60–80% express mammaglobin. In the workup of metastases of unknown primary or metastases from a TNBC, a panel of these three immunostains is suggested for a thorough evaluation.

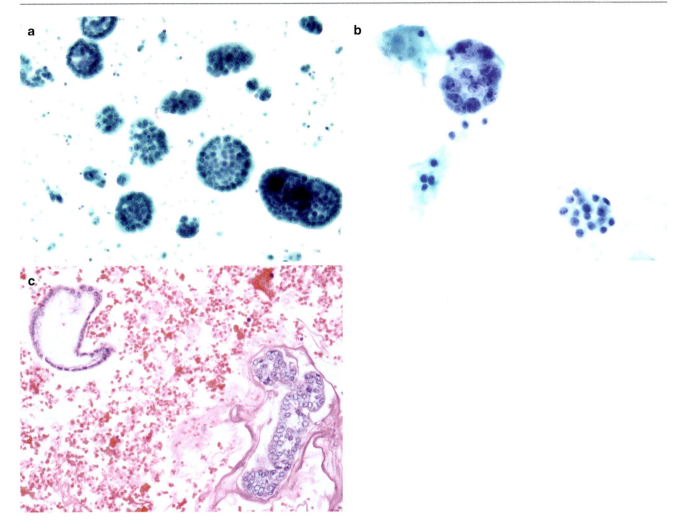

Fig. 4.18 Metastatic ductal carcinoma of breast in pleural effusion: (**a**) In body cavity fluids, including pleural, pericardial, and peritoneal effusions and cerebrospinal fluid (CSF), metastatic breast carcinoma may reveal several patterns. Tumor cells of metastatic ductal carcinoma may form a 3-D "cannon ball" clusters or "morula," as seen here. The cells in the periphery of these tumor cell clusters have a columnar configuration. The contours of the cell spheres are smooth (community borders) in contrast to the scalloped borders seen in mesothelial cell proliferations. In this SurePath LBP, the background shows some inflammatory cells and benign mesothelial cells, in a different plane of focus than the tumor cells (Pap stain); (**b**) Another case of metastatic ductal carcinoma of breast in pleural effusion on ThinPrep LBP shows similar cohesive clusters of tumor cells or morula with markedly enlarged nuclei, hyperchromasia, and prominent nucleoli. Compare the nuclear size of the malignant tumor cells with those of the lymphocytes and benign mesothelial cells in the background. Note that the background elements are present on the similar plane of focus as the tumor cells. These tumor cell clusters lack the "windows" between the cells, which is a feature typically seen in benign mesothelial cell clusters (Pap stain); (**c**) Metastatic ductal carcinoma of breast in pleural effusion on the CB section shows a group of metastatic ductal carcinoma cells (bottom right) with similar cytomorphology as described previously. Also appreciate the benign mesothelial cell cluster (top left) (H&E)

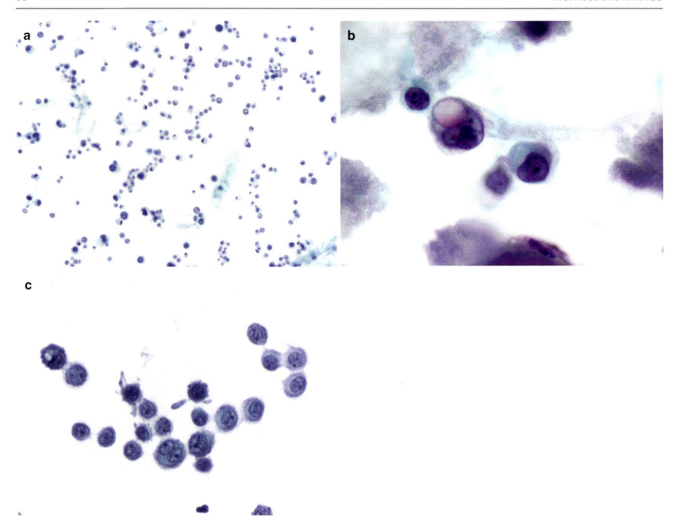

Fig. 4.19 Metastatic lobular carcinoma of breast in peritoneal effusion: (**a**) Lobular carcinoma in body cavity fluids have a predominant single-cell appearance as seen here with hyperchromatic enlarged nuclei, scanty cytoplasm, and conspicuous nucleoli. Single-file configuration and bull's-eye arrangement serve as basic patterns. The low cellularity of lobular carcinoma in fluid could lead to a potential pitfall in diagnosis due to bland cytology of tumor cells. Lobular carcinoma cells may be difficult to distinguish from reactive mesothelial cells or inflammatory cells (TP, Pap). (**b**) On higher magnification one can appreciate occasional cells with signet ring-like morphology with eccentrically placed enlarged and hyperchromatic nuclei and a prominent mucin vacuole. The background shows moderately abundant blood (TP, Pap). (**c**) Metastatic lobular carcinoma in CSF presents mostly as single cells with similar cytology as seen in lobular carcinoma elsewhere. The cytologic features include linear cell arrangement, enlarged hyperchromatic nuclei, increased N;C ratio, irregular nuclear membranes and a vacuolated cytoplasm (Cytospin, Pap stain)

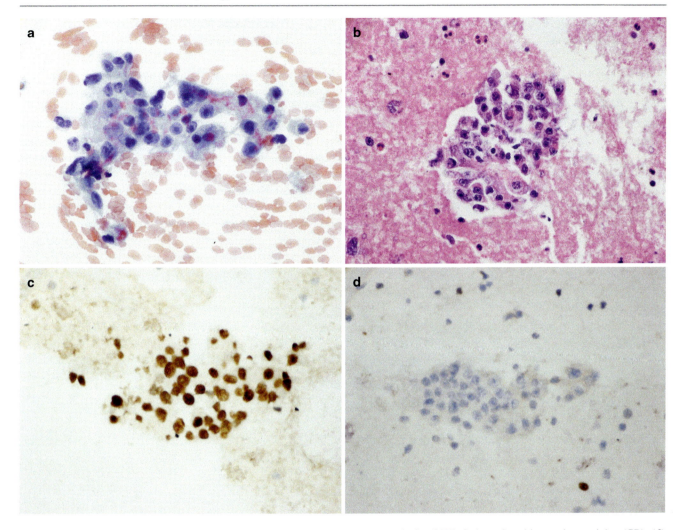

Fig. 4.20 Metastatic apocrine carcinoma of breast to thyroid gland: (**a**) Morphology is similar to that described for apocrine carcinoma of the breast (Fig. 4.12a). In this case, the differential diagnosis was primary Hurthle cell neoplasm of thyroid. However, the clinical history and type of breast carcinoma were known (CS, Pap stain); (**b**) CB section showing similar features to those described before in Fig. 4.12b; (**c**) Immunostain for GATA-3 showed positive nuclear staining (CB); (**d**) Immunostain for TTF-1 was negative (CB). Thyroid molecular test, ThyroSeq (University of Pittsburgh Medical Center, Pittsburgh, PA and CBLPath, Rye Brook, NY, collaborative test) failed to show any thyroid neoplasm-associated genes and the genetic abnormalities supported metastasis to thyroid

4.10.2 Predictive/Prognostic Markers in Breast Carcinoma

With therapeutic advances, breast cancer patients are having better survival, with some showing late recurrences. As pathologists play an increasing role in the era of personalized medicine, it has become more common to test for estrogen receptor (ER), progesterone receptor (PR), and HER2/neu expression in patients with known recurrent or metastatic breast carcinoma. Testing for ER, PR, and HER 2 by IHC has been developed and optimized for use on formalin-fixed paraffin-embedded (FFPE) tissue obtained by incisional/excisional biopsies or resection specimens. HER 2/neu and the ER and PR status are important prognostic and predictive factors in the management of patients with breast carcinoma. Studies on the immunocytochemical analysis of ER, PR, and HER 2/neu on conventional smears, touch preparations, cytospins, and LBP, with different fixation methods and with different antibodies, have shown conflicting results, particularly for HER 2/neu. The prevailing recommendations and contemporary practices of breast FNA caution against the use of cytology smears and cytospins for ancillary testing unless the laboratory has specific protocols for IHC on cytologic material and they recommend use of CB sections, as they are analogous to surgical pathology material. Studies have shown that IHC for HER 2/neu, ER, and PR performed on FFPE cell blocks, prepared from fresh FNA and serous effusions, is reliable in predicting the expression of these markers when correlated with IHC and/or FISH performed on the corresponding histological specimens [20].

4.10.3 Distinguishing Between NST Versus Lobular Carcinoma

Lobular and NST type of carcinomas have distinctly different clinical behaviors and prognostic implications; distinguishing these lesions on cytology is therefore critical for patient management. The most common molecular alteration in lobular carcinoma is the complete loss of E-Cadherin expression [21]. More than 85% of NST type of carcinoma cells show strong membranous staining, whereas more than 85% of lobular carcinoma cells show loss of E-Cadherin. In addition, reduced or impaired E-Cadherin expression is associated with reduced disease-free interval and overall survival. Another marker useful in this distinction between lobular versus NST type of carcinoma is p120 catenin, which binds within the internal surface of the cell membrane to form a cadherin-catenin complex. p120 catenin demonstrates membranous staining in NST type lesions and diffuse cytoplasmic staining in lobular lesions and is very helpful especially in lobular carcinoma manifesting as single cells in the preparation.

4.11 Metastatic Non-mammary Tumors to the Breast

Metastases to breast account for approximately 1.3–3% of malignant mammary tumors [1, 22]. The most commonly reported primary tumors to metastasize to the breast include hematopoietic neoplasms, malignant melanoma, and small cell carcinoma of the lung. The average interval between non-mammary (primary) tumor diagnosis and development of metastatic disease in the breast is around 2 years. In approximately one-third of patients, a breast mass may be the initial clinical presentation of the non-mammary primary. It is more common for a disseminated tumor to involve the breast as a component of systemic spread. An accurate diagnosis of breast metastases is important for optimal therapy and avoidance of unnecessary surgery. Clinical history and knowledge of prior non-mammary malignancy are very important factors in establishing a diagnosis of a metastatic tumor. The radiologic feature of microcalcifications favors a breast primary. Pathological assessment on FNA and NCB with immunohistochemistry are important in distinguishing between metastatic versus breast primary (Fig. 4.21) [1, 22].

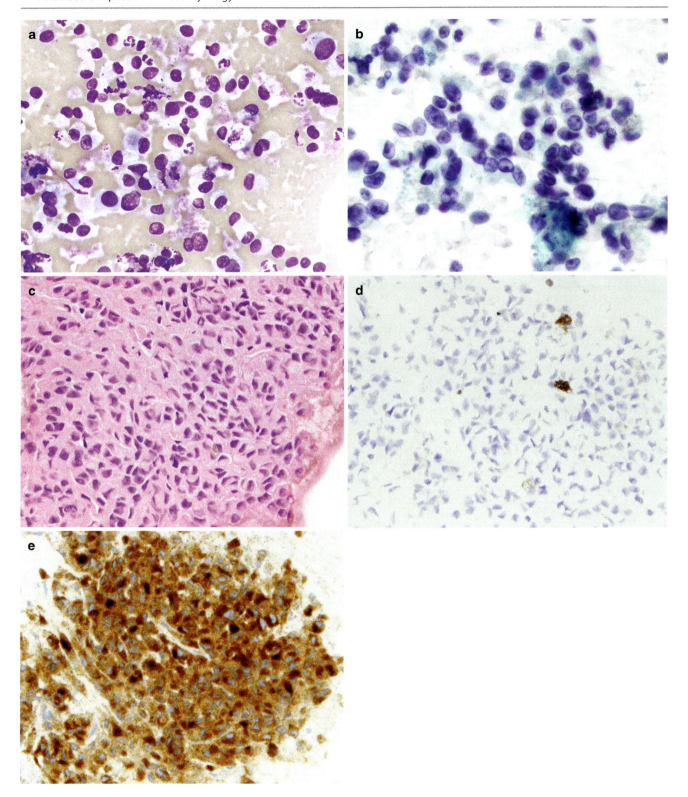

Fig. 4.21 Metastatic melanoma to the breast: (**a**) Isolated cells with eccentrically placed, enlarged and irregular nuclei with prominent nucleoli and finely vacuolated-to-dense cytoplasm. Occasional binucleated cells are present. A linear pattern of cell arrangement is noted at bottom right of the image. Differential diagnoses include pleomorphic lobular carcinoma and high-grade lymphoma (CS, DQ stain); (**b**) Note the macronucleoli and an intranuclear inclusion at the 8 o'clock position. N:C ratio is high (CS, Pap stain); (**c**) Histology of melanoma (resection, H&E); (**d**) The infiltrating tumor was cytokeratin negative (CB); (**e**) The tumor was immunoreactive for melanoma markers, HMB-45, S-100, SOX-10 and Melan-A (CB, HMB-45)

References

1. Hoda SA, Brogi E, Koerner FC, Rosen PP. Rosen's diagnosis of breast pathology by needle core biopsy. 4th ed. Philadelphia, PA: Lippincott Williams & Wilkins; 2016.
2. Dong J, Ly A, Arpin R, Ahmed Q, Brachtel E. Breast fine needle aspiration continues to be relevant in a large academic medical center: experience from Massachusetts General Hospital. Breast Cancer Res Treat. 2016;158:297–305.
3. Ly A, Ono JC, Hughes KS, Pitman MB, Balassanian R. Fine-needle aspiration biopsy of palpable breast masses: patterns of clinical use and patient experience. J Natl Compr Cancer Netw. 2016;14:527–36.
4. Topps AR, Barr SP, Pikoulas P, Pritchard SA, Maxwell AJ. Preoperative axillary ultrasound-guided needle sampling in breast cancer: comparing the sensitivity of fine needle aspiration cytology and core needle biopsy. Ann Surg Oncol. 2018;25:148–53.
5. Kwak JY, Kim EK, Park HL, Kim JY, Oh KK. Application of the breast imaging reporting and data system final assessment system in sonography of palpable breast lesions and reconsideration of the modified triple test. J Ultrasound Med. 2006;25:1255–61.
6. Hoda RS. Non-gynecologic cytology on liquid-based preparations: a morphologic review of facts and artifacts. Diagn Cytopathol. 2007;35:621–34.
7. Alwahaibi NY, Alsubhi MS, Aldairi N, Alshukaili A, Bai UR. Comparison of ultrafast papanicolaou stain with the standard papanicolaou stain in body fluids and fine needle aspiration specimens. J Lab Phys. 2016;8:19–24.
8. Arul P, Masilamani S. Application of National Cancer Institute recommended terminology in breast cytology. J Cancer Res Ther. 2017;13:91–6.
9. Field AS. Breast FNA biopsy cytology: current problems and the International Academy of Cytology Yokohama standardized reporting system. Cancer. 2017;125:229–30.
10. Ly TY, Barnes PJ, MacIntosh RF. Fine-needle aspiration cytology of mammary fibroadenoma: a comparison of ThinPrep® and Cytospin preparations. Diagn Cytopathol. 2011;39:181–7.
11. Heymann JJ, Halligan AM, Hoda SA, Facey KE, Hoda RS. Fine needle aspiration of breast masses in pregnant and lactating women:
12. Yu SN, Li J, Wong SI, Tsang JYS, Ni YB, Chen J, et al. Atypical aspirates of the breast: a dilemma in current cytology practice. J Clin Pathol. 2017;70:1024–32.
13. Haji BE, Das DK, Al-Ayadhy B, Pathan SK, George SG, Mallik MK, et al. Fine-needle aspiration cytologic features of four special types of breast cancers: mucinous, medullary, apocrine, and papillary. Diagn Cytopathol. 2007;35:408–16.
14. Jha A, Agrawal V, Tanveer N, Khullar R. Metaplastic breast carcinoma presenting as benign breast lump. J Cancer Res Ther. 2017;13:593–6.
15. Green KM, Turyan HV, Jones JB, Hoda RS. Metastatic lobular carcinoma in a ThinPrep Pap test: cytomorphology and differential diagnosis. Diagn Cytopathol. 2005;33:58–9.
16. Ohashi R, Matsubara M, Watarai Y, Yanagihara K, Yamashita K, Tsuchiya SI, et al. Pleomorphic lobular carcinoma of the breast: a comparison of cytopathological features with other lobular carcinoma variants. Cytopathology. 2017;28:122–30.
17. Michael CW, Buschmann B. Can true papillary neoplasms of breast and their mimickers be accurately classified by cytology? Cancer. 2002;96:92–100.
18. Plonczak AM, DiMarco AN, Dina R, Gujral DM, Palazzo FF. Breast cancer metastases to the thyroid gland – an uncommon sentinel for diffuse metastatic disease: a case report and review of the literature. J Med Case Rep. 2017;11:269.
19. Rao R, Hoda SA, Marcus A, Hoda RS. Metastatic breast carcinoma in cerebrospinal fluid: a cytopathological review of 15 cases. Breast J. 2017;23:456–60.
20. Shabaik A, Lin G, Peterson M, Hasteh F, Tipps A, Datnow B, et al. Reliability of Her2/neu, estrogen receptor, and progesterone receptor testing by immunohistochemistry on cell block of FNA and serous effusions from patients with primary and metastatic breast carcinoma. Diagn Cytopathol. 2011;39:328–32.
21. Peng Y, Butt YM, Chen B, Zhang X, Tang P. Update on immunohistochemical analysis in breast lesions. Arch Pathol Lab Med. 2017;141(8):1033–51.
22. Georgiannos SN, Chin J, Goode AW, Sheaff M. Secondary neoplasms of the breast: a survey of the 20th century. Cancer. 2001;92:2259–66.

experience with 28 cases emphasizing ThinPrep findings. Diagn Cytopathol. 2015;43:188–94.

Inflammatory and Reactive Lesions of the Breast

5

Simona Stolnicu

A variety of inflammatory and reactive processes can occur in the breast. Some inflammatory processes have an infectious cause; other lesions are manifestations of systemic diseases or of an autoimmune reaction. In some cases, the etiology cannot be accurately determined. Most of these lesions require a breast biopsy to confirm the diagnosis and to exclude a malignancy. Most inflammatory and reactive lesions are rare; the exceptions are subareolar abscess and fat necrosis, which can be encountered more frequently.

5.1 Breast Inflammations

Inflammations of the breast are generally called *mastitis*. These rare lesions occur more frequently in patients under the age of 50 years. There is a spectrum of inflammatory lesions in the breast, from acute mastitis (usually associated with lactation) to chronic mastitis. Most are associated with an infectious cause, but for some, the etiology is not well understood or may reflect an idiopathic process [1].

5.1.1 Acute Mastitis

Acute mastitis, also called *puerperal mastitis*, is a lesion associated with lactation and favored by stagnation of mammary secretion. The passage of the infectious agent is represented by nipple damage, particularly nipple fissures. Onset of the lesion usually occurs 2–3 weeks after the start of lactation. Clinically, it is associated with pain and cutaneous signs of inflammation, as the overlying skin becomes swollen, red, and hot (Fig. 5.1). If the inflammatory process is caused by *Staphylococcus aureus*, an abscess develops over time, which macroscopically appears as a well-defined cavity, full of a creamy yellow substance. Microscopically, the breast tissue is destroyed and replaced by a collection of neutrophils, bordered by a pyogenic membrane (Figs. 5.2 and 5.3). Of note, acute inflammation can be associated with severe, reactive epithelial atypia in the remaining ducts and acini in the vicinity of the abscess. When these changes are present, interpretation should be conservative [2]. At a chronic stage, fistula can develop (Fig. 5.4). The differential diagnosis particularly includes inflammatory breast carcinoma, both clinically and pathologically. In cases of inflammatory breast carcinoma, the skin lesions include more than two thirds of the breast and is usually associated with a palpable mass, which is demonstrated on ultrasound and/or mammogram; pathologically, the presence of tumor emboli can be seen in the lymphatic vessels of the dermis (Fig. 5.5).

S. Stolnicu, MD, PhD
Department of Pathology, University of Medicine and Pharmacy, Tîrgu Mureş, Romania

© Springer International Publishing AG, part of Springer Nature 2018
S. Stolnicu, I. Alvarado-Cabrero (eds.), *Practical Atlas of Breast Pathology*, https://doi.org/10.1007/978-3-319-93257-6_5

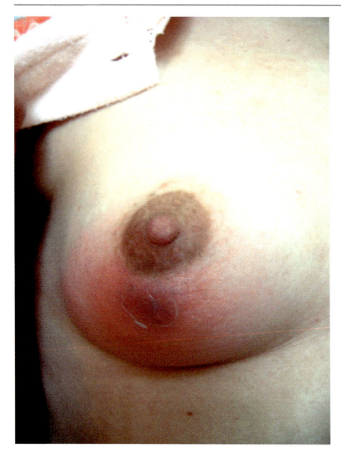

Fig. 5.1 Breast abscess: The overlying skin becomes swollen, red, and hot. (*Courtesy of* Dr. M. F. Coros)

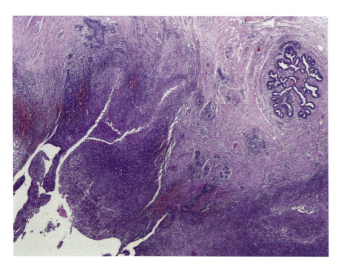

Fig. 5.2 The breast tissue is destroyed and replaced by a collection of neutrophils

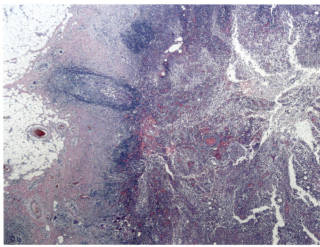

Fig. 5.3 The abscess is bordered at the periphery by a pyogenic membrane and numerous multinucleated cells

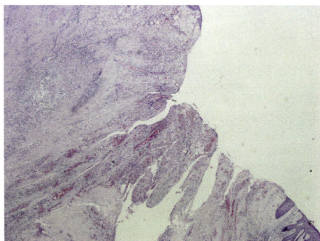

Fig. 5.4 At a chronic stage, the abscess develops fistula to the skin

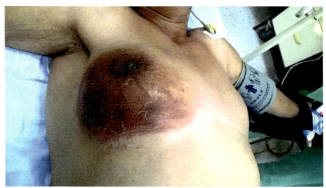

Fig. 5.5 Abscess can be confused with Inflammatory carcinoma on clinical examination; in contrast to the abscess, the inflammatory carcinoma is represented by cutaneous signs of inflammation comprising most of the breast skin, and it is associated with a malignant tumor in the breast tissue (*not shown*)

5.1.2 Subareolar Abscess

Subareolar abscess can occur during the reproductive period, but also in postmenopausal women; rare cases are reported in males. *Staphylococcus*, *Streptococcus*, and *Proteus* are the etiologic agents involved. Congenital or acquired nipple inversion and retraction may be associated in some cases. Inflammatory skin signs are sometimes present and make diagnosis easier. An imprecisely demarcated area with increased density can be noticed on mammography. The lesion develops from galactophorous ducts, whose glandular epithelium is gradually replaced by squamous metaplasia

(Figs. 5.6, 5.7, and 5.8). The result is obstruction and extension of the duct by keratinous and cellular debris. The extended duct breaks, and the surrounding stroma may develop an abscess, with numerous multinucleated, foreign-body giant cells (Figs. 5.9 and 5.10). The lesion may be associated with the formation of a cutaneous fistula. Over time, this area is replaced by granulation tissue and fibrosis (Fig. 5.11). In some cases, a sinus tract may develop from the abscess to the overlying skin. The differential diagnosis includes an epithelial inclusion cyst, which is usually unassociated with inflammation.

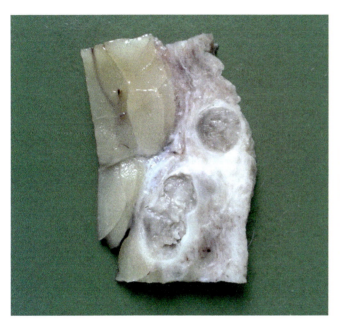

Fig. 5.6 Subareolar abscesses: Breast surgical specimen with multiple round and well-delineated cavities filled with pus on the cut surface

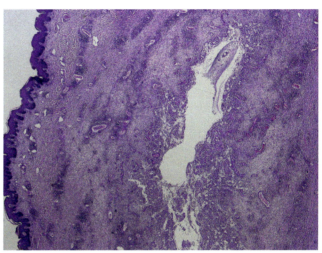

Fig. 5.8 Subareolar abscess. An abscess with numerous neutrophils developed around a galactophorous duct with squamous metaplasia

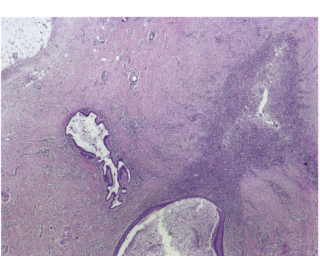

Fig. 5.7 Breast subareolar abscesses develop from galactophorous ducts whose glandular epithelium is gradually replaced by squamous metaplasia

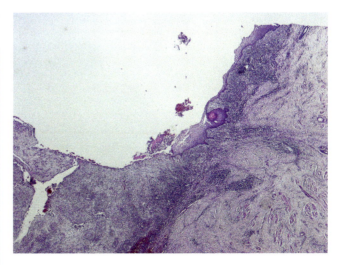

Fig. 5.9 Subareolar abscess. The cavity of the abscess is lined by squamous epithelium

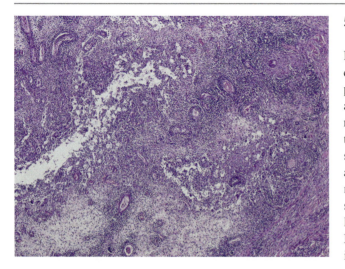

Fig. 5.10 Subareolar abscess, showing numerous neutrophils and multinucleated, foreign-body giant cells

5.1.3 Plasma Cell Mastitis

Plasma cell mastitis represents a diffuse reactive process characterized by an abundant inflammatory infiltrate rich in plasma cells, which affects the ducts and acini, as well as the adjacent stroma. It develops in postmenopausal women as a result of the presence of a lipid-rich material in the acini and the lumen ducts, which sometimes enters the periductal stroma. Clinically, it causes leakage and nipple retraction associated with the presence of an indurated and ill-defined mass, usually located at the periphery of the breast or in the subareolar area and often associated with enlarged axillary lymph nodes. This mass can mimic a carcinoma. Microscopically, the ducts are moderately dilated, containing histiocytes within the lumen, but also lipid material and desquamated epithelium. The surrounding area contains an inflammatory infiltrate with numerous plasma cells and few lymphocytes and neutrophils. Because of the presence of lipid material in the stroma, multinucleated, foreign-body giant cells may appear, in addition to plasma cells and lymphocytes. The differential diagnosis includes ductal ectasia (which affects the galactophorous ducts and not the terminal duct/lobular unit) and granulomatous mastitis (which microscopically shows the presence of granulomas).

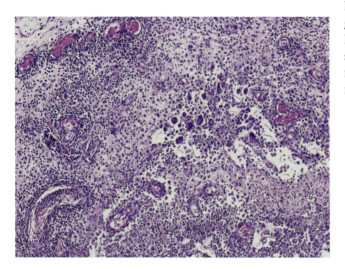

Fig. 5.11 Subareolar abscess. Over time, the abscess area is replaced by granulation tissue and fibrosis

5.1.4 Lymphocytic Mastopathy

Lymphocytic mastopathy (also called *diabetic mastopathy*) is characterized by a painless, imprecisely bordered formation. It can occur at any age and in both sexes, but it usually affects young to middle-aged women. It is considered an autoimmune reaction, which occurs in patients with Hashimoto's thyroiditis, Sjögren's syndrome, systemic lupus erythematosus, arthropathy, and diabetes (type I, insulin-dependent). Clinically, patients present with a palpable or mammographically detected breast mass, which may be bilateral in some cases. A biopsy is required to confirm benignity (Fig. 5.12). Microscopically, an inflammatory infiltrate rich in polyclonal B lymphocytes is localized around the acini in the center of the lobules, but also around ducts and vessels; it is usually accompanied by epithelioid myofibroblasts. The inflammatory infiltrate is very well-circumscribed. Germinal centers are rarely formed (Fig. 5.13). Sclerotic changes (due to stromal fibrosis with keloidal features and increased concentration of stromal spindle cells) and obliteration of acini may occur over time. The lymphocytes sometimes migrate into the epithelial layer of the acini and ducts, appearing as a lymphoepithelial lesion. In some cases, lymphocytic mastopathy has been observed in combination with *in situ* or invasive breast carcinoma or malignant lymphoma. Some authors have even suggested that lymphocytic mastopathy is the precursor of malignant lymphoma.

A number of conditions are included in the differential diagnosis:

- Plasmocytic mastitis (characterized by the presence of large numbers of plasma cells and few lymphocytes)
- Duct ectasia (the ducts are cystically dilated; it is accompanied by inflammation and fibrosis)
- Fibrocystic disease (inflammation; cystically dilated, hyperplastic ducts and acini; apocrine metaplasia of their epithelium)
- Pseudolymphoma (mixed population of inflammatory cells, forming reactive follicles with germinal centers)
- Malignant lymphoma (proliferation of atypical lymphoid cells, which destroy the acini and ducts)
- Infiltrating lobular breast carcinoma (atypical proliferation of invasive tumor cells, usually arranged in an "Indian file" pattern, sometimes with intracytoplasmic mucin or intracytoplasmic lumina with eosinophilic material and positive for cytokeratin)
- Granular cell tumor (epithelioid myofibroblasts are present, but the tumor is positive for S-100 protein)

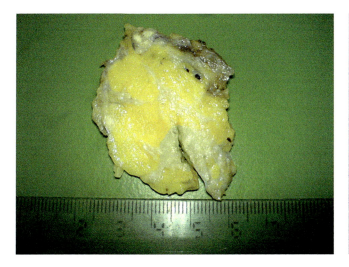

Fig. 5.12 Lymphocytic mastopathy: Surgical specimen of an ill-defined palpable mass, suspected on mammographic examination

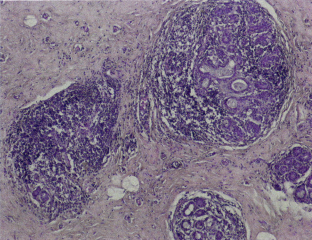

Fig. 5.13 Lymphocytic mastopathy. Well-circumscribed inflammatory infiltrate rich in lymphocytes is localized around the acini in the center of the lobules; germinal centers are lacking

5.1.5 Specific Infections

Rarely, the breast parenchyma may develop specific infections. These can include fungal infections (especially in severely immunocompromised patients), such as histoplasmosis, blastomycosis, cryptococcosis, aspergillosis, chromomycosis, or coccidioidomycosis; parasitic infections, such as filariasis, cysticercosis, sparganosis, or echinococcosis (Fig. 5.14); mycobacterial infections, especially infection by *Mycobacterium tuberculosis* (see below); other bacterial infections, such as actinomycosis and cat scratch disease (see below); and viral infections such as *Herpes simplex* infection. These lesions may present as a mass, abscess, or cyst, or they may be asymptomatic lesions detected mammographically. The clinical presentation and morphological changes induced by these organisms are highly variable. Many are associated with a granulomatous reaction, whereas others mimic a carcinoma.

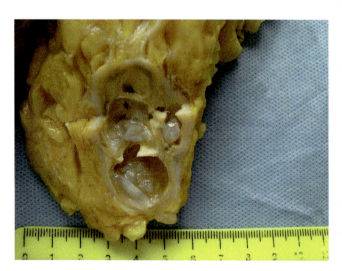

Fig. 5.14 Breast echinococcosis: large cyst filled with small vesicles containing a serous fluid

5.2 Breast Granulomatous Reactions

5.2.1 Idiopathic Granulomatous Lobular Mastitis

Idiopathic granulomatous lobular mastitis is a rare inflammatory condition of the breast of unknown etiology. This granulomatous inflammatory process may affect the breast in the absence of infection, trauma, or foreign material. The pathogenesis has not yet been fully elucidated. Most authors point to a localized autoimmune response to the presence of mammary secretion (rich in lipids and proteins) extravasated in the stroma. However, more recent papers suggest an association with *Corynebacterium*, a gram-positive bacillus in some of the cases. Granulomatous lobular mastitis occurs in patients at a mean age of 30 years, sometimes after pregnancy or lactation. A connection with drug-induced hyperprolactinemia or a prolactinoma has sometimes been highlighted. Studies have failed to prove any link between lesion development and the prolonged use of oral contraceptives. Clinically, it is characterized by a nodular, palpable mass about 3 cm in diameter, which may be confused with a malignancy (Fig. 5.15). The nodular formation is not usually located in the subareolar area. Microscopically, the lesion is characterized by multiple granulomas located within the intralobular mammary stroma, producing distortion of acini and ducts (Fig. 5.16). These granulomas are composed of multinucleated giant cells, neutrophils, lymphocytes, plasma cells, and eosinophils (Fig. 5.17). Microabscesses and squamous metaplasia can sometimes be noticed. Also, in some cases, the granulomas present cysts in the central area, lined by neutrophils and gram-positive bacilli representing *Corynebacterium* can be seen within the cystic spaces. The progression of the lesion leads to a larger, granulomatous, confluent process that eventually progresses to the interlobular stroma and will transform into fibrosis. The differential diagnosis includes other granulomatous inflammatory processes such as tuberculosis (recognized by special stains and specific tests) and sarcoidosis (Kveim test, chest X-ray), as well as a granulomatous reaction that may occur within a carcinoma.

5.2.2 Tuberculous Mastitis

Tuberculous mastitis is rarely encountered in developed countries. It occurs mostly in Africa, in young patients in combination with breast carcinoma, Hodgkin's disease, or HIV infection. Tuberculous mastitis has a predilection for lactating breast, the infection inoculating dilated milk ducts, but it can also occur in males. Breast infection may rarely be the first manifestation of tuberculosis, but typically it occurs as a secondary lesion; the axillary lymph nodes are usually considered the source of the breast disease through a retrograde lymphatic spread. Clinically, it is characterized by a firm mass that can be confused with carcinoma, especially when it is associated with axillary lymphadenopathy. The nodular mass can sometimes cause ulceration of the overlying skin, and it may occasionally be associated with nipple discharge. Microscopically, numerous granulomas may be observed, which damage the lobular architecture. They are accompanied by central necrosis and surrounded by epithelioid and multinucleated giant cells and a bordering lymphocytic crown (Fig. 5.18). Special stains (Ziehl-Nielsen) may reveal *Mycobacterium tuberculosis* within the lesion, but most of the published cases were not associated with the presence of the acid-fast bacilli, even though some authors required very rigid diagnostic criteria [3]. The differential diagnosis includes granulomatous reactions caused by tularemia, syphilis, cryptococcosis, cysticercosis, hydatid cyst, injection of foreign material, trauma, and cat scratch disease as well as idiopathic granulomatous mastitis (see above). Clinical symptoms associated with clinical investigations and special stains allow differentiation between these lesions and tuberculosis. A malignant tumor may be ruled out by the microscopic examination of the lesion.

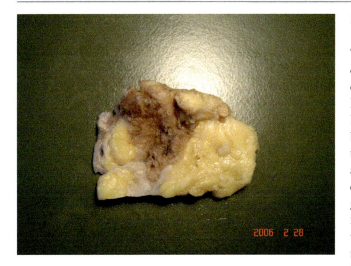

Fig. 5.15 Granulomatous lobular mastitis. A nodular, palpable mass about 3 cm in diameter may be confused with a malignancy because of the presence of central necrosis

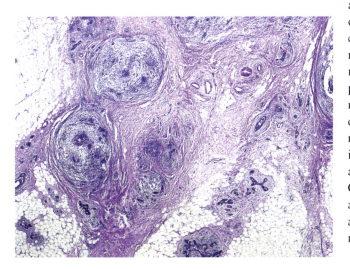

Fig. 5.16 Granulomatous lobular mastitis. Microscopically, the lesion is characterized by multiple granulomas located within the intralobular mammary stroma

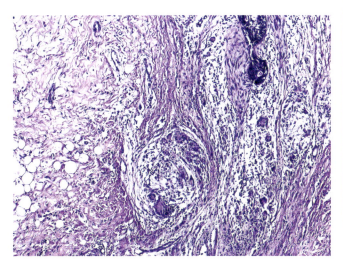

Fig. 5.17 Granulomatous lobular mastitis. The granuloma is composed of multinucleated giant cells, neutrophils, lymphocytes, plasma cells, and eosinophils

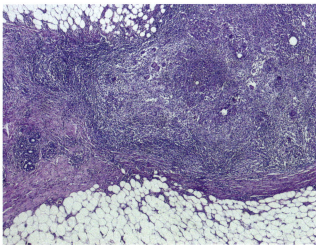

Fig. 5.18 Tuberculous mastitis. Numerous granulomas damage the lobular architecture and are accompanied by central necrosis and surrounded by epithelioid and multinucleated giant cells and a bordering lymphocytic crown

5.2.3 Sarcoidosis

Sarcoidosis is rarely located in the mammary gland; it usually refers to the impairment of the breast in a systemic disease. It occurs in young women as solitary or multiple nodules, sometimes with severe bilateral involvement simulating a carcinoma. Microscopically, characteristic granulomas are usually located in the interlobular stroma, but they also may be intralobular. They have a tendency to confluence, with no central necrosis, and are composed of variable number of epithelioid cells and multinucleated giant cells (which may have asteroid corpuscles), with a peripheral lymphocyte area. The differential diagnosis involves tuberculous mastitis (granulomas with central caseous necrosis, with a tendency for confluence and without a tendency for progression to fibrosis); idiopathic granulomatous mastitis; other infectious mammary granulomas; foreign-body granuloma; and noncaseous granulomas of ductal ectasia, in which granulomas are found in the vicinity of the dilated ducts. Of note, sarcoid-type granulomatous reaction of the mammary gland can sometimes occur in association with breast carcinoma (in both breast tissue and axillary lymph nodes), but in this case, the clinical and radiological picture generally does not indicate sarcoidosis.

5.2.4 Cat Scratch Disease

This zoonotic disease originates from *Bartonella henselae*. It usually occurs as a regional, localized granulomatous lymphadenopathy near the site of inoculation after a cat scratch. This disease rarely involves the axillary lymph nodes and the breast parenchyma, but when it occurs, it may mimic a malignant tumor. Histologically, the breast lesion is composed of granulomas with histiocytes and occasional multinucleated giant cells, extensive inflammatory infiltration at the periphery, and necrotizing inflammation in the center, usually with a star shape. A similar picture is observed in the axillary lymph nodes, in which the presence of granulomatous lesions does not disturb the normal architecture (Figs. 5.19 and 5.20). An accurate anamnestic investigation may reveal that the patient had contact with domestic animals and had observed the appearance of an erythematous papule on the breast skin prior to the breast lesion. In most cases, the specific serological test is positive for *Bartonella henselae* [4].

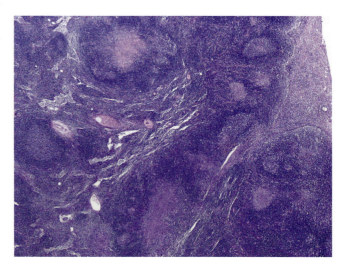

Fig. 5.19 Cat scratch disease involving an axillary lymph node, showing preserved normal architecture of the lymph node but with the presence of multiple granulomas

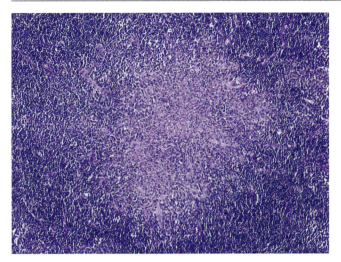

Fig. 5.20 Cat scratch disease involving an axillary lymph node. The granuloma has numerous epithelioid cells, with occasional multinucleated giant cells and extensive inflammatory infiltration at the periphery. The center is represented by a necrotizing inflammation, with a characteristic star shape

5.2.5   Suture Granuloma

Suture granuloma is a foreign-body giant cell inflammatory reaction that develops around unabsorbed surgical sutures after a biopsy or quadranectomy. Grossly, the lesion appears as a small, firm lump. Microscopically, it is characterized by a noncaseous granuloma composed of birefringent foreign material, around which numerous multinucleated, foreign-body giant cells appear, admixed with lymphocytes and histiocytes (Figs. 5.21 and 5.22).

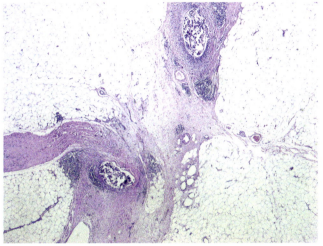

Fig. 5.21 Suture granuloma, microscopically characterized by two noncaseous granulomas involving the breast tissue

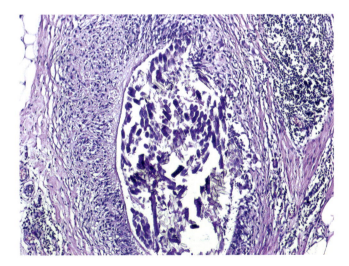

Fig. 5.22 Suture granuloma. The granuloma is composed of foreign material, around which numerous epithelioid cells and multinucleated foreign-body giant cells appear, admixed with lymphocytes and histiocytes

5.2.6 Silicone Granuloma

As a result of the increasingly frequent use of silicone breast implants, breast pathologists can often encounter breast lesions related to silicone. The changes in breast tissue due to silicone implantation are usually limited to the vicinity of the implant and may be represented by the presence of an adherent, fibrous capsule, macroscopically showing as a firm, gray to tan structure adherent to the implant. Microscopically, it is lined by a single layer of flattened macrophages and consists of myofibroblasts, fibroblasts, histiocytes, T-type lymphocytes, plasma cells, and multinucleated foreign-body giant cells containing birefringent material. The presence of the capsule may cause distortion and firmness of the breast parenchyma and can complicate with contraction, infection, or rupture.

Also, in patients with silicon gel implants, silicone may protrude within the capsule or outside, within the breast parenchyma, producing numerous round microcyst spaces. These spaces vary in size and appear empty (when the silicone is lost during the technical process). They are lined by a thick, eosinophilic film material or contain a pale (birefringent) material, surrounded by histiocytes and multinucleated giant cells, which mimic an adipose necrosis. In some cases, the silicone may enter the lumens of acini and ducts. The presence of the silicone may also produce fat necrosis. A granulomatous lesion similar to the one in breast tissue can also occur in regional axillary lymph nodes or other sites of the body, to which the silicone can diffuse through lymphatic or hematic vessels (Figs. 5.23 and 5.24).

In other patients with implants, fibrous scar, microcalcifications, and synovium-like metaplasia can occur. The metaplasia is represented by a lining epithelium resembling normal synovium but composed of multiple layers of histiocytes with an epithelioid appearance in a reticulin network, sometimes also presenting a papillary hyperplasia (which can occasionally be difficult to differentiate from papillary carcinoma) [5]. The cell linings are positive for Vimentin, CD68, alpha1-antichymotrypsin, and lysozyme, but negative for cytokeratin and factor VIII [2]. Cases in which squamous metaplasia is present have been reported. The nipple can be affected by nipple inversion or nipple discharge of silicone. Of note, the changes associated with the presence of the silicone can microscopically mimic a liposarcoma, and in these cases, knowing the clinical history of the patient is essential. In general, all these alterations associated with silicone implants make the detection of breast carcinomas (especially those of small size) difficult, so careful follow-up of these patients is advised.

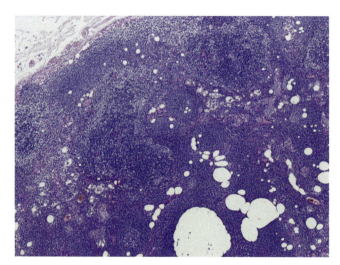

Fig. 5.23 Silicone granuloma in axillary lymph node, showing areas of inflammatory cells and multinucleated, foreign-body giant cells surrounding numerous round microcyst spaces that are variable in size and appear empty because the silicone is lost during the technical process

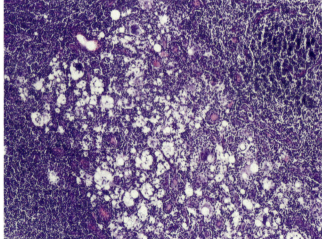

Fig. 5.24 Silicone granuloma in axillary lymph node: numerous microcysts and multinucleated foreign-body giant cells

5.3 Fat Necrosis

Fat necrosis develops as a result either of trauma (accidental or surgical, including biopsies) or of a ductal ectasia or fibrocystic disease (in which the breaking of dilated cysts leads to stromal extravasation of the luminal content). Fat necrosis after radiation therapy for breast carcinoma has also been described. In some cases, however, no history of injury or other previous lesion can be elicited. Clinically and macroscopically, the lesion appears as a painless, hard, yellow-brown or sometimes yellow-gray, solid or cystic mass, sometimes with focal hemorrhage. The cysts are a consequence of liquefactive necrosis and contain oily fluid or necrotic fat.

The lesions are imprecisely demarcated and sometimes cause skin retraction or thickening (Figs. 5.25, 5.26, and 5.27). As a consequence, the lesion can be confused with a malignancy. The differential diagnosis of fat necrosis is even more difficult clinically in patients previously diagnosed with a breast carcinoma who were treated with conservative surgery and radiotherapy, in whom a recurrent malignant lesion is usually suspected. The lesion can be confused with a carcinoma on mammography, because most fat necrosis lesions are spiculated, poorly defined, and may contain calcifications. The location of the lesion is usually superficial in the subareolar or periareolar region, but any region of the breast can be involved. On microscopy, it is characterized by adipose necrosis due to disruption of fat cells (which gives a multicystic appearance of the area) and inflammatory reaction composed of lymphocytes, plasma cells, macrophages with foamy cytoplasm or full of hemosiderin, multinucleated foreign-body giant cells, hemorrhagic infiltrate, and deposits of cholesterol crystals (Figs. 5.28, 5.29, 5.30, and 5.31). Over time, the lesion is replaced by a fibrosis process, which can be associated with areas of calcification and collagen deposits (Figs. 5.32 and 5.33) [6]. As a reactive process, a squamous metaplasia can occur, involving the epithelium of the ducts and lobules in the affected area.

The differential diagnosis for a malignancy is made clinically and on mammography. Fat necrosis is differentiated microscopically from an inflammatory process, in which usually no adipose necrosis can be observed, and from silicon granuloma, in which a history of breast implant is known. On microscopic examination, an inexperienced pathologist may confuse the process with a lipoma, but the lipoma is composed of adipose cells presenting eccentric nuclei, whereas the fat necrosis is represented by necrotic adipose cells without nuclei (Figs. 5.34 and 5.35).

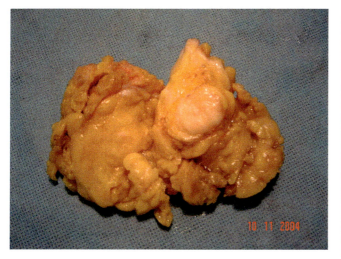

Fig. 5.25 Fat necrosis: a painless, hard, yellow-gray solid nodule, which was suspicious on mammography. Microscopic examination demonstrated fat necrosis (*not shown*)

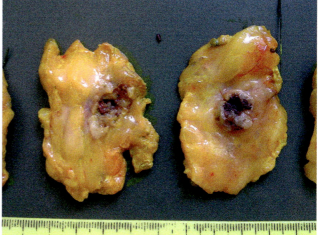

Fig. 5.26 Fat necrosis: a solid yellow nodule with focal hemorrhage and cystic areas, very suspicious for malignancy

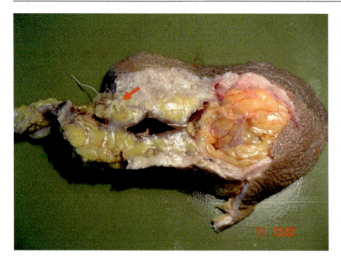

Fig. 5.27 Fat necrosis: surgical specimen of mastectomy after a quadranectomy for invasive carcinoma with a gray, solid yellow nodule suspicious for recurrence (*arrow*). Microscopic examination proved it to be fat necrosis (*not shown*)

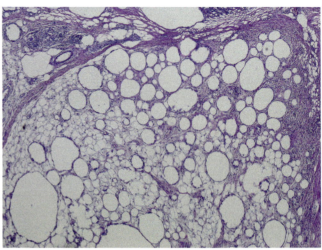

Fig. 5.30 Fat necrosis. Multiple cysts are surrounded by an inflammatory reaction composed predominantly of macrophages with foamy cytoplasm. At the periphery, lymphocytes and plasma cells can also be detected

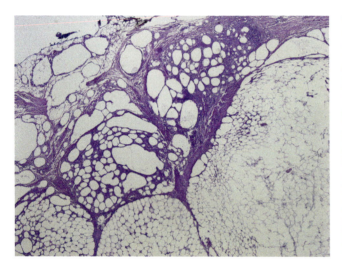

Fig. 5.28 Fat necrosis: adipose necrosis due to disruption of fat cells, which gives a multicystic appearance

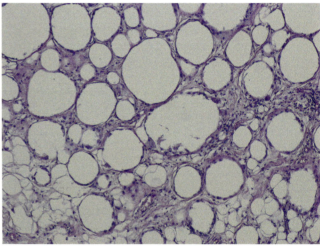

Fig. 5.31 Fat necrosis: multiple cysts surrounded by macrophages and multinucleated, foreign-body giant cells

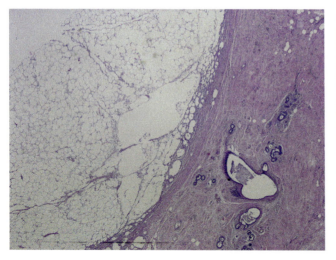

Fig. 5.29 Fat necrosis: multiple cysts, some large

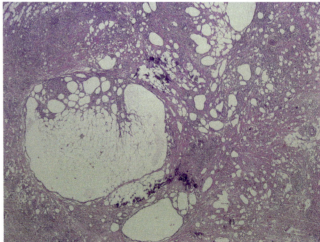

Fig. 5.32 Fat necrosis: cysts associated with areas of calcification

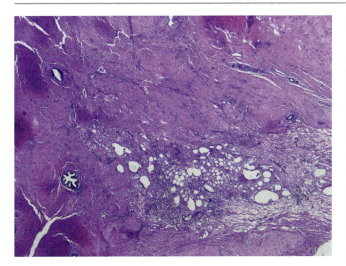

Fig. 5.33 Fat necrosis. Over time, the lesion is replaced by a fibrosis process, which can be associated with areas of collagen deposits

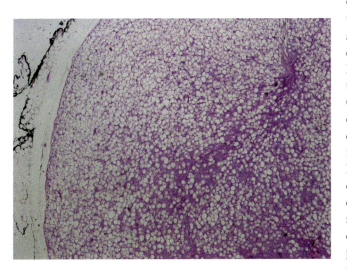

Fig. 5.34 Lipoma. On microscopic examination, fat necrosis can also be confused with a lipoma

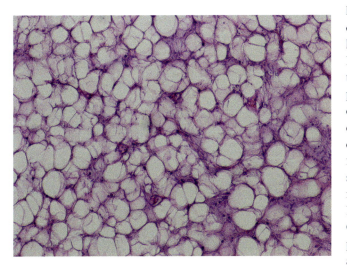

Fig. 5.35 Lipoma. This tumor is composed of adipose cells presenting an eccentric nucleus; fat necrosis is represented by necrotic adipose cells without nuclei

5.4 Mammary Duct Ectasia

Also called *periductal mastitis*, mammary duct ectasia is a distinct lesion characterized by dilated galactophorous ducts in the subareolar area, associated with inflammation and progressive periductal fibrosis. The exact etiology or pathogenesis of the lesion is unknown. Some authors believe that the lesion starts with duct dilatation and consecutive stasis, while others consider that the initial stage consists of the inflammatory process. Most authors believe that the lesion is due to atrophy and involution of the ducts associated with stagnation of the secretion in the lumen of older patients, but duct ectasia occurs at any age, including in children and males. The mean age at which it typically occurs is 50 years. Clinically, it can mimic a breast carcinoma; it can be associated with nipple retraction or discharge, pain, fistula, subareolar abscess, or pseudotumoral appearance due to a mass. On palpation, the clinician can detect the dilated ducts as a wormlike mass beneath the areola. Radiologically, it may also mimic a carcinoma of ductal *in situ* type, as the calcifications can be seen in a ductal pattern on mammography. Many pathologists microscopically confuse it with fibrocystic disease originating in the terminal duct/lobular unit. Grossly, during the sampling of the surgical specimen, dilated, thick-walled ducts can be observed; these contain a creamy secretion within the lumen, similar to the one found in ductal carcinoma *in situ* (Figs. 5.36 and 5.37). Microscopically, the galactophorous ducts are dilated and contain a secretory eosinophilic material in the lumen. The ducts are surrounded by an inflammatory infiltrate represented by lymphocytes and plasma cell, which can be abundant in several cases (Fig. 5.38 and 5.39). As the lesion progresses, macrophages with a foamy cytoplasm migrate into the lumen of the duct, or migrate within the epithelium (causing an abnormal distribution of the remaining epithelial cells into small nests that can be confused with epithelial hyperplasia by less experienced pathologists) or within the duct wall (Figs. 5.40 and 5.41) [7]. However, epithelial hyperplasia never occurs in ductal ectasia. Over time, epithelial cells can exfoliate or may flatten. There is an inflammatory infiltrate around the duct, composed of lymphocytes, plasma cells, histiocytes, multinucleated foreign-body giant cells, and ochrocytes (histiocytes containing yellow-brown ceroid pigment). Less frequently, the inflammatory infiltrate can be of the granulomatous type, or it can be of an acute form, with the presence of abscesses or fistulae. In advanced stages, a process of fibrosis replaces the periductal inflammation (Fig. 5.42). Sometimes the granulation tissue and later the fibrosis can lead to the obliteration of the ducts. Other times, the lumen can be obliterated by remnants of persisting epithelium, which may proliferate to form secondary glands, creating a pattern that resembles a recanalized thrombus of a blood vessel.

The differential diagnosis includes plasmacytic mastitis and fibrocystic disease, both of which are located at the level of the terminal duct/lobular unit. Sometimes, duct ectasia can extend deep into the breast tissue, in which case differential diagnosis is made with the presence of elastic lamina in the wall of the dilated ducts, which does not occur in the acini. (Elastic tissue stain is helpful.)

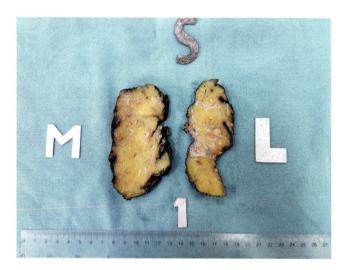

Fig. 5.36 Mammary duct ectasia: grossly, surgical specimen with dilated thick-walled ducts, which contain a creamy secretion within the lumen

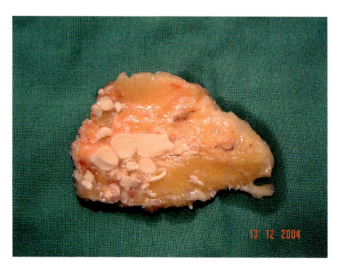

Fig. 5.37 Mammary duct ectasia: This surgical specimen with dilated, thick-walled ducts with a creamy secretion within the lumen is similar to the specimen found in ductal carcinoma in situ

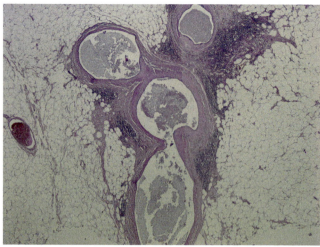

Fig. 5.38 Mammary duct ectasia: dilated galactophorous ducts containing a secretory eosinophilic material in the lumen

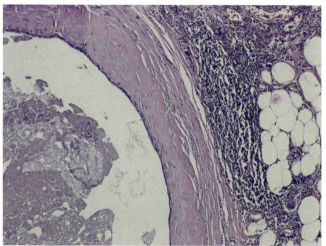

Fig. 5.39 Mammary duct ectasia: a dilated duct, surrounded by an inflammatory infiltrate represented by lymphocytes and plasma cells

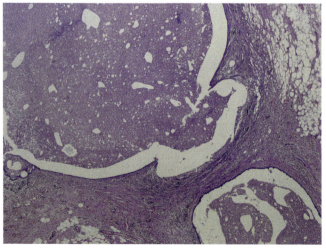

Fig. 5.40 Mammary duct ectasia: dilated galactophorous ducts containing an eosinophilic secretion and surrounded by macrophages with a foamy cytoplasm

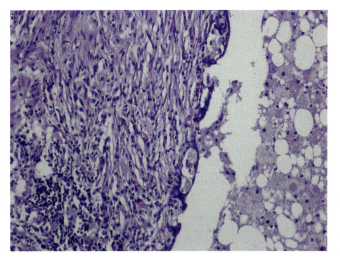

Fig. 5.41 Mammary duct ectasia. Macrophages with a foamy cytoplasm migrate into the lumen of the duct and migrate within the epithelium, causing an abnormal distribution of the remaining epithelial cells into small nests, which can be confused with epithelial hyperplasia

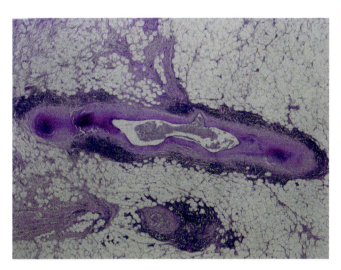

Fig. 5.42 Mammary duct ectasia. In advanced stages, a process of fibrosis replaces the periductal inflammation; later, the fibrosis can obliterate the ducts

5.5 Gouty Tophus

Gouty tophus develops in female patients with gout, but it may sometimes occur in a massive process of necrosis. The lesion may be multinodular or bilateral. Macroscopically, the white mass is well-defined. Microscopically, the breast tissue presents a nodular mass composed of feathery-shaped spaces occupied by urate crystals, surrounded by a foreign-body giant cell inflammatory reaction (Fig. 5.43) [1]. In addition to microscopic examination, the examination of the lesion should be performed using polarized light, because urate crystals are birefringent. Gouty tophus is different microscopically from a cholesterol granuloma, in which cholesterol crystals dissolve during technical processing, so that only the optical needle-shaped, empty space occupied by them can be observed during the microscopic examination (Fig. 5.44).

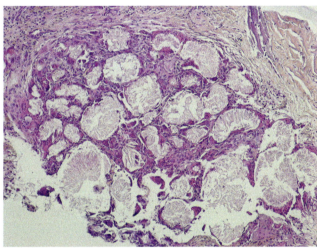

Fig. 5.43 Gouty tophus: nodular mass composed of feathery-shaped spaces occupied by urate crystals, surrounded by a foreign-body giant cell inflammatory reaction

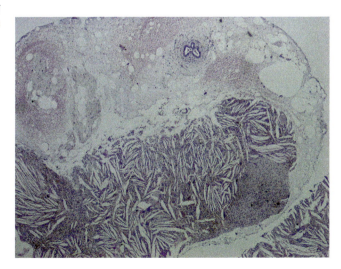

Fig. 5.44 Cholesterol granuloma. Cholesterol crystals dissolve during technical processing, so only the optical needle-shaped, empty space occupied by them can be observed during the microscopic examination

5.6 Amyloidosis

Amyloid deposits rarely occur in the breast. They are associated with benign or malignant breast lesions in patients with both systemic and localized amyloidosis, raising questions of clinical, mammographic, and microscopic diagnosis because their appearance can be confused with a process of fibrosis or elastosis. Microscopically, amyloid is deposited as a homogeneous, eosinophilic, amorphous material that is found periductally (which can lead to obstruction and atrophy of the ducts), interstitially, or vascularly. The deposits are associated with lymphoplasmacytic infiltrate, along with giant cells, but special stains (Congo red) can confirm the presence of the amyloid material, which is also birefringent in polarizing lenses.

5.7 Breast Infarct

Breast infarct is a rare lesion that clinically may be confused with carcinoma of the breast. Lesion pathogenesis is still unclear, suggesting increased metabolic activity of the breast parenchyma. Most patients who develop such lesions are middle-aged, obese, and have undergone anticoagulant therapy. It can also occur as a complication of intraductal papilloma, fibroadenoma, phylloides tumor, pregnancy or lactation (in patients who are younger), and in diabetic patients. Clinically, the lesion is associated with pain and tenderness, cutaneous ecchymosis, skin rash, and sometimes cutaneous edema (mimicking an inflammatory carcinoma). Sometimes the lesion in the breast is associated with enlargement of axillary lymph nodes, due to a reactive process. Macroscopically, the area of necrosis is purple-red. Microscopically, there is an extensive area of coagulative necrosis (where only the outlines of cells can be recognized, but the architecture is preserved), associated with hemorrhagic infiltrate, and inflammatory-type cells at the periphery. In some cases, intravascular thrombus may occur at the border of the necrosis area. Over time, a process of fibrosis replaces the affected area. The differential diagnosis includes necrotic processes with other causes, such as caseous necrosis, tumor necrosis, or fat necrosis.

5.8 Inflammatory Pseudotumor

Inflammatory pseudotumor is a very rare benign condition of unknown etiology, presenting with variable and nonspecific imaging features that may mimic a benign or malignant neoplasm. It most commonly arises in the lung, although it may also develop in various organs such as the pancreas; head and neck; thoracic, hepatic, and biliary organs; and the retroperitoneum. It has an autoimmune etiology, associated with the development of a fibrotic tumor-like lesion composed of a proliferation of spindle cells with a fascicular and vaguely storiform architecture. The spindle cells show no nuclear atypia, and mitotic figures are spare (Fig. 5.45). A prominent vascular proliferation is usually identified throughout the lesion, with some vasocentric inflammatory cells obliterating the vessels. The prominent inflammatory infiltrate consists of both diffusely distributed lymphocytes and plasma cells, as well as aggregates of inflammatory cells with rare lymphoid follicles. The architecture of the follicles may mimic a stroma-rich and vascular-rich Castleman disease, a peculiar form of immune reaction of unknown cause, characterized by lymphoid and vascular hyperplasia of the lymph nodes, but also found in the mediastinum or retroperitoneum [8]. The lesion must fulfil published criteria for IgG4-related disease [9]:

- Elevated IgG4 levels in serum (>135 mg/dL)
- Presence of an organ enlargement as a mass or nodular lesion
- Pathological examinations with the presence of numerous IgG4-positive plasma cells in the lesion tissue

The microscopic diagnosis is difficult even for an experienced breast pathologist, not only because the lesion is very rare in the breast but also because it may mimic other conditions. Immunohistochemical stain, however, shows negativity of cells for actin and desmin (excluding a peculiar leiomyoma or an inflammatory myofibroblastic tumor), for CD34 and CD31 (discarding a benign vascular tumor), for kappa and lambda (excluding a plasmacytoma), and for CD21 and CD35 (excluding a follicular dendritic cell sarcoma).

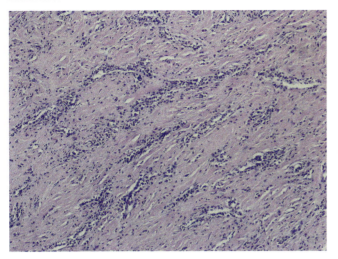

Fig. 5.45 Inflammatory pseudotumor of the breast: proliferation of spindle cells with a fascicular and vaguely storiform architecture, showing no nuclear atypia; mitotic figures are spare. A prominent vascular proliferation can be identified throughout the lesion, with some vasocentric inflammatory cells obliterating the vessels

5.9 Vasculitis

Various forms of vasculitis in a variety of systemic disorders (such as giant cell arteritis, Wegener's granulomatosis, polyarteritis, scleroderma, or dermatomyositis) may also involve the breast [5]. The breast is affected as an isolated manifestation or as part of multiorgan involvement. Of note, the breast lesions may mimic a breast carcinoma, especially from a clinical and/or radiological point of view; the biopsy is of great help in these situations.

Necrotizing granulomatous vasculitis is a nonneoplastic, inflammatory-type lesion of different tissues; breast involvement can occur in Wegener's granulomatosis, although it is very unusual. The breast lesion may present as single or multiple nodules. Some case reports have demonstrated an association of a breast mass and lung nodules at the time of diagnosis. Some authors have described the radiological appearance as an ill-defined, irregular mass or focal, asymmetric density on a mammogram that is suspicious for carcinoma, and as an irregular, hypoechoic nodular mass or a mass with parenchymal mixed echogenicity, consistent with mastitis or abscess on ultrasound examination. In very rare cases, microcalcifications are present within a suspicious breast mass on mammography [10]. Microscopically, multiple areas of necrotizing granulomatous vasculitis associated with macrophages and inflammatory cells can be detected (Figs. 5.46 and 5.47). Wegener's granulomatosis of the breast must be considered in the differential diagnosis of a single breast mass associated with microcalcifications and multiple associated lung nodules.

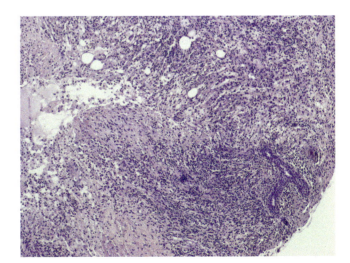

Fig. 5.46 Wegener's granulomatosis. Areas of necrotizing granuloma associated with macrophages and inflammatory cells can be detected in the vicinity of normal acini

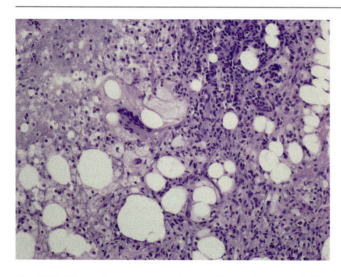

Fig. 5.47 Wegener's granulomatosis: central necrosis surrounded by inflammatory cells and foreign-body giant cells

References

1. Tavassoli FA. Pathology of the breast. 2nd ed. New York, NY: Appleton and Lange; 1999.
2. Moinfar F. Essentials of diagnostic breast pathology. Berlin: Springer-Verlag; 2007.
3. Symmers W, McKeown KC. Tuberculosis of the breast. Br Med J. 1984;289:48–9.
4. Iannace C, Lo Conte D, Di Libero L, Varricchio A, Testa A, Vigorito R, et al. Cat scratch disease presenting as breast cancer: a report of an unusual case. Case Rep Oncol Med. 2013;2013:507504.
5. Rosen PP. Rosen's breast pathology. 3rd ed. Philadelphia, PA: Lippincott Williams & Wilkins; 2009. p. 47.
6. Schnitt SJ, Collins LC. Biopsy interpretation of the breast. Philadelphia, PA: Lippincott Williams & Wilkins; 2009. p. 22.
7. O'Malley FP, Pinder SE. Breast pathology. London: Churchill Livingstone; 2006. p. 68.
8. Gerald W, Kostianovsky M, Rosai J. Development of vascular neoplasia in Castleman's disease. Report of seven cases. Am J Surg Pathol. 1990;14:603–14.
9. Zen Y, Nakanuma Y. IgG4-related disease: a cross-sectional study of 114 cases. Am J Surg Pathol. 2010;34:1812–9.
10. Georgescu R, Podeanu MD, Colcer I, Grigorescu G, Coroş MF, Moldovan C. Wegener's granulomatosis of the breast with peculiar radiological aspects mimicking breast carcinoma. Breast J. 2015;21:550–2.

Papillary Tumors of the Breast

Helenice Gobbi and Marina De Brot

The evaluation and classification of papillary lesions of the breast are one of the most challenging areas of mammary pathology. The difficulties are even greater when the samples are small, such as those obtained by core-needle biopsy. There are different terminologies for the various entities included under the designation of papillary lesions of the breast, which makes it even more difficult to standardize diagnoses and better understand the biological evolution of these lesions. Papillary lesions comprise a broad spectrum of lesions in terms of their clinical presentation, morphologic appearance, malignant potential, and clinical behavior. Papillary lesions of the breast have in common a pattern of growth characterized by arborescent fibrovascular cores covered by epithelium. The spectrum of papillary lesions ranges from benign to atypical to malignant based on the presence and extent of atypia in the epithelium component along with loss of myoepithelial cells within fibrovascular cores and at the periphery of the lesion. The papillary lesions include central and peripheral papillomas, papillomas with atypical ductal hyperplasia, papillomas with ductal carcinoma in situ, intraductal papillary carcinoma, encapsulated papillary carcinoma, solid papillary carcinoma, and invasive papillary carcinoma. Usually, pathologists find it easy to recognize a papillary lesion of the breast through observation of the proliferation of the digitiform structures covered by epithelium. However, it may be difficult to classify the tumor as benign, atypical, or malignant, and when malig-

nant, there is the challenge of recognizing whether the tumor is in situ or invasive, or if the lesion includes both in situ and invasive components. Recent reviews on diagnostic aspects and biological significance of papillary lesions are available in the literature and are cited in the text and included in the references for those interested. Morphologic features are the most important criteria in evaluating papillary tumors of the breast. However, immunohistochemistry may be useful as an adjunct to diagnosis, both on core-needle biopsy and excisional biopsy. The presence and distribution of myoepithelial cells in the lesion is one of the most helpful features to make the correct diagnosis. In some cases, it may require the use of immunohistochemistry for myoepithelial cell markers. If a papillary lesion is suspected owing to imaging, core biopsy, or macroscopic examination, frozen sections should be avoided because the differential diagnosis between papilloma, atypical, or malignant papillary lesion on frozen sections can be problematic. In addition, the freezing may produce artifacts and distortions that will hamper the definitive classification of the lesion on paraffin sections. In this chapter, we will discuss the definitions, diagnostic criteria, and use of the immunohistochemical markers to aid in the differential diagnosis of papillary lesions. The nomenclature and definitions adopted in this chapter will be those recommended by the 2012 classification of the World Health Organization (WHO) for tumors of the breast.

H. Gobbi, MD, PhD (✉)
Department of Surgery, Institute of Health Sciences, Federal University of Triangulo Mineiro, Uberaba, MG, Brazil

M. De Brot, MD, PhD
Department of Anatomic Pathology, A. C. Camargo Cancer Center, Sao Paulo, Brazil

© Springer International Publishing AG, part of Springer Nature 2018
S. Stolnicu, I. Alvarado-Cabrero (eds.), *Practical Atlas of Breast Pathology*, https://doi.org/10.1007/978-3-319-93257-6_6

6.1 Papilloma

Papillomas are benign lesions characterized by finger-like fibrovascular cores covered by epithelial and myoepithelial cells. They are divided into two groups: central (solitary) and peripheral (multiple) papillomas [1]. The central papillomas originate in the large ducts of the subareolar region, such as the segmental or subsegmental duct, without involving the terminal-duct lobular unit. They are typically solitary. The peripheral papillomas in turn start in the terminal-duct lobular unit and may extend to the ducts. Central and peripheral papillomas are primarily a disease of middle-aged women, most frequently found in women 40–50 years of age [2–4]. Clinically solitary papillomas are located beneath the areola, usually present with unilateral sanguineous, or sero-sanguineous, nipple discharge, and less often as palpable mass. Multiple papillomas are often peripherally located and clinically occult, but they can also present with nipple discharge. Usually they are discovered incidentally by mammographic calcifications or manifest as an enhancing mass on magnetic resonance imaging [5, 6]. Central papillomas are generally <1 cm in diameter, and occasionally may measure four or five centimeters. Grossly, they are often visible and appear as tan-pink, circumscribed nodules, within a cystically dilated duct (Fig. 6.1). Papillary fronds may be seen in large lesions, but more frequently the lesion has a bosselated or verrucous surface [5, 6].

Histologically, the arborizing fronds of both types of papillomas are typically broad and covered by epithelial (outer layer) and myoepithelial cells (inner layer) (Figs. 6.2, 6.3, and 6.4). The myoepithelial cell layer is always present in the papillae and at the periphery of the involved ducts. However, its visualization is variable and sometimes it is necessary to use immunohistochemistry for myoepithelial cell markers such as calponin (Fig. 6.5), actin, smooth muscle myosin heavy chain, actin, p63, or others [1, 7–12].

The myoepithelial component may be prominent (Fig. 6.6) or hyperplastic, sometimes resembling adenomyoepithelioma [6, 13]. Apocrine metaplasia is frequently present in the epithelium of benign papillomas (Fig. 6.7). Squamous metaplasia may also be seen, most often associated with infarction (Fig. 6.8). Areas of hemorrhage or infarction may occur spontaneously or secondary to fine-needle aspiration or core-needle biopsy procedures (Figs. 6.9 and 6.10). Collagenous spherulosis can also involve the epithelium of intraductal papillomas and should not be misinterpreted as an area of atypical ductal hyperplasia or ductal carcinoma in situ [5, 6, 13]. Recognition of the intraluminal eosinophilic material basement membrane surrounded by flattened myoepithelial cells is crucial to differentiate it from cribriform ductal carcinoma in situ (Figs. 6.11 and 6.12).

A variable amount of stromal fibrosis of the papillary fronds and the surrounding duct wall is another common finding associated with papillomas, especially in large and central lesions. These lesions are called sclerosing intraductal papillomas. The fibrous tissue may contain epithelial cell nests or entrapped glands [2, 13]. Microcalcifications are commonly associated with sclerosing papillomas (Fig. 6.13).

The luminal epithelial component is composed of a layer of cuboidal or columnar cells. Nonetheless, varied degrees of epithelial proliferation, sometimes excessive, makes the differential diagnosis between papilloma and malignant papillary lesions difficult [2, 13]. The criteria used to classify epithelial proliferation within a papilloma are similar to those occurring in ducts and terminal-duct lobular units. Usual ductal hyperplasia involving papilloma is characterized by proliferation of epithelial cells with imprecise cell boundaries, forming irregular secondary slit-like lumens or fenestrations (Figs. 6.14 and 6.15). The hyperplasia may be extreme and may grow in a contiguous pattern between adjacent papillae [2, 5]. The cell population is heterogeneous, with nuclei of varying sizes and shapes (Fig. 6.16), sometimes with formation of nuclear grooves and pseudo-inclusions. The benign nature of the epithelial proliferation involving a papilloma can be confirmed by immunostainings for CK5/6 (Fig. 6.17) and estrogen receptor (Fig. 6.18), which typically show a patchy, mosaic staining pattern. The pattern of immunostaining for estrogen receptor in epithelial cells of usual hyperplasia is different from the homogeneous staining usually seen in atypical ductal hyperplasia and low-grade ductal carcinoma in situ. The malignant counterpart shows lack of CK5/6 expression and a more homogeneous and stronger staining for estrogen receptor [1, 7–12].

Some intraductal papillomas may have areas of atypical ductal epithelial proliferation, previously referred as "atypical papillomas." Atypia may involve the papilloma to a varying extent, but features of a benign papilloma remain evident in part of the lesion. Peripheral papillomas more often show foci of atypical ductal hyperplasia (ADH) or ductal carcinoma in situ (DCIS) than that of solitary, central papillomas [1–3]. There are no universally accepted criteria for distinguishing ADH involving a papilloma and papilloma with DCIS from each other [1, 6, 13]. The terminology proposed by the WHO classification of breast tumors (2012) designate these lesions based on the extent of atypical epithelium whereas some authorities have previously applied the proportion criteria using a cut-off of 30% [1, 14]. These lesions are designated as papilloma with ADH or papilloma with DCIS if the epithelial proliferation fulfills the criteria for ADH or DCIS outside of the context of a papillary lesion. The extent cut-off according to some authors is 3 mm. When the extent of atypia is less than

3 mm, the lesion is diagnosed as papilloma with ADH (Fig. 6.19), while DCIS within a papilloma is diagnosed when this atypical population is ≥3 mm (Fig. 6.20). When DCIS is present, it is most often of low or intermediate nuclear grade, with solid, cribriform and/or micropapillary patterns [1, 13, 14]. Small foci of necrosis may be seen. The foci of ADH and DCIS have few or no myoepithelial cells (Figs. 6.21 and 6.22), lack expression of high-molecular weight keratins (Figs. 6.23 and 6.24), and show strong and diffuse staining for estrogen (Fig. 6.25) and progesterone receptors [7–12].

A benign central papilloma without atypical change is associated with a twofold increase in the risk of subsequent breast carcinoma; this risk is threefold for peripheral papillomas [1, 15].

The clinical significance of ADH or DCIS in a papilloma is not well-defined. Page et al. have reported an increased risk (7.5-fold) for the subsequent development of breast cancer, and this risk was almost exclusively confined to the ipsilateral breast in patients with lesions they categorized as papillomas with atypia using the definitions described above [15]. The risk of subsequent carcinoma and local recurrence associated with an atypical papilloma does not appear to be related to the extent of ADH or DCIS within the papilloma. In such cases, the concurrent presence of ADH or DCIS within the surrounding breast parenchyma is more important than the extent of atypia within the papilloma itself [1, 13, 15]. Based in this information, papillomas with atypia and/or DCIS should be managed by complete excision. In cases of atypia or DCIS in papilloma, the adjacent breast tissue should be carefully examined to rule out the possibility of finding atypia or DCIS. The finding of these associated lesions seems to be the most important factor in influencing the therapeutic decisions for the patient [1, 13].

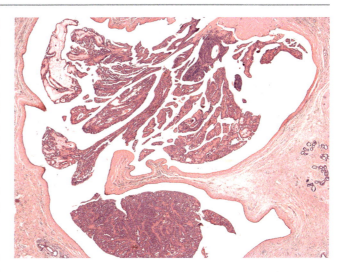

Fig. 6.2 Solitary central papilloma

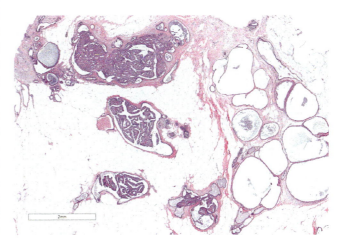

Fig. 6.3 Peripheral papillomas

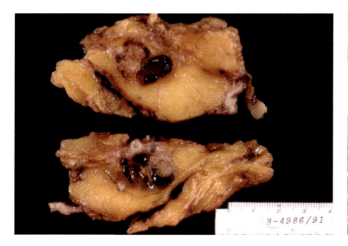

Fig. 6.1 Gross view of an intraductal papilloma. A white lobulated mass projects into a cystically dilated duct

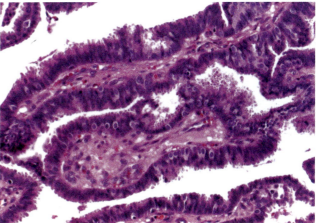

Fig. 6.4 Papillary fronds of an intraductal papilloma consist of fibrovascular cores covered by an outer epithelial cell layer surrounded by an inner myoepithelial cell layer

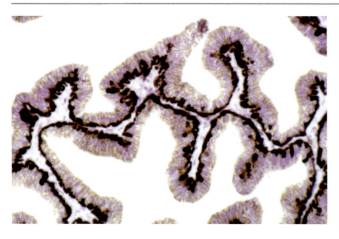

Fig. 6.5 Calponin immunostain highlights the myoepithelial cell layer

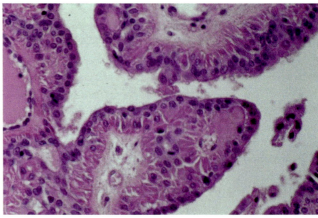

Fig. 6.6 Papilloma with prominent myoepithelial cells

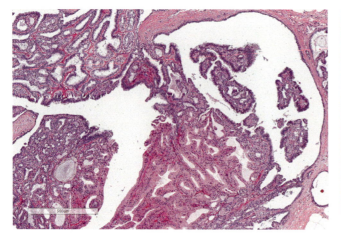

Fig. 6.7 Apocrine metaplasia in an intraductal papilloma

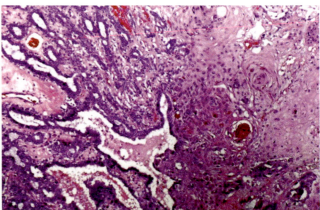

Fig. 6.8 Squamous metaplasia in an intraductal papilloma

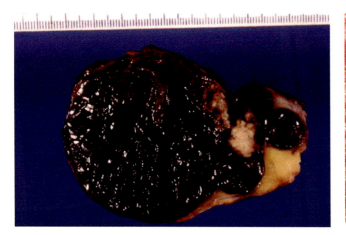

Fig. 6.9 Gross view of a papilloma with hemorrhage post-core needle biopsy procedure

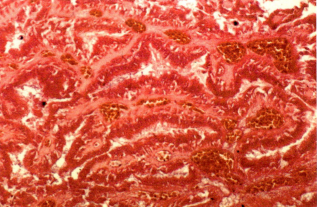

Fig. 6.10 Necrosis of intraductal papilloma

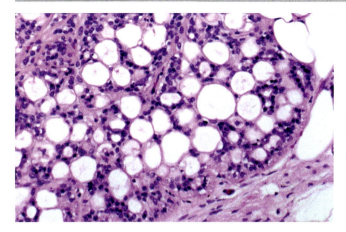

Fig. 6.11 Intraductal papilloma with collagenous spherulosis

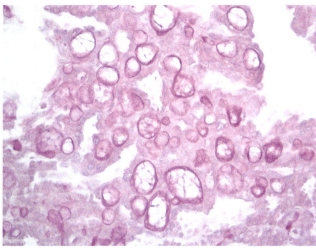

Fig. 6.12 Intraductal papilloma with collagenous spherulosis highlighted by PAS stain

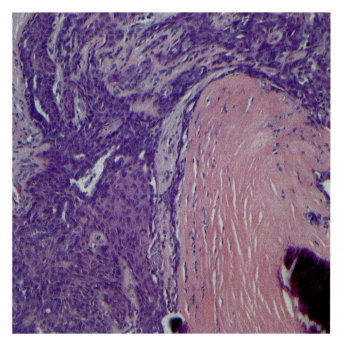

Fig. 6.13 Intraductal papilloma with sclerosis and microcalcification

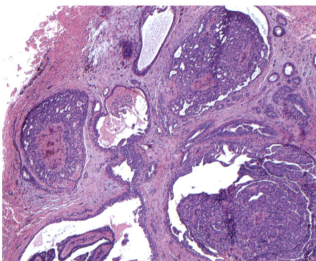

Fig. 6.14 Clustered peripheral papillomas involved by usual ductal hyperplasia

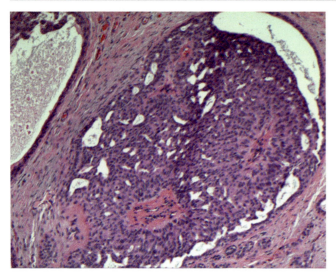

Fig. 6.15 Peripheral papilloma with usual ductal hyperplasia. The epithelial cells are arranged around slit-like spaces and show crowed overlapping nuclei

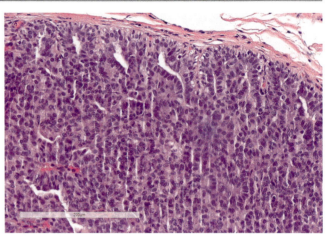

Fig. 6.16 Intraductal papilloma with florid epithelial proliferation that fills the spaces between papillae. The proliferation has the architectural and cytologic features of usual ductal hyperplasia

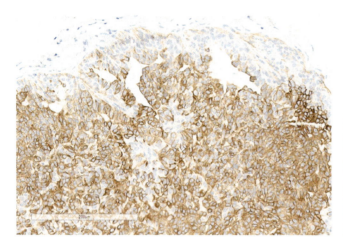

Fig. 6.17 Immunostaining for cytokeratin 5/6 shows a patchy pattern in the proliferating epithelial cells of usual ductal hyperplasia involving a papilloma

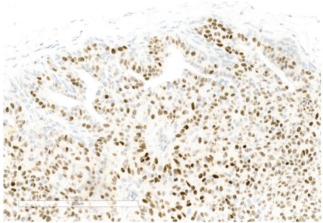

Fig. 6.18 Usual ductal hyperplasia involving papilloma shows a patchy of mosaic immunostaining pattern for estrogen receptor with variable staining intensity

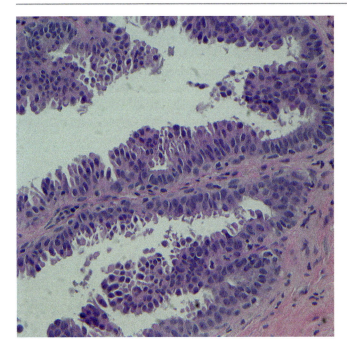

Fig. 6.19 Micropapillary atypical ductal hyperplasia (<3 mm) partially involving a papilloma

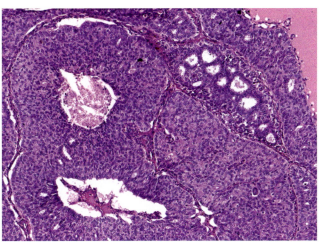

Fig. 6.20 Papilloma with extensive area of monotonous cell proliferation (>3 mm) with architectural and cytologic features characteristic of ductal carcinoma in situ

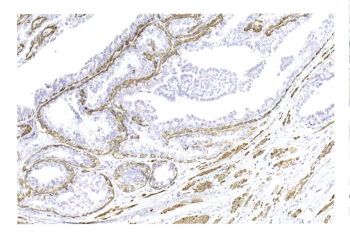

Fig. 6.21 Calponin immunostain highlights myoepithelial cells lining papillary fronds of a papilloma. Small focus of micropapillary atypical ductal hyperplasia (<3 mm) lacks myoepithelial cells and is negative for calponin

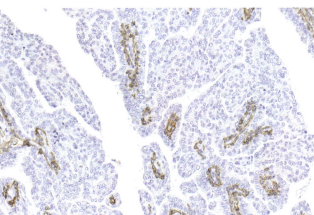

Fig. 6.22 Calponin immunostains few myoepithelial cells of fibrovascular cores of residual benign papilloma. Myoepithelial cells are not present within the areas of ductal carcinoma in situ

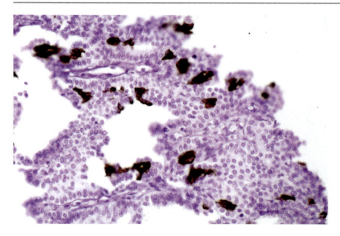

Fig. 6.23 Papilloma with micropapillary atypical ductal hyperplasia (ADH) immunostained for high molecular weight cytokeratin (CK5/6). The epithelial cells of ADH are negative for CK 5/6

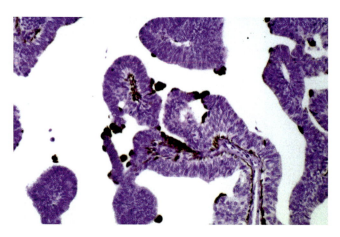

Fig. 6.24 Papilloma with ductal carcinoma in situ immunostained for high molecular weight cytokeratin (CK5/6). The neoplastic epithelial cells are negative for CK 5/6; CK5/6 highlights residual myoepithelial cells

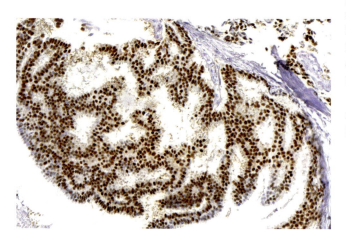

Fig. 6.25 The neoplastic cells of ductal carcinoma in situ involving a papilloma are strongly positive for estrogen receptor

6.2 Intraductal Papillary Carcinoma

Intraductal papillary carcinoma, also known as papillary ductal carcinoma in situ and noninvasive papillary carcinoma, is a malignant non-invasive neoplastic epithelial proliferation with papillary architectural features arising and growing within the lumen of the ductal-lobular system [16]. They are distinguished by the complete or near-complete absence of myoepithelial cells in the papillary fronds of the intraductal neoplastic proliferation. Clinically, nipple discharge or a palpable mass may be present, depending on location and size of the lesion [2, 3, 6, 16]. Microscopically, intraductal papillary carcinomas are characterized by variably dilated ductal-lobular spaces filled with slender or branching fibrovascular cores covered by a single cell population of neoplastic epithelial cells. The neoplastic cells can be arranged in one or several layers of bland columnar cells overlying the fibrovascular stalks [2, 3, 12, 17]. The papillae are thin and delicate with minimal fibrosis compared with those of the intraductal papillomas (Figs. 6.26, 6.27, and 6.28).

Rare myoepithelial cells are seen within the papillae or admixed with the epithelial proliferation. A myoepithelial cell layer is retained at the periphery of the involved duct wall, defining the in situ nature of the lesion. However, the myoepithelial cell layer may be more or less attenuated at the periphery of larger lesions [5, 8, 13]. Some cases may show a dual cell population of malignant cells, with the presence of a second type of cell with clear cytoplasm adjacent to the basal membrane, and may be confused with myoepithelial cells and cause an erroneous diagnosis. A negative immunohistochemical staining for myoepithelial cell markers helps in the differential diagnosis [7, 8]. The neoplastic cells can proliferate and form additional architectural patterns such as solid, cribriform, and micropapillary. When the proliferation is extensive, it may obliterate the spaces between the papillary fronds. The majority of the lesions show low or intermediate nuclear features, although rare high-grade lesions have been described [2, 3, 6].

The prognosis of patients with intraductal papillary carcinoma is similar to that of ductal carcinoma in situ in general [13, 16].

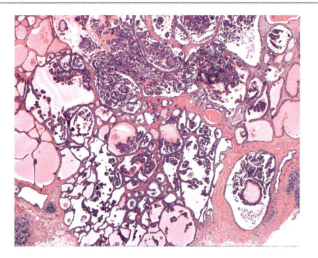

Fig. 6.26 Low-power view of intraductal papillary carcinoma. The terminal-duct lobular units show thin fibrovascular stalks covered by atypical epithelium

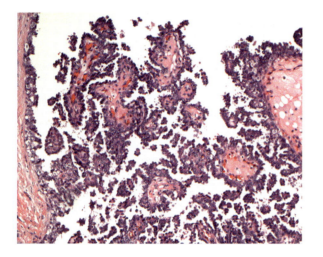

Fig. 6.27 Medium-power view of intraductal papillary carcinoma showing papillary fronds covered by low-grade atypical cells arranged in a micropapillary pattern. Myoepithelial cells are not seen

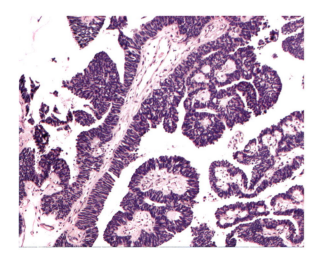

Fig. 6.28 Intraductal papillary carcinoma showing branching fibrovascular stalks covered by a single population of columnar, tall, neoplastic cells. No myoepithelial cells are present

6.3 Encapsulated Papillary Carcinoma

This tumor is a variant of papillary carcinoma, characterized by fine fibrovascular cores covered by neoplastic epithelial cells of low or intermediate nuclear grade and surrounded by a fibrous capsule [14, 18–20]. In the majority of cases, there is no myoepithelial cell layer within the papillae and at the periphery of the lesion. Encapsulated papillary carcinoma (EPC) is a recently proposed term to describe papillary carcinoma occurring within a cystically dilated duct [18–20]. EPCs were previously considered a variant of papillary ductal carcinoma in situ and called intracystic papillary carcinoma or encysted papillary carcinoma owing to their discrete nodular growth, lack of stromal reaction, and indolent clinical behavior [6, 14, 17]. The finding that these lesions typically lack myoepithelial cells at their periphery has raised questions about their true nature [13, 18, 19]. EPCs are mainly found in older women and usually appear as a retroareolar circumscribed mass, with or without nipple discharge. On gross examination, these lesions appear as a circumscribed, friable mass, within a cystically dilated space. Histologically, EPCs are characterized by one or more nodules of papillary carcinoma surrounded by a thick fibrous capsule (Fig. 6.29). The papillary fronds are lined by neoplastic epithelial proliferation arranged in various patterns, including solid and cribriform (Fig. 6.30). Most of the EPCs have low- or intermediate-grade nuclei (Fig. 6.31), but rarely high nuclear grade lesions may be seen. The low- and intermediate-grade EPCs are diffusely positive for estrogen receptor while in the high-grade tumors the estrogen receptor staining is less consistent [8–10, 18]. Myoepithelial cells are not present in the papillae and at the periphery of the tumor nodules of encapsulated papillary carcinomas on hematoxylin-eosin stained sections, nor are they detected with immunohistochemistry for myoepithelial markers (Figs. 6.32, 6.33, and 6.34). In contrast, papillary ductal carcinomas in situ show myoepithelial cells at the periphery of the involved spaces [8–10, 18]. Encapsulated papillary carcinoma may occur alone, but more often the surrounding breast tissue contains foci of low- or intermediate-nuclear grade DCIS, usually with a cribriform (Fig. 6.31) or micropapillary pattern [6, 13, 18, 19].

Many encapsulated papillary carcinomas, long considered variants of papillary ductal carcinoma in situ, may in fact be a form of low-grade invasive carcinoma with an expansive growth pattern or part of a spectrum from in situ to invasive neoplasm. Axillary node metastasis has been reported in encapsulated papillary carcinoma with no evidence of frank stromal invasion or associated invasive carcinoma, and provides further support for this concept [2, 13, 19].

Encapsulated papillary carcinoma has a favorable prognosis with adequate local excision when no DCIS or invasive carcinoma is noted in the surrounding breast parenchyma. However, there is a higher risk of local recurrence when DCIS is present in the adjacent breast tissue. A small proportion of encapsulated papillary carcinomas may be associated with an invasive component, which is usually of non-special type, with no papillary features. The associated invasive component can range from microinvasive to larger foci [2, 13, 19]. Notably, after needle procedures, benign and malignant epithelial cells can be displaced into the biopsy site and the needle tract. To avoid misinterpretation of epithelial displacement and entrapped epithelium as areas of true invasive carcinoma, one has to recognize this iatrogenic artefact and the putative invasion should be clearly present beyond the fibrous capsule of the lesion. There are controversies regarding the classification of these encapsulated papillary carcinoma, and there is no universal agreement on how to stage encapsulated papillary carcinoma in this situation. To prevent overtreatment, the 2012 WHO classification of breast tumors recommends that encapsulated papillary carcinomas that lack areas of conventional invasive carcinoma should be staged according to the greatest dimension of the invasive component only [14, 18]. Outcome studies have demonstrated that the encapsulated papillary carcinomas are associated with an excellent prognosis with adequate local therapy alone. Given their indolent clinical course and good prognosis, lesions without an invasive component rarely metastasize and should be managed as DCIS given their indolent clinical course and good prognosis [13, 14, 19].

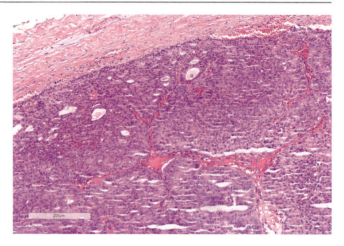

Fig. 6.30 Papillary fronds of encapsulated papillary carcinoma lined by a single uniform cell proliferation. Myoepithelial cells are not seen within the papillae and at periphery of the lesion

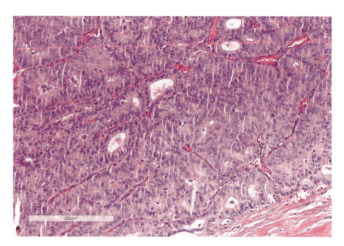

Fig. 6.31 Encapsulated papillary carcinoma showing low-grade atypical neoplastic cells growing in solid and cribriform pattern, supported by thin fibrovascular cores

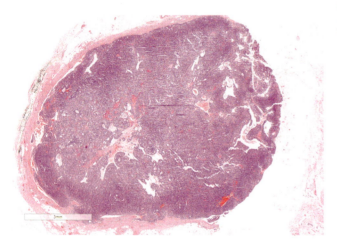

Fig. 6.29 Low-power view of encapsulated papillary carcinoma characterized by papillary proliferation surrounded by a thick fibrous capsule

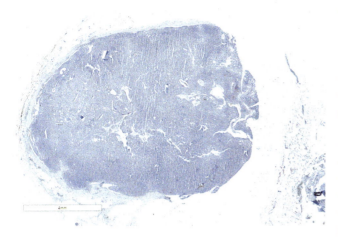

Fig. 6.32 Low-power view of encapsulated papillary carcinoma double immunostained for calponin and p63. Myoepithelial cells are not present within the papillae and at the periphery of nodule

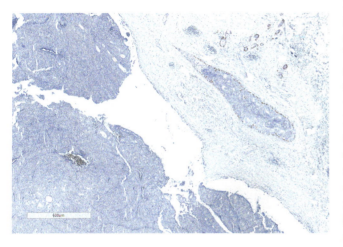

Fig. 6.33 Encapsulated papillary carcinoma immunostained for p63. No myoepithelial cells are seen within the papillae or at the periphery of nodule. An adjacent focus of ductal carcinoma is surrounded by a layer of p63-positive myoepithelial cells

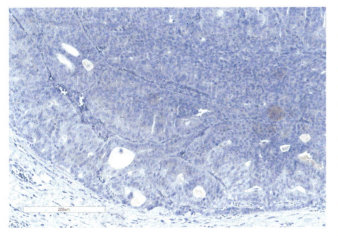

Fig. 6.34 High-power view of encapsulated papillary carcinoma double immunostained for calponin and p63. Myoepithelial cells are not present within the papillae and at the periphery of nodule

6.4 Solid Papillary Carcinoma

The term solid papillary carcinoma describes a type of papillary carcinoma characterized by closely apposed expansile, solid cellular nodules. Fibrovascular cores within the nodules are delicate and can be inconspicuous; hence the growth pattern appears solid at low magnification [14, 21–23]. They were historically considered to be variants of DCIS, and the majority occur in postmenopausal, older women (seventh to eighth decades). Solid papillary carcinomas often exhibit neuroendocrine differentiation and have been called neuroendocrine breast carcinoma, spindle cell DCIS, neuroendocrine DCIS, and endocrine DCIS [2, 21–23]. Clinically they present as palpable mass or occur with bloody nipple discharge. At gross examination, a well circumscribed, soft, multinodular, whitish-grey mass may be seen. Size may range from a few millimeters to several centimeters [14, 21]. Low-power examination shows multiple circumscribed, rounded, aggregated, solid nodules of neoplastic epithelial cells, lacking cribriform or discrete papillary architecture. The delicate fibrovascular network, devoid of myoepithelial cell layer, is discernible at high magnification (Figs. 6.35 and 6.36). The fibrovascular cores can be variably collagenized, with peripheral palisading of tumor cells forming perivascular rosettes. The neoplastic cells are ovoid- or spindle-shaped and often exhibit neuroendocrine features, with granular eosinophilic cytoplasm and immunoreactivity for cromogranin and/or synaptophysin in at least half of the cases [6, 8, 9, 12]. The densely cellular neoplastic cells may form a streaming appearance like that seen in usual ductal hyperplasia, and may be mistaken for intraductal papilloma extensively involved by usual ductal hyperplasia. The cells have usually low- to intermediate-grade nuclei, stain strongly for estrogen and progesterone receptor, and are negative for HER2, CK5/6, and CK14 [4, 8, 9, 12]. Solid papillary carcinomas may also exhibit intracellular and extracellular mucin production, and may be associated with a frank invasive component often with mucinous, neuroendocrine features though other histological patterns occur [8, 9].

A heterogeneous staining pattern is typical for myoepithelial markers. Some nodules show an intact layer of myoepithelial cells at their periphery, and some show few myoepithelial cells, suggesting attenuation of the duct wall. The absence of myoepithelial cells within the cellular proliferation is characteristic, but they are sometimes focally retained. Some solid nodules with slightly irregular margins lack myoepithelial cells at the periphery, raising the possibility that at least some of these tumors represent circumscribed nests of invasive carcinoma and not a variant of DCIS [9, 14, 21]. It is very difficult to determine, based solely on histological sections stained by hematoxylin and eosin, whether a solid papillary carcinoma is only in situ, or if it has both in situ and invasive areas. Immunostains for myoepithelial markers may be helpful to differentiate these lesions. In some tumors, however, the precise classification of solid papillary carcinomas is difficult and controversial even using immunostains for myoepithelial markers. In the absence of conventional invasive carcinoma, the solid papillary carcinomas have an indolent clinical course similar to that of DCIS [6, 9, 14]. According to the 2012 WHO classification of breast tumors, if there is uncertainty about the presence of invasion, the lesion should be regarded as in situ for staging and management purposes [14, 21].

6.5   Invasive Papillary Carcinoma

Pure invasive papillary carcinomas are exceptionally rare, and are characterized by predominantly papillary structures (>90% of tumor) with fibrovascular cores lined by malignant epithelial cells in the invasive component [14, 24]. Since the lesion is very uncommon, diagnostic criteria are not well-documented. The majority of cases of invasive papillary carcinomas are seen admixed with another special type or a carcinoma of no special type. More often, areas of conventional types of invasive carcinoma (such as invasive ductal or mucinous) are seen in association with papillary DCIS, encapsulated papillary carcinoma, or solid papillary carcinomas; these lesions should not be classified as invasive papillary carcinomas [6, 13]. The main differential diagnosis is a metastatic papillary tumor originating from another organ, most frequently from ovary or lung [13, 24].

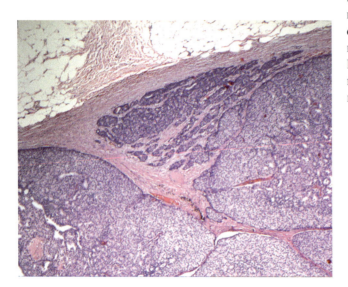

Fig. 6.35 Low-power view showing multiple nodules of solid papillary carcinoma comprising irregular nests with adjacent focus of pseudoinvasion within the dense, fibrotic stroma

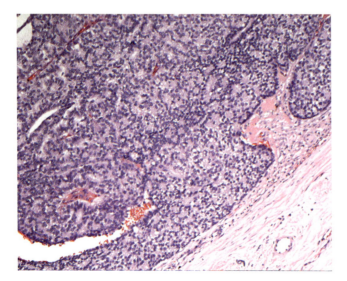

Fig. 6.36 High-power view of solid papillary carcinoma showing uniform population of low-grade neoplastic cells growing in a solid pattern, with focal rosette formation. Fibrovascular cores are evident. Myoepithelial cells are absent within the nodule and at the periphery

6.6   Fine-Needle Aspiration Cytology of Papillary Lesions

Cytological interpretation of papillary lesions of breast is challenging and represents a gray zone in fine-needle aspiration cytology (FNAC) of the breast. Different authors reported a low diagnostic accuracy of FNAC for papillary lesions of the breast [25, 26]. An unequivocal cytological diagnosis of papillary carcinoma is extremely difficult because clear distinction between benign and malignant lesions cannot be made on cytology alone. These lesions top the list of conditions in which there is a risk of false-positive diagnosis on FNAC. Many cytological criteria have been used to distinguish papillary lesions and include: overall cellularity, degree of atypia of the epithelial cells and clusters that are present, atypia of the individual cells in the background, and papillary fragments (Fig. 6.37). Other useful cytological features that can assist in the differentiation of malignant from benign papillary lesions is the presence of a greater number of single cells with atypia in the background, plasmacytoid cells in the background, and the presence of papillary fragments with ramifying edges with long and slender papillae. However, there is significant overlap in terms of architecture and cytological atypia, which is usually mild, and cytomorphological features alone are not sufficient for the precise diagnosis of papillary lesions of the breast [25]. If a papillary lesion is suspected in the FNAC, prompt histological evaluation is warranted for accurate diagnosis [25, 26].

6.7   Papillary Lesions on Core-Needle Biopsy

Evaluation of papillary lesions of the breast can be difficult, and in core-needle biopsy specimens, where under-sampling can be a problem, accurate diagnosis can be even more challenging [27–29]. There is an agreement that surgical excision is required when an atypical papillary lesion or papillary carcinoma is present on a core-needle biopsy. However, the need for surgical excision in patients in whom a benign intraductal papilloma is found on core-needle biopsy sample is an unresolved issue [6]. There is some controversy in the literature about whether the size of the core biopsy device correlates with complete evaluation of the lesion and the need for excision. In limited samples, the question is whether there will be associated areas of atypical hyperplasia or ductal carcinoma in situ, if complete excision of the lesion is not performed, in cases in which the limited sample afforded by core-needle biopsy showed benign papilloma (Fig. 6.38). As literature data are limited and retrospective, some authors recommend that benign papillomas diagnosed on the core biopsy should be completely excised due to risk of upgrade in the excision specimen [2, 6, 29].

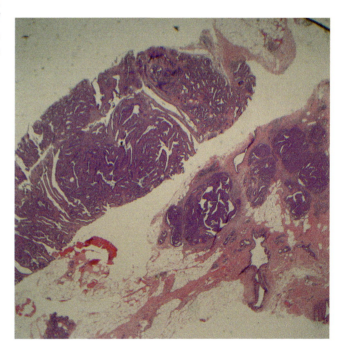

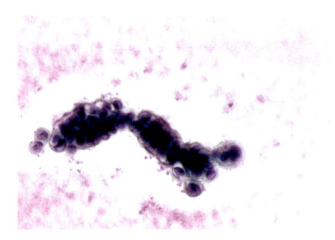

Fig. 6.37 Fine needle aspiration cytology showing a papillary fragment composed by bland epithelial cells

Fig. 6.38 Low-power view of large-gauge vacuum biopsy with benign papillomas

6.8   Epithelial Displacement

Mechanical displacement of epithelium may occur following needling procedures such as core-needle biopsy and fine-needle aspiration of papillary lesions [2, 5, 13]. These lesions are inherently friable, and the excisional specimen often shows foci of displaced epithelium within the core-needle biopsy site (Figs. 6.39 and 6.40). It is important to be aware of its occurrence and to recognize it histologically to avoid erroneous diagnosis of invasive carcinoma in patients with intraductal papilloma or in situ carcinoma [5]. The displaced epithelium is characterized by nests of epithelium with varying degrees of degenerative changes and squamoid features associated with a spectrum of biopsy site changes such as organizing hemorrhage, acute and chronic inflammation, foreign body reaction (i.e., foamy histiocytes, giant cells, and cholesterol clefts), fat necrosis, granulation tissue, or scarring. The absence of associated myoepithelial cells in the epithelial clusters is not, by itself, sufficient for a diagnosis of invasive carcinoma [6]. A diagnosis of invasive carcinoma should be considered only if epithelial cell nests are involved by desmoplastic stroma and in an area away from the needle biopsy site, and there is no prior diagnosis of invasive carcinoma [2].

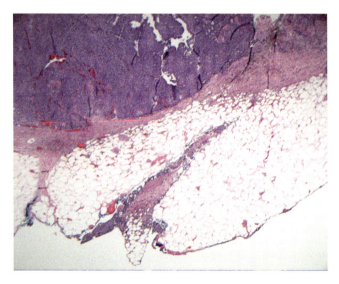

Fig. 6.39 Low-power view of excision specimen following core needle biopsy of encapsulated papillary carcinoma showing needle tract with entrapped epithelium

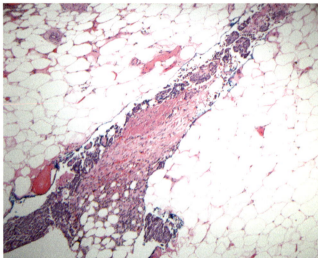

Fig. 6.40 Displaced epithelial cell nests within the biopsy site

References

1. O'Malley F, Visscher D, MacGrogan G, Tan PH, Ichihara S. Intraductal papilloma. In: Lakhani SR, Ellis IO, Schnnitt SJ, Tan PH, van de Vijver MJ, editors. WHO classification of tumours of the breast. 4th ed. Lyon: IARC Press; 2012. p. 100–2.
2. Wei S. Papillary lesions of the breast: an update. Arch Pathol Lab Med. 2016;140:628–43.
3. Jorns JM. Papillary lesions of the breast: a practical approach to diagnosis. Arch Pathol Lab Med. 2016;140:1052–9.
4. Agoumi M, Giambattista J, Hayes MM. Practical considerations in breast papillary lesions: a review of the literature. Arch Pathol Lab Med. 2016;140:770–90.
5. Mulligan AM, O'Malley FP. Papillary lesions of the breast: a review. Adv Anat Pathol. 2007;14:108–19.
6. Collins LC, Schnitt SJ. Papillary lesions of the breast: selected diagnostic and management issues. Histopathology. 2008;52:20–9.
7. Hill CB, Yeh IT. Myoepithelial cell staining patterns of papillary breast lesions: from intraductal papillomas to invasive papillary carcinomas. Am J Clin Pathol. 2005;123:36–44.
8. Tse GM, Ni YB, Tsang JY, Shao MM, Huang YH, Luo MH, et al. Immunohistochemistry in the diagnosis of papillary lesions of the breast. Histopathology. 2014;65:839–53.
9. Moritani S, Ichihara S, Kushima R, Okabe H, Bamba M, Kobayashi TK, et al. Myoepithelial cells in solid variant of intraductal papillary carcinoma of the breast: a potential diagnostic pitfall and a proposal of an immunohistochemical panel in the differential diagnosis with intraductal papilloma with usual ductal hyperplasia. Virchows Arch. 2007;450:539–47.
10. Grin A, O'Malley FP, Mulligan AM. Cytokeratin 5 and estrogen receptor immunohistochemistry as a useful adjunct in identifying atypical papillary lesions on breast needle core biopsy. Am J Surg Pathol. 2009;33:1615–23.
11. Ichihara S, Fujimoto T, Hashimoto K, Moritani S, Hasegawa M, Yokoi T. Double immunostaining with p63 and high-molecular-weight cytokeratins distinguishes borderline papillary lesions of the breast. Pathol Int. 2007;57:126–32.
12. Collins LC, Carlo VP, Hwang H, Barry TS, Gown AM, Schnitt SJ. Intracystic papillary carcinomas of the breast: a reevaluation using a panel of myoepithelial cell markers. Am J Surg Pathol. 2006;30:1002–7.
13. Schnitt SJ, Collins LC. Papillary lesions. In: Schnnitt SJ, Collins LC, editors. Biopsy interpretation of the breast. 2nd ed. Philadelphia, PA: Lippincott Williams & Wilkins; 2013. p. 228–66.
14. Tan PH, Schnitt SJ, van de Vijver MJ, Ellis IO, Lakhani SR. Papillary and neuroendocrine breast lesions: the WHO stance. Histopathology. 2015;66:761–70.
15. Page DL, Salhany KE, Jensen RA, Dupont WD. Subsequent breast carcinoma risk after biopsy with atypia in a breast papilloma. Cancer. 1996;78:258–66.
16. MacGrogan G, Tse G, Collins L, Tan PH, Chaiwun B, Reis-Filho JS. Intraductal papillary carcinoma. In: Lakhani SR, Ellis IO, Schnnitt SJ, Tan PH, van de Vijver MJ, editors. WHO classification of tumours of the breast. 4th ed. Lyon: IARC Press; 2012. p. 103–5.
17. Ni YB, Tse GM. Pathological criteria and practical issues in papillary lesions of the breast – a review. Histopathology. 2016;68:22–32.
18. Collins L, O'Malley F, Visscher D, Moriya T, Ichihara S, Reis-Filho JS. Encapsulated papillary carcinoma. In: Lakhani SR, Ellis IO, Schnnitt SJ, Tan PH, van de Vijver MJ, editors. WHO classification of tumours of the breast. 4th ed. Lyon: IARC Press; 2012. p. 106–7.
19. Mulligan AM. Encapsulated papillary carcinoma of the breast. Surg Pathol Clin. 2009;2:319–50.
20. Mulligan AM, O'Malley FP. Metastatic potential of encapsulated (intracystic) papillary carcinoma of the breast: a report of 2 cases with axillary lymph node micrometastases. Int J Surg Pathol. 2007;15:143–7.
21. Visscher D, Collins L, O'Malley F, Badve S, Reis-Filho JS. Solid papillary carcinoma. In: Lakhani SR, Ellis IO, Schnnitt SJ, Tan PH, van de Vijver MJ, editors. WHO classification of tumours of the breast. 4th ed. Lyon: IARC Press; 2012. p. 108–9.
22. Tan BY, Thike AA, Ellis IO, Tan PH. Clinicopathologic characteristics of solid papillary carcinoma of the breast. Am J Surg Pathol. 2016;40:1334–42.
23. Tacchini D, Vassallo L, Butorano MA, Mancini V, Megha T. Solid papillary carcinoma of the nipple: an in situ carcinoma or an expansive growth tumor? Pathologica. 2016;108:136–9.
24. Tse G, Moriya T, Niu Y. Invasive papillary carcinoma. In: Lakhani SR, Ellis IO, Schnnitt SJ, Tan PH, van de Vijver MJ, editors. WHO classification of tumours of the breast. 4th ed. Lyon: IARC Press; 2012. p. 64.
25. Prathiba D, Rao S, Kshitija K, Joseph LD. Papillary lesions of breast – an introspect of cytomorphological features. J Cytol. 2010;27:12–5.
26. Tse GM, Ma TK, Lui PC, Ng DC, Yu AM, Vong JS, et al. Fine needle aspiration cytology of papillary lesions of the breast: how accurate is the diagnosis? J Clin Pathol. 2008;61:945–9.
27. Seely JM, Verma R, Kielar A, Smyth KR, Hack K, Taljaard M, et al. Benign papillomas of the breast diagnosed on large-gauge vacuum biopsy compared with 14 gauge core needle biopsy – do they require surgical excision? Breast J. 2017;23:146–53.
28. Armes JE, Galbraith C, Gray J, Taylor K. The outcome of papillary lesions of the breast diagnosed by standard core needle biopsy within a Breast Screen Australia service. Pathology. 2017;49:267–70.
29. Jakate K, De Brot M, Goldberg F, Muradali D, O'Malley FP, Mulligan AM. Papillary lesions of the breast: impact of breast pathology subspecialization on core biopsy and excision diagnoses. Am J Surg Pathol. 2012;36:544–51.

Benign Lesions (Proliferations) and Tumors of the Breast

Simona Stolnicu

Most of the lesions included in this chapter are frequently encountered in breast pathology and easy to diagnose. Some of them, however, may mimic radiologically, clinically, and pathologically an invasive carcinoma (the so-called pseudoinfiltrative lesions of the breast). Especially in these cases, the experience of the pathologist together with ancillary studies allow a correct diagnosis, while management requires a breast tumor board approach. Also, some of these lesions increase the risk of developing a malignancy, and closer follow-up should be considered in these patients.

7.1 Fibrocystic Changes

Fibrocystic changes are an extremely important finding in breast pathology, due to their high frequency, their ability to mimic carcinoma clinically, radiologically, and morphologically, and the possible relationships between some of their forms and the development of a breast carcinoma. Currently, it is considered that fibrocystic changes are represented by a very heterogeneous spectrum of processes, some physiologic and some pathologic, with widely varying cancer risks [1–3]. It originates in the terminal duct/lobular unit (TDLU). Several names have been proposed for this lesion (fibrous mastopathy, mammary dysplasia, etc.), but the terms fibrocystic disease or fibrocystic changes are currently in use (in the latter case, the histopathological report should specify and describe all the changes detected within the biopsy or surgical specimen).

Fibrocystic changes occur more frequently during the reproductive period (ages 20–45); more than one-third of women aged between these two limits develop fibrocystic disease [4]. Its emergence is favored by hormonal disorders (change in the estradiol-progesterone ratio), while prolonged treatment with oral contraceptives or methylxanthines (coffee, tea, chocolate) have not been proved to be definitively involved in the pathogenesis of fibrocystic changes.

Clinically, the lesion is frequently multifocal and bilateral, and especially occurs in the upper-outer quadrant of the breast. Associated symptoms are the following: breast discomfort; and a feeling of heaviness or pain that is sometimes associated with nipple discharge. About 20% of the patients present axillary adenopathy associated with sensitivity (due to axillary lymph node reaction to the inflammatory process of the breast, as a result of a cyst rupture). After menopause, the lesions gradually regress (excluding patients who either receive estrogen replacement therapy or are obese). The changes can be detected by ultrasound examination,

S. Stolnicu, MD, PhD
Department of Pathology, University of Medicine and Pharmacy,
Tîrgu Mureş, Romania

© Springer International Publishing AG, part of Springer Nature 2018
S. Stolnicu, I. Alvarado-Cabrero (eds.), *Practical Atlas of Breast Pathology*, https://doi.org/10.1007/978-3-319-93257-6_7

especially because of the presence of the cysts, or by mammography (which detects microcalcifications associated with cysts, but characteristically a diffuse density secondary to the extensive stromal fibrosis can be detected). Tru-Cut Biopsy replaced fine-needle aspiration (FNA) as the method to diagnose palpable and non-palpable fibrocystic changes, and in most of the cases a portion of the cyst together with other associated lesions can be detected on microscopic examination.

Macroscopically, the lesion has ill-defined margins and it is usually represented by a gray-white fibrous tissue with elastic consistency, which on the cut surface has numerous cysts with a variable diameter of 2–20 mm, filled with clear or blue, yellow, sometimes hemorrhagic fluid (Figs. 7.1, 7.2, 7.3, and 7.4). However, in cases with small cysts identified on ultrasound or mammography, the macroscopic examination may disclose only an area of fibrosis and the microscopic examination will be necessary to reveal additional findings.

Microscopically, fibrocystic changes are characterized by a series of changes that are usually associated with one another:

- Hyperplasia of mammary ducts and acini, which retain their round shape and are lined by two characteristic cell layers (epithelial and myoepithelial cells).
- Cystic dilatation of the ducts and acini, forming micro- and macrocysts containing an acellular eosinophilic material in the lumina (Figs. 7.5, 7.6, 7.7, and 7.8); the lumina may also contain exfoliated epithelial cells or histiocytes with vacuolated cytoplasm (due to lipid content) and a small round nucleus, centrally located, called lamprocytes which, due to the hemorrhage, may contain hemosiderin pigment (Figs. 7.9 and 7.10); the migration of these cells from the lumina into epithelial layer can mimic a pseudo-pagetoid appearance (Fig. 7.11) that should not be mistaken for a precursor or a malignant lesion (immunohistochemical positivity of lamprocytes for CD-68 as well as negativity for pan-Cytokeratin can help to differentiate the two lesions); the cysts are lined by a cuboidal, cylindrical, or flattened epithelium (the latter condition occurs due to the containing contents of the cyst) (Figs. 7.12 and 7.13); if only one single cyst is identified in the breast tissue, it is called a *solitary cyst*; if more cysts are identified, fibrocystic changes diagnosis is preferable; the solitary cyst is usually unique with a diameter of over 10 mm; some of the cysts may contain calcifications of varying types including calcium, calcium phosphate, apatite, or calcium oxalate (Fig. 7.14).
- Apocrine metaplasia, which involves both acini and intralobular ducts (but sometimes also the extralobular ones); it represents a transformation of the cells of normal cuboidal/cylindrical epithelium into apocrine cells, which are characterized by a larger size, rounded or cylindrical shape, with abundant eosinophilic granular cytoplasm, a round nucleus, and a centrally located prominent nucleolus (Fig. 7.15); apocrine metaplasia may involve the epithelium of acini or ducts, without their cystic dilatation (in this case the term *apocrine adenosis* can be used), or it can involve cystically dilated ducts or acini; also, apocrine metaplasia can occur in the absence of any other changes, within normal acini or ducts, without any clinical/pathological significance (Fig. 7.16); the epithelium of apocrine metaplasia may sometimes be flat or may present a complex proliferation with small papillae centered around a fibro-vascular axis or forming arches and bridges (Figs. 7.17, 7.18, and 7.19); apocrine metaplasia cells may sometimes exhibit atypia represented by nuclear enlargement (more than threefold nuclear size variation), nuclear pleomorphism, prominent nucleolus, and mitotic figures; also, apocrine metaplastic cells may sometimes show intracytoplasmic microvacuoles, cells which are similar to the sebaceous cells (sebocrine metaplasia); immunohistochemically, apocrine cells are usually negative for estrogen receptors (ER) and progesterone receptors (PR) while they are positive for androgen receptors (AR) [5].
- Chronic inflammatory process due to the rupture of cysts and release of their contents into the surrounding stroma; the inflammatory infiltrate is usually composed of lymphocytes, plasma cells, and histiocytes (Figs. 7.20 and 7.21).
- Fibrosis of the stroma, which varies quantitatively from one lesion to the other and also from one field to another within the same lesion; the intralobular stroma is sclerotic, sometimes indistinguishable from the interlobular stroma; myxoid changes or microcalfications may occur (Figs. 7.22 and 7.23).
- Fibroadenomatoid changes similar to those that occur in fibroadenomas, but being diffuse and not circumscribed, forming a mass in fibrocystic changes (Fig. 7.24).
- Epithelial hyperplasia, which occurs only in some fibrocystic changes and which is the most important component because its presence increases the relative risk to the development of breast carcinoma. Therefore, in 1986, the College of American Pathologists [2] distinguished between *functional fibrocystic changes*, with no epithelial hyperplasia associated, and *proliferative fibrocystic changes*, with epithelial hyperplasia prone to carcinoma development (Figs. 7.25, 7.26, 7.27, 7.28, 7.29, 7.30, 7.31, 7.32, and 7.33). The two entities should be separated from a pathological point of view and treated differently. If the epithelium of apocrine metaplasia is accompanied by hyperplasia, the lesion is designated as proliferative fibrocystic changes and reported accordingly. The same rule applies to the solitary cyst if it is accompanied by epithelial hyperplasia.

Differential diagnosis is made with the following:

- Ductal ectasia (which has a different location and affects extralobular ducts, and a chronic inflammatory infiltrate can be observed periductally, as well as the presence of elastic tissue).
- Galactocele (a cavity beneath the areola filled with milk, due to the abrupt suppression of lactation; the cavity is usually lined by a secretory epithelium and the surrounding tissue may present areas of lipogranuloma due to the leakage of the cyst content consisting especially of a collection of foamy histocytes containing milk intracytoplasmatically) (Fig. 7.34).
- Hydatic cyst (produced by Echinococcus, very rare in the breast, presenting as usually unilocular cyst fluid filled but also containing daughter cysts and microscopically lined by three layers: germinal internal layer, laminated membrane beneath the germinal layer, and outer layer of dense fibrovascular tissue with chronic inflammatory infiltrate and variable calcifications) (Fig. 7.35).
- Pseudocyst cavity after surgical removal of breast lesions (the cavity is not lined by an epithelium and is surrounded by inflammatory infiltrate and numerous histiocytes) (Fig. 7.36).
- Cystic atrophy in postmenopausal patients (originating in intralobular acini and ducts, which are lined by an atrophic epithelium and surrounded by intralobular stroma while there is no association with the other conditions of fibrocystic changes).
- Flat atypia (the ducts and acini involved in such a lesion are usually distended, have a smooth contour, and may contain secretory material and microcalcifications mimicking fibrocystic changes at low-power; however, at high-power, they are lined by one-to-several epithelial cells lacking polarity with round nuclei presenting low atypicality and sometimes apical snouts while the myoepithelial cells are present but attenuated and barely visible at the periphery) (Figs. 7.37 and 7.38).
- Cystic hypersecretory hyperplasia or ductal carcinoma *in situ* (represented by cysts filled with secretory material which on microscopic examination resemble the thyroid colloid; the cysts are lined by epithelium showing various degrees of hyperplasia and/or ductal carcinoma *in situ*, with areas showing evidence of secretory activity resembling the lactating breast) (Figs. 7.39, 7.40, and 7.41).
- Blunt duct adenosis (distension of acini and ducts, with rounded or irregular contour, lined by both epithelial cells with columnar features and prominent myoepithelial cells, with various secretions within the lumina; some authors consider blunt duct adenosis as part of the spectrum of fibrocystic changes since the TDLU expands without ductal and/or lobular proliferation) (Figs. 7.42 and 7.43).
- Fibroadenoma (a nodular mass of more than 10 mm in diameter, surrounded by a capsule at the periphery and not associated with cysts or inflammation).
- *In situ* breast carcinoma of ductal or lobular type or atypical ductal or lobular hyperplasia (in the presence of atypical epithelial hyperplasia); as well as with Swiss-cheese tumor (also called juvenile papillomatosis, typically occurring in children—unlike fibrocystic changes—as a grossly distinct multinodular mass with clustering of cystic formations; microscopically, multiple cysts are associated with epithelial hyperplasia and papillomatosis usually without atypia) as well as multiple papillomatosis (multiple cysts involved by a papillary proliferation of fibro-vascular axes lined both epithelial and myoepithelial cells without atypia; other microscopic findings of fibrocystic changes are missing) (Figs. 7.44, 7.45, and 7.46) [6].

Changes such as fibrosis, dilatation of acini and ducts (only visible microscopically), involution or enlargement of lobules, when unaccompanied by other changes characteristic for fibrocystic changes, should be reported as normal changes because they are not considered benign pathological changes. In the final histopathological report, one must list all the changes or lesions found within the specimen, in the descending order of importance with regard to their potential level of breast cancer risk, including microcalcifications (even if these were associated with normal breast tissue).

If the fibrocystic changes are not associated with epithelial proliferation, the risk of subsequent development of invasive carcinoma is extremely low (0.89 relative risk), increasing with a positive family history (1.2 relative risk) and presence of larger cysts (1.3 relative risk); therefore, no specific follow-up is recommended for these patients other than for the normal population [6, 7]. Prognosis of fibrocystic changes without proliferation is excellent whether the prognosis of the proliferative lesion depends to the degree of the proliferation and/or atypia. No surgical treatment is indicated for patients with non-proliferative disease while hormonal treatment for providing symptomatic relief may be of use. For patients with large cysts, evaluation of the cysts using fine-needle aspiration (FNA) guided by ultrasound may be an option. The cytological assessment of the fluid is generally performed when the appearance of the fluid is bloody or turbid, or in cases in which the cyst does not collapse completely after aspiration; in some centers, however, the fluid is routinely cytologically examined. Also, when the lesion is associated with epithelial hyperplasia without atypia, a good radiological-pathological correlation is needed, and radiological follow-up is recommended. However, when proliferative changes are associated with atypia, surgical excision is indicated, and further treatment is based on the type and extent of the atypical proliferation.

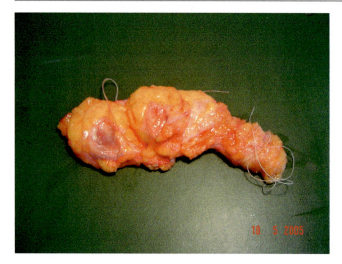

Fig. 7.1 Fibrocystic changes: surgically removed breast quadrant presenting an area of fibrosis and multiple cysts of various sizes

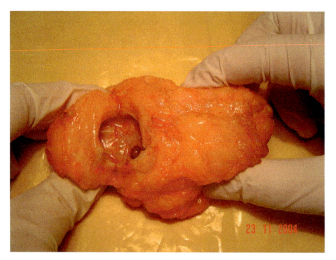

Fig. 7.2 Fibrocystic changes: on the cut surface, one of the cysts has smooth internal wall and the content is partially hemorrhagic

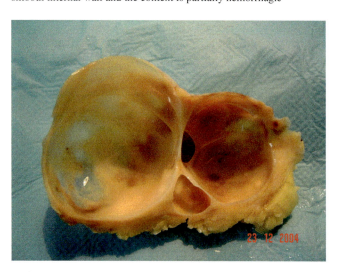

Fig. 7.3 Fibrocystic changes: surgical specimen with multiple cysts of various sizes with smooth contour

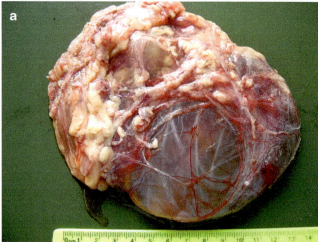

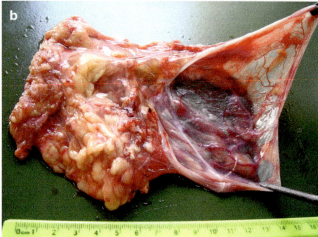

Fig. 7.4 Fibrocystic changes: (**a**) Surgical specimen with multiple cysts, one of which is large size. (**b**) On the cut surface, the largest cyst has smooth and thin wall due to the large amount of content

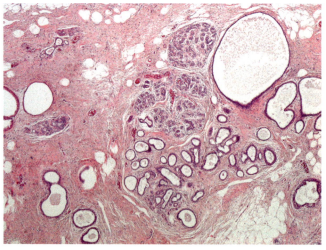

Fig. 7.5 Functional fibrocystic changes: hyperplasia of mammary ducts and acini, some of them cystically dilated

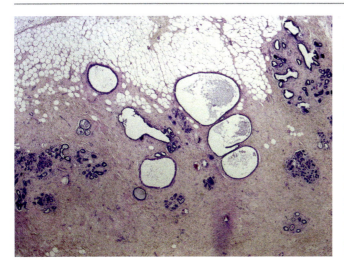

Fig. 7.6 Functional fibrocystic changes: hyperplasia of mammary ducts and acini, some of them cystically dilated

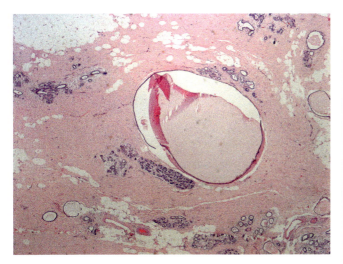

Fig. 7.7 Functional fibrocystic changes: multiple cysts containing an acellular eosinophilic material in the lumina

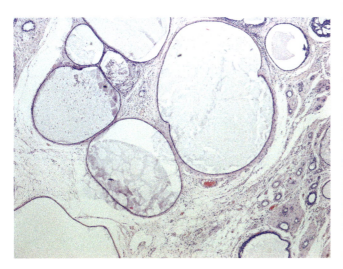

Fig. 7.8 Fibrocystic changes: multiple cysts, most of them containing an acellular eosinophilic material in the lumina

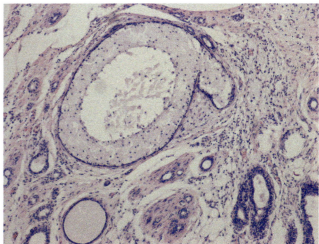

Fig. 7.9 Fibrocystic changes: the lumina of the cysts contain exfoliated epithelial cells and histiocytes with vacuolated cytoplasm (due to lipid content) and a small round nucleus, centrally located (called lamprocytes)

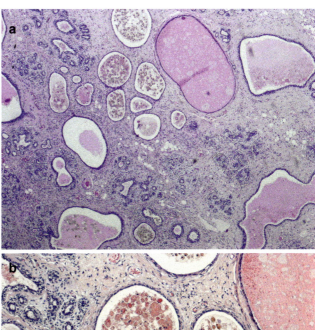

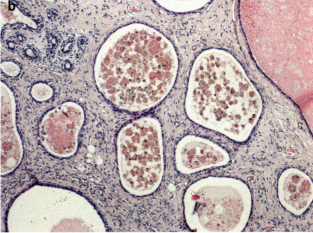

Fig. 7.10 Fibrocystic changes: (**a**) The lumina of the cysts contains numerous lamprocytes, (**b**) which due to the hemorrhage contain hemosiderin pigment intracytoplasmatically

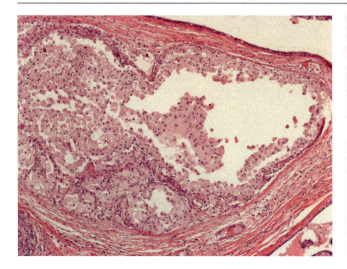

Fig. 7.11 Fibrocystic changes: the migration of lamprocytes from the lumina into epithelial layer can mimic a pseudo-pagetoid appearance

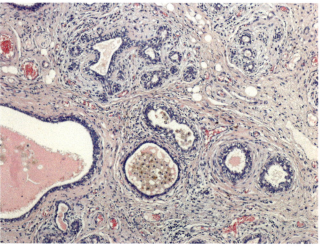

Fig. 7.12 Functional fibrocystic changes: hyperplasia of mammary ducts and acini, which retain their round shape and are lined by two characteristic cell layers (inner epithelial and outer myoepithelial cells)

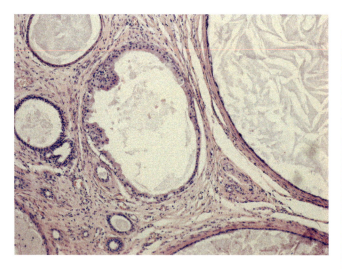

Fig. 7.13 Functional fibrocystic changes: some of the cysts have cuboidal epithelium, some have flattened epithelium, and some have epithelium with apocrine metaplasia

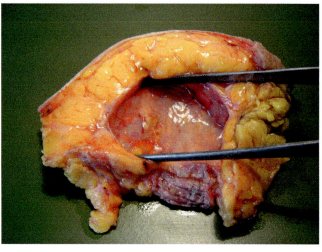

Fig. 7.14 Surgical specimen with one single cyst, called solitary cyst

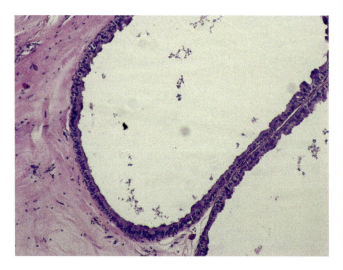

Fig. 7.15 Functional fibrocystic changes: two cysts lined by cylindrical epithelium with apocrine metaplasia

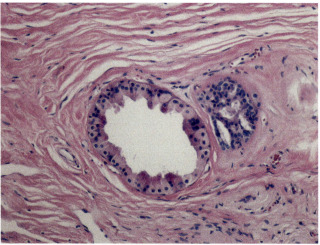

Fig. 7.16 Apocrine metaplasia involves the epithelium of acini, without their cystic dilatation; the cells are of larger size, rounded or cylindrical shape, with abundant eosinophilic granular cytoplasm and a round nucleus

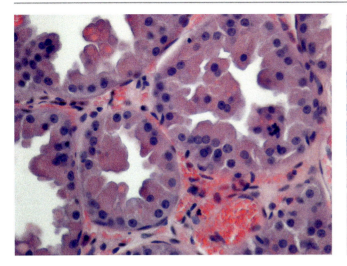

Fig. 7.17 Apocrine metaplasia; cylindrical cells with abundant eosinophilic granular cytoplasm and nuclei with prominent nucleoli

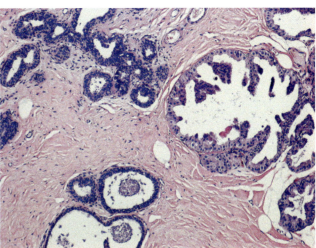

Fig. 7.18 Apocrine metaplasia with complex proliferation without atypia: cysts lined by metaplastic apocrine epithelium forming papillae and micropapillae

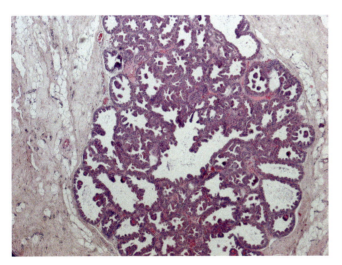

Fig. 7.19 Apocrine metaplasia with complex proliferation without atypia: cysts lined by metaplastic apocrine epithelium forming papillae (with a fibro-vascular axis) and micropapillae (without a fibro-vascular axis)

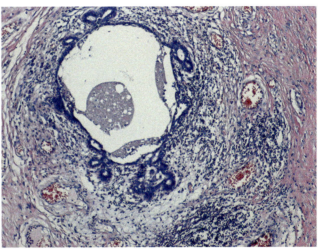

Fig. 7.20 Functional fibrocystic changes: chronic inflammatory process around the cyst

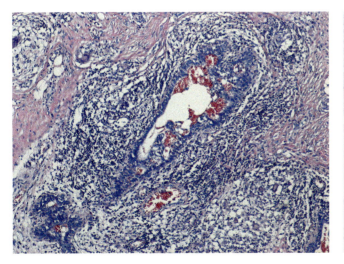

Fig. 7.21 Fibrocystic changes: chronic inflammatory process around the cyst represented by lymphocytes, plasma cells, and histiocytes, some of them multinucleated

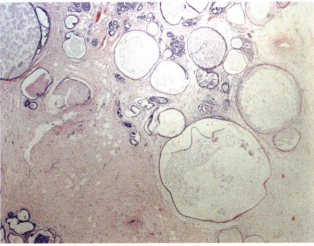

Fig. 7.22 Fibrocystic changes with fibrosis with a sclerotic appearance

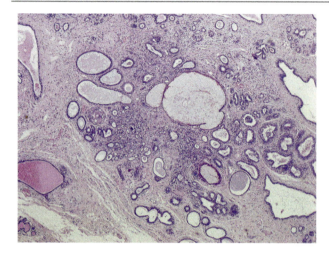

Fig. 7.23 Fibrocystic changes: microcalcifications into the stroma adjacent to the cysts

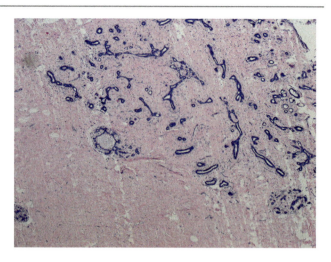

Fig. 7.24 Fibrocystic changes with fibroadenomatoid changes: they are similar in morphologic appearance to fibroadenoma, but have a diffuse character

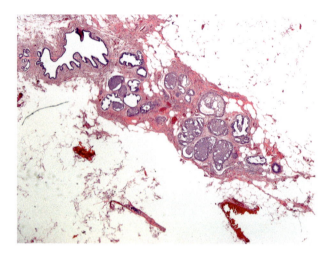

Fig. 7.25 Proliferative fibrocystic changes: multiple acini of the TDLU involved by a luminal proliferation without atypia while the duct is not affected

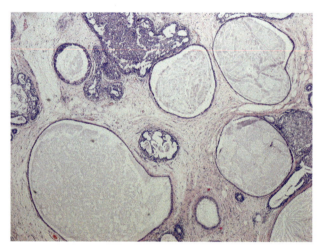

Fig. 7.26 Proliferative fibrocystic changes: some of the cysts are lined by a double layer of cells while others have intraluminal proliferation without atypia

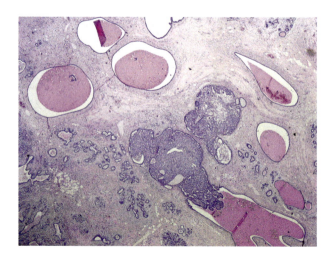

Fig. 7.27 Proliferative fibrocystic changes: some of the cysts are lined by a double layer of cells while others have intraluminal proliferation without atypia which involves partially or entirely the cysts

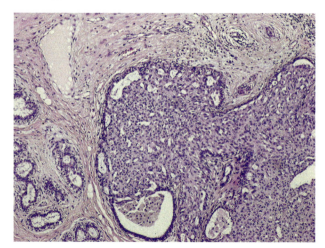

Fig. 7.28 Proliferative fibrocystic changes: high-power examination reveals that intraluminal proliferation is represented by a mixed population of cells with spindle shaped overlapping nuclei, syncytial appearance of the cytoplasm, and secondary lumina at the periphery of the cyst (usual ductal hyperplasia, without atypia)

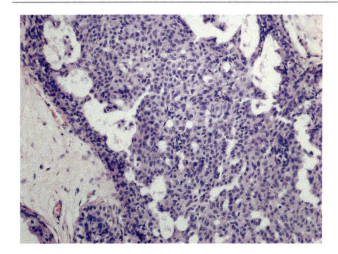

Fig. 7.29 Proliferative fibrocystic changes with usual ductal hyperplasia without atypia: most of the secondary lumina are located at the periphery of the cyst

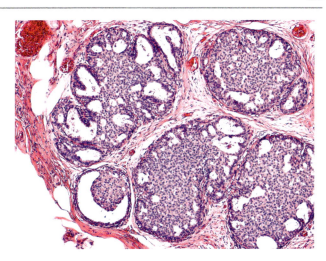

Fig. 7.30 Proliferative fibrocystic changes with usual ductal hyperplasia without atypia displaying various architecture appearance, including glomeruloid-type

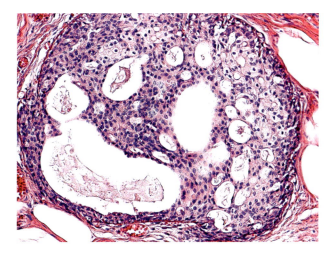

Fig. 7.31 Proliferative fibrocystic changes with usual ductal hyperplasia without atypia: high-power examination reveals a mixed population of epithelial, myoepithelial, and apocrine cells

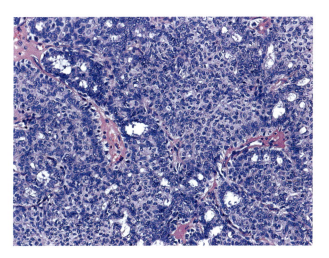

Fig. 7.32 Proliferative fibrocystic changes with usual ductal hyperplasia without atypia: high-power examination reveals a mixed population of epithelial and myoepithelial cells

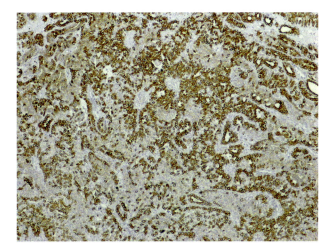

Fig. 7.33 Proliferative fibrocystic changes with usual ductal hyperplasia without atypia: the cells are Cytokeratin 18-positive (which is not helpful for differential diagnosis with atypical ductal hyperplasia since the later lesion is also positive for this marker)

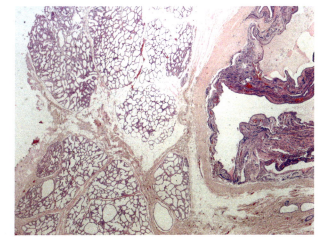

Fig. 7.34 Galactocele: a cavity lined by a cuboidal to flattened epithelium, surrounded by inflammatory infiltrate and breast parenchyma with secretory features (lactational changes)

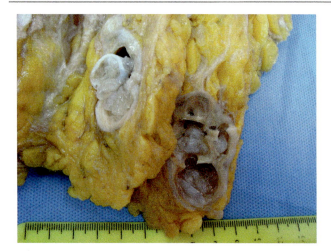

Fig. 7.35 Hydatic cysts within breast parenchyma: especially when this lesion is represented by multiple cysts it can be confused with fibrocystic changes; on cut surface one can appreciate the presence of the daughter cysts

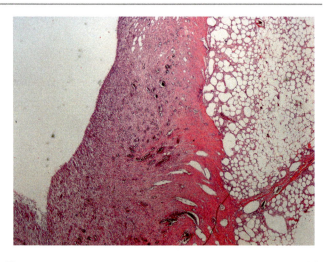

Fig. 7.36 Pseudocyst: the cavity is not lined by an epithelium and it is surrounded by granulation tissue and fat necrosis areas

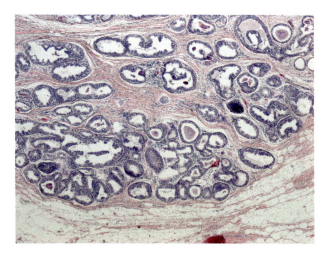

Fig. 7.37 Flat atypia: distended ducts and acini with smooth contour mimicking fibrocystic changes at low-power examination

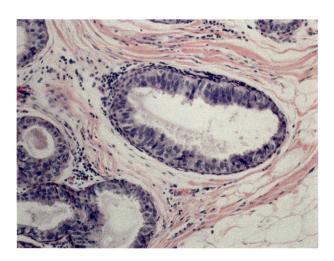

Fig. 7.38 Flat atypia: at high-power examination, the ducts and acini are lined by one to several epithelial cells lacking polarity, with round nuclei presenting low-atypicallity, apical snouts while the myoepithelial cells are present but attenuated and barely visible at the periphery

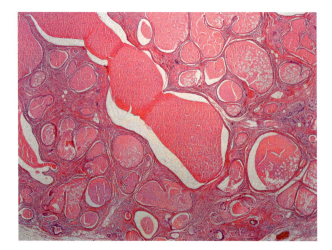

Fig. 7.39 Cystic hypersecretory hyperplasia: multiple cysts filled with secretory material which on microscopic examination, unlike in fibrocystic changes, resemble the thyroid colloid

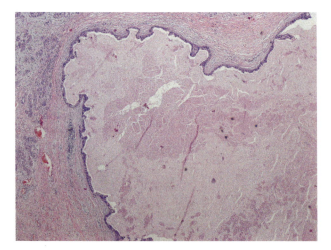

Fig. 7.40 Cystic hypersecretory hyperplasia with atypia: cysts filled with secretory material and lined by mostly flat atypical epithelium

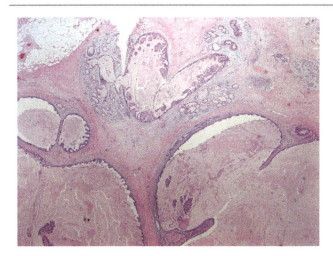

Fig. 7.41 Cystic hypersecretory hyperplasia with atypia: multiple cysts lined by atypical epithelium with various architecture like flat, papillary, micropapillary; areas of microinvasion can be detected as well in the upper part of the picture

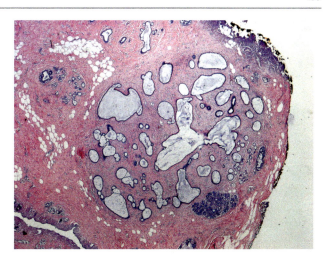

Fig. 7.42 Blunt duct adenosis: distension of acini and ducts, with rounded or irregular contour, lined by both epithelial cells and prominent myoepithelial cells

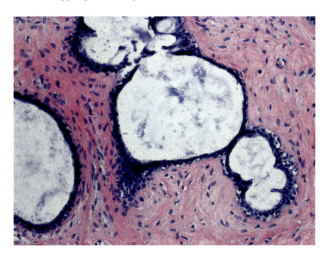

Fig. 7.43 Blunt duct adenosis: characteristically, the epithelial cells have columnar features and the myoepithelial cells are visible and prominent

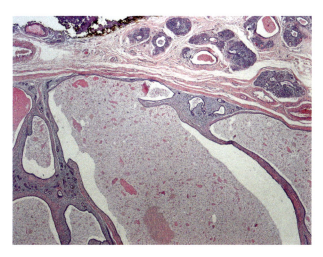

Fig. 7.44 Juvenile papillomatosis: distinct nodular mass within breast parenchyma, with smooth contour at the periphery

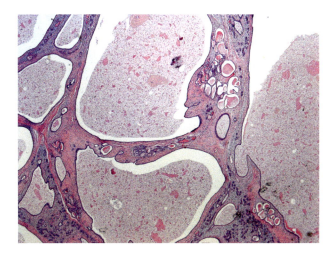

Fig. 7.45 Juvenile papillomatosis: multiple cystic spaces containing a secretory eosinophilic material within the lumina; no areas of intraepithelial proliferation can be detected in this picture

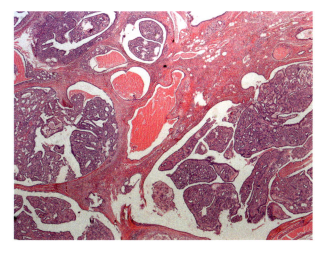

Fig. 7.46 Multiple papillomatosis: multiple cysts involved by a papillary proliferation of fibro-vascular axes lined both epithelial and myoepithelial cells without atypia

7.2   Radial Scar

First described by Semb in 1928, radial scar is a benign breast lesion which consists of a central area of fibro-elastosis surrounded by radially oriented ducts and acini [8]. The average age of occurrence is 55 years and the lesion can be multicentric (especially when it is small) and bilateral, and is often associated with fibrocystic changes or other lesions like adenosis, microcalcifications, apocrine metaplasia, collagenous sferulosis, papilloma, usual or atypical ductal hyperplasia, or *in situ* carcinoma of ductal or lobular type, invasive carcinoma. Regarding the pathogenesis of the lesion, some authors argue that it forms due to the obliteration of ducts within ductal ectasia, while others argue that it is due to a reactive process resulting from fine-needle biopsies performed for diagnostic purposes or from any other trauma through the breast parenchyma that may lead to a scar. The incidence is very variable (1.7–43% of cases) in relation with the sampling method and the type of the associated lesion. The radial scar may mimic an invasive carcinoma clinically, radiologically, and morphologically, especially for inexperienced pathologists. Radiologically, the lobular normal architecture is distorted and usually one can appreciate a stellate lesion with irregular configuration on mammography (like a "star in the sky"), simulating an invasive carcinoma; microcalcifications are, however, an uncommon finding (Fig. 7.47). Clinically, if it is larger in size, it can be confused, on palpation, with a carcinoma. Grossly, its diameter is typically under 1 cm and is not evident, being identified only microscopically (Fig. 7.48). When it is larger, it has a stellate, rarely nodular appearance, with a hard-white core, whitish, resembling a scar from which fibrous bands originate in the surrounding tissues. Radial scar is the most frequent, represented by a small lesion, less than 10 mm in diameter, usually with no hyperplasia associated. However, complex sclerosing lesion (also called infiltrative epitheliosis, a term that is not encouraged because it is very confusing for the clinicians) is a similar lesion but with a diameter of more than 10 mm, associated with hyperplasia (without atypia, or *in situ* ductal or lobular type); being larger, this lesion is less organized than the radial scar [9]. In routine practice, both lesions (radial scar and complex sclerosing lesion) can be misinterpreted on gross examination as an infiltrating carcinoma, and especially on frozen sections and pathologists are advised to wait for the permanent sections whenever a correct diagnosis cannot be established with confidence.

Microscopically, the central area is composed of fibrous and collagenous tissue, in a small quantity or which can be extended, in some cases covering the entire lesion. Also, massive areas of elastosis can be identified within the central area. Around it, within the midzone, radially arranged acini and ducts can be observed. Those in the central area are more compressed and distorted (raising concern for an invasive carcinoma), while those located in the peripheral area are round. They are bordered by two layers of cells (epithelial and myoepithelial) and can exhibit epithelial hyperplasia. Sometimes, ducts and acini can display apocrine metaplastic epithelium (a situation in which the diagnosis is very difficult even for more experienced pathologists). Another characteristic feature is that the epithelial cells seem to be retracted from the myoepithelial cells and the surrounding stroma, due to real retraction of the stroma but also to vacuolization of the cytoplasm of the myoepithelial cell. When this phenomenon occurs, a slit-like space is identified next to the epithelial cells and only small picnotic nuclei of the myoepithelial cells can be observed at the periphery of the distorted ducts. Especially in these cases, the use of ancillary stains for myoepithelial cells is of great help. Of interest, pathologists should use nuclear myoepithelial markers (such as p63) since cytoplasmic markers or membrane markers would not highlight the myoepithelial cells. At the periphery of the lesion, distended ducts forming cysts are highly characteristic (Figs. 7.49, 7.50, 7.51, 7.52, 7.53, 7.54, 7.55, 7.56, 7.57, 7.58, 7.59, 7.60, 7.61, 7.62, and 7.63). Less characteristic features are the following: presence of necrosis in the lumina of the tubules; presence of massive, usually ductal, hyperplasia in the center of the lesion rather than in the midzone; presence of vascular or perineural invasion (not clinically significant); presence of a malignant transformation (especially at the periphery of the lesion; this phenomenon may alter the symmetry of the scar, and is associated with reactive desmoplastic stroma and the myoepithelial cells are absent) (Figs. 7.64, 7.65, 7.66, 7.67, 7.68, 7.69, 7.70, 7.71, 7.72, 7.73, 7.74, 7.75, and 7.76).

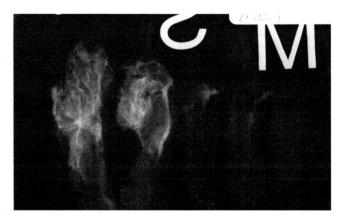

Fig. 7.47 Radial scar: lobular normal architecture is distorted on mammography and the lesion has a stellate shape, simulating an invasive carcinoma

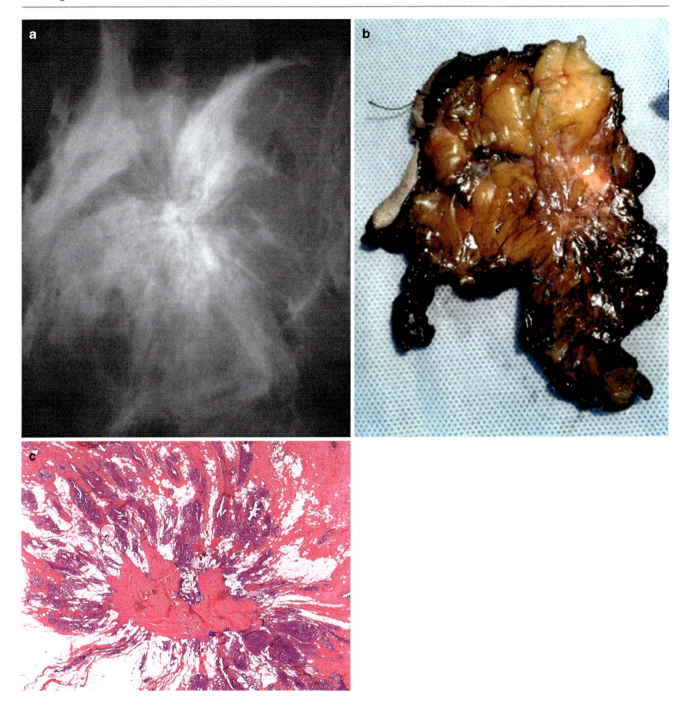

Fig. 7.48 Radial scar: (**a**) 53-year-old patient with a suspicious stellate lesion on mammography and (**b**) macroscopically with (**c**), a diameter of 10 mm, which at microscopic examination was diagnosed as a radial scar

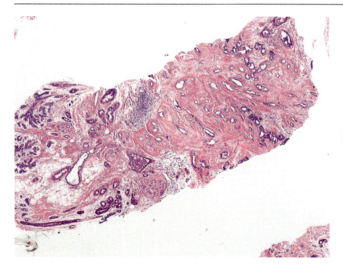

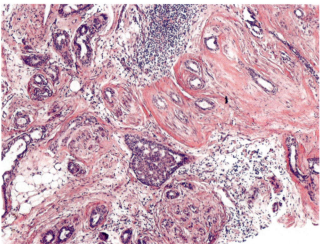

Fig. 7.49 Radial scar: on a biopsy one can appreciate three distinct areas—central area (right side), middle area and peripheral area (right side)

Fig. 7.50 Radial scar (high-power examination of the same lesion from Fig. 7.49): central area is characterized by entrapped tubular structure within a sclerotic tissue (left side), middle area is represented by inflammatory infiltrate and cysts with usual ductal hyperplasia, and at the periphery (right side) one can appreciate small round cysts

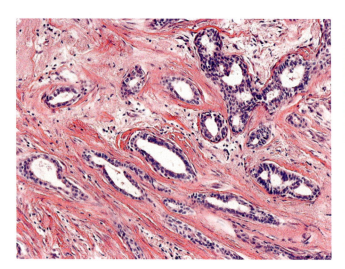

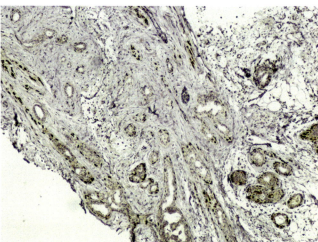

Fig. 7.51 Radial scar (high-power examination of the same lesion from Fig. 7.49): distorted angulated tubular structures lined by two layers of cells; areas of cribriform appearance raising concern of an infiltrative process can be appreciated

Fig. 7.52 Radial scar (high-power examination of the same lesion from Fig. 7.49): the presence of the myoepithelial layer is highlighted on p63 stain at the periphery of the angulated tubular structures

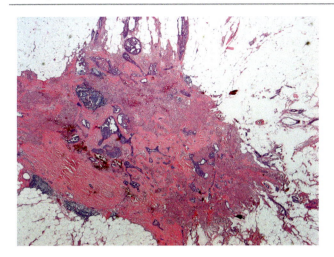

Fig. 7.53 Radial scar (surgical specimen followed the Tru-Cut biopsy from Fig. 7.49): a stellate-shape lesion with a central area of elastosis, midzone of inflammatory infiltrate and ducts with usual ductal hyperplasia and areas of hemorrhage due to the previous biopsy

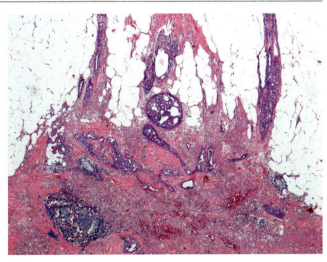

Fig. 7.54 Radial scar (surgical specimen followed the Tru-Cut biopsy from Fig. 7.49): high-power examination reveals usual ductal hyperplasia involving the midzone

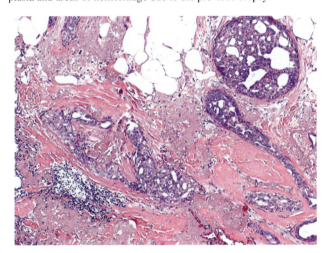

Fig. 7.55 Radial scar (surgical specimen followed the Tru-Cut biopsy from Fig. 7.49): high-power examination reveals central area of fibrosis and elastosis

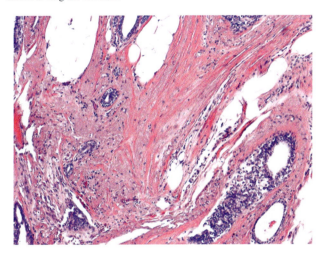

Fig. 7.56 Radial scar (surgical specimen followed the Tru-Cut biopsy from Fig. 7.49): entrapped tubules lined by epithelial and myoepithelial cells

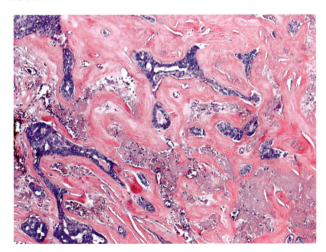

Fig. 7.57 Radial scar (surgical specimen followed the Tru-Cut biopsy from Fig. 7.49): high-power examination reveals that the epithelial cells seem to be retracted from the surrounding stroma; this phenomenon makes difficult the identification of the myoepithelial cells

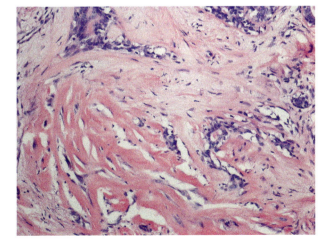

Fig. 7.58 Radial scar (surgical specimen followed the Tru-Cut biopsy from Fig. 7.49): high-power examination reveals that the epithelial cells seem to be retracted from the myoepithelial cells and the surrounding stroma and a slit-like space is identified next to the epithelial cells; only small picnotic nuclei of the myoepithelial cells can be observed at the peryphery of the dirtorted ducts

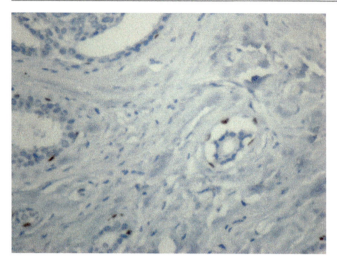

Fig. 7.59 Radial scar (surgical specimen followed the Tru-Cut biopsy from Fig. 7.49): the presence of the myoepithelial cells is highlighted with p63, a myoepithelial nuclear marker

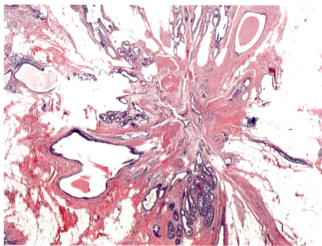

Fig. 7.60 Radial scar with a star-like shape at low power

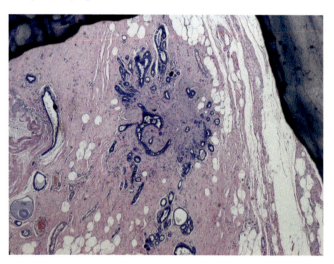

Fig. 7.61 Radial scar with a star-like shape and microcalcifications

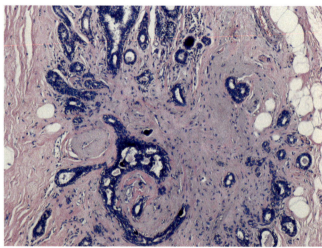

Fig. 7.62 Radial scar with a star-like shape and microcalcifications (same lesion as Fig. 7.62): high-power examination allows the detection of two cell layers

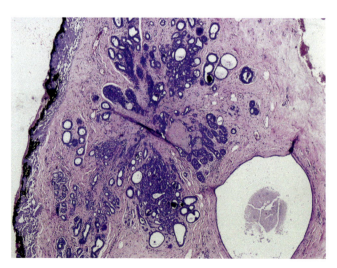

Fig. 7.63 Radial scar associated with microcalcifications and areas of adenosis

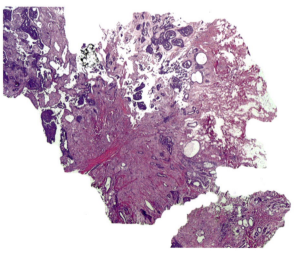

Fig. 7.64 Complex sclerosing lesion: 41-year-old patient with a palpable nodule for which frozen section examination was performed; at macroscopic examination a 21 mm stellate lesion was detected and two tissue fragments were sampled; first tissue fragment shows a central area of fibrosis with entrapped tubular structures and cysts with epithelial proliferation at the periphery

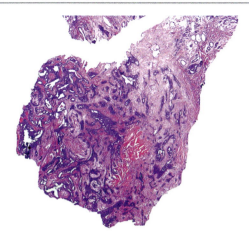

Fig. 7.65 Complex sclerosing lesion: lesion from Fig. 7.64 second tissue fragment at frozen section examination is more suspicious for a malignant process since it has only a small area of fibrosis in the center while the majority of the tissue presents nests of various sizes and shapes infiltrating the breast parenchyma

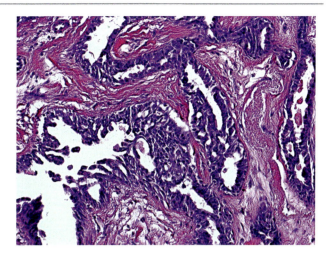

Fig. 7.66 Complex sclerosing lesion: lesion from Fig. 7.64 on high-power examination shows irregular and angulated nests of epithelial cells with secondary lumina and micropapillae; due to the dense stroma, the detection of the myoepithelial cells is difficult

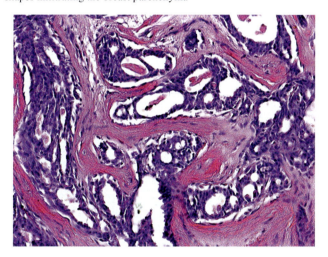

Fig. 7.67 Complex sclerosing lesion: lesion from Fig. 7.64 on high-power examination—other areas of epithelial cells with rounded contour and cribriform morphology; myoepithelial cells are difficult to detect

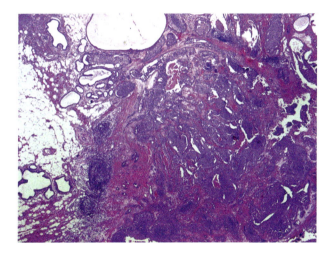

Fig. 7.68 Complex sclerosing lesion: lesion from Fig. 7.64 on permanent section examination has only a small area of fibrosis and elastosis, while the majority of the lesion is represented by nests of epithelial cells; cystic dilated ducts may be seen at the periphery of the lesion

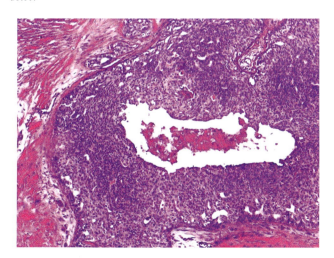

Fig. 7.69 Complex sclerosing lesion: lesion from Fig. 7.64 on permanent section examination with central area of necrosis involving some of the epithelial nests

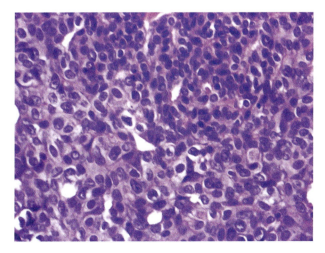

Fig. 7.70 Complex sclerosing lesion: lesion from Fig. 7.64 on permanent section. High-power examination detects a mixed population of epithelial and myoepithelial cells with ovoid nuclei and syncytial cytoplasm lacking atypical mitotic figures (usual ductal hyperplasia without atypia)

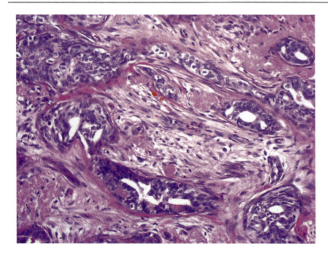

Fig. 7.71 Complex sclerosing lesion: lesion from Fig. 7.64 on permanent section examination—due to the fibrosis, one cannot easily appreciate the presence of the myoepithelial cells

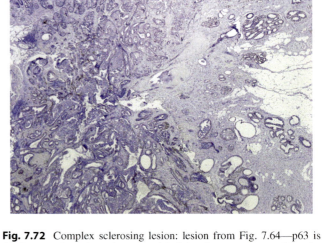

Fig. 7.72 Complex sclerosing lesion: lesion from Fig. 7.64—p63 is the best marker since the myoepithelial cells are attenuated by the fibrosis

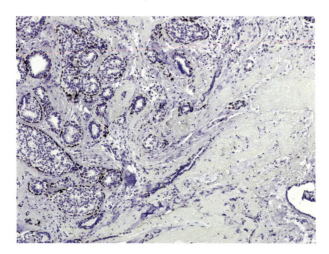

Fig. 7.73 Complex sclerosing lesion: lesion from Fig. 7.64—p63 marks a myoepithelial cell layer at the periphery of all the tubular structures and epithelial nests, including those with central necrosis

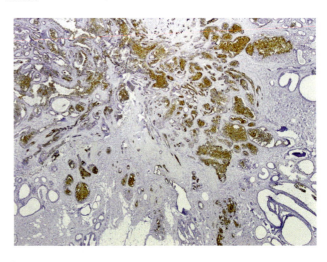

Fig. 7.74 Complex sclerosing lesion: lesion from Fig. 7.64—Cytokeratin 5/6 is mosaic-like positive distinguishing the usual ductal hyperplasia from atypical ductal hyperplasia or DCIS; final diagnosis was complex sclerosing lesion with usual ductal hyperplasia and areas of necrosis (due to the large size of the lesion—more than 10 mm—the complexity and its lack of classic organization like in a radial scar); no further treatment was indicated

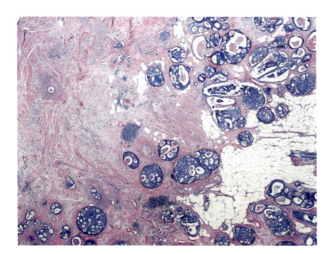

Fig. 7.75 Radial scar with areas of extensive grade 1 DCIS at the periphery (ER was positive in 100% of the epithelial cells in the areas of DCIS—not shown)

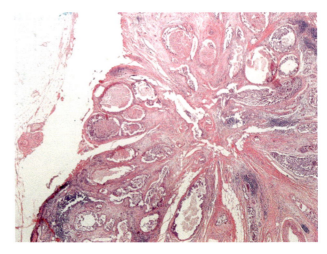

Fig. 7.76 Radial scar with areas of extensive grade 3 DCIS of comedonecrosis type at the periphery

Differential diagnosis is made with malignant lesions (tubular carcinoma, grade 1 invasive carcinoma of NST—no special type and invasive tubulo-lobular carcinoma) or benign lesions (microglandular adenosis, sclerosing adenosis, syringomatous adenoma and sclerosing papilloma). The most important differential diagnosis, however, is made with tubular carcinoma (Table 7.1). Radial scar has a stellate configuration while tubular carcinoma is represented by a nodule with infiltrative margins. Radial scar has a fibro-elastotic central part while tubular carcinoma has desmoplastic stroma throughout the lesion (central area with fibro-elastosis is not present). The ducts and acini that form the scar are distorted and entrapped in the central part of the lesion and lined by epithelial and myoepithelial cells, surrounded by a distinct basal membrane, elements that can be observed in both routine staining and through immunohistochemical analysis. In tubular carcinoma, tubules are angulated, lined only by epithelial cells, sometimes with apical snouts, and are located peripherally and/or centrally (Figs. 7.77, 7.78, 7.79, 7.80, 7.81, 7.82, and 7.83). To detect the presence of the myoepithelial cells in the radial scar, a panel of myoepithelial markers may be used such as p63, Calponin, SMA (smooth muscle actin), SMMHC (smooth muscle myosin heavy chain) [10] and, to confirm the presence of the basal membrane, Collagen IV and Laminin are of great help. Recall that myoepithelial antigens are often attenuated in sclerosing lesions (similar to DCIS), and one should not change the diagnosis if myoepithelial cells can be identified on H-E sections; but if the immunohistochemical stain is negative, one should try to perform immunohistochemical

stains with other myoepithelial markers (the best would be a panel of markers) and one should examine the whole lesion.

Moreover, radial scar is associated with epithelial proliferation usually without atypia (rarely with *in situ* ductal or lobular carcinoma), while in the tubular carcinoma, the association with atypical ductal hyperplasia or low-grade ductal carcinoma *in situ* is common. Grade 1 NST infiltrating carcinoma can also display tubular structures with open lumina of round and/or angulated shape. However, the proliferation of the atypical epithelial cells in grade 1 NST infiltrating carcinoma tend to be more florid, with more than one cell layer lining the tubular structures and associated with micropapillae, transluminal bridging forming secondary microglandular structures (features not characteristic for tubular carcinoma). Also, the other characteristics of the radial scar are not found within a grade 1 NST infiltrating carcinoma. In the tubulo-lobular infiltrating carcinoma (a subtype of lobular infiltrating carcinoma) small and rounded glands with open lumina are admixed with the classic "Indian-file" pattern and the tumor cells are more uniform, less cohesive than in the tubular carcinoma or grade 1 NST type carcinoma, while E-Cadherin is usually negative. Also, the characteristic central hyalinized area, entrapped tubular structures and other characteristics of the radial scar are absent (Fig. 7.84 and 7.85).

Another differential diagnosis is made with adenosis, especially with sclerosing adenosis and microglandular adenosis. These have a pseudoinfiltrative pattern. Sclerosing adenosis does not have a stellate appearance. The lesion is round and lobulo-centric, this being the most important microscopic parameter. In contrast to the radial scar, the lesion is composed of a proliferation of (rather than entrapped) tubular structures, which are compressed by a fibrous stroma (rather than collagenized and associated with elastosis). Also, the tubular structures are lined by two types of cells (similar to the radial scar) and there are dilated cysts at the periphery of the lesions. Microglandular adenosis is a rare lesion characterized by a haphazardly infiltrative pattern of round and small tubules in which the myoepithelial cells are lacking. Also, the lesion does not have a stellate configuration and the center of the lesion lacks fibrosis and elastosis. The morphology together with the myoepithelial markers may help in differentiating from a radial scar. The syringomatous adenoma is a benign tumor always located within the nipple and with a nodular appearance, although with infiltrative margins. Syringomatous adenoma does not have a characteristic central area with hyaline and elastotic appearance. Sclerosing papilloma may resemble a radial scar (and some radial scars may represent the late stage of development of a sclerosing papilloma, according to some authors), both sharing the fibrotic center and dilated ducts at the periphery. At low power, however, the sclerosing papilloma does not have a stellate configuration.

Table 7.1 Differential diagnosis between radial scar and tubular carcinoma

	Radial scar	Tubular carcinoma
Origin	TDLU	TDLU
Size	Usually less than 10 mm	Usually less than 20 mm
Shape	Stellate	Infiltrative/stellate
Stroma	Fibroelastic within the central area	Desmoplastic throughout the lesion
Tubules	Entrapped, distorted, centrally located, open lumina	Proliferative, angulated, throughout the lesion, open lumina
Apical snouts	Absent	Present
Myoepithelial cells	Present	Absent
Basal membrane	Present	Absent
Associated lesions	UDH, very rare ADH or DCIS, LN	DCIS or ADH common
Detection method	Incidental finding usually	Screening programme in most of the cases

ADH atypical ductal hyperplasia, *DCIS* ductal carcinoma *in situ*, *LN* lobular neoplasia, *TDLU* terminal duct-lobular unit, *UDH* usual ductal hyperplasia

Data suggesting that the radial scar is a premalignant lesion that should be surgically excised derive from the radiological literature, while pathological publications demonstrated contradictory results and that the risk of malignant transformation is low unless the lesion is associated with atypical ductal hyperplasia or ductal carcinoma *in situ* or lobular neoplasia [6, 11–13]. Also, some data showed that the presence of multiple radial scars increases the risk of malignant transformation [12]. Radial scars without epithelial atypia can be managed by vacuum-assisted core-needle biopsy and follow-up with meticulous radiological-pathological correlation, although some centers still recommend surgical excision [14–16]. Radial scars with epithelial atypia need to be excised. The final pathological report should contain data about the number of radial scar-type lesions and associated lesions.

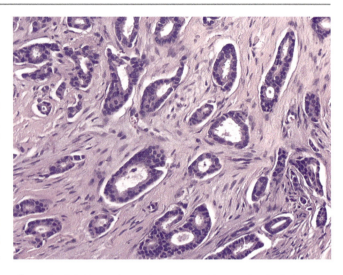

Fig. 7.79 Tubular carcinoma is represented by angulated tubular structures lined by only low-grade atypical epithelial cells with apical snouts

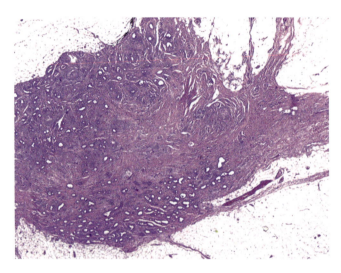

Fig. 7.77 Tubular carcinoma may present a stellate shape as in the radial scar

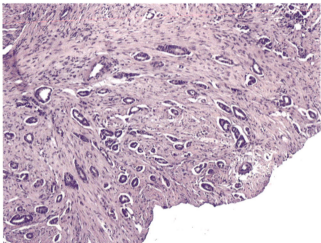

Fig. 7.80 Tubular carcinoma: desmoplastic stroma is present

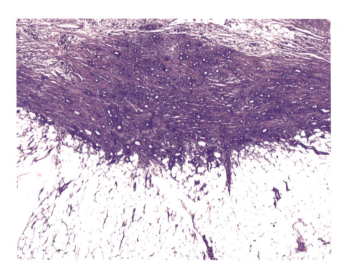

Fig. 7.78 Tubular carcinoma: tubular structures are infiltrating the fat tissue at the periphery of the lesion

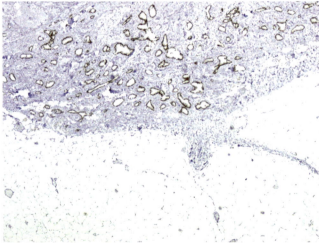

Fig. 7.81 Tubular carcinoma: most of the epithelial cells are positive for ER

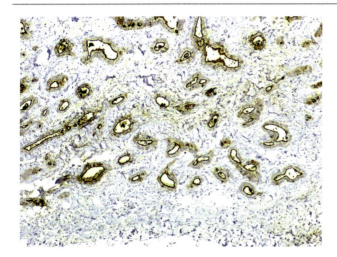

Fig. 7.82 Tubular carcinoma: atypical epithelial cells are positive for EMA

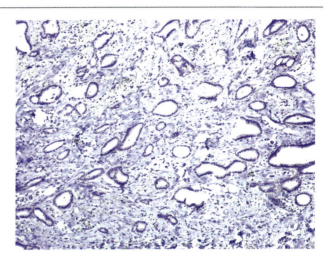

Fig. 7.83 Tubular carcinoma: p63 is negative as myoepithelial cells are absent

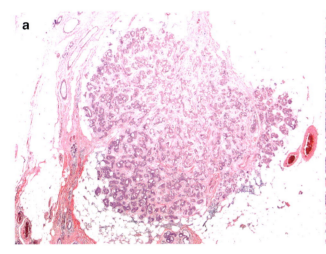

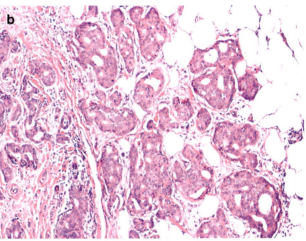

Fig. 7.84 Grade 1 infiltrating carcinoma of no special type: (**a**) The tumor displays tubular structures with open lumina, of round and/or angulated shape, together with more cribriform rounded shape areas; (**b**) the proliferation of the atypical epithelial cells in grade 1 NST infil-trating carcinoma is more florid, with more than one cell layer lining the tubular structures associated with bridges and secondary lumina; the other characteristics of the radial scar are not found

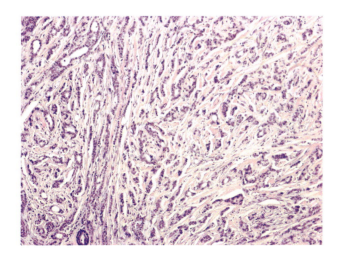

Fig. 7.85 Tubulo-lobular carcinoma: small and rounded glands with open lumina are admixed with the classic "Indian-file" pattern; the tumor cells are uniform; E-Cadherin is usually negative (not shown); the characteristic central hyalinized area, entrapped tubular structures and other characteristics of the radial scar are absent

7.3 Adenosis

Adenosis is represented by a proliferation of the acini resulting in enlargement of the lobules. It is a relatively common lesion that can have several microscopic versions with different clinical-pathological significance. The multiplication of the acini is accompanied by a process of fibrosis in most cases. The lesion can be detected microscopically, but it may sometimes appear as a palpable tumor mass, causing confusion with carcinoma (especially when it is also associated with microcalcifications). Adenoses occur mainly in the third and fourth decades of life, most often in association with fibrocystic changes.

7.3.1 Simple Adenosis

Simple adenosis is a multiplication of the acini that leads to enlargement of the lobules. It is rarely associated with a fibrosis process, so there is no distortion of lobular architecture. The acini are bound by two layers of typical cells exhibiting no atypia (Figs 7.86 and 7.87). This subtype is detected in most cases on microscopic examination, and does not form a visible mass. Sometimes the epithelial cells may undergo apocrine metaplasia, the lesion being diagnosed as *apocrine simple adenosis* (Fig. 7.88). When examining at low power, one can appreciate two main characteristics of the lesion: the rounded contour of the lobules and the uniformity of the appearance. In most cases, the diagnosis is easy and does not require ancillary examinations. Simple adenosis can be associated with various benign conditions of the breast, and if there is no atypia, the lesion does not require surgical excision.

Secretory adenosis is a variant of simple adenosis, represented by a proliferation of round acini, containing an eosinophilic secretory material (similar to the thyroid colloid, but with a more granular appearance). The structures are lined by both epithelial cells (which may have vacuolated cytoplasm) and flattened myoepithelial cells, surrounded by basement membrane. The presence of myoepithelial cells can be highlighted by immunohistochemical examination for Actin or p63, which differentiates it from microglandular adenosis. The epithelial cells are positive for S-100 Protein. Another differential diagnosis is made with secretory carcinoma (a very rare subtype of invasive carcinoma, usually developed in children, in which signs of atypia and stromal invasion are present). Finally, cystic hypersecretory hyperplasia is characterized by similar colloid-like material within the lumina, but the structures forming the lesion are cystically dilated.

Blunt duct adenosis is a controversial variant of simple adenosis. Some authors consider it as a minor alteration of lobular architecture, which develops within physiological limits. Some other authors call it *columnar cell change*. The lobular architecture is usually preserved, as is the intralobular specialized stroma, but the acini are dilated, with rounded ends and bordered by cylindrical epithelial cells with apical snouts, but lacking atypia. The epithelial cells are usually single-layered, but can sometimes be multilayered. The lumen of the acini frequently comprises round calcifications, resembling psammoma bodies. The myoepithelial cell layer is present and hypertrophic, so that these cells are easily identified during the microscopic examination at high power, as well as the basement membrane (Figs. 7.89, 7.90, 7.91, 7.92, 7.93, 7.94, 7.95, and 7.96). Differential diagnosis is made with fibrocystic changes, in which the architecture of the normal lobule is missing (but other changes are present) as well as with flat atypia in which the dilated acini are lined by several layers of low atypical epithelial cells, while the myoepithelial cells are present but attenuated. Also, blunt duct adenosis must be differentiated from columnar cell hyperplasia, a lesion with preserved architecture similar to that of blunt duct adenosis but in which the distended acini are lined by more than four layers of epithelial cells with elongated nuclei, oriented perpendicular to the basement membrane; cellular crowding, however, may give the impression of nuclear hypercromasia, the hyperplastic epithelial cells may form small tufts, and apical snouts may be present.

7.3.2 Sclerosing Adenosis

Sclerosing adenosis is the most frequent type of adenosis and is represented by the multiplication of acini associated with proliferation of a dense fibrous connective tissue (different from the normal intralobular connective tissue) that compresses the acini. It usually represents an incidental microscopic finding since the lesion is microscopic in size, but may also appear as a palpable gray nodule of varying sizes, increased consistency, with lobular or imprecisely defined edges. If the lesion has the appearance of a nodule, it can be called nodular sclerosing adenosis, a term that has been used incorrectly for other types of adenoses. Also, such a lesion can be termed *adenosis tumor*, which refers to the fact that the lesion becomes palpable, resembling a tumor formation (Fig. 7.97). Microscopic diagnosis is sometimes difficult, as the lesion can be confused with a malignant lesion owing to its pseudoinfiltrative pattern. Microscopic appearance is characteristic of a more cellular lesion in the center than on the periphery. One of the most important characteristics is the lobulo-centric appearance of the lesion when examined at low power (Figs. 7.98 and 7.99). It is round or oval and is constituted by a multiplication of acini, which are round or cystically dilated on the edge, but elongated or compressed in the center of the lesion due to the fibrosis. Therefore, sometimes the center of the lesion looks pseudoinvasive and very cellular. When compressed, the acini lose the lumina and transform into cords or solid structures (Figs. 7.100 and 7.101). Some areas may display confluent growth of these structures, with cribriform areas, very suspicious for invasion (of great help in these areas is the identification of myoepithelial cells together with the examination at low power) (Figs. 7.102 and 7.103). Often it is notable that the proliferation of acini is arranged around the intralobular duct, sometimes extending into its lumen, thus, the focus of sclerosing adenosis appears intracystically (Fig. 7.104). The acini are bound by a basement membrane and the two characteristic layers (epithelial and myoepithelial) with no evidence of atypia. These acini structures may sometimes contain an eosinophilic secretion. The stroma is dense, fibrous, and can present foci of elastosis. Also, rarely, the lesion may have an infiltrative pattern at the periphery, with benign-looking proliferative acini infiltrating the fat tissue, which can be mistaken for an invasive carcinoma. In some of the lesions, especially in late stage of evolution, massive fibrosis and spindle-shaped myoepithelial cells may also lead to a pseudoinfiltrative area in the center of the lesion (Figs. 7.105 and 7.106). In these situations, it is essential to look at the lesion at low power. Sometimes calcification foci may appear, as well as apocrine metaplasia (Figs. 7.107 and 7.108). Apocrine cells may display various features, from conventional abundant granular pink cytoplasm with round nuclei and prominent nucleoli, but they may also have more enlarged and atypical nuclei, which should not be confused with a carcinoma (Figs. 7.109 and 7.110). When all or almost all the acinic structures are involved by apocrine metaplasia, the lesion is called *sclerosing apocrine adenosis* (Figs. 7.111 and 7.112). Only significant atypia should be considered for a diagnosis of atypical apocrine adenosis or DCIS involving sclerosing adenosis (the distinction between these two lesions is not clear cut yet) (Fig. 7.113). It is important, however, not to over-diagnose these lesions, but, on the other hand, to recognize them properly since atypical apocrine adenosis with severe atypia has a significant increased relative risk for malignant transformation. Some sclerosing adenosis may display intraductal or intralobular epithelial hyperplasia with or without atypia; more rarely, acini may be arranged perineurally or perivascularly with no clinical significance [17]. Therefore, these two latter elements should not be regarded as indicators of malignancy. In some cases, intralobular or intraductal carcinoma may occur in a sclerosing adenosis (in these cases, looking at low power would prompt a correct diagnosis due to the lobulo-centric appearance of the lesion; also, immunohistochemical stains with E-Cadherin and Cytokeratin 5/6 would be of much help to differentiate between these lesions and usual ductal hyperplasia) (Fig. 7.114). Of interest, sclerosing adenosis can be very florid and cellular in pregnant patients (when mitoses are more numerous, degenerative cells and areas of geographic necrosis may occur).

In all these difficult situations, ancillary stains are of great help, particularly the use of p63. Since the acini are compressed by the sclerosing process and the myoepithelial cells are compressed and attenuated, a nuclear marker is better than a cellular marker or a membrane marker (Fig. 7.115). The presence of a continuous or discontinuous myoepithelial layer at the periphery of acinary structures is in favor of a diagnosis of sclerosing adenosis.

The variant called *tubular adenosis* is a form of sclerosing adenosis in which the acini multiply, branch, and extend into the surrounding adipose tissue (Fig. 7.116). Due to the peculiar arrangement of the acini, in which most of them are cut longitudinally in the plane of the section and the branching phenomenon, they have pointed or rounded ends and compressed lumina. The lumina sometimes contain eosinophilic or basophilic secretion, occasionally with calcification foci. They are bordered by two characteristic layers and a basement membrane at the periphery, which may sometimes be thickened. The epithelial layer is represented by cuboid cells with round or oval nuclei, fine chromatin, eosinophilic cytoplasm and lacking apical snouts. The outer layer consists of flattened myoepithelial cells with small and hyperchromatic nuclei. The surrounding stroma may be sclerosing or hypocellular. However, tubular adenosis lacks the circumscription of sclerosing adenosis and its cellularity in the center of the lesion.

The differential diagnosis of sclerosing adenosis is made with other types of adenosis (microglandular adenosis in particular), as well as with radial scar, tubular adenoma, ductal adenoma, and, especially tubular carcinoma. Within microglandular adenosis, the acini are disposed irregularly, they are small, have a round shape, with an eosinophilic secretion into the lumen. They are bordered by a single layer of epithelial cells and basement membrane, the myoepithelial layer being absent. The epithelial cells are positive for Cytokeratin, S-100 protein, and the basement membrane is positive for laminin in PAS staining. The stroma is hypocellular and composed mainly of collagen fibers. The radial scar has a stellate appearance (in contrast to the rounded appearance of sclerosing adenosis), with a central area of fibrosis and elastosis, and it is sometimes associated with epithelial hyperplasia at the periphery. Tubular adenoma consists of small uniform, tubular structures, with reduced stroma, but the lesion has a circumscribed character, sometimes a capsule at the periphery, and a diameter over 1 cm. Ductal adenoma is also well-circumscribed, sometimes growing into a ductal lumen. In tubular carcinoma, the tubules are distributed irregularly and infiltrate the fat tissue, in association with a desmoplastic stroma. The neoplastic tubules are angulated, with open lumina, sometimes with apical snouts, and are delimited by a single layer of epithelial cells with minimal atypia. The myoepithelial layer and basement membrane are absent (Fig. 7.117). The most important characteristics of the two lesions are shown in Table 7.2. A difficult differential diagnosis is between sclerosing adenosis associated with intraductal or intralobular carcinoma and invasive carcinoma. In this case, the lesion should be initially examined at low power because a process of fibrosis and elastosis often appears in the center of a sclerosing adenosis, which compresses the acini, while the acini are cystically dilated on the edge. In an invasive carcinoma, the stroma is desmoplastic (with the exception of tubular carcinoma, in which the stroma may also be hyalinized in some cases). On the other hand, immunohistochemical examinations for Actin or p63 differentiate the two lesions, because myoepithelial cells are missing in the invasive carcinoma.

The risk of malignant transformation in a sclerosing adenosis is slightly increased compared to normal population, similar to the risk in usual ductal hyperplasia [18]. The presence of sclerosing adenosis in a core biopsy does not require surgical excision unless there is radiological suspicion, association with microcalcifications, a spiculated contour, or presence of atypia. In the absence of suspicion, clinical-radiological follow-up may be advisable for the patient. Pathologists, especially those with limited experience, should be very careful with this type of lesion when a frozen section examination is required by the clinician; and when all the criteria for a positive diagnosis are lacking, one should wait for permanent sections.

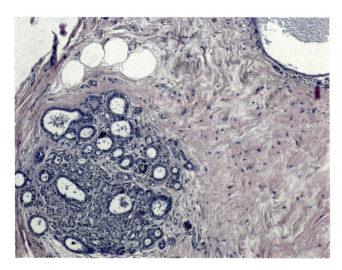

Fig. 7.86 Simple adenosis: multiplication of the acini and enlargement of the lobules without an associated process of fibrosis and no distortion of the lobular architecture

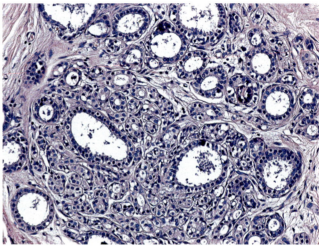

Fig. 7.87 Simple adenosis: the acini are lined by two characteristic cell layers and are associated with microcalcifications

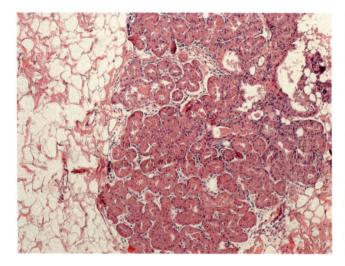

Fig. 7.88 Apocrine simple adenosis: characteristic lobular architecture preserved with multiplication of the acini which undergone apocrine metaplasia without atypia

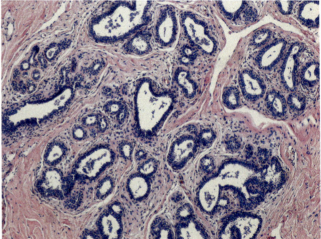

Fig. 7.89 Blunt duct adenosis: the lobular architecture is usually preserved, as well as the intralobular specialized stroma

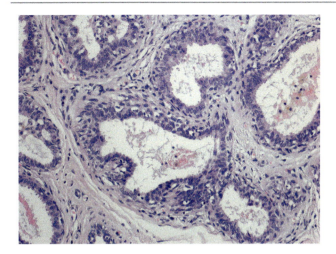

Fig. 7.90 Blunt duct adenosis: the acini are dilated, with rounded ends

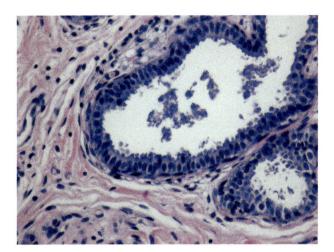

Fig. 7.92 Blunt duct adenosis: another example with distended acini and preserved architecture

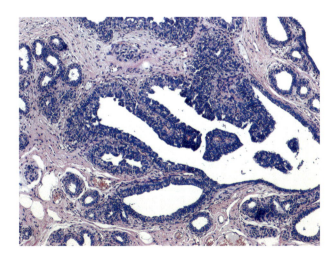

Fig. 7.94 Columnar cell hyperplasia: similar preserved architecture as in blunt duct adenosis but the distended acini are lined by several layers of epithelial cells with elongated nuclei, oriented perpendicular to the basement membrane; cellular crowding may, however, give the impression of nuclear hypercromasia and the hyperplastic epithelial cells may form small tufts; apical snouts may be present

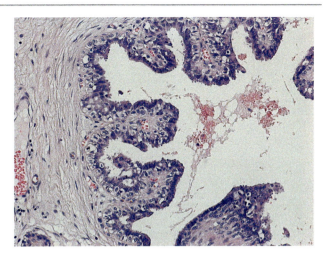

Fig. 7.91 Blunt duct adenosis: the acini are lined by cylindrical epithelial cells with ovoid-to-elongated nuclei, oriented in perpendicular fashion to the basement membrane, with evenly dispersed chromatin and rare mitotic figure, with apical snouts, lacking atypia; hypertrophic myoepithelial cells are visible even at low-power magnification

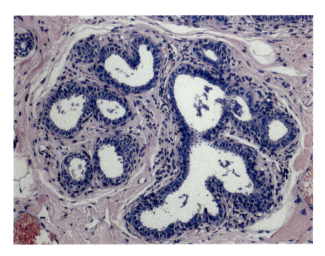

Fig. 7.93 Blunt duct adenosis: in this case (similar to Fig. 7.92), some of the acini have attenuated myoepithelial cells, but still present

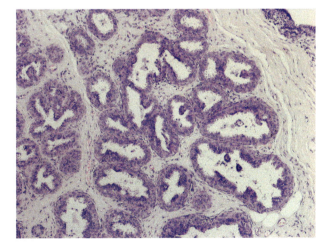

Fig. 7.95 Flat atypia: lobular architecture is preserved like in blunt duct adenosis and acini are dilated

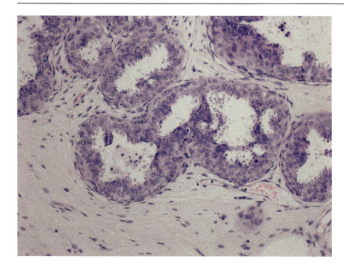

Fig. 7.96 Flat atypia (similar to lesion in Fig. 7.95): acini are lined by several layers of low atypical epithelial cells with rather rounded nuclei (as opposed to elongated) and visible nucleoli; the nuclei are not perpendicular to the basement membrane; myoepithelial cells are present but attenuated

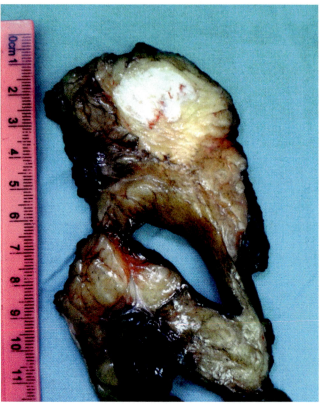

Fig. 7.97 Adenosis tumor: a sclerosing adenosis with large size, forming a palpable tumor-like mass within the breast parenchyma

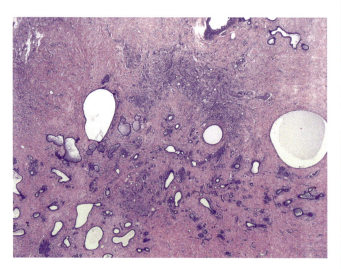

Fig. 7.98 Sclerosing adenosis: lobulo-centric appearance of the lesion at low-power examination; at the periphery, the acini are cystic-dilated

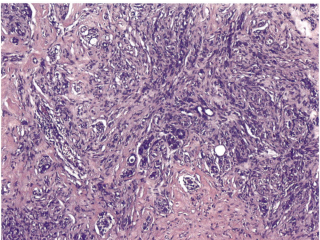

Fig. 7.99 Sclerosing adenosis: the lesion is characteristically more cellular in the center (elongated or compressed acini in the center of the lesion due to the fibrosis) than on the periphery—pseudoinvasive pattern mimicking an infiltrating carcinoma

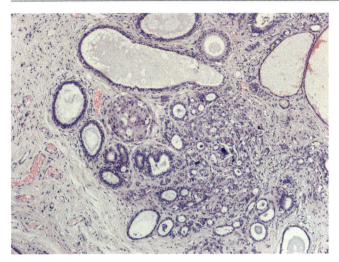

Fig. 7.100 Sclerosing adenosis: hyperplastic and compressed acini in the center of the lesion, forming cords, while at the periphery, they are dilated forming cysts, associated with apocrine metaplasia, inflammatory infiltrate into the stroma and microcalcifications

Fig. 7.101 Sclerosing adenosis: the lesion is more cellular in the middle zone than at the periphery and is associated with microcalcifications

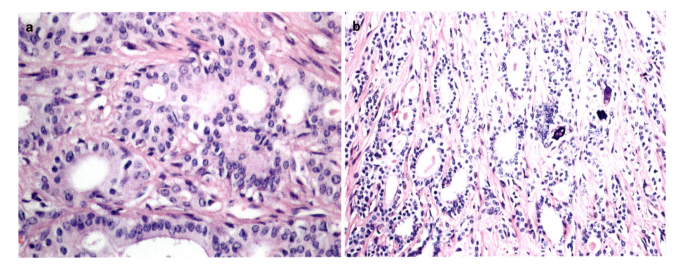

Fig. 7.102 Sclerosing adenosis: some areas may display confluent growth of these structures, with **a**, tubular and **b**, cribriform areas, very suspicious for invasive

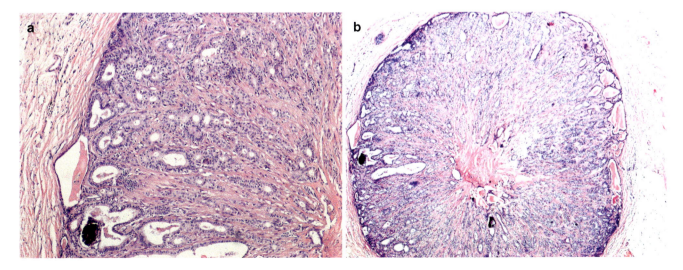

Fig. 7.103 Sclerosing adenosis: (**a**, **b**) Of great help in these areas is the identification of myoepithelial cells together with the examination at low power

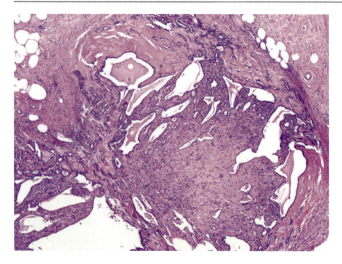

Fig. 7.104 Sclerosing adenosis: the proliferation of acini is arranged around the intralobular duct, sometimes extending into its lumen, thus, the focus of sclerosing adenosis appears intracystically

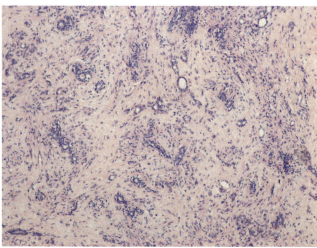

Fig. 7.105 Sclerosing adenosis: in late stage of evolution, massive fibrosis and spindle-shape myoepithelial cells may also lead to a pseudoinfiltrative area in the center of the lesion

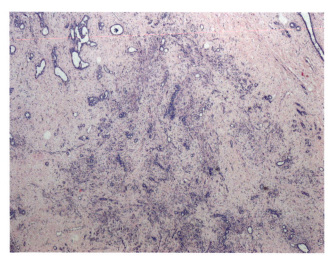

Fig. 7.106 Sclerosing adenosis: for this type of lesion (like in Fig. 7.105), it is advisable to examine the lesion at low power

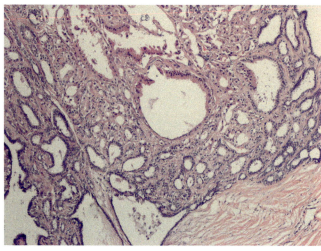

Fig. 7.107 Sclerosing adenosis with focus of apocrine metaplasia

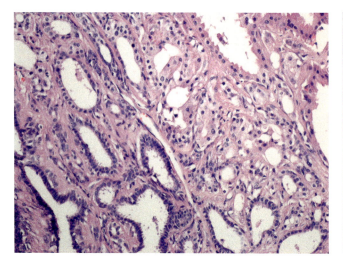

Fig. 7.108 Sclerosing adenosis: high-power examination of the same lesion as in Fig. 7.107 reveals lack of atypia within the apocrine metaplasia; the cells have round nuclei and prominent nucleoli (not enough features to diagnose the lesion as atypical)

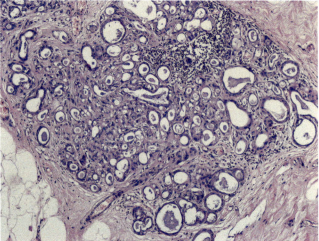

Fig. 7.109 Sclerosing adenosis with areas of apocrine metaplasia displaying more enlarged and atypical nuclei

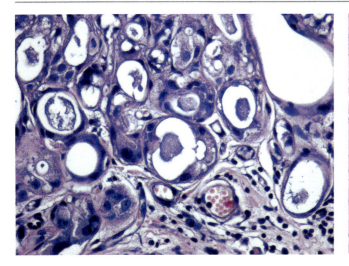

Fig. 7.110 Sclerosing adenosis with areas of apocrine metaplasia displaying more enlarged and atypical nuclei, which should not be confused with a carcinoma

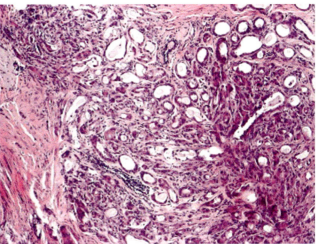

Fig. 7.111 Sclerosing apocrine adenosis: a sclerosing adenosis in which almost all the acinic structures are involved by apocrine metaplasia

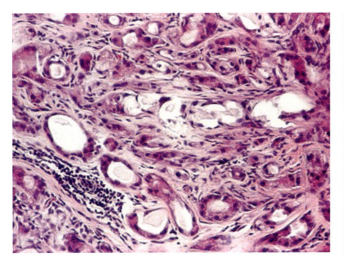

Fig. 7.112 Sclerosing apocrine adenosis: even if the apocrine metaplasia displays slightly more pleomorphic cells, it is advisable not to over-diagnose these type of lesions as atypical apocrine adenosis or DCIS unless there is significant atypia

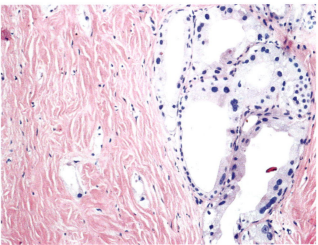

Fig. 7.113 Acini with significant apocrine atypia: the nuclei are four times more enlarged as the normal apocrine cells and are hyperchromatic

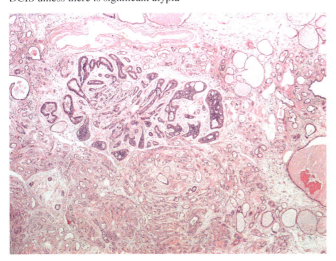

Fig. 7.114 Sclerosing adenosis with focus of DCIS of low-grade: examination at low power would prompt a correct diagnosis due to the lobulo-centric appearance of the lesion

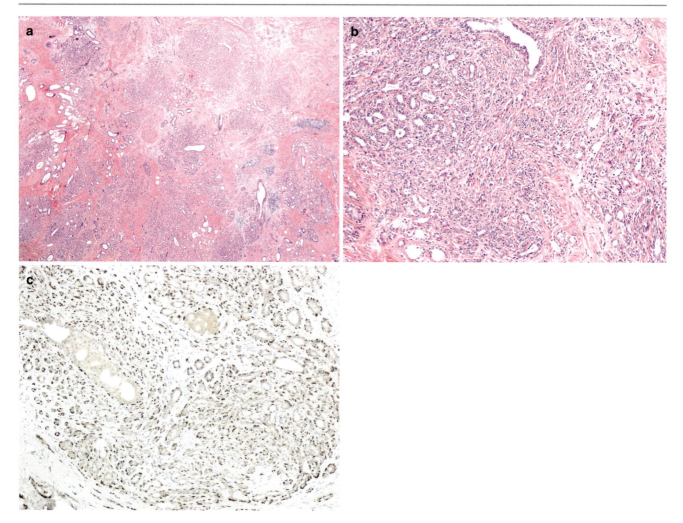

Fig. 7.115 Sclerosing adenosis: (**a**) Low-power examination reveals a lobulo-centric lesion in which (**b**), all the acini are lined by two cells layers; however, (**c**) more cellular areas and areas with compressed acini are difficult to diagnose and myoepithelial cells are not easy not be identified; their presence can be demonstrated with p63 stain

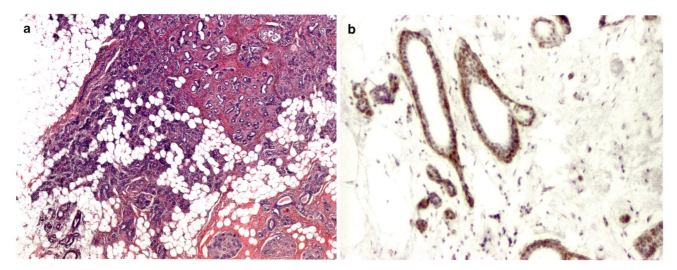

Fig. 7.116 Tubular adenosis: (**a**) Hyperplastic acini multiply, branch, and extend into the surrounding adipose tissue; this lesion lacks the circumscription of sclerosing adenosis and its cellularity in the center; however, the acini are lined by two cell layers. (**b**) Smooth Muscle Actin stain demonstrates that a layer of myoepithelial cells is present

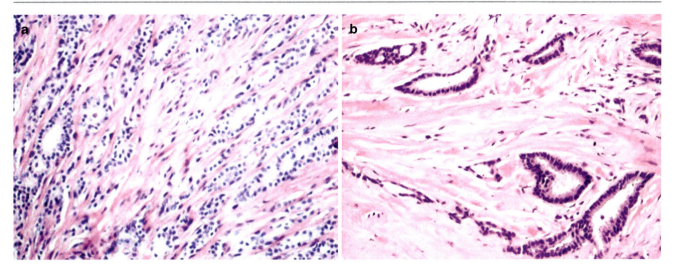

Fig. 7.117 (**a**) Differential diagnosis between compressed tubular structures in sclerosing adenosis lined by two cell types and (**b**) angulated tubules lined by one cell type in tubular carcinoma

Table 7.2 Main differences between sclerosing adenosis and tubular carcinoma

	Sclerosing adenosis	Tubular carcinoma
Shape	Lobulocentric	Infiltrative, stelate
Relation with adipose tissue	Respects adipose tissue	Infiltrates adipose tissue
Stroma	Sclerotic	Desmoplastic
Tubular structures	Compressed in the center, obliterated lumina, cystically dilated at periphery	Open lumina, angulated shape
Myoepithelial cells	Present	Absent
Basal membrane	Present	Absent
In situ component	Absent	Present

7.3.3   Microglandular Adenosis

Microglandular adenosis is a rare lesion characterized by irregular proliferation of small tubular structures arranged in a hypocellular hyalinized stroma [19–21]. The mean age of occurrence is 50 years, but it can occur at any age. Grossly, the lesion can be very small or can form a palpable firm and gray nodular mass with a mean diameter of 3–4 cm and ill-defined margins. No specific radiological findings are associated with microglandular adenosis. Microscopically, tubular structures haphazardly infiltrate the surrounding tissue (no lobulo-centric pattern is present), mimicking a low-grade infiltrating carcinoma. However, no stromal desmoplasia is present. The tubular structures are round, open, and their lumen contains a PAS-positive (sometimes Alcian-positive) eosinophilic secretory material (similar to the colloid material found within the thyroid gland), and are lined by a layer of cuboidal or flat epithelial cells without nuclear atypia. The cells have round nuclei with indistinct nucleoli, whereas the cytoplasm may be clear, eosinophilic, or granular. The epithelial cells are positive for Cytokeratin 8, 18, 7, HMW-CK (such as CK 34beta E12), EGFR, and S-100 protein. The epithelial cells are, however, negative for ER, PR, HER2, EMA, CK20, CK 5/6, and p63 [22, 23]. The myoepithelial cell layer is absent, microglandular adenosis being the only benign breast lesion in which myoepithelial cells are lacking. Therefore, the myoepithelial markers are negative. However, the basement membrane is present (demonstrable by immunohistochemical examination for Laminin and Collagen IV, or electron microscopy examination). The basement membrane in microglandular adenosis surrounding ductal type structures is thick and layered; it is therefore always obvious on special stains or immunostaining (Fig. 7.118). The lesion may present microcalcification foci or apocrine metaplasia. Perineural or vascular invasion has not been observed in any of these lesions. Differential diagnosis is made with tubular carcinoma (composed of tubular structures, lined by a layer of epithelial cells with mild atypia, but arranged in a desmoplastic stroma, without myoepithelial cells and basement membrane). The main differences between microglandular adenosis and tubular carcinoma are listed in Table 7.3. Another differential diagnosis is made with tubular adenosis, which has a myoepithelial layer (myoepithelial cells are positive for Actin and p63). Sometimes, microglandular adenosis can display atypia (*atypical microglandular adenosis,* in which the glands become more complex, with luminal bridges and cribriform areas, while atypia is present and cells are multilayered), and there are publications suggesting that these lesions represent a precursor and can transform into invasive carcinomas such as adenoid-cystic or metaplastic carcinoma [23]. It is particularly difficult to differentiate between *in situ* carcinoma developed in a background of a microglandular adenosis and invasive carcinoma developed on microglandular adenosis, because both lack myoepithelial cells; the microglandular adenosis with *in situ* carcinoma, however, has a basal membrane surrounding the round tubular structures, and lacks coalescent and solid epithelial growth (Fig. 7.119).

Microglandular adenosis lacking atypia is treated with local excision. Incomplete excision may lead to recurrence and, in consequence, a complete surgical excision is required. In the cases with atypia present, negative surgical margins and performing sentinel lymph node excision is advisable together with a close correlation with the radiological settings, discussing the case in the tumor board and close follow-up of the patient.

7.3.4　Adenomyoepithelial Adenosis

Adenomyoepithelial adenosis is an extremely rare breast entity. Microscopically, the lesion is usually diffuse and infiltrative, composed of round tubular structures, arranged irregularly, containing eosinophilic secretion, and bordered by a layer of cuboidal or cylindrical epithelial cells, sometimes with apocrine or squamous metaplasia. The outer tubular structures are bordered by a layer of myoepithelial cells and basement membrane. The myoepithelial cells can be very prominent, with clear cytoplasm, and sometimes hyperplastic. The lesion shows no atypia. Differential diagnosis is made with microglandular adenosis (where the myoepithelial cells are absent) and adenomyoepithelioma (a benign tumor with the same microscopic appearance, but forming a nodule and with a diameter of more than 1 cm).

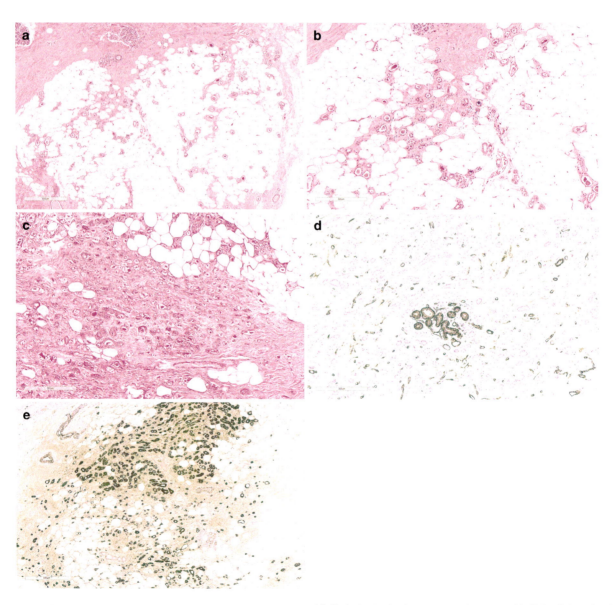

Fig. 7.118 Microglandular adenosis: (**a**) Tubular structures haphazardly infiltrate the breast tissue mimicking a low-grade infiltrating carcinoma; (**b**) the tubular structures are round, open, and their lumen contains an eosinophilic secretory material (**c**) which is PAS-positive. (**d**) Stain for Actin demonstrates that myoepithelial cell layer is absent compared to normal acini; (**e**) The tubular structures are lined by epithelial cells, positive for S-100 Protein and the basement membrane positive for PAS

Table 7.3 Major differences between microglandular adenosis and tubular carcinoma

	Microglandular adenosis	Tubular carcinoma
Pattern of growth	Infiltrative	Infiltrative, stellate
Tubules	Small and round	Angulated
Apical snouts	Absent	Present
Luminal secretion	Present	Absent
Epithelial cells	Present	Present and atypical
Myoepithelial cells	Absent	Absent
Basal membrane	Present	Absent
Stroma	No desmoplasia	Demoplastic
Immunohistochemical stains	ER, PR, EMA-; S 100 protein, Laminin, Colagen IV+	ER, PR, EMA+; S100 protein, Laminin, ColagenIV-
Associated DCIS	Not present	Present

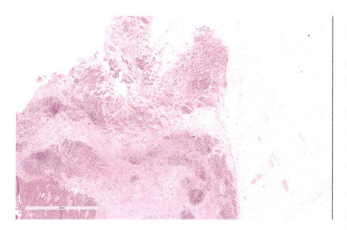

Fig. 7.119 Invasive carcinoma developed on microglandular adenosis is difficult to differentiate from *in situ* carcinoma developed in a background of a microglandular adenosis: both lack myoepithelial, but the former lesion illustrated in this picture has an obvious infiltrative component with coalescent and solid epithelial growth

7.4 Pregnancy-Like Changes

Pregnancy-like changes, also called pseudolactational changes (or pseudolactational metaplasia, pseudolactational hyperplasia) are similar to those which occur in the mammary gland during pregnancy or breastfeeding, but they occur in patients who are not pregnant or breastfeeding. The etiology is unknown. Some of the patients have never been pregnant and others are postmenopausal. Exceptionally, the lesion has also been described in men. The mechanism of development of this lesion is widely debated, in some cases considered a persistence of lactational changes from a previous pregnancy, but in most cases the lesion is considered to be caused by an exogenous hormonal intake or by the administration of other drugs such as antihypertensive or neuroleptic medication. Pseudolactational changes never form a palpable mass. The lesion is identified on microscopy and usually affects several lobules, but when it occurs within one lobule, only a few acini are affected. It can present in two microscopic forms, both associated with the preservation of the normal architecture of the lobule. The first form, called *classic type*, has dilated acini, with abundant secretory material in the lumen and lined by a cylindrical epithelium (Figs. 7.120 and 7.121). Epithelial cells have abundant, granular, or vacuolated cytoplasm, and small and round nuclei. The cytoplasm is positive for S-100 protein and α-lactalbumin. The second variant, called *hobnail-type*, has the same architecture and the cytoplasmic vacuolization is minimal, but the epithelial cells have different sizes and hyperchromatic, irregular nuclei, which are located in the apical part of the cell and create a "hobnail" appearance (Figs. 7.122, 7.123, and 7.124). The secretory material within the dilated structures is minimal. It may contain detached cells, some of which are multinucleated. This appearance is very similar to the changes called Arias-Stella in the endometrium or cervix. In both variants, the cells are negative for Mucicarmine and Alcian blue, but they contain PAS-positive intracytoplasmic granules, and the intraluminal secretion is positive for Mucicarmin and Alcian blue. In some cases, calcifications also appear in the lumen of the cysts. These changes can sometimes also affect the ducts.

Differential diagnosis is made with lactation and pregnancy changes (which affect all lobules and all the acini within a lobule; it is mandatory, however, to know the clinical history and age of the patients), with hypersecretory cystic hyperplasia (cystic cavities lined by a cylindrical or flat epithelium consisting of cells without atypia and containing an eosinophilic material in the lumen, of colloid-type), as well as various microscopic mammary carcinoma variants (all associated with cytological atypia). Of note, a rare lesion called *pregnancy-like hyperplasia* may occur. It is similar to pregnancy-like changes, but has a multilayered epithelium with papillary fronds composed entirely of epithelial cells lining the dilated acini. The secretion within the lumina may contain microcalcification; the lesion can therefore be detected radiologically. Also, hyperplasia can sometimes be associated with atypia, most of the cases occurring in association with cystic hypersecretory hyperplasia [24].

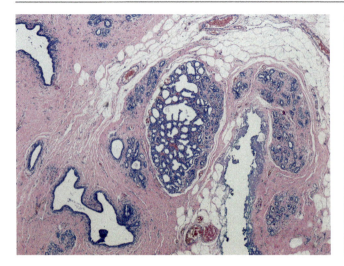

Fig. 7.120 Pregnancy-like changes: the lesion only affects several lobules and some but not all the acini within a lobule

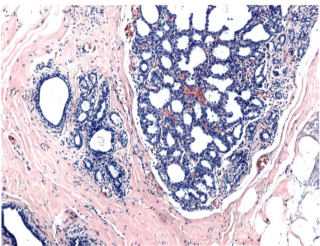

Fig. 7.121 Pregnancy-like changes: in the classic type, one can appreciate the preservation of the normal lobule, dilated acini lined by a cuboidal/cylindrical epithelium with vacuolated cytoplasm and small, round nuclei

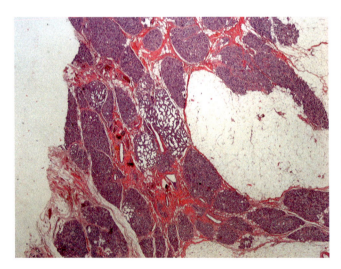

Fig. 7.122 Pregnancy-like changes: the lesion is represented by lactational metaplasia involving some but not all the lobules

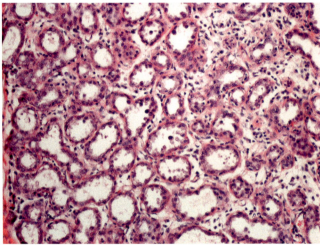

Fig. 7.123 Pregnancy-like changes: hobnail-type with epithelial cells having different sizes, hyperchromatic, irregular nuclei, which are located in the apical part of the cell

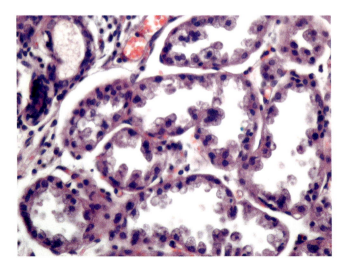

Fig. 7.124 Pregnancy-like changes: hobnail-type

7.5 Epithelial Metaplasia

7.5.1 Apocrine Metaplasia

Apocrine Metaplasia is the most frequent form of epithelial metaplasia encountered within the breast. It is represented by the transformation of the epithelial cells lining both ducts and acini into larger, cuboidal or columnar cells, with large amount of granular eosinophilic cytoplasm, apical snouts, round nuclei, and visible nucleoli. Lipofuscin granules and iron pigment can be seen intracytoplasmatically. It does not have a clinical significance itself unless associated with atypia and/or other pathological breast conditions. The most frequent association is with fibrocystic changes. Apocrine metaplasia is not detectable with radiological investigations and is not visible to the naked eye. It can be detected e only via microscopic examination, and in this particular case it may involve a few structures or sometimes may be more extensive.

Simple apocrine metaplasia (represented by a single layer of apocrine cells) has to be differentiated from *hyperplastic apocrine changes* (multiple layers of cells) and *atypical apocrine metaplasia* (nuclei enlarged more than three times than normal and pleomorphic) (Fig. 7.125).

7.5.2 Clear Cell Metaplasia

Clear cell metaplasia may occur in the acini and ducts and is occasionally detected under microscopic examination. It occurs, however, much less frequently than apocrine metaplasia. It is seen especially in patients in pre- and postmenopause, with no relation to the pregnancy or exogenous hormonal use. It is a focal lesion with partial or complete involvement of a lobule, but most often, multiple lobules are affected. The architecture of the lobule does not change, but it increases in size due to the increase in volume of metaplastic epithelial cells. The epithelial cells have clear, abundant cytoplasm, sometimes foamy or vacuolated (Fig. 7.126). The cytoplasm sometimes contains PAS-positive granules, but is negative for Alcian blue and Mucicarmin. The nuclei are located eccentrically and are small and round, with no obvious nucleolus. The lumen of the acini is usually open, but it can also be obliterated; however, the acini are never cystically dilated. Differential diagnosis should be made with pregnancy-like changes (presenting a typical secretion located at the luminal border of the cells), myoepithelial cell hyperplasia (metaplastic clear cells are not positive for S-100 protein, Actin or any other myoepithelial markers), as well as primary or metastatic clear cell carcinoma (clear cells show signs of atypia, infiltration of the stroma, and stromal response; in the metastases, the clinical history information

is very helpful). Clear cell metaplasia is not associated with an increased risk for developing a breast carcinoma.

7.5.3 Squamous Metaplasia

Squamous metaplasia occurs mainly in infarction areas within an intraductal papilloma or on a previous biopsy site, sometimes within a fibroadenoma (Figs. 7.127, 7.128, 7.129, and 7.130). Also, the lactiferous ducts may undergo extensive squamous metaplasia, which may obliterate the duct and produce a cyst eventually associated with inflammation (subareolar abscess). Recent papers suggest however that the myoepithelial cell appears to be the cell of origin of metaplastic squamous epithelium. Differential diagnosis includes metaplastic carcinoma (especially low-grade adenosquamous carcinoma but in which, besides the areas of squamous cells with low atypicality, tubules embedded in a desmoplastic stroma with infiltrative margins are seen).

7.5.4 Mucinous Metaplasia

Mucinous metaplasia occurs either within a papilloma or associated with pregnancy-like changes [25]. Rarely, it can be seen in association with collagenous spherulosis (it is also called mucinous spherulosis, but there is an associated proliferation of myoepithelial cells within this lesion) (Fig. 7.131). It must be differentiated from a mucinous breast carcinoma (which has atypia and stromal invasion).

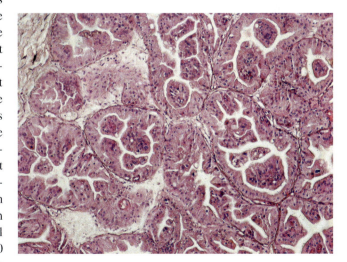

Fig. 7.125 Apocrine metaplasia: ducts and acini are distended, lined by a simple cylindrical apocrine epithelium in some of the areas but mostly by hyperplastic apocrine epithelium forming papillae and micropapillae; however, no atypia is detected

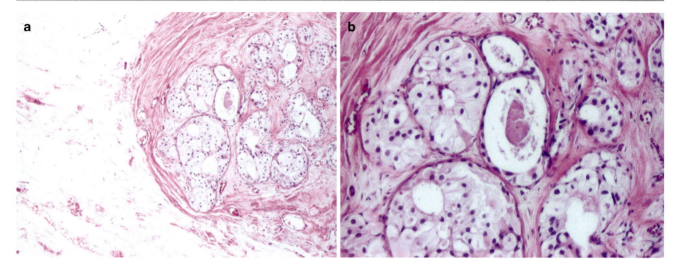

Fig. 7.126 Clear cell metaplasia: (**a**) The architecture of the lobule is not changed, but it increases in size due to the increase in volume of metaplastic epithelial cells: (**b**) the epithelial cells have clear, abundant cytoplasm, with small, round, nuclei located eccentrically

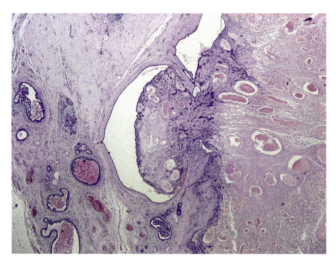

Fig. 7.127 Sclerosing papilloma with massive area of necrosis—consequently, foci of squamous metaplasia can be detected

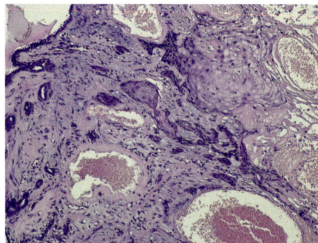

Fig. 7.128 Sclerosing papilloma with massive area of necrosis (same lesion as in Fig. 7.127)—high-power examination allows detection of benign foci of squamous metaplasia

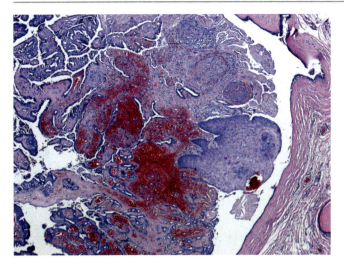

Fig. 7.129 Intraductal papilloma with areas of hemorrhage and squamous metaplasia

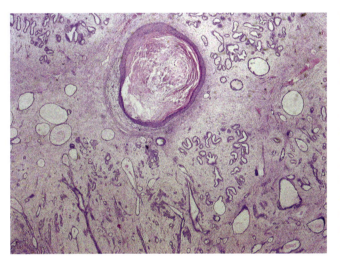

Fig. 7.130 Fibroadenoma with central area of squamous metaplasia

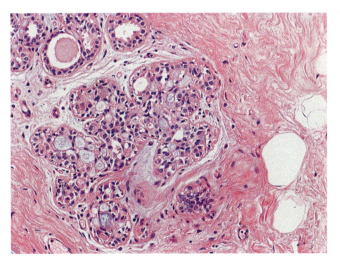

Fig. 7.131 Mucinous metaplasia can be seen in association with collagenous spherulosis (it is also called mucinous spherulosis)

7.6 Microcalcifications

Microcalcifications are calcium deposits that can occur in benign and malignant lesions, but also in association with normal breast tissue, especially in menopause or after lactation. In benign lesions, microcalcifications occur more frequently in sclerosing adenosis and fibrocystic changes. In malignant lesions, comedocarcinoma type of DCIS and NST-infiltrating carcinoma are the most frequent associations. The presence of microcalcifications is an important finding on mammography, because, depending on size, shape, number, and distribution, they allow the differentiation between benign and malignant lesions (Figs. 7.132 and 7.133). They occur due to either tumor necrosis or calcification of the secretion product from the mammary acini and ducts. The mammographic appearance of microcalcifications in benign lesions is round, punctuated, and regular, while in malignant ones microcalcifications are polymorphic, irregular, and branched. Since some forms of microcalcification are characteristic of both benign and malignant lesions, it is always advisable that mammographic diagnosis be followed by a biopsy and a microscopic diagnosis be established.

Sometimes, besides calcium, microcalcifications may also contain small amounts of aluminum, potassium, iron, silicon, titanium, and sulphides. Such layered deposits, usually occurring inside cysts and rarely in the adjacent stroma, are called Liesegang rings and should not be confused with the parasites on microscopy. Also, crystalline deposits with an eosinophilic appearance may occur within the cyst. These usually accompany benign lesions, but have also been recorded in atypical intraductal hyperplasia or *in situ* ductal carcinomas. Crystals can be few or extremely numerous inside a cyst or may involve several cysts. Their size is variable, and they can have various shapes: triangular, quadrangular, pentagonal, or hexagonal. The chemical composition and ultrastructural appearance suggest that they are made up of condensed protein material.

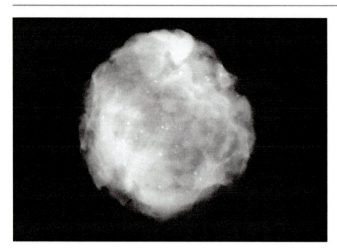

Fig. 7.132 Mammography in a 38-year-old patient reveals multiple benign-looking microcalcifications after a lactation period of 2 years

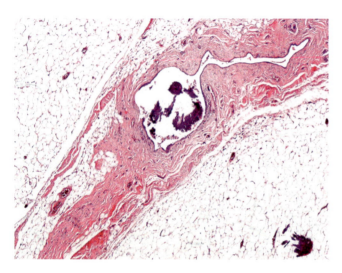

Fig. 7.133 Microscopic examination reveals multiple areas of micro-calcifications associated with normal breast tissue (same patient as in Fig. 7.132)

7.7 Hypersecretory Cystic Hyperplasia

Hypersecretory cystic hyperplasia is a rare, macroscopically well-defined lesion that consists of a various number of cysts with a diameter between 0.5 and 2 cm, smooth wall, and a greenish jelly material inside. Microscopically, the lesion consists of numerous dilated cystic ducts, surrounded by a fibrous stroma. The ducts are delimited by a unilateral, cuboidal, or flattened epithelium. The epithelial cells have round, uniform nuclei and moderate eosinophilic cytoplasm (Fig. 7.134). Rarely, the epithelium may be layered or have papillary (arranged on a fibro-vascular axis) or micropapillary (lacking a fibro-vascular axis) growths. If there is a nuclear pleomorphism in these situations, the lesion is called *atypical hypersecretory cystic hyperplasia*. The cysts contain an eosinophilic, PAS-positive acellular material, retracted from the cyst walls, with smooth or scalloped margins and showing characteristic slits, folds, linear cracks, or small punched-out holes. The secretion is not associated with necrosis or microcalcifications. These elements are very similar to thyroid colloid. If one or more cysts rupture, the secretion that reaches the adjacent stroma produces a chronic inflammatory reaction. The lesion must be distinguished from fibrocystic changes (the cysts have a different content and are associated with other changes as well). In young patients, juvenile papillomatosis can occur, but it forms a macroscopic mass, while microscopically it is characterized by multiple cysts and ectatic ducts with intraluminal secretion and foamy histiocytes. Of note, in some cases, cystic hypersecretory hyperplasia may coexist with pregnancy-like hyperplasia [18]. Also, the lesion must be distinguished from secretory carcinoma (characterized by atypical features and invasion into the stroma) (Fig. 7.135).

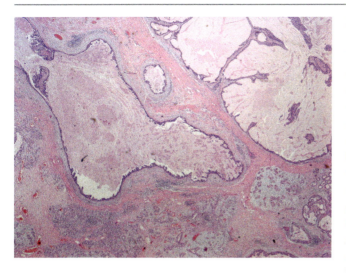

Fig. 7.134 Cystic hypersecretory hyperplasia: multiple cysts filled with secretory material resembling the colloid; cysts are line by atypical epithelium in this case

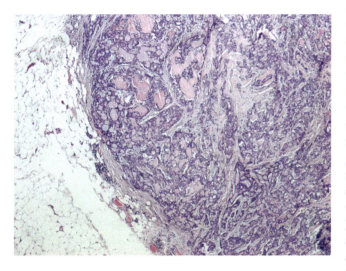

Fig. 7.135 Secretory carcinoma is characterized by atypical features and invasion into the stroma, unlike cystic hypersecretory hyperplasia

7.8   Mucocele-Like Tumor

The mucocele-like tumor is a benign rare lesion, usually microscopic in size; in some lesions, however, it may form a well-demarcated palpable mass identified on radiological examinations. Macroscopically, the lesion consists of many cysts of various sizes on the cut surface, containing a gelatinous material. Microscopically, it consists of cystic cavities lined by a single-layer cuboidal, cylindrical, or flattened epithelium, without signs of atypia and containing an abundant secretory material (Fig. 7.136). The epithelium may present papillary stratification or micropapillary growths. Some cavities are ruptured, and the mucinous material is extravasated into the adjacent stroma, forming mucin pools of different sizes, similar to the same lesion within the salivary glands. This material can lack epithelial cells, although sometimes they have epithelial cell groups that "float" in the mucus. These groups are the epithelial cells that delineate the cysts and which, by rupturing, reach the surrounding stroma. These cell groups *must* contain myoepithelial cells for a diagnosis for mucocele-like tumor. If it is difficult to identify them on Hematoxylin-Eosin stains, immunohistochemical examination for myoepithelial markers are of real use. The secretory material has the same histochemical characteristics as mucinous carcinoma (PAS- and Alcian blue-positive), suggesting the possibility of a continuous spectrum of alterations, including both mucocele-like tumor at one end of the spectrum, and mucinous carcinoma at the other end [6]. This theory suggests that the mucocele-like tumor is a precursor lesion of mucinous carcinoma. However, most invasive mucinous carcinomas derive from *in situ* ductal carcinoma, which sometimes can be detected at the periphery of the lesion. Mucocele-like tumor has also to be distinguished from hypocellular invasive mucinous carcinoma (the distinction is very challenging; however, in the latter, myoepithelial cells are lacking and also, coarse and granular microcalcifications are usually absent, while they are characteristically present in the former), mucinous cystadenocarcinoma (a mucin-producing type of invasive carcinoma) and from other lesions of the breast with a myxoid stroma (for example, myxoid fibroadenoma) (Figs. 7.137, 7.138, 7.139, and 7.140).

Excisional biopsy is recommended for mucocele-like tumor, especially if it was diagnosed on a Tru-Cut biopsy and/or it is associated with atypia or a breast mass.

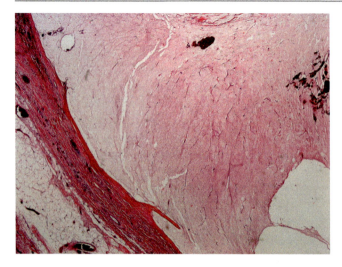

Fig. 7.136 Mucocele-like tumor: cystic cavity lined by a single layer of flattened epithelium, without signs of atypia and containing an abundant secretory material lacking epithelial or myoepithelial cells

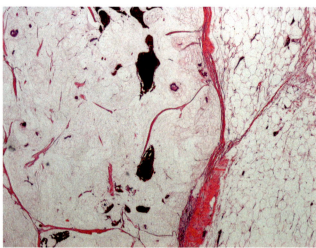

Fig. 7.137 Mucinous infiltrating carcinoma of hypocellular type: pools of mucin with rare groups of low-atypical epithelial cells in which myoepithelial cells are lacking

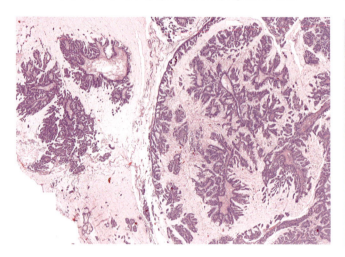

Fig. 7.138 Mucinous cystadenocarcinoma: cystic dilated spaces containing massive amounts of mucin, lined by stratified atypical cells; pools of mucin with floating papillae lined by atypical cells can be also detected at the left side of the picture; the myoepithelial cells are missing through the entire lesion

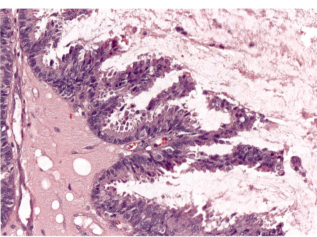

Fig. 7.139 Mucinous cystadenocarcinoma: the cysts are lined by several layers of atypical columnar cells producing mucin

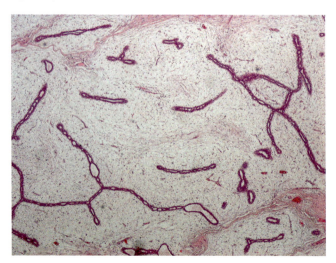

Fig. 7.140 Fibroadenoma with myxoid stroma

7.9   Benign Tumors of the Breast

7.9.1   Tubular Adenoma

Tubular adenoma is a rare benign breast tumor that occurs mainly in young patients (although it may occur at any age) in the form of a single, well-defined, firm, yellow-gray lesion. It has a mean diameter of 3 cm, mobile on superficial and deep planes. Rarely, the tumor may be bilateral or multiple. Radiologically, it resembles a fibroadenoma. Microscopically, it is composed of small tubular, rounded structures with little stoma between them, sometimes containing a minimal lymphocytic infiltrate (Figs. 7.141, 7.142, 7.143, 7.144, 7.145, and 7.146). These structures are lined by an internal epithelial layer represented by uniform cells (lacking atypia and presenting very few mitoses) and peripherally surrounded by a myoepithelial layer. The tubules have a small lumina that may be empty or may contain an eosinophilic proteinaceous material or mucin. The tubules are sometimes larger in size and may be branched. At the periphery, the tumor is surrounded by a fibrous capsule, but in some cases no capsule can be seen. Sometimes, a combined microscopic appearance of adenoma and fibroadenoma can be observed, suggesting that the two processes are related; some authors consequently consider that tubular adenoma should not be distinguished from fibroadenoma, although the latter is a biphasic tumor with a prominent mesenchymal component, while the former has little intervening stroma. There is no association with the development of tubular carcinoma with pregnancy (although some authors report the appearance of these tumors during pregnancy), or oral contraceptives. In a tubular adenoma, infarcted areas, apocrine metaplasia, atypical intraepithelial hyperplasia, atypical intralobular hyperplasia, secretory, and lactation changes may occur. Very rarely, cases of *in situ* or invasive carcinoma developed in a tubular adenoma have been described. Rarely, cases of stromal proliferation have been described in a tubular adenoma, the stromal component being formed of spindle cells with nuclear pleomorphism and mitotic activity. This is not surprising, given the link between a tubular adenoma, a fibroadenoma, and a phyllodes tumor. For the diagnosis of tubular adenoma, some authors request a size of more than 1 cm or presence of the capsule in lesions under 1 cm, since the tubular structures present within the tumor are identical to the acini in normal breast tissue or in adenosis [25].

Differential diagnosis is made with tubular adenosis (the lesion does not have the appearance of a nodule delimited by a capsule, being characterized by an infiltrating appearance) and tubular carcinoma (tubular structures infiltrate the surrounding tissue, are angulated, delimited by a layer of atypical epithelial cells without the presence of myoepithelial cells and basal membrane and are associated with a desmoplastic stroma).

Tubular adenoma does not increase the risk for developing a breast carcinoma, and surgical excision is curative.

7.9.2   Lactating Adenoma

Lactating adenoma is a benign tumor that develops in younger patients only during pregnancy or breastfeeding. It appears in the mammary gland and more rarely in ectopic mammary tissue of the axilla, thoracic wall, or vulva. Macroscopically, it is a well-defined nodular tumor with lobulated contour, a gray-yellow color, and soft consistency. Rarely, lactation adenoma may be multiple. Microscopically, the lesion is well-delimited by the adjacent tissue, but most often it does not have a proper capsule. It consists of multiple lobes surrounded by delicate fibrous bands. The lobes are formed by numerous round acini with varied secretory activity depending on the duration of pregnancy or breastfeeding. Thus, during pregnancy, the acini are only slightly distended, containing a small amount of secretion, while the epithelial cells have a small number of cytoplasmic vacuoles (Figs. 7.147, 7.148, 7.149, and 7.150). Tumors developed during lactation have distended acini containing abundant secretion, and the epithelial cells have many vacuoles intracytoplasmatically and hyperchromatic nuclei ("hobnail cells"), which have a similar appearance to the Arias-Stella changes. The secretory material contains lipids and is associated with degenerated cells or cellular debris. Myoepithelial cells are present but flattened. They can be identified by immunohistochemical examinations with myoepithelial markers. In a small number of cases, infarction areas may occur. Of interest, some tumors may contain a higher number of mitoses. The breast tissue adjacent to the tumor exhibits gestational or lactational hyperplasia. Differential diagnosis is made with gestational and lactational hyperplasia (both of which have a diffuse character) as well as fibroadenoma and tubular adenoma (which do not show lactation type secretion changes in the epithelium). Lactating adenoma is a benign tumor that does not increase the risk of developing a carcinoma and surgical excision is curative. However, lactating adenoma may occur simultaneously with a carcinoma during pregnancy or lactation.

7.9.3   Apocrine Adenoma

Apocrine adenoma is a benign, nodular, well-defined tumor, microscopically constituted by a proliferation of acini surrounded by a reduced stroma and exhibiting apocrine metaplasia of the epithelium. It appears in younger patients and is a rare lesion. Microscopically, the acini are lined by cylindrical metaplastic epithelial cells with abundant eosinophilic granular cytoplasm and a round nucleus with prominent nucleolus. This epithelium is usually single-layered, but can also exhibit papillary or micropapillary hyperplasia without or with atypia. Differential diagnosis is made with tubular adenoma, lactating adenoma, and fibroadenoma, which may present focal apocrine metaplasia but does not involve the epithelial component entirely in most of the cases. Also, differential diagnosis is made with apocrine adenosis, which does not constitute a nodule but is rather a microscopic lesion. The lesion is benign and does not increase the risk for developing a carcinoma unless it is associated with atypia.

7.9.4 Pleomorphic Adenoma

Pleomorphic adenoma is a rare tumor, similar to that developing in the salivary glands. It may occur at any age (mean age 65 years), usually as a single tumor, rarely multifocal, with cases also reported in men. Some authors consider that pleomorphic adenoma is a variant of intraductal papilloma with extensive cartilaginous metaplasia or a variant of adenomyoepithelioma. Macroscopically, it has the appearance of a well-defined and lobulated nodule, with an average diameter of 2 cm, firm consistency, and alternating elastic or soft white-gray areas. It is usually located in the subareolar or juxta-areolar area and is sometimes associated with nipple discharge. Microscopically, the tumor is well-delimited, with expansive margins, and consists of epithelial and myoepithelial cell groups, arranged in a myxochondroid stroma, which frequently has osseous foci. Epithelial and myoepithelial cells form tubular structures, cords, or islands. Sometimes, myoepithelial cells have a spindle shape, but most of the time they are rounded. Immunohistochemical stains can highlight both epithelial and myoepithelial cell populations (Figs. 7.151, 7.152, 7.153, and 7.154). Differential diagnosis is made with intraductal papilloma (it can have a chondroid or bone component, but no myoepithelial cell islands, and it has a classic papillary architecture that is missing in the pleomorphic adenoma), carcinoma of NST type with small areas of chondroid or osseous differentiation (the carcinomatous component with atypia and invasive areas is obvious), metaplastic carcinoma (atypical cells and areas of invasive carcinoma), benign mesenchymal breast tumors or malignant such as osteosarcoma and chondrosarcoma (both represented by high atypical cells, lacking the epithelial and myoepithelial component) (Figs. 7.155, 7.156, and 7.157).

Pleomorphic adenoma is a benign lesion, but which can cause local recurrences.

7.9.5 Ductal Adenoma

Ductal adenoma is a benign tumor that develops in the lumen of a cystically dilated duct (synonymous with *sclerosing papilloma*). The mean age of occurrence is 40 years. It is sometimes associated with pain and nipple discharge. Mammographically, it has well-defined margins and can present microcalcifications. Macroscopically, it appears as a single or multiple nodular formation of approximately 2 cm in diameter and located intracystically. Microscopically, glandular structures on the periphery are delimited by the two characteristic layers and may be distended, while in the center of the lesion there is a fibrotic and hyalinization area, which compresses the adjacent glandular structures, with a pseudoinfiltrating appearance. The wall of the duct where the lesion occurs may be thickened. At the periphery of the lesion, one can sometimes detect remnants of the cystic duct space in which the lesion developed. Areas of apocrine or squamous metaplasia may occur, and only through multiple sections can the presence of papillary axes within the lesion be determined (Figs. 7.158, 7.159, 7.160, and 7.161). When these can be highlighted, the term of sclerosing papilloma is preferred. Differential diagnosis is made with sclerosing adenosis (usually, it does not develop within a duct), central or peripheral papilloma (proliferation of fibro-vascular axes delimited by two atypical cell layers without the central areas of hyalinization), adenomyoepithelioma (when the myoepithelial cell proliferation is prominent), and infiltrating carcinoma of NST type (glandular structures delimited by atypical epithelial cells, without myoepithelial cells and which infiltrate the stroma) (Figs. 7.161, 7.162, 7.163, 7.164, and 7.165). Ductal adenoma does not increase the risk of developing a malignant lesion and does not lead to local recurrences after surgical excision.

7.9.6 Other Types of Benign Tumors

Salivary-gland and skin adnexal type of tumors, such as cylindroma and clear cell hidradenoma, may occur, very rarely, in the breast. They are morphologically identical to their counterparts that occur in the skin or salivary glands.

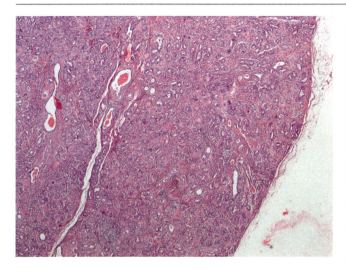

Fig. 7.141 Tubular adenoma: nodular tumor surrounded by a thin fibrous capsule at the periphery

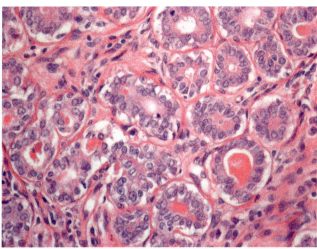

Fig. 7.142 Tubular adenoma: rounded structures, containing an eosinophilic proteinaceous material, lined by two cell layers, with little stoma between them

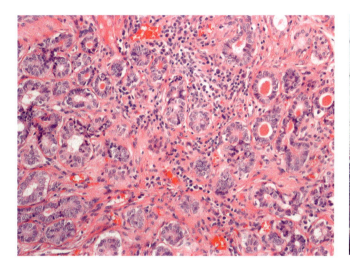

Fig. 7.143 Tubular adenoma: the stroma contains a minimal lymphocytic infiltrate

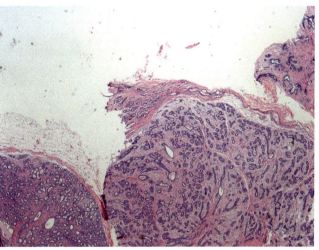

Fig. 7.144 Tubular adenoma: a combined microscopic appearance of adenoma and fibroadenoma can be observed in this lesion

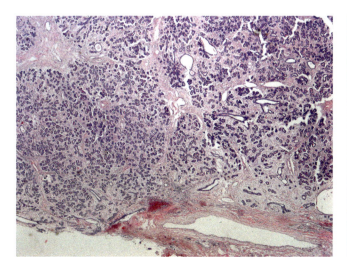

Fig. 7.145 Tubular adenoma: no capsule at the periphery of the tumor can be detected in this lesion

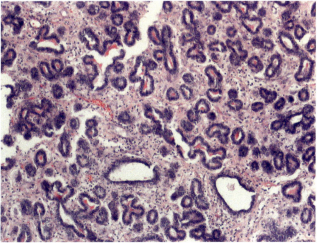

Fig. 7.146 Tubular adenoma: the round tubular structures are lined by an internal epithelial layer and peripherally surrounded by a myoepithelial layer

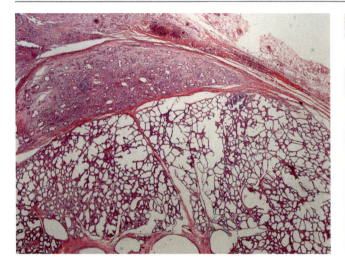

Fig. 7.147 Lactating adenoma: nodular tumor surrounded by a fibrous capsule at the periphery

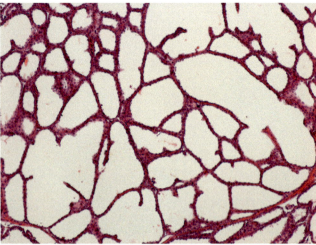

Fig. 7.148 Lactating adenoma: numerous round and distended acini lined by flattened epithelium

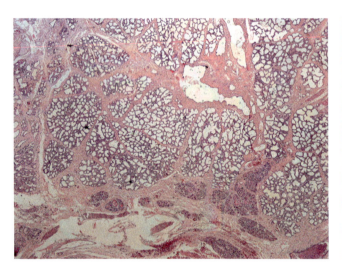

Fig. 7.149 Lactating adenoma: nodule without a capsule at the periphery, consisting of multiple lobes surrounded by delicate fibrous bands

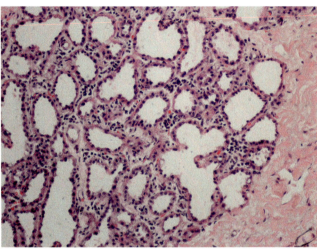

Fig. 7.150 Lactating adenoma developed during pregnancy: the acini are only slightly distended, lined by epithelial cuboidal cells with small number of cytoplasmic vacuoles

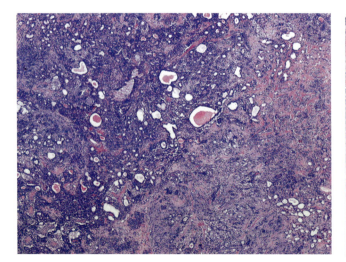

Fig. 7.151 Pleomorphic adenoma: mixed epithelial and myoepithelial proliferation

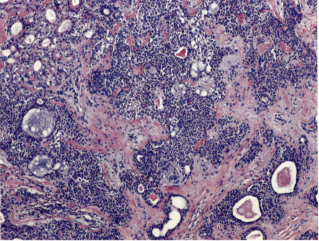

Fig. 7.152 Pleomorphic adenoma: epithelial and myoepithelial cells form tubular structures, cords, or islands

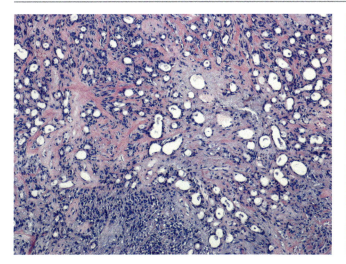

Fig. 7.153 Pleomorphic adenoma: tubular structures are predominant in this area of the tumor

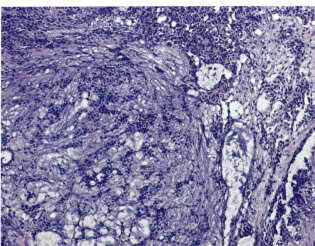

Fig. 7.154 Pleomorphic adenoma: the myxochondroid stroma is predominant in this area of the tumor; the myoepithelial cells have spindle shape

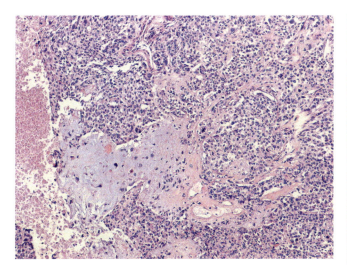

Fig. 7.155 Infiltrating carcinoma of no special (NST) type with small areas of chondroid differentiation (the carcinomatous component with atypia and invasive areas are obvious)

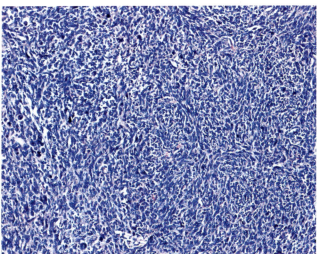

Fig. 7.156 Metaplastic carcinoma of spindle type: highly pleomorphic spindle atypical cells infiltrating the stroma

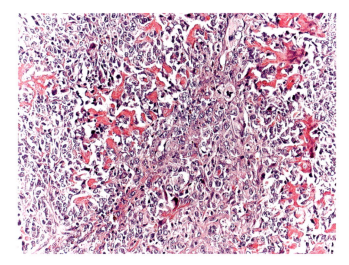

Fig. 7.157 Primary osteosarcoma of the breast represented by highly atypical cells with osteoid atypical areas, lacking the epithelial and myoepithelial component

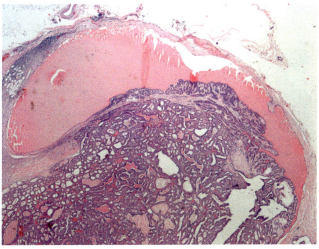

Fig. 7.158 Ductal adenoma: the tumor is located within a cystic duct space presenting a thickened wall

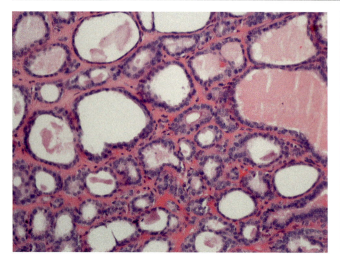

Fig. 7.159 Ductal adenoma: the tubular structures are delimited by the two characteristic layers

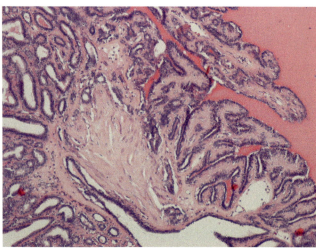

Fig. 7.160 Ductal adenoma: fibrotic and hyalinization area, which compresses the adjacent glandular structures, with a pseudoinfiltrating appearance

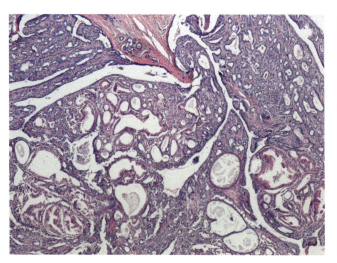

Fig. 7.161 Ductal adenoma: area of apocrine metaplasia

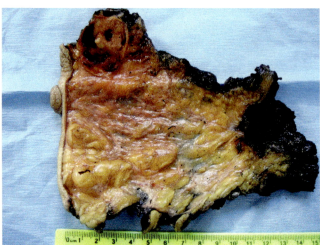

Fig. 7.162 Adenomyoepithelioma: macroscopic appearance of a nodular lesion developed within a cystic space; on the cut surface, the nodule has yellow color and soft consistency

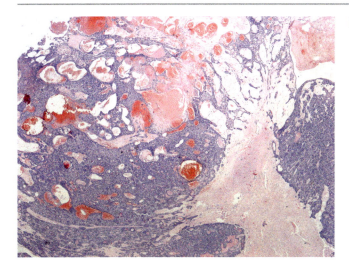

Fig. 7.163 Adenomyoepithelioma (same lesion as in Fig. 7.162): microscopic examination reveals proliferation of solid areas within a cystic space admixed with fibrosis and hemorrhage

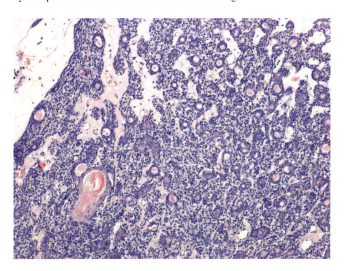

Fig. 7.164 Adenomyoepithelioma (same lesion as in Fig. 7.162): tubular structures lined by epithelial and myoepithelial cells; the myo-epithelial component is more prominent, forming nests of clear cells surrounding the tubules

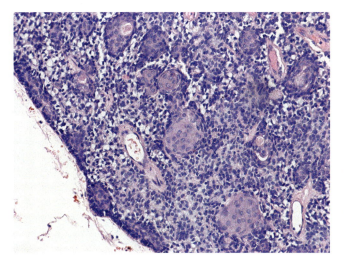

Fig. 7.165 Adenomyoepithelioma (same lesion as in Fig. 7.162): areas of benign squamous metaplasia

References

1. Moinfar F. Essentials of diagnostic breast pathology. New York, NY: Springer; 2007. p. 16.
2. Hutter RVP. Consensus meeting: is "fibrocystic disease" of the breast precancerous? Arch Pathol Lab Med. 1986;110:171–3.
3. Stolnicu S, Mocan S, Radulescu D, Podeanu MD. Diagnosticul morfologic al leziunilor mamare. Lanham, MD: University Press; 2005.
4. Leis HP Jr. Fibrocystic disease of the breast. J Med Assoc Alabama. 1962;32:97–104.
5. Tavassoli FA, Purcell CA, Bratthauer GL, Man Y-G. Androgen receptor expression along with loss of bcl-2, ER and PR expression in benign and malignant apocrine lesions of the breast: implications for therapy. Breast J. 1996;4:261–9.
6. Tavassoli FA, Eusebi V. Tumors of the mammary gland. AFIP Atlas of tumor pathology, series 4. Washington, DC: American Registry of Pathology; 2009.
7. Dupont WD, Page DL. Risk factors for breast cancer in women with proliferative disease. N Engl J Med. 1985;312:146–51.
8. Semb C. Pathologico-anatomical and clinical investigations of fibroadenomatosis cystica mammae and its relation to the other pathological conditions in mamma, especially cancer. Acta Chir Scand. 1928;64:1–484.
9. Anderson TJ, Battersby S. Radial scars and complex sclerosing lesions. Histopathology. 1994;24:296–7.
10. Hilson JB, Schnitt SJ, Collins LC. Phenotypic alterations in myoep-ithelial cells associated with benign sclerosing lesions of the breast. Am J Surg Pathol. 2010;34(6):896–900.
11. Lakhani SR, Schnitt SJ, Tan PH, van de Vijver MJ. WHO classifica-tion of tumors of the breast. IARC: Lyon; 2012.
12. Jacobs TW, Byrne C, Colditz G, Connolly JL, Schnitt SJ. Radial scar in benign breast-biopsy specimens and the risk of breast can-cer. N Engl J Med. 1999;340(6):430–6.
13. Sanders ME, Page DL, Simpson JF, Schuyler PA, Dale Plummer W, Dupont WD. Interdependence of radial scar and proliferative disease with respect to invasive breast carcinoma risk in patients with benign breast biopsies. Cancer. 2006;106(7):1453–61.
14. Resetkova E, Edelweiss M, Albarracin CT, Yang WT. Management of radial sclerosing lesions of the breast diagnosed using percuta-neous vacuum-assisted core needle biopsy: recommendations for excision based on seven years of experience at a single institution. Breast Cancer Res Treat. 2011;127(2):335–43.
15. Bianchi S, Giannotti E, Vanzi E, Marziali M, Abdulcadir D, Boeri C, et al. Radial scar without associated atypical epithelial prolifera-tion on image-guided 14-gauge needle core biopsy: analysis of 49 cases from a single—center and review of the literature. Breast. 2012;21(2):159–64.
16. Ferreira AI, Borges S, Sousa A, Ribeiro C, Mesquita A, Martins PC, et al. Radial scar of the breast: is it possible to avoid surgery? Eur J Surg Oncol. 2017;43(7):1265–72.
17. Carter DJ, Rosen PP. Atypical apocrine metaplasia in scleros-ing lesions of the breast. A study of 51 patients. Mod Pathol. 1991;4:1–5.
18. Rosen PP. Rosen's breast pathology. 3rd ed. Philadelphia, PA: Lippincott Williams and Wilkins; 2009.
19. Tavassoli FA, Norris HJ. Microglandular adenosis of the breast. A clinicopathologic study of 11 cases with ultrastructural observa-tions. Am J Surg Pathol. 1983;7(8):731–7.
20. Clement PB, Azzopardi JG. Microglamdular adenosis of the breast—a lesion simulating tubular racinoma. Histopathology. 1983;7(2):169–80.
21. Rosen PP. Microglandular adenosis. A benign lesion simulating invasive mammary carcinoma. Am J Surg Pathol. 1983;7(2):137–44.

22. Geyer FC, Lacroix-Triki M, Colombo PE, Patani N, Gauthier A, Natrajan R, et al. Molecular evidence in support of the neoplastic and precursor nature of microglandular adenosis. Histopathology. 2012;60:E115–30.
23. Khalifeh IM, Albarracin C, Diaz LK, Symmans FW, Edgerton ME, Hwang RF, et al. Clinical, histopathologic and immunohistochemical features of mucroglandular adenosis and transition into in situ and invasive carcinoma. Am J Surg Pathol. 2008;32(2):544–52.
24. Shin SJ, Rosen PP. Pregnancy-like (pseudolactational) hyperplasia: a primary diagnosis in mammographically detected lesions of the breast and its relationship to cystic hypersecretory hyperplasia. Am J Surg Pathol. 2000;24:1670–4.
25. Tavassoli FA. Pathology of the breast. 2nd ed. Appleton and Lange: Stamford, CT; 1999.

Myoepithelial Lesions and Tumors of the Breast

Michael Z. Gilcrease

Myoepithelial cells contain actin and myosin filaments that enable the cells to contract and thereby assist in moving secretory material through the duct lumen [1–4]. A stellate network of branching myoepithelial cells forms a net-like boundary between the luminal epithelial cells and the basement membrane, with many large gaps that allow direct contact between the glandular luminal epithelial cells and the basement membrane [5–7]. A number of conditions can lead to metaplastic or proliferative changes in the myoepithelial cell layer, resulting in a variety of benign and malignant myoepithelial cell lesions.

Nonneoplastic myoepithelial lesions are common, often observed as an incidental finding in the breast, and include myoepithelial hyperplasia, sclerosing adenosis, and collagenous spherulosis. Myoepithelial neoplasms are uncommon and include adenomyoepithelioma, malignant adenomyoepithelioma, and myoepithelial carcinoma.

8.1 Myoid and Squamous Metaplasia

Myoepithelial cells can occasionally acquire a muscle-like appearance, often in association with otherwise normal terminal duct-lobular units [8]. Myoid metaplasia doesn't constitute a lesion per se but represents one end of the spectrum of the dual epithelial-myoepithelial phenotype of myoepithelial cells (Fig. 8.1). Some proliferative lesions such as adenosis and sclerosing adenosis infrequently appear to have a prominent smooth muscle cell component. Such lesions have been referred to as myoid hamartomas [9], but electron microscopy suggests that the apparent smooth muscle cell component is likely derived from myoid metaplasia of myoepithelial cells, so such lesions do not represent true hamartomas [8, 10].

The myoepithelial cell also appears to be the cell of origin of metaplastic squamous epithelium [11]. Squamous metaplasia commonly occurs at sites of trauma, such as biopsy sites or in the breast tissue immediately surrounding surgical cavities, where it replaces the normal epithelium of ducts and lobules (Fig. 8.2). Squamous metaplasia is sometimes observed contiguous with myoepithelial hyperplasia, where the metaplastic squamous cells (which share the p63 and high-molecular-weight keratin expression of myoepithelial cells) have been observed to express muscle-specific actin and vimentin, consistent with their derivation from the adjacent myoepithelial cells [1].

M. Z. Gilcrease, MD, PhD
Division of Pathology and Laboratory Medicine, Department of
Pathology, The University of Texas M. D. Anderson Cancer Center,
Houston, TX, USA
e-mail: mgilcrease@mdanderson.org

© Springer International Publishing AG, part of Springer Nature 2018
S. Stolnicu, I. Alvarado-Cabrero (eds.), *Practical Atlas of Breast Pathology*, https://doi.org/10.1007/978-3-319-93257-6_8

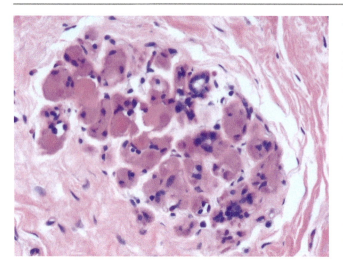

Fig. 8.1 Myoid metaplasia. The myoepithelial cells exhibit increased, brightly eosinophilic cytoplasm

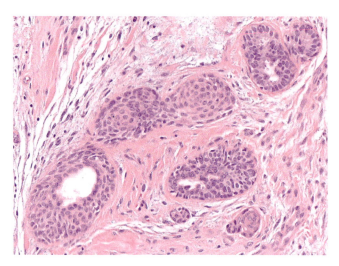

Fig. 8.2 Squamous metaplasia involving a duct. The squamous cells often appear to arise from or replace the myoepithelial cell layer

8.2 Myoepithelial Hyperplasia

Myoepithelial hyperplasia can be associated with a variety of benign and malignant lesions of the breast, or it may occur in otherwise unremarkable ducts [4]. When present in isolation, myoepithelial hyperplasia is sometimes referred to as myoepitheliosis [12]. It sometimes produces small nodular lesions, but often has no distinct clinical or gross pathologic features. It has no known risk for the development of breast cancer. It most often occurs in the periphery of the breast in association with terminal duct-lobular units, where the proliferating myoepithelial cells surround one or multiple ducts (Fig. 8.3). The associated ducts can be either distended or occluded. The degree of myoepithelial proliferation can range from a mildly increased number of myoepithelial cells to solid sheets of proliferating cells. Sometimes a papillary growth pattern is observed, in which the proliferating myoepithelial cells expand the fibrovascular cores of microscopic papillae. The individual myoepithelial cells can appear cuboidal, plasmacytoid, or spindled, with clear-to-eosinophilic cytoplasm. Mitotic activity and cytologic atypia are absent.

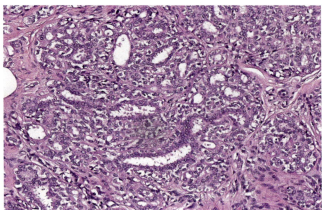

Fig. 8.3 Myoepithelial hyperplasia. The proliferating myoepithelial cells extend from below the luminal layer into the adjacent stroma

8.3   Sclerosing Adenosis

Sclerosing adenosis is a lobulocentric proliferation of small glands that is often observed in association with other fibrocystic changes. Each of the small glands in sclerosing adenosis maintains the epithelial, myoepithelial, and basement membrane components [13, 14]. In contrast to adenosis, in which acini or tubules are embedded in a loose connective tissue stroma, sclerosing adenosis has a dense fibrous stroma that compresses and distorts the associated glands. The resulting thin elongated epithelial structures often have attenuated luminal epithelium and conspicuous or hyperplastic myoepithelial cells (Fig. 8.4).

Sclerosing adenosis may form a mass lesion when it is a component of fibrocystic change, but in isolation it usually does not form a discrete mass. It is often an incidental lesion, but it is frequently associated with microcalcifications and, thus, it may lead to a stereotactic biopsy for indeterminate calcifications identified mammographically [15]. On occasion, histologically similar lesions may produce a palpable mass or a mass lesion detected radiographically. Such lesions are sometimes referred to as adenosis tumors or nodular sclerosing adenosis [16]. In patients with sclerosing adenosis, there is a small but significant risk for the subsequent development of breast cancer, similar to that observed for usual ductal hyperplasia [17].

Histologically, the luminal epithelial cells in sclerosing adenosis often become attenuated, and the myoepithelial cells appear as short linear arrays of epithelioid cells, mimicking an invasive carcinoma. When there is clearing of the myoepithelial cell cytoplasm, the linear arrays of myoepithelial cells can be mistaken for an invasive lobular carcinoma. Rarely, sclerosing adenosis can involve nerves (Fig. 8.5) [18].

Atypical lobular hyperplasia (ALH), lobular carcinoma in situ (LCIS), or ductal carcinoma in situ (DCIS) may become superimposed on sclerosing adenosis, making the distinction from invasive carcinoma even more difficult (Fig. 8.6) [19, 20]. Recognition of a lobulocentric arrangement at low power and the presence of myoepithelial cells at high power are features that allow such lesions to be distinguished from an invasive carcinoma. When carcinoma in situ is superimposed over sclerosing adenosis, one can generally see additional areas of uninvolved sclerosing adenosis in the surrounding tissue. In problematic cases, immunohistochemical staining for myoepithelial markers, such as muscle-specific actin, p63, or calponin, can reveal the presence of myoepithelial cells and rule out an invasive carcinoma.

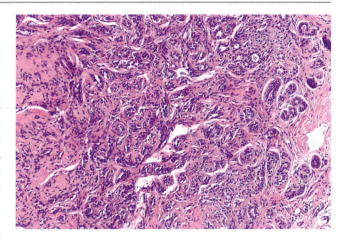

Fig. 8.4 Sclerosing adenosis. In contrast to adenosis, the small glands in sclerosing adenosis have compressed lumens

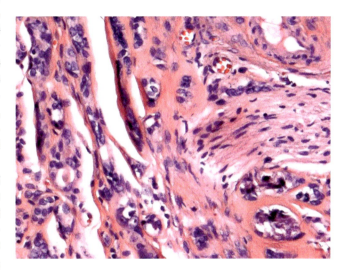

Fig. 8.5 Perineural invasion by sclerosing adenosis. Sometimes the two cell layers may not be clearly seen when the small glands are compressed against the nerve

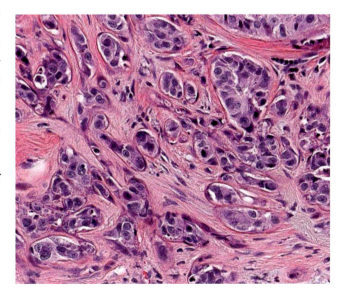

Fig. 8.6 DCIS involving sclerosing adenosis. The carcinoma cells appear to have an infiltrative pattern, but the myoepithelial cell layer of the underlying sclerosing adenosis is maintained

8.4 Collagenous Spherulosis

Collagenous spherulosis is a benign intraductal lesion that is often an incidental finding. However, it may have associated microcalcifications and thus may be observed in stereotactic biopsy specimens obtained for indeterminate or suspicious calcifications. It is sometimes observed in association with papillomas, usual ductal hyperplasia, and adenosis [21].

Histologically, collagenous spherulosis appears to have round, punched-out spaces surrounded by epithelial and myoepithelial hyperplasia (Fig. 8.7). These punched-out areas superficially resemble those in cribriform DCIS, but they are not actual spaces. They contain basophilic myxoid material or eosinophilic basement membrane-like material admixed with collagen, elastin, and acid mucin, and represent pseudolumina or spherules of extracellular stroma, similar to the pseudolumina or invaginations of extracellular stroma observed in adenoid cystic carcinoma [22]. The spherules are surrounded by a basement membrane that separates the extracellular material within the spherules from adjacent myoepithelial cells, which appear to produce the material that forms the spherules. Thus, in contrast to true glandular lumina that are lined by luminal epithelial cells with the apical portions forming the lumina, the pseudolumina in collagenous spherulosis are surrounded by a basement membrane and an adjacent myoepithelial cell layer at the basal aspect of the glandular epithelial cells [23].

This lesion has a distinctive appearance that is easy to recognize when one becomes familiar with it, but when ALH or LCIS becomes superimposed over collagenous spherulosis, the resulting lesion may be easily confused with low-grade cribriform DCIS (Fig. 8.8) [21].

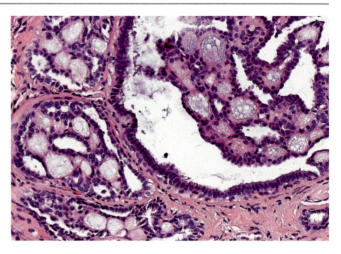

Fig. 8.7 Collagenous spherulosis. The cribriform structures do not have true glandular lumina, but instead contain pseudolumina with extracellular myxoid or eosinophilic material

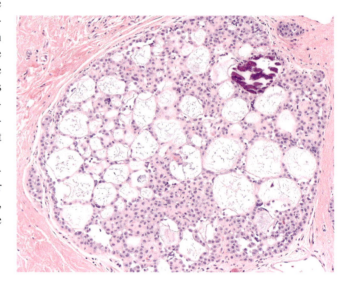

Fig. 8.8 LCIS involving collagenous spherulosis. The neoplastic lobular cells adjacent to pseudolumina may mimic DCIS

8.5 Adenomyoepithelioma

Adenomyoepitheliomas are uncommon benign neoplasms composed of both luminal epithelial cells and myoepithelial cells. They may be identified on routine breast imaging as an irregularly shaped mass with lobulated borders, or they may present clinically as a nontender, palpable mass. They can occur either centrally or peripherally in the breast, and they usually present as a solitary lesion. They can measure up to 8 cm, but the mean size is 2–3 cm. The mean age at presentation is 59 years [12, 24, 25].

Histologically, adenomyoepitheliomas are composed of varying numbers of small round or oval glands lined by bland cuboidal epithelial cells and surrounded by proliferating myoepithelial cells (Fig. 8.9). The myoepithelial cells can be polygonal or spindled. Often there is a papillary component, which is sometimes prominent (Fig. 8.10). Some authors, in fact, consider adenomyoepitheliomas to be variants of intraductal papillomas. The diagnosis of adenomyoepithelioma is made when the myoepithelial cell proliferation is extensive and present diffusely throughout the lesion. Immunohistochemical staining for myoepithelial cell markers can be helpful in highlighting the extent of the myoepithelial cell proliferation (Fig. 8.11). Depending on the overall histologic pattern and cytologic appearance of the cells, adenomyoepitheliomas can be categorized as tubular, lobulated, or spindle cell variants [12].

The tubular variant is made up of a collection of small round ducts, superficially resembling a tubular adenoma, but the myoepithelial cells surrounding the small ducts are more prominent (Fig. 8.12). The hyperplastic myoepithelial cells can compress and sometimes occlude the adjacent ducts. The entire lesion is generally well circumscribed with focal irregular areas at the borders, where the ducts surrounded by myoepithelial cells protrude into surrounding breast tissue (Fig. 8.13).

The lobulated variant contains solid areas of proliferating myoepithelial cells with interspersed compressed tubules (Fig. 8.14). The solid areas of myoepithelium are often divided into lobules by interspersed fibrous septa. The lesions are often encapsulated, but the proliferating myoepithelial cells can extend beyond the fibrous capsule. These lesions are sometimes centrally infarcted, or they may have areas of hyaline degeneration. Sometimes there are associated calcifications.

In the spindle cell variant, the spindled myoepithelial cells are usually the predominant cell type, with only occasional interspersed ducts (Fig. 8.15). The spindled cells form sheets that compress the ducts, sometimes making the interspersed ducts difficult to see. The spindled cells can have clear or eosinophilic cytoplasm, and sometimes have a plasmacytoid appearance. The spindle cell variant of adenomyoepitheliomas can mimic a leiomyoma, which is quite rare in the breast, but the spindle cells in spindled adenomyoepitheliomas are strongly S-100 positive and exhibit some weak staining for cytokeratin.

The epithelial component of adenomyoepitheliomas can undergo apocrine, mucinous, or squamous metaplasia [26]. Sebaceous cells are sometimes observed. When squamous metaplasia is present, it sometimes has an atypical appearance, but if not frankly malignant, this does not appear to be clinically significant (Fig. 8.16). Some adenomyoepitheliomas are sclerotic, and the glandular component can mimic an invasive carcinoma in areas where the myoeptihelial cells are attenuated.

Up to 3 mitotic figures per 10 high-power fields may be observed in adenomyoepitheliomas. Cytologic atypia and/or necrosis may also be observed [12]. Such findings in isolation are not associated with malignant behavior. Adenomyoepitheliomas are nevertheless prone to local recurrence, perhaps because they often have small satellite foci adjacent to but separate from the main lesion (Fig. 8.17). These small satellite foci generally resemble the main lesion, but are not as fully developed. Complete surgical excision with a margin of normal tissue has generally been recommended to minimize the risk of local recurrence [12, 27].

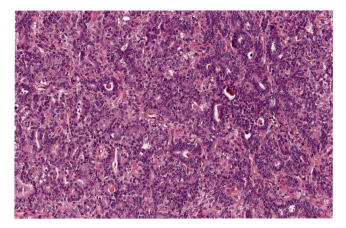

Fig. 8.9 Adenomyoepithelioma. The lesion is composed of small round or oval glands lined by bland cuboidal epithelial cells and surrounded by proliferating myoepithelial cells

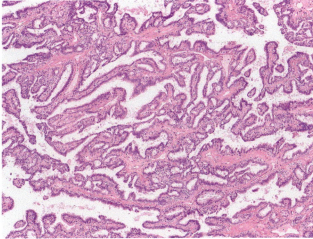

Fig. 8.10 Adenomyoepithelioma. A focal or prominent papillary architecture is often present, with myoepithelial cells proliferating within the fibrovascular cores

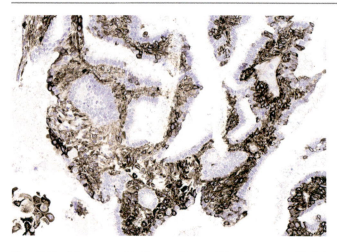

Fig. 8.11 Adenomyoepithelioma. The proliferating myoepithelial cells in this case are highlighted by immunohistochemical staining for cytokeratin 5/6 (Immunoperoxidase with DAB chromogen)

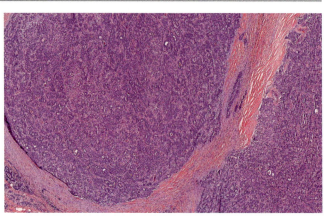

Fig. 8.12 Adenomyoepithelioma, tubular variant. The collection of small round ducts superficially resembles a tubular adenoma, but the myoepithelial cells are more prominent

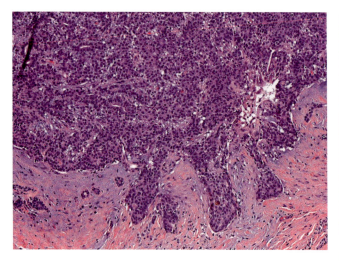

Fig. 8.13 Adenomyoepithelioma, tubular variant. Focal irregular borders may be seen, with small areas of the lesion protruding into surrounding breast tissue

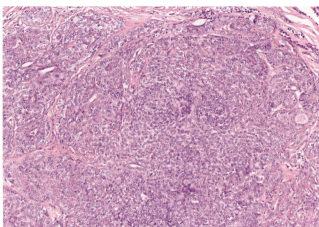

Fig. 8.14 Adenomyoepithelioma, lobular variant. Much of the lesion contains near-solid areas of proliferating myoepithelial cells

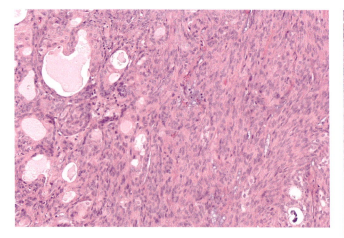

Fig. 8.15 Adenomyoepithelioma, spindle cell variant. The spindle cell areas, when dominant, may resemble a smooth muscle neoplasm with entrapped ducts

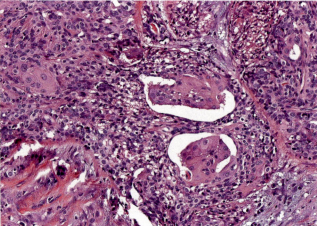

Fig. 8.16 Adenomyoepithelioma with squamous metaplasia. The glandular component in some areas can be partially or completely replaced with metaplastic squamous cells

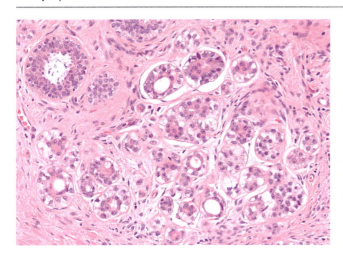

Fig. 8.17 Satellite focus of adenomyoepithelioma. The lesion resembles the adjacent adenomyoepithelioma but is not as fully developed. It may contribute to local recurrence

8.6   Malignant Adenomyoepithelioma

Adenomyoepitheliomas can undergo malignant transformation. Either the epithelial component, the myoepithelial component, or both can become malignant [25, 28–32]. Sometimes, the malignant component is observed to arise only focally within an adenomyoepithelioma. Although minimum criteria for malignancy have not been clearly defined, the malignant component generally shows a combination of severe cytologic atypia, high mitotic activity (generally 4 or more mitotic figures per 10 high-power fields), necrosis, and an infiltrative growth pattern (Figs. 8.18 and 8.19).

It is important to recognize that an infiltrative pattern is often observed in benign adenomyoepitheliomas, as well as cystic degeneration and necrosis. For a diagnosis of malignant adenomyoepithelioma to be made, severe cytologic atypia and/or high mitotic activity must also be present. The malignant lesions, like their benign counterparts, often have microscopic foci surrounding the main tumor (Fig. 8.20). A wide excision to include a rim of grossly normal tissue should be performed to minimize the risk of local recurrence.

Malignant adenomyoepitheliomas can produce distant metastases and, like metaplastic carcinomas and centrally necrotizing carcinomas of the breast, these metastases often spread to the brain and the lungs [29, 33–35].

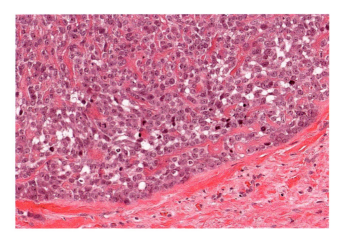

Fig. 8.18 Malignant adenomyoepithelioma. The myoepithelial component in this lesion shows increased nuclear atypia and mitotic activity

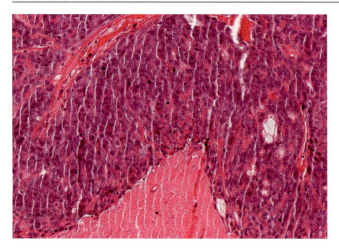

Fig. 8.19 Malignant adenomyoepithelioma. This lesion has greater nuclear pleomorphism, mitotic activity, and necrosis

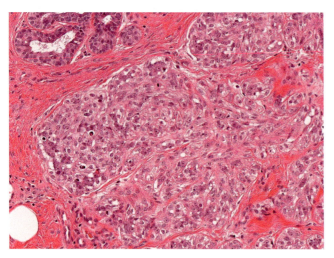

Fig. 8.20 Malignant adenomyoepithelioma. Microscopic foci adjacent to the main lesion also show increased nuclear atypia and mitotic activity

8.7 Myoepithelial Carcinoma

Myoepithelial carcinomas are, by definition, composed of a pure population of malignant myoepithelial cells [36, 37]. It is quite rare for myoepithelial carcinomas to arise de novo. More often, they occur as the malignant component of a malignant adenomyoepithelioma. They almost always present as a mass lesion. The mean tumor size is 2.6 cm, and the mean age at presentation is 69.5 years [37].

Histologically, myoepithelial carcinomas are most often composed of spindled cells, but they may also have round, ovoid, or epithelioid cells. The cytoplasm may be indistinct, eosinophilic, clear, or vacuolated (Figs. 8.21 and 8.22). The neoplastic cells often appear to emanate from the myoepithelial layer of entrapped benign ducts [37]. Mitotic activity is variable (up to 9 mitoses per 10 high-power fields have been reported), and necrosis may occur but is uncommon.

When the myoepithelial cells in a malignant myoepithelial carcinoma are entirely spindled, the distinction between a spindle cell metaplastic carcinoma and a myoepithelial carcinoma has been made on the basis of a myoepithelial morphology in the latter, such as plump spindled cells with clear cytoplasm, as well as markers of myoepithelial differentiation. However, spindle cell metaplastic carcinomas can have varying degrees of myoepithelial differentiation, including p63, S-100 and muscle-specific actin expression, so the distinction between the two at times may be arbitrary [37].

Both spindle cell metaplastic carcinomas and myoepithelial carcinomas may behave aggressively and metastasize hematogenously to the brain and the lungs (Fig. 8.23). The current WHO Classification of Tumors of the Breast states that there are currently no definitive criteria to differentiate these lesions. Nor do they appear to have distinct clinical behavior. Therefore, under the current WHO classification, myoepithelial carcinoma is grouped together with metaplastic carcinoma [38].

Malignant adenomyoepitheliomas, myoepithelial carcinomas, and spindle cell metaplastic carcinomas are generally triple-negative carcinomas that are treated like other triple-negative breast cancers [37]. However, growing evidence of characteristic molecular changes in metaplastic carcinomas of the breast, such as activating PIK3CA mutations and other aberrations of the PI3K pathway, have led to therapeutic strategies targeting this pathway in metaplastic carcinomas, and such therapies might also be effective for malignant adenomyoepitheliomas and myoepithelial carcinomas [39]. One patient with a malignant adenomyoepithelioma was included on a clinical trial targeting the PI3K pathway in metaplastic carcinomas, and the patient with the malignant adenomyoepithelioma did achieve a partial response [40]. Further studies are needed to establish the efficacy of such treatments for patients with malignant adenomyoepitheliomas and myoepithelial carcinomas.

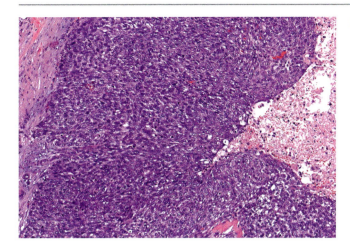

Fig. 8.21 Myoepithelial carcinoma. The cells resemble myoepithelial cells with inconspicuous to clear cytoplasm, but there is increased atypia, mitotic activity, and necrosis

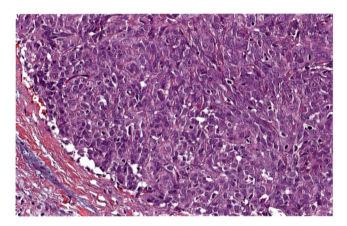

Fig. 8.22 Myoepithelial carcinoma. This example has plump round-to-spindled cells with eosinophilic cytoplasm and mitotic activity

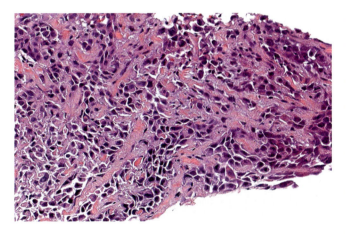

Fig. 8.23 Myoepithelial carcinoma, metastatic to lung. The metastatic lesion contains atypical epithelioid and plasmacytoid cells with eosinophilic cytoplasm

References

1. Deugnier MA, Teuliere J, Faraldo MM, Thiery JP, Glukhova MA. The importance of being a myoepithelial cell. Breast Cancer Res. 2002;4(6):224–30.
2. Clarke C, Sandle J, Lakhani SR. Myoepithelial cells: pathology, cell separation and markers of myoepithelial differentiation. J Mammary Gland Biol Neoplasia. 2005;10(3):273–80.
3. Gudjonsson T, Adriance MC, Sternlicht MD, Petersen OW, Bissell MJ. Myoepithelial cells: their origin and function in breast morphogenesis and neoplasia. J Mammary Gland Biol Neoplasia. 2005;10(3):261–72.
4. Hamperl H. The myothelia (myoepithelial cells). Normal state; regressive changes; hyperplasia; tumors. Curr Top Pathol. 1970;53:161–220.
5. Yaziji H, Gown AM, Sneige N. Detection of stromal invasion in breast cancer: the myoepithelial markers. Adv Anat Pathol. 2000;7(2):100–9.
6. Dewar R, Fadare O, Gilmore H, Gown AM. Best practices in diagnostic immunohistochemistry: myoepithelial markers in breast pathology. Arch Pathol Lab Med. 2011;135(4):422–9.
7. Corben AD, Lerwill MF. Use of myoepithelial cell markers in the differential diagnosis of benign, in situ, and invasive lesions of the breast. Surg Pathol Clin. 2009;2(2):351–73.
8. Eusebi V, Cunsolo A, Fedeli F, Severi B, Scarani P. Benign smooth muscle cell metaplasia in breast. Tumori. 1980;66(5):643–53.
9. Daroca PJ Jr, Reed RJ, Love GL, Kraus SD. Myoid hamartomas of the breast. Hum Pathol. 1985;16(3):212–9.
10. Shepstone BJ, Wells CA, Berry AR, Ferguson JD. Mammographic appearance and histopathological description of a muscular hamartoma of the breast. Br J Radiol. 1985;58(689):459–61.
11. Raju GC. The histological and immunohistochemical evidence of squamous metaplasia from the myoepithelial cells in the breast. Histopathology. 1990;17(3):272–5.
12. Tavassoli FA. Myoepithelial lesions of the breast. Myoepitheliosis, adenomyoepithelioma, and myoepithelial carcinoma. Am J Surg Pathol. 1991;15(6):554–68.
13. Urban JA, Adair FE. Sclerosing adenosis. Cancer. 1949;2(4):625–34.
14. Foote FW, Stewart FW. Comparative studies of cancerous versus noncancerous breasts. Ann Surg. 1945;121(2):197–222.
15. MacErlean DP, Nathan BE. Calcification in sclerosing adenosis simulating malignant breast calcification. Br J Radiol. 1972;45(540):944–5.
16. Nielsen BB. Adenosis tumour of the breast—a clinicopathological investigation of 27 cases. Histopathology. 1987;11(12):1259–75.
17. Jensen RA, Page DL, Dupont WD, Rogers LW. Invasive breast cancer risk in women with sclerosing adenosis. Cancer. 1989;64(10):1977–83.
18. Davies JD. Neural invasion in benign mammary dysplasia. J Pathol. 1973;109(3):225–31.
19. Fechner RE. Lobular carcinoma in situ in sclerosing adenosis. A potential source of confusion with invasive carcinoma. Am J Surg Pathol. 1981;5(3):233–9.
20. Eusebi V, Collina G, Bussolati G. Carcinoma in situ in sclerosing adenosis of the breast: an immunocytochemical study. Semin Diagn Pathol. 1989;6(2):146–52.
21. Resetkova E, Albarracin C, Sneige N. Collagenous spherulosis of breast: morphologic study of 59 cases and review of the literature. Am J Surg Pathol. 2006;30(1):20–7.
22. Clement PB, Young RH, Azzopardi JG. Collagenous spherulosis of the breast. Am J Surg Pathol. 1987;11(6):411–7.
23. Grignon DJ, Ro JY, Mackay BN, Ordonez NG, Ayala AG. Collagenous spherulosis of the breast. Immunohistochemical and ultrastructural studies. Am J Clin Pathol. 1989;91(4):386–92.

24. Rosen PP. Adenomyoepithelioma of the breast. Hum Pathol. 1987;18(12):1232–7.

25. Loose JH, Patchefsky AS, Hollander IJ, Lavin LS, Cooper HS, Katz SM. Adenomyoepithelioma of the breast. A spectrum of biologic behavior. Am J Surg Pathol. 1992;16(9):868–76.

26. Cai RZ, Tan PH. Adenomyoepithelioma of the breast with squamous and sebaceous metaplasia. Pathology. 2005;37(6):557–9.

27. Young RH, Clement PB. Adenomyoepithelioma of the breast. A report of three cases and review of the literature. Am J Clin Pathol. 1988;89(3):308–14.

28. Pauwels C, De Potter C. Adenomyoepithelioma of the breast with features of malignancy. Histopathology. 1994;24(1):94–6.

29. Rasbridge SA, Millis RR. Adenomyoepithelioma of the breast with malignant features. Virchows Arch. 1998;432(2):123–30.

30. Ahmed AA, Heller DS. Malignant adenomyoepithelioma of the breast with malignant proliferation of epithelial and myoepithelial elements: a case report and review of the literature. Arch Pathol Lab Med. 2000;124(4):632–6.

31. Fan F, Smith W, Wang X, Jewell W, Thomas PA, Tawfik O. Myoepithelial carcinoma of the breast arising in an adenomyoepithelioma: mammographic, ultrasound and histologic features. Breast J. 2007;13(2):203–4.

32. Noel JC, Simon P, Aguilar SF. Malignant myoepithelioma arising in cystic adenomyoepithelioma. Breast J. 2006;12(4):386.

33. Simpson RH, Cope N, Skalova A, Michal M. Malignant adenomyoepithelioma of the breast with mixed osteogenic, spindle cell, and carcinomatous differentiation. Am J Surg Pathol. 1998;22(5):631–6.

34. Chen PC, Chen CK, Nicastri AD, Wait RB. Myoepithelial carcinoma of the breast with distant metastasis and accompanied by adenomyoepitheliomas. Histopathology. 1994;24(6):543–8.

35. Michal M, Baumruk L, Burger J, Manhalova M. Adenomyoepithelioma of the breast with undifferentiated carcinoma component. Histopathology. 1994;24(3):274–6.

36. Behranwala KA, Nasiri N, A'Hern R, Gui GP. Clinical presentation and long-term outcome of pure myoepithelial carcinoma of the breast. Eur J Surg Oncol. 2004;30(4):357–61.

37. Buza N, Zekry N, Charpin C, Tavassoli FA. Myoepithelial carcinoma of the breast: a clinicopathological and immunohistochemical study of 15 diagnostically challenging cases. Virchows Arch. 2010;457(3):337–45.

38. Tan PH, Ellis IO. Myoepithelial and epithelial-myoepithelial, mesenchymal and fibroepithelial breast lesions: updates from the WHO classification of tumours of the breast 2012. J Clin Pathol. 2013;66(6):465–70.

39. Moulder S, Moroney J, Helgason T, Wheler J, Booser D, Albarracin C, et al. Responses to liposomal doxorubicin, bevacizumab, and temsirolimus in metaplastic carcinoma of the breast: biologic rationale and implications for stem-cell research in breast cancer. J Clin Oncol. 2011;29(19):e572–5.

40. Moulder S, Helgason T, Janku F, Wheler J, Moroney J, Booser D, et al. Inhibition of the phosphoinositide 3-kinase pathway for the treatment of patients with metastatic metaplastic breast cancer. Ann Oncol. 2015;26(7):1346–52.

Danielle Fortuna, Adam Toll, and Juan P. Palazzo

Fibroepithelial lesions of the breast are a group of biphasic neoplasms, lesions characterized by proliferation of both mesenchymal and epithelial elements. On the whole, these lesions constitute one of the most commonly encountered neoplasms in routine practice and span the spectrum of biological significance from benign to malignant. Prototypic examples of these neoplasms include the fibroadenoma (FA) and phyllodes tumor (PT), with the phyllodes tumor requiring further subtyping into benign, borderline/intermediate, and malignant in accordance with the World Health Organization (WHO) recommendations [1]. These specific lesions within this group have diverse clinical behavior, natural history, and therapeutic implications, despite showing considerable morphologic overlap at times. Since many of the initial diagnoses are rendered in core biopsies, this can potentially compound a diagnostic challenge, and clinical-pathological correlation is imperative. Here, we present a review of fibroepithelial lesions with an emphasis on morphology and distinguishing features. Hamartomas, also considered a fibroepithelial lesion, is discussed below under the differential diagnosis section of fibroadenoma.

9.1 Fibroadenoma

The clinical presentation of the fibroadenoma (FA) mirrors its natural history. Fibroadenomas usually occur in women less than 30 years of age. Additionally, immunosuppressive therapy with cyclosporine has been associated with increased development of fibroadenomas [2, 3]. Typically, fibroadenomas are well-demarcated, mobile, round, and rubbery lesions [4]. Although the average diameter is 2 cm, larger fibroadenomas may occur; fibroadenomas greater than 10 cm are sometimes referred to as "giant fibroadenomas" [4]. The larger fibroadenomas are usually encountered in adolescents. They can be single or present as multiple nodules in one or both breasts in a synchronous or metachronous fashion (Fig. 9.1). Current work suggests that the growth of fibroadenomas is hormonally-dependent and influenced by estrogen-status [5, 6]. This helps to explain why most fibroadenomas may regress with time and the quality of the stroma changes with patient age. The presence of FAs in older women outside of the range of childbearing years may

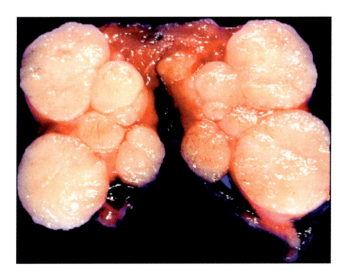

Fig. 9.1 Gross appearance of fibroadenoma shows lobulation and nodularity. It is sharply demarcated from the small amount of attached tissue

D. Fortuna, MD
Department of Pathology, Thomas Jefferson University, Philadelphia, PA, USA
e-mail: Danielle.fortuna@jefferson.edu

A. Toll, MD
Department of Pathology, St. Luke's University Health Network, Bethlehem, PA, USA
e-mail: adam.toll@sluhn.org

J. P. Palazzo, MD (✉)
Department of Pathology, Thomas Jefferson University Hospital, Philadelphia, PA, USA
e-mail: juan.palazzo@jefferson.edu

© Springer International Publishing AG, part of Springer Nature 2018
S. Stolnicu, I. Alvarado-Cabrero (eds.), *Practical Atlas of Breast Pathology*, https://doi.org/10.1007/978-3-319-93257-6_9

be related to exogenous hormone therapy (estrogen replacement) or obesity.

Radiographically, fibroadenomas typically appear as well-circumscribed or lobulated masses (Fig. 9.2). Frequently calcifications are present, and the most common calcification pattern shows initial small peripheral, punctate dots which coalesce over time with coarser features [7]. Occasionally, dystrophic or pleomorphic calcifications may be associated with fibroadenomas, especially when accompanying extensive stromal hyalinization.

Similar to their radiographic appearance, fibroadenomas at the gross bench are well-circumscribed nodules with occasional lobulation (Fig. 9.1). Stromal variations, such as myxoid change and hyalinization, are reflected in its gross texture and appearance of the cut surface. Calcifications impart a gritty surface.

Although biphasic, the stromal component of the FA typically predominates over the epithelial component, but the overall ratio of the two components is variable, not only among FAs but even in a single lesion. On low power, the initial histologic impression is classically described by the pattern by which the stroma grows around the ductal structures: intracanalicular (circumferential stromal proliferation) or pericanalicular (stromal proliferation which compresses the ductal structures into cleft-like spaces) (Figs. 9.3 and 9.4). The distinction between these two growth patterns is not of prognostic significance, but these patterns are important in that they form the underlying structure of the fibroadenoma onto which many stromal and epithelial changes can be subsequently applied. Additionally, both patterns can be present within the same lesion.

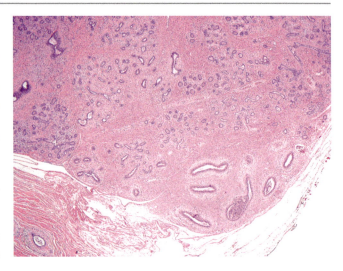

Fig. 9.3 Growth patterns of fibroadenoma. The pericanalicular pattern is comprised of stroma growing around round, open tubules

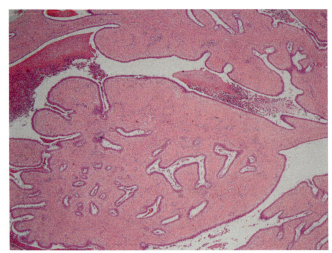

Fig. 9.4 Growth patterns of fibroadenoma. The intracanalicular pattern features stroma growing with compression of tubules

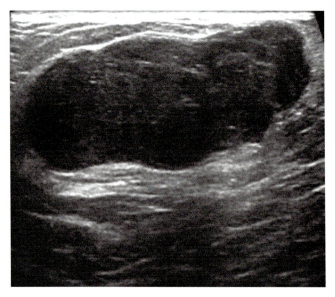

Fig. 9.2 Ultrasound image of a fibroadenoma shows an oval, lobulated, but circumscribed hypoechoic mass

The mesenchymal aspect of the FA has two major components with variable features: the cellular component and the background stromal component. The cellular component consists of bland spindle cells with infrequent mitoses. Cellularity ranges from sparse (hypocellular) to focally/extensively hypercellular ("cellular fibroadenoma," discussed below). Stromal giant cells can also be seen; however, close inspection will reveal the degenerative quality of the nuclei. Importantly, these changes also do not qualify as stromal atypia. The stromal background can be myxoid, fibrous, or hyalinized. Calcifications are common in hyalinized FAs. Heterologous and homologous breast differentiation includes lipomatous, smooth muscle, and osteochondroid elements, and is an uncommon finding [8]. Hormonal changes seen in young or pregnant patients can yield mitoses or infarction. However, neither of these changes denote malignancy in a typical fibroadenoma as mitoses are generally less than 3 per 10 high-power fields, even in cellular fibroadenomas [9], and infarction is secondary to ischemia, in contrast to true tumor necrosis. Figures 9.5, 9.6, 9.7, 9.8, 9.9, 9.10, 9.11, and 9.12 highlight the stromal features of fibroadenomas.

The epithelial component of the FA consists of glandular structures embedded within a stromal proliferation. The low-power appearance is quite informative as the epithelial structures are relatively uniformly distributed throughout the lesion (i.e., not haphazard). It is important to keep in mind that the epithelial component of the FA is subject to all of the epithelial changes that can be seen in background breast tissue. This includes, but is not limited to, varying degrees of epithelial proliferation with or without atypia, adenosis, and metaplasias. The low-power appearance is again helpful to

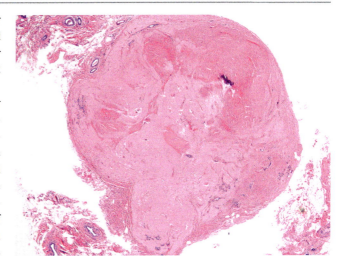

Fig. 9.7 Despite extensive stromal hyalinization and the paucity of glandular elements, the lesion maintains the low-power silhouette of a fibroadenoma

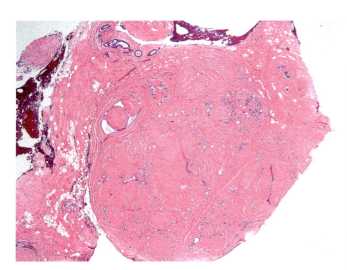

Fig. 9.5 The low-power appearance of a fibroadenoma shows a well-circumscribed and lobulated nodule. The epithelial elements are regularly distributed within the lesion

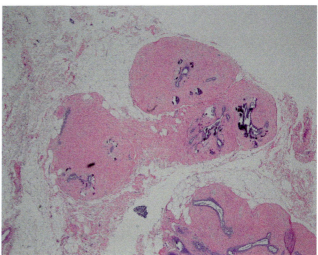

Fig. 9.8 At this magnification, the hyalinized nodules, scattered epithelial elements, and calcifications are appreciated

appreciate the overall architecture, as well as to identify areas with epithelial changes. Figures 9.13, 9.14, 9.15, 9.16, and 9.17 show various epithelial changes seen in fibroadenomas.

Fibroadenoma variants are the followings:

- **Cellular FA** (Fig. 9.18). "Cellular" refers to the stromal component. Despite the hypercellularity of the stroma here, there is no atypia of the stromal cells, no significant increase in mitotic figures present, and maintenance of the well-circumscribed border. The presence of stromal atypia or increased mitoses in what appears to be a "cellular FA" may suggest a phyllodes tumor. (See below for further discussion.)
- **Juvenile FA** (Fig. 9.19). The term "juvenile FA" refers to fibroadenomas occurring in young patients, which often

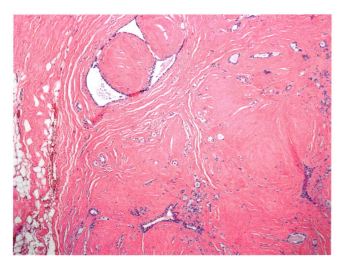

Fig. 9.6 The presence of both pericanalicular and intracanalicular patterns can be appreciated

grow as large masses with occasional breast distortion. This FA variant is characterized by increased stromal cellularity with prominent stromal fascicles, pericanalicular growth pattern, and usual ductal hyperplasia. Micropapillary ductal architecture, also seen in juvenile FAs, bears a striking resemblance to the hyperplastic features seen in gynecomastia. Significant stromal nuclear atypia is lacking [10].

- **Complex fibroadenoma** (Fig. 9.20). Epithelial proliferations may occur including sclerosing adenosis, apocrine changes, and cysts greater than 0.3 cm. These changes can be prominent enough to obscure the presence of a fibroadenoma or even simulate invasive ductal carcinoma (Fig. 9.14). These are defining features of "complex fibroadenoma" which have a slight increase in the relative risk for carcinoma [11].

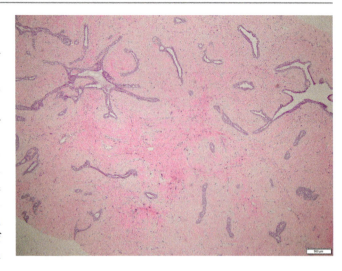

Fig. 9.11 Low-power view of a fibroadenoma showing stromal giant cells

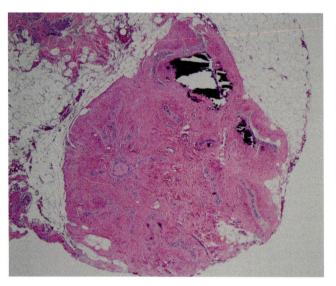

Fig. 9.9 Notice the well-demarcated and sharp margins of the fibroadenoma

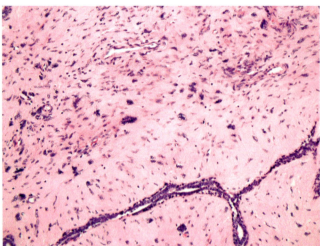

Fig. 9.12 On higher power, these cells can be further characterized as degenerative-type changes, showing a smudgy quality of the nuclei. Notice the lack of any other evidence of malignancy

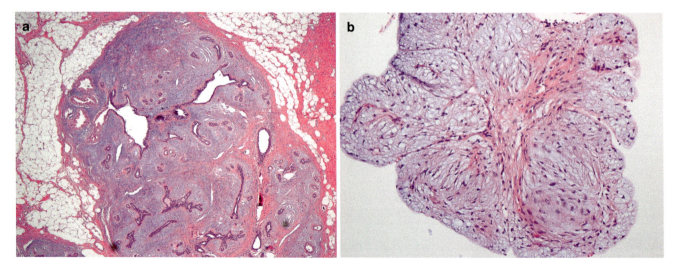

Fig. 9.10 (**a, b**) Myxoid stromal changes within fibroadenomas are common and can be the predominant finding in a core biopsy

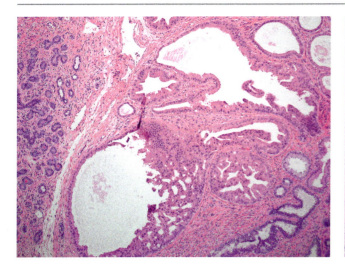

Fig. 9.13 Fibroadenoma with apocrine metaplasia, usual ductal hyperplasia (bottom), and prominent pericanalicular pattern (left)

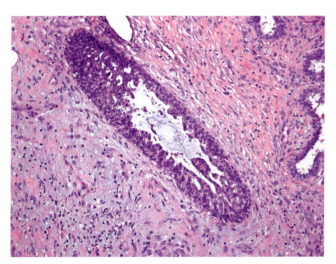

Fig. 9.14 Fibroadenoma with usual ductal hyperplasia

- **FA with atypia and malignancy** (Figs. 9.21 and 9.22). As previously mentioned, FAs are subject to epithelial proliferations encountered routinely in breast tissue, including atypia. Although considered a benign neoplasm, FAs can harbor atypical and frankly malignant ductal and lobular proliferations with the incidence of malignancy reported as 0.1–0.3%. Lobular carcinoma seems to occur more frequently than ductal carcinoma in this setting [4]. The extent of FA involvement is variable. The atypical lesion may be entirely confined to the fibroadenoma, or, on the other hand, the fibroadenoma may have been colonized by the malignancy present outside the nodule from the surrounding breast tissue. Radiographic and clinical correlation is of utmost importance in these circumstances, as its impact on clinical management is quite significant. Examples of fibroadenomas involved by these lesions are illustrated in Figs. 9.15 and 9.16.

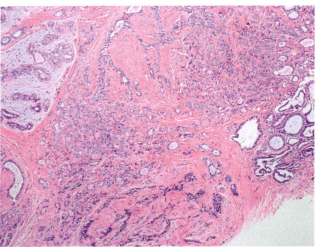

Fig. 9.15 Fibroadenoma with sclerosing adenosis. On low power, the lesion maintains the characteristic lobulation and, peripherally, typical areas of a fibroadenoma. The entire central portion of the image shows an epithelial proliferation occupying the center of the image. It is important to recognize the lobulo-centric architecture of the proliferation, a key feature of adenosis

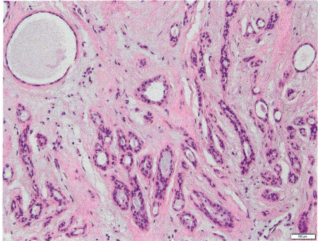

Fig. 9.16 On higher-power view of the lesion shown in Fig. 9.15, tubules lined by an attenuated myoepithelial layer can be appreciated. Immunohistochemistry for myoepithelial cell markers (p63/Calponin, S-100, CK 5/6) will demonstrate the presence of these cells in the areas of adenosis

- **Tubular adenoma** (Fig. 9.23). Tubular adenoma histologically shows a compact arrangement of uniform tubules lined by a dual cell bilayer of inner epithelial and outer myoepithelial cells. Similar to the conventional FA, these lesions are always well-circumscribed radiologically and lack a capsule. Some lesions may show areas of otherwise conventional fibroadenomas admixed with tubular adenoma areas. This supports the notion that many of these entities in fact lie on a spectrum of fibroepithelial lesions of the breast.

Fig. 9.17 Fibroadenoma with atypical ductal hyperplasia (left). Atypical architectural features are beginning to emerge within the epithelial elements of this fibroadenoma

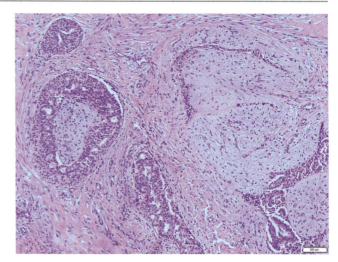

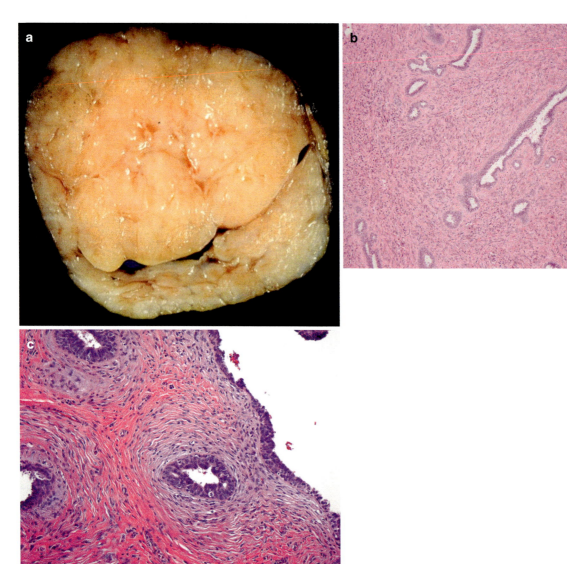

Fig. 9.18 (**a**) Cellular fibroadenoma showing a tan-yellow appearance owing to its increased cellularity. (**b**) The cleft-like space in the lower portion of the image corresponds to an intracanalicular growth pattern in that area. Histologically, there is stromal hypercellularity. (**c**) Focal areas of stromal condensation around the epithelium; however, this is typically focal. Note that there is no stromal nuclear atypia or obvious mitoses

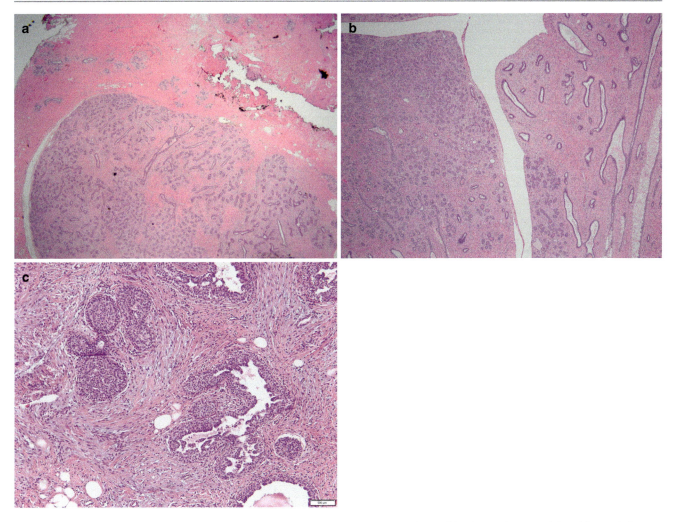

Fig. 9.19 (**a**, **b**) Juvenile fibroadenomas are well-circumscribed and, like conventional fibroadenomas, can show a mix of both pericanalicular and intracanalicular growth patterns. (**c**) These lesions often harbor areas of epithelial proliferation such as usual ductal hyperplasia seen here and micropapillary hyperplasia (bottom) with tapering papillae reminiscent of that seen in gynecomastia

- **Lactating adenoma (nodular gestational hyperplasia)** (Fig. 9.24). Depending on the author's preference, nodular gestational hyperplasia (lactating adenoma) is sometimes considered a variant of fibroadenoma showing physiologic, secretory epithelial changes. This lesion may occur during pregnancy or the postpartum period. Histologically, it shows compact arrangement and hyperplasia of true acini arranged in the alveolar pattern of the lactating breast. The luminal cells are enlarged with vacuolated cytoplasm. These lesions can become quite large, and due to their rapid growth during pregnancy can have a concerning, clinical presentation; however, they are benign. Because of this, lactating adenomas are encountered in routine biopsies. Due to their rapid proliferation, necrosis may be noted in the lesions and should not be regarded as an atypical finding [12].
- **Fibroadenomatoid changes**. "Fibroadenomatoid changes" is the term used to describe parenchymal changes which resemble a fibroadenoma, but collectively do not form a discrete, well-circumscribed mass lesion. This entity is considered to represent non-neoplastic, stromal hyperplastic changes, unlike fibroadenomas which are benign neoplasms.

Fibroadenomas are benign lesions, and after the core biopsy diagnosis, they are typically managed surgically by complete excision or non-surgically with monitoring by imaging. Fibroadenomas with a history of rapid growth in size are typically excised completely for a full histologic evaluation [13, 14]. Regarding the inherent risk of cancer harbored by FAs, when confined to the FA, the presence of atypical ductal or lobular proliferations does not denote an increase in subsequent cancer risk. Complex fibroadenomas, however, have been reported to be associated with a higher relative risk for cancer development [15].

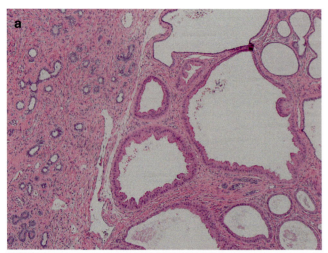

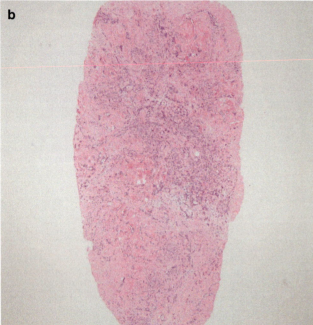

The phyllodes tumor is an important entity in the differential diagnosis because of its impact on clinical management and outcomes. Although the different features will be discussed below, it has been recently postulated that fibroadenomas and phyllodes tumors may not be entirely mutually exclusive. For example, a study of the long-term outcome of malignant phyllodes tumors showed that a considerable proportion of patients with phyllodes tumors had a clinical history of previous fibroadenoma, suggesting that fibroadenomas can potentially undergo malignant transformation to a phyllodes tumor [16]. Also, areas of fibroadenomatoid changes are not uncommon in phyllodes tumors, which not only complicates the diagnostic challenge but also suggests a possible relationship between these fibroepithelial lesions (Fig. 9.25).

Differential diagnosis in fibroadenoma is done with the following lesions:

- **Hamartomas** of the breast show a similar clinical presentation to that of FA: a mobile, well-circumscribed mass. Compared to the fibroadenoma, the histology shows a *dis-*

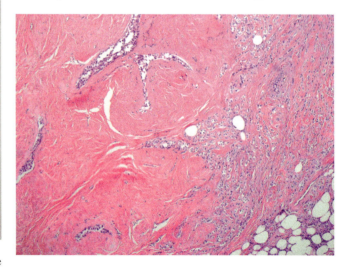

Fig. 9.20 (**a**) Complex fibroadenoma with cystic spaces, apocrine metaplasia, and (**b**) sclerosing adenosis

Fig. 9.22 Fibroadenoma with invasive lobular carcinoma

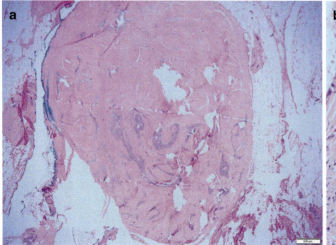

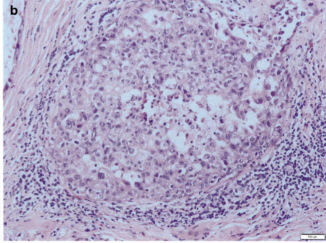

Fig. 9.21 (**a**, **b**) Fibroadenoma with DCIS. Aside from the focus of epithelial proliferation in the center of the image, this fibroadenoma is extensively hyalinized with few other epithelial elements. Higher power shows high grade DCIS with central necrosis

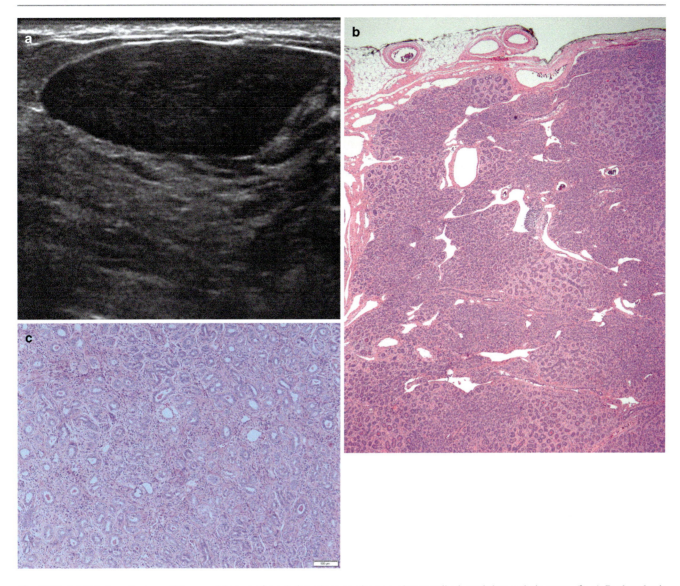

Fig. 9.23 (**a**) Tubular adenoma. Ultrasound image of a tubular adenoma shows a circumscribed, oval, hypoechoic mass. (**b**, **c**) Back-to-back tubules characterize this variant of fibroadenoma

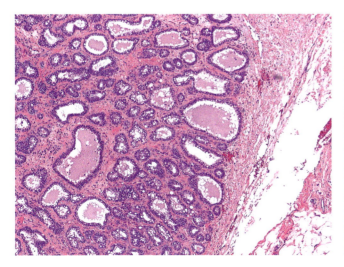

Fig. 9.24 Lactating adenoma showing numerous tubules with luminal eosinophilic secretions, lined by cells with vacuolated cytoplasms and minimal nuclear atypia

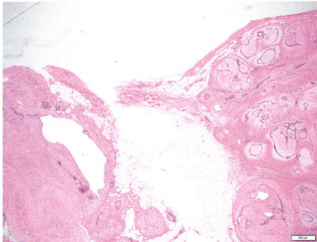

Fig. 9.25 Fibroadenoma (right) with area of phyllodes tumor (left). The bottom left (adjacent to the phyllodes tumor) shows areas of fibro-adenomatoid change

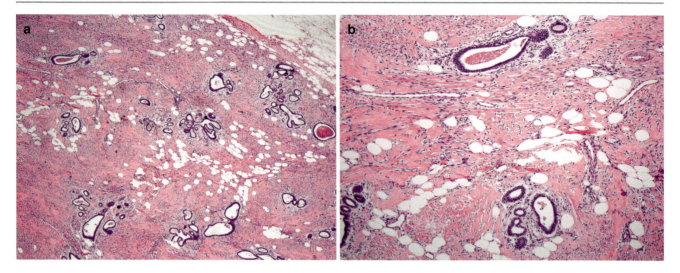

Fig. 9.26 (**a, b**) Breast hamartoma. This lesion is a well-circumscribed nodule of haphazardly arranged breast elements. Hamartomas frequently contain adipose tissue and pseudoangiomatoid stromal hyperplasia, both helpful features when diagnosing this entity

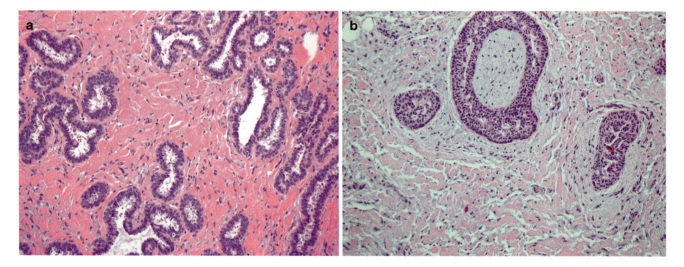

Fig. 9.27 (**a**) Pseudoangiomatous stromal hyperplasia can be a mass-forming lesion or can be seen within fibroepithelial lesions, such as in these high-power images of a hamartoma and (**b**) fibroadenoma. The fibroadenoma also shows usual ductal hyperplasia

ordered combination of histologically normal ductal and lobular structures (Fig. 9.26). This contrasts the regularly distributed epithelial components seen in a FA. On core biopsy, the well-demarcated border initially helps to identify the hamartoma as lesional breast tissue, as opposed to sampling of normal parenchyma that would lack the sharp margins seen in an hamartoma. Although hamartomas can show stromal changes similar to those seen in a FA, such as hyalinization and occasional myoid differentiation, hamartomas are not typically stroma-predominant lesions. The frequent presence of adipose tissue within the hamartoma helps to distinguish this from a FA.

- **Pseudoangiomatous stromal hyperplasia (PASH)** is a proliferation of interlobular myofibroblasts, imparting

small, cleft-like spaces in the stroma reminiscent of vascular spaces (Fig. 9.27). PASH can form a well-circumscribed lesion alone; however, it is also a common finding in the stroma of fibroepithelial lesions, such as fibroadenomas and hamartomas.

- **Nodular sclerosing adenosis** is characterized by a marked proliferation of compressed, slit-like glandular structures, embedded in a background of hyalinized stroma (Fig. 9.28). Low-power magnification is critical to this diagnosis. This lesion is unencapsulated; however, the crowded glands of nodular sclerosing adenosis conform to the architecture of an expanded, but well-defined lobule. On core biopsy, this can be challenging, as the differential includes both tubular adenoma and

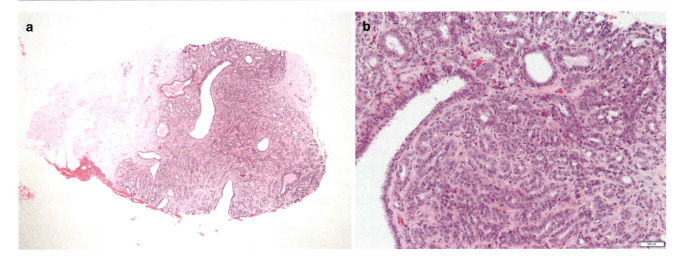

Fig. 9.28 (**a**) Nodular sclerosing adenosis as seen in a core biopsy. The lesion is relatively well-circumscribed with open and closed tubules that frequently extend beyond the main nodule. (**b**) Notice the proliferation of round and slit-like glandular spaces

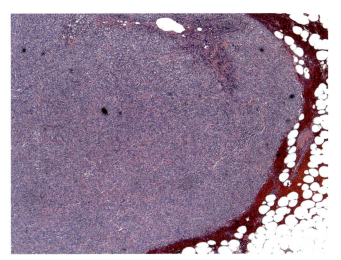

Fig. 9.29 Solitary fibrous tumors showing a well-circumscribed border. The spindle cells proliferation and dense bands of hyaline sclerosis can be appreciated

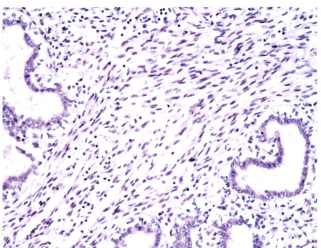

Fig. 9.30 Breast adenomyoepitheliomas are biphasic tumors with epithelial and spindle cells. They can have a variegated appearance owing in part to the morphologic spectrum of myoepithelial cells

carcinoma. The patent, round lumens of a tubular adenoma help distinguish it from nodular sclerosing adenosis. Carcinoma can be excluded with the use of myoepithelial markers as they will demonstrate the intact myoepithelial cells of nodular sclerosing adenosis.

- Although the stroma of a **solitary fibrous tumor** (SFT) can resemble a fibroadenoma, SFT fundamentally lacks an epithelial component (Fig. 9.29). SFT shows varying cellularity within the lesion, scattered bands of sclerosis, and occasionally its characteristic staghorn vasculature.
- **Adenomyoepithelioma** is a biphasic tumor with both a glandular and mesenchymal proliferation; however, its cellular stroma is comprised of myoepithelial cells, which

demonstrate diffuse expression of myoepithelial cell markers with IHC. The adenomyoepithelioma has various histologic patterns, as myoepithelial cells display a wide spectrum of cellular morphology (i.e., spindled, plasmacytoid, and abundant clear cytoplasm) (Fig. 9.30). Recognizing the prominent proliferation of myoepithelial cells is key to the diagnosis.

- Although **intraductal papillomas** alone intrinsically lack the classic features of a fibroadenoma, rarely, papillomas can be a part of a fibroadenoma's epithelial component, especially in the juvenile fibroadenoma. It is imperative to correlate biopsy findings with imaging. For example, if there is a discrepancy between the size of the intraductal papilloma and the size of the mass on imaging, carefully study the background parenchyma for stromal features suggestive of a fibroadenoma. This is to be distinguished from juvenile papillomatosis, a rather uncommon mass-like lesion composed of cysts and epithelial proliferation. This entity lacks the predominant stromal proliferation and nodular growth pattern of fibroadenomas.

- FA with prominent myxoid stroma tend be hypocellular lesions with decreased stromal cells and epithelial components. On core biopsy, the presence of only myxoid stroma could raise the possibility of a myxoma, but myxomas are uncommon lesions of the breast. However, the more important consideration when faced with acellular myxoid stroma is a **mucinous lesion**, such as a mucocele or mucinous carcinoma. Both mucocele and mucinous carcinoma can have a well-circumscribed appearance. Evaluation of the entire lesion may be necessary to resolve this distinction. In general, histologic evaluation of a mucinous lesion in its entirety is strongly encouraged to exclude mucinous carcinoma.

9.2 Phyllodes Tumor

In contrast to the patient demographics typical of fibroadenomas, phyllodes tumor (PT) characteristically presents one to two decades later and is heralded by a rapidly growing mass or sudden increased size of a pre-existing mass [17]. By imaging, phyllodes tumors present as large, multilobulated lesions that may show cleft like cystic spaces (Figs. 9.31 and 9.32).

Grossly, the cut surface is lobulated with cleft-like spaces, a reflection of its classic "leaf-like" architecture (Fig. 9.33). Necrosis may be present, secondary to either ischemic or tumor necrosis (Fig. 9.34). Overlying skin changes are not uncommon and range from discoloration to skin ulceration (Fig. 9.35). Nipple retraction can occur but is a less common physical finding [18].

As in fibroadenomas, the stromal component of a PT predominates over the epithelial component. Phyllodes tumors are diagnosed based on the presence of the following stromal features: stromal cellularity, stromal cytologic atypia, stromal mitotic activity, and prominence of stromal overgrowth [1]. Additionally, the degree to which the above diagnostic

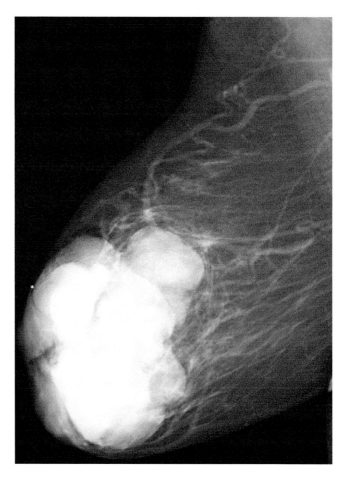

Fig. 9.31 Mammogram of a Phyllodes tumor shows a large circumscribed, multilobulated dense mass

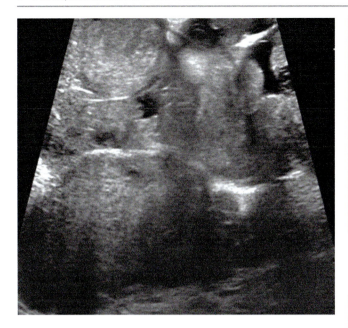

Fig. 9.32 Ultrasound, corresponding to Fig. 9.31, shows the cleft-like cystic spaces

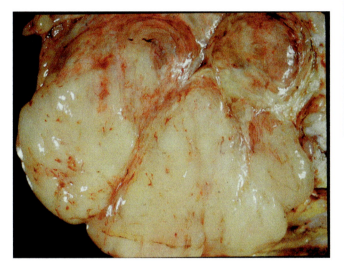

Fig. 9.33 Gross image of a benign Phyllodes tumor showing sharply accentuated nodules and deep grooves. A gelatinous cut surface suggests myxoid changes within the lesion

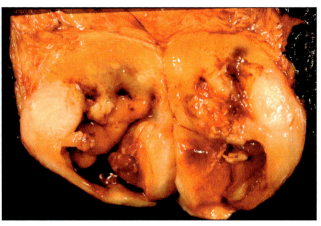

Fig. 9.34 Malignant Phyllodes tumor with a centrally hemorrhagic, friable area, consistent with necrosis

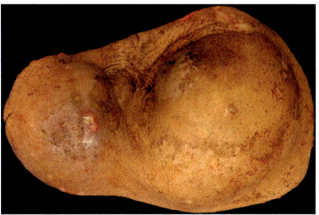

Fig. 9.35 Phyllodes tumor that has ulcerated the overlying skin

features are present further stratify PTs into the following major histologic subtypes: benign, borderline, and malignant. This histologic classification is based on recommendations from the World Health Organization [1]. These histologic subtypes carry important prognostic value and clinical implications (Table 9.1).

In addition to the three features used in the tumor subtyping, it is important to understand the fundamental characteristics of PT. The classic leaf-like silhouette of the PT is created by the stromal proliferation compressing the ductal elements into thin, slit-like spaces. This is an exaggerated intracanalicular pattern of growth. The other growth pattern

is pericanalicular, in which the stroma grows circumferentially around the epithelial structures without compression. (These patterns are analogous to those described in fibroadenomas, contributing to the extensive morphologic overlap of these lesions.) In PT, both intracanalicular and pericanalicular growth patterns are usually present.

- **Stromal overgrowth** is a feature limited to the borderline and malignant phyllodes subtypes. To assess for the presence of stromal overgrowth, one should see stromal proliferation without epithelial elements in at least one low-power field (×4) [9]. This feature is rarely observed in fibroadenoma.
- **Subepithelial stromal condensation** describes the distinct enhancement of stromal hypercellularity immediately beneath the epithelial component (Fig. 9.36). This creates a "cambium layer" similar conceptually to that seen in the embryonal rhabdomyosarcoma. The "cambium layer" can be seen in all subgroups of PT and serves as a good predictor of PT in biopsies when present [10].

Table 9.1 Phyllodes tumor subtyping into benign, borderline, and malignant

Subtype	Stromal hypercellularity	Stromal cytologic atypia	Mitotic activity (stromal) per 10 high-power fields (hpf)	Tumor border	Comments
Benign	Mild	Minimal	<5	Pushing border (well-defined)	Stromal overgrowth not present
Borderline	Moderate/high	Moderate	Frequent (5–9)	Pushing ± focal infiltrative	Features intermediate between benign and malignant
Malignant	High	Marked; + pleomorphism	>10	Infiltrative	High-grade sarcoma features with marked stromal overgrowth; ± focal fibrosarcoma-like appearance; ± heterologous elements

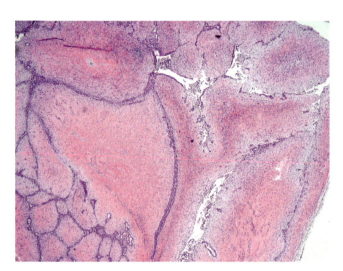

Fig. 9.36 Low-power magnification of a Phyllodes tumor showing stromal overgrowth and subepithelial stromal condensation (cambium layer)

- **Stromal atypia** refers to the nuclear membrane irregularity, degree and variation in nuclear size, and presence of nucleoli (Fig. 9.37). Frank nuclear pleomorphism is generally restricted to the malignant phyllodes. Scattered multinucleated, degenerative atypia (like stromal giant cells seen in FA, see above) is not considered pleomorphism.

In an attempt to standardize some of the above grading/subtyping criteria, previous studies have proposed different measuring sticks to grade **stromal hypercellularity**. A study by Jacobs et al. [19] used normal perilobular stroma cellularity as a reference for grading stromal hypercellularity. For instance, twice the cellularity of normal perilobular stroma along with no overlapping of stromal cells is considered mild hypercellularity. High cellularity shows stromal cells with extensive overlapping, and moderate hypercellularity is in between mild and high (Fig. 9.38).

Another informative feature included in the table is the **tumor border**: the interface between the tumor and adjacent parenchyma. As the lesion advances in histologic grade, there is a greater propensity for an invasive border, a factor which can complicate surgical excision and predispose to recurrence. Focal areas of an invasive tumor border in what appears to be a benign PT or cellular fibroadenoma warrants a careful consideration of borderline PT (Fig. 9.39).

Figures 9.40, 9.41, 9.42, and 9.43 show examples of PTs of various subtypes.

Histologic subtype (grade) of the PT is currently the major factor in predicting clinical outcome. The malignant PT carries the highest risk for recurrence and metastasis; however, all grades of PT harbor the potential (albeit of variable degrees) for local recurrence and metastasis. Overall, the rates of metastatic disease are related to histologic subtype and have been reported with much variability, ranging from 0% to 28.6% of patients. Local recurrence ranges from 10% to 30% [10, 20]. Benign PTs behave in a similar clinical fashion to FA; however, as indicated in the previous statement, a small subset of benign PT can recur and/or metastasize. Consequently, the mainstay for management of a PT of any histologic grade includes excision with clear margins. The role for chemotherapy and radiation is not entirely elucidated for malignant PT, most likely due to its uncommon occurrence. Sentinel lymph node biopsy and/or excision is not routinely performed in this setting, since metastasis of PT is generally via the hematogenous route with the common sites of metastasis being the lung and bone. Axillary lymphadenopathy is common but is frequently secondary to reactive lymph node changes; however, axillary lymph node metastasis is a rare event [18, 21].

As mentioned above, the standard of care for PT is surgical excision with clear margins. Efforts are being made in recent literature to define the adequacy of a negative margin (i.e., 1.0 cm versus narrower). Given the wide range of tumor recurrence frequency, margin status and adequacy are being

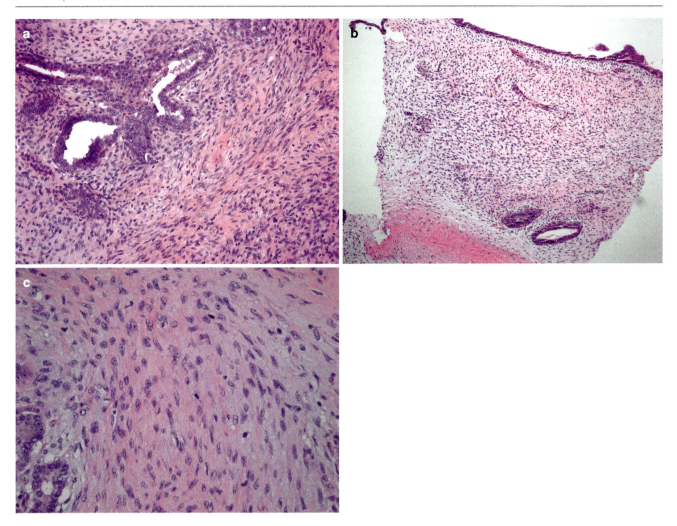

Fig. 9.37 (a–c) Phyllodes tumor demonstrating stromal hypercellularity with stromal cells showing nuclear atypia with irregular nuclear contours, variability in nuclear size, and nucleoli

studied in terms of the true correlation with recurrence rate. Conflicting data has emerged on this topic with new studies finding that a positive surgical margin does not predict recurrence [22]. Additional studies have looked at adequacy of negative margins, with a 1-cm margin showing no advantage over narrower negative margins [23]. A major discrepancy between the lack of correlation with margin status and recurrence may be related to multifocality of the tumor, as well as background fibroadenomatoid change, a potential precursor of new fibroepithelial tumor foci [23].

Within the class of fibroepithelial lesions, perhaps the most challenging distinction is between fibroadenoma and the benign and borderline PT. As previously mentioned, these biphasic tumors exhibit the same stromal growth patterns—intracanalicular and pericanalicular. The intracana-

licular pattern, which contributes to the PT's classic leaf-like architecture, can also be seen in FA; however, it is usually focal and not as well developed and exaggerated as in PT. In a biopsy, this feature is sometimes present as "stromal fragmentation," in which a fragment of stroma is peripherally lined by epithelium, representing the exaggerated cleft-like spaces [9]. The cellular fibroadenoma presents a unique difficulty on core biopsy, as its increased stromal hypercellularity mimics that of PT. Recent studies have aimed to evaluate various features that may help distinguish these two entities on biopsy [9, 24]. For instance, mitotic activity in cellular FA is usually less than 3 per 10 high-power field. In other words, cellular fibroadenomas exhibit an inappropriately low mitotic rate compared to what would be expected for a PT of comparable stromal hypercellularity. Stromal overgrowth, when

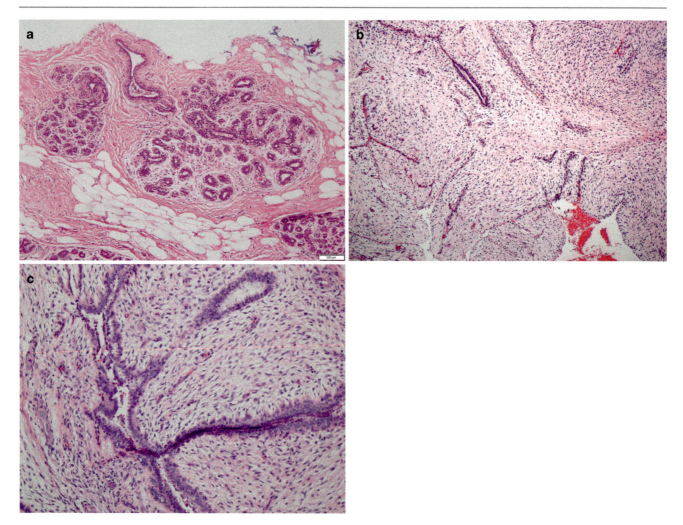

Fig. 9.38 (**a**) Normal perilobular stroma for comparison used in gauging stromal hypercellularity. (**b**, **c**) Examples of stromal hypercellularity in Phyllodes tumors

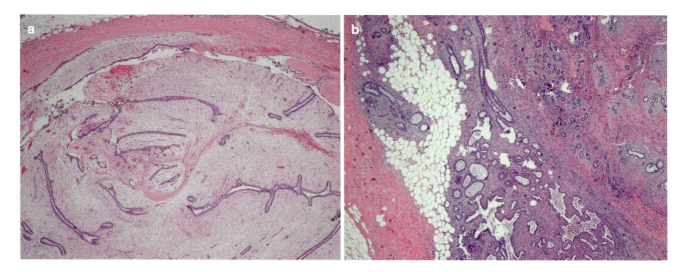

Fig. 9.39 (**a**) Benign Phyllodes tumor showing a pushing border/interface with the adjacent parenchyma. (**b**) Borderline tumors can show foci of invasion at their border

present, is strongly suggestive of a PT, as this is rarely observed in the fibroadenoma regardless of stromal cellularity. The tumor border can be very informative when examining fibroepithelial lesions. Fibroadenomas, regardless of cellularity, will show a well-defined border, unlike borderline PT, which can show focal areas of invasion. In the context of hypercellularity and stromal overgrowth, adipose tissue within the stroma has also been shown to be more frequent in PT [9, 24]. It is most important to evaluate all the aforementioned features when assessing a fibroepithelial lesion. At least three mitoses per 10 high-power fields generally favor a PT. In the absence of increased mitotic, a combination of the above helps favor PT over cellular FA [9, 24].

Despite the aforementioned features to discriminate between these two neoplasms, on core biopsies the distinction may still not be possible. The pathologist may make a

diagnosis of "fibroepithelial lesion" with a qualifying statement that the differential includes both fibroadenomas and PT. The natural history of these indeterminate core biopsies has been studied with roughly one-third of patients being diagnosed with PT following surgical excision [25].

With only stromal components present in biopsy material, fibromatosis and metaplastic carcinoma, including the fibromatosis-like/spindle cell type, are in the differential diagnosis (Fig. 9.44). Cytokeratin (CK) positivity with immunohistochemistry supports metaplastic carcinoma, as borderline PT are typically negative for CK. Histologically, fibromatosis exhibits bland spindle cells that are arranged in long, sweeping fascicles with scattered bands of hyalinized collagen. Fibromatosis consistently displays an infiltrative border. Although phyllodes tumors can show occasional fascicular stromal pattern, fibromatosis is not a biphasic lesion,

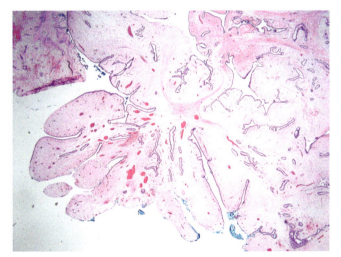

Fig. 9.40 Benign phyllodes tumor with classic leaf-like architecture, an exaggerated intracanalicular pattern of stromal growth

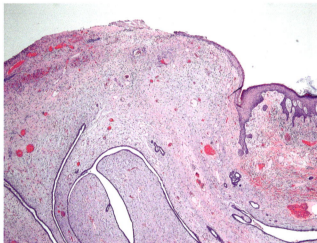

Fig. 9.42 Phyllodes tumors can cause skin changes ranging from discoloration to ulceration of overlying skin, as seen here

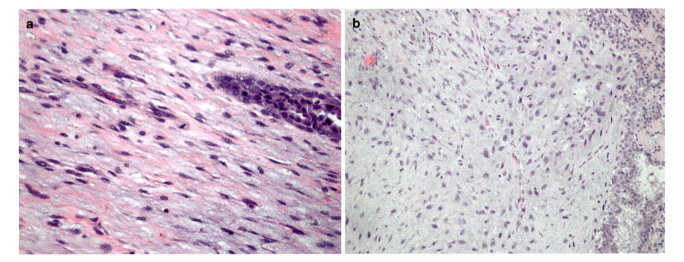

Fig. 9.41 (**a, b**) Mitotic figures are readily seen in the stroma of phyllodes tumors

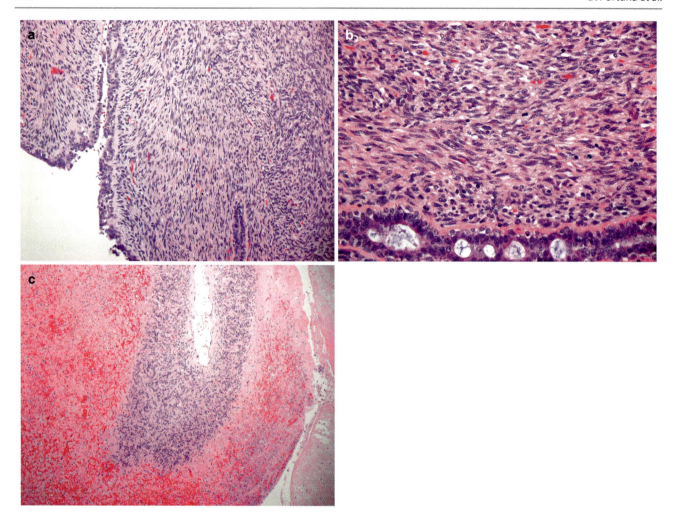

Fig. 9.43 (**a**, **b**) Malignant Phyllodes tumor. Stromal hypercellularity, mitotic figures and nuclear atypia are readily seen even at low power. (**c**) The tumor shows a peritheliomatous pattern of necrosis—prominent tumor necrosis with sparing of the tumor, which immediately surrounds a large blood vessel

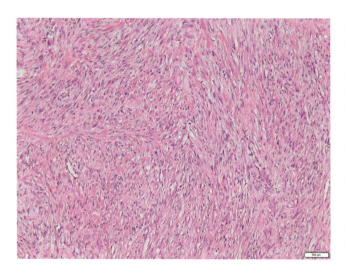

Fig. 9.44 Breast metaplastic carcinoma with spindle cells. Small fragments of tumor in a core biopsy raise the possibility of the stroma of a Phyllodes tumor. Immunohistochemical stains can be helpful in this differential

and, therefore, will not have a closely associated epithelial component other than the entrapment of the surrounding breast tissue. Beta-catenin nuclear positivity can be seen in both fibromatosis and PT [26]; therefore, morphology will be most helpful in distinguishing these two entities, and clinical and radiologic correlation are imperative.

The entity "periductal stromal tumor" refers to a low-grade, malignant fibroepithelial tumor that shows considerable morphologic overlap with phyllodes tumor. It is a rare entity and is characterized by its lack of the exaggerated intracanalicular ("leaf-like") architecture seen in PT, and instead shows a predominantly pericanalicular pattern of stromal growth [1]. Transformation to phyllodes tumor has been reported in cases of this lesion [27]. According to the WHO classification of breast tumors, this entity may represent part of the PT disease spectrum.

Malignant PT. On a core biopsy, a malignant PT will typically present as a high-grade malignancy with

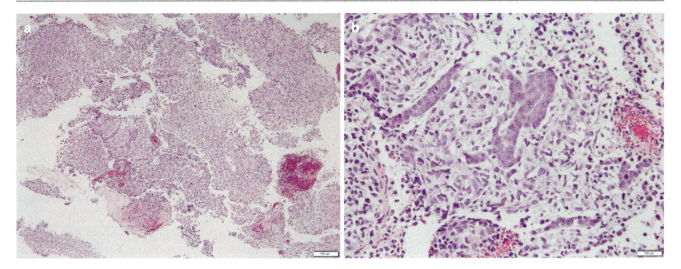

Fig. 9.45 (**a**) Breast metaplastic carcinoma. Low-power magnification shows fragments of a high grade sarcomatoid neoplasm. (**b**) Higher power shows frankly malignant ductal elements, which is highly suggestive of a carcinoma rather than a Phyllodes tumor

sarcomatous features. If a core biopsy shows a high-grade malignancy with sarcomatous features without an epithelial component, the pathologist should exclude the possibility of a malignant PT with scant evidence of the epithelial component (e.g., stromal overgrowth). Malignant PT is more common than primary or metastatic sarcomas of the breast; however, malignant PT is less common than carcinoma. With these histologic features, the most likely primary carcinoma would be a metaplastic carcinoma, sarcomatoid type. A very helpful morphologic feature favoring malignant PT is identifying the characteristic leaf-like architecture created by the intracanalicular growth of stroma. Abundant stromal overgrowth, a prominent feature of malignant PT, may make finding these areas difficult; therefore, extensive sampling of the tumor is required [10]. The findings of in situ carcinoma (DCIS) or associated malignant epithelial elements favor a metaplastic carcinoma (Fig. 9.45).

Immunohistochemistry can be a useful in this differential diagnosis. Although cytokeratins are used in routine practice to resolve the issue of carcinoma with ease, malignant PT can show some stromal CK positivity [28]. This staining is typically focal, compared to the more diffuse cytokeratin positivity in carcinoma, but keep in mind that the extent of staining may be difficult to assess with limited biopsy material. A panel of CKs is recommended if the differential diagnosis favors a metaplastic carcinoma. An example CK panel includes: pan-CK (AE1/AE3), high molecular weight CK (CK903 / cytokeratin 34βE12), CAM 5.2, CK7 [29]. CD34, a marker that is commonly positive in the stromal cells of PT, is usually negative in metaplastic carcinomas. However, CD34 positivity is only seen in approximately 50% of malignant PT [28]. In light of the above discussion, it may not be possible to render a definitive diagnosis on core biopsy. The distinction should then be made on excision as the treatment for these entities is quite different.

9.3 Immunohistochemistry in the Diagnosing of Fibroepithelial Lesions

There is no single marker that can help in the distinction between fibroadenomas and PT; therefore, this distinction relies on the clinical, radiologic, and pathologic features of the lesion. The most significant role for immunohistochemistry in fibroepithelial lesions is in the exclusion process of various entities in the differential diagnosis. When faced with a core biopsy showing a sarcomatoid process with no epithelial elements present, whether high- or intermediate-grade lesions, the use of multiple cytokeratin stains (including high molecular weight CK) and p63 to exclude a carcinoma should be considered, especially metaplastic carcinoma (sarcomatoid types). See the above differential diagnoses sections for more details on the staining patterns of respective entities. Regarding hormone receptors in fibroepithelial lesions, the stromal component of fibroadenomas shows estrogen-dependent growth. Estrogen receptor positivity is inversely related to histologic grade of PT (malignant PTs shows low positivity). While interesting in a pathophysiologic perspective, hormone receptor status does not currently play a role in routine clinical practice [30].

Conclusion

Fibroadenomas, in fact, will constitute the majority of fibroepithelial lesions seen in routine practice. However, the purpose of the core biopsy in this setting is to exclude the more biologically significant process: the phyllodes tumor. Despite considerable morphologic overlap, the clinical management and implications are quite different. A diagnosis of PT will result in surgical excision, whereas other fibroepithelial lesions may be managed conservatively. Occasionally, a lesion may show features indeterminate between fibroadenoma and PT. In these cases, it may be appropriate to diagnose a fibroepithelial lesion, noting PT cannot be excluded. Clinical and radiologic correlation is critical in all cases.

References

1. Tan P, Tse G, Lee A, Simpson J, Hanby A. Fibroepithelial tumors. In: Lakhani S, Ellis I, Schnitt S, Tan P, van de Vijver M, editors. WHO classifications of tumors of the breast. 4th ed. Lyon: IARC Press; 2012. p. 142–7.
2. Darwish A, Nasr AO, El Hassan LA, Fahal AH. Cyclosporine-A therapy-induced multiple bilateral breast and accessory axillary breast fibroadenomas: a case report. J Med Case Rep. 2010;4:267.
3. Weinstein SP, Orel SG, Collazzo L, Conant EF, Lawton TJ, Czerniecki B. Cyclosporin A-induced fibroadenomas of the breast: report of five cases. Radiology. 2001;220(2):465–8.
4. Yang X, Kandil D, Cosar EF, Khan A. Fibroepithelial tumors of the breast: pathologic and immunohistochemical features and molecular mechanisms. Arch Pathol Lab Med. 2014;138(1):25–36.
5. Cericatto R, Pozzobon A, Morsch DM, Menke CH, Brum IS, Spritzer PM. Estrogen receptor-alpha, bcl-2 and c-myc gene expression in fibroadenomas and adjacent normal breast: association with nodule size, hormonal and reproductive features. Steroids. 2005;70(3):153–60.
6. Sapino A, Bosco M, Cassoni P, Castellano I, Arisio R, Cserni G, et al. Estrogen receptor-beta is expressed in stromal cells of fibroadenoma and phyllodes tumors of the breast. Mod Pathol. 2006;19(4):599–606.
7. Goel NB, Knight TE, Pandey S, Riddick-Young M, de Paredes ES, Trivedi A. Fibrous lesions of the breast: imaging-pathologic correlation. Radiographics. 2005;25(6):1547–59.
8. Kuijper A, Mommers EC, van der Wall E, van Diest PJ. Histopathology of fibroadenoma of the breast. Am J Clin Pathol. 2001;115(5):736–42.
9. Yasir S, Gamez R, Jenkins S, Visscher DW, Nassar A. Significant histologic features differentiating cellular fibroadenoma from phyllodes tumor on core needle biopsy specimens. Am J Clin Pathol. 2014;142(3):362–9.
10. Tan BY, Acs G, Apple SK, Badve S, Bleiweiss IJ, Brogi E, et al. Phyllodes tumours of the breast: a consensus review. Histopathology. 2016;68(1):5–21.
11. Diaz NM, Palmer JO, McDivitt RW. Carcinoma arising within fibroadenomas of the breast. A clinicopathologic study of 105 patients. Am J Clin Pathol. 1991;95(5):614–22.
12. Sanders M, Brooks J, Palazzo J. Mesenchymal lesions of the breast. In: Palazzo JP, editor. Difficult diagnoses in breast pathology. New York, NY: Demos Medical; 2011. p. 172–95.
13. Guray M, Sahin AA. Benign breast diseases: classification, diagnosis, and management. Oncologist. 2006;11(5):435–49.
14. Greenberg R, Skornick Y, Kaplan O. Management of breast fibroadenomas. J Gen Intern Med. 1998;13(9):640–5.
15. Dupont WD, Page DL, Parl FF, Vnencak-Jones CL, Plummer WD Jr, Rados MS, et al. Long-term risk of breast cancer in women with fibroadenoma. N Engl J Med. 1994;331(1):10–5.
16. Abe M, Miyata S, Nishimura S, Iijima K, Makita M, Akiyama F, et al. Malignant transformation of breast fibroadenoma to malignant phyllodes tumor: long-term outcome of 36 malignant phyllodes tumors. Breast Cancer. 2011;18(4):268–72.
17. Krishnamurthy S, Ashfaq R, Shin HJ, Sneige N. Distinction of phyllodes tumor from fibroadenoma: a reappraisal of an old problem. Cancer. 2000;90(6):342–9.
18. Mishra SP, Tiwary SK, Mishra M, Khanna AK. Phyllodes tumor of breast: a review article. ISRN Surg. 2013;2013:361469.
19. Jacobs TW, Chen YY, Guinee DG Jr, Holden JA, Cha I, Bauermeister DE, et al. Fibroepithelial lesions with cellular stroma on breast core needle biopsy: are there predictors of outcome on surgical excision? Am J Clin Pathol. 2005;124(3):342–54.

20. Mituś JW, Blecharz P, Walasek T, Reinfuss M, Jakubowicz J, Kulpa J. Treatment of patients with distant metastases from phyllodes tumor of the breast. World J Surg. 2016;40(2):323–8.

21. Telli ML, Horst KC, Guardino AE, Dirbas FM, Carlson RW. Phyllodes tumors of the breast: natural history, diagnosis, and treatment. J Natl Compr Cancer Netw. 2007;5(3):324–30.

22. Cowan ML, Argani P, Cimino-Mathews A. Benign and low-grade fibroepithelial neoplasms of the breast have low recurrence rate after positive surgical margins. Mod Pathol. 2016;29(3):259–65.

23. Jang JH, Choi MY, Lee SK, Kim S, Kim J, Lee J, et al. Clinicopathologic risk factors for the local recurrence of phyllodes tumors of the breast. Ann Surg Oncol. 2012;19(8):2612–7.

24. Lee AH, Hodi Z, Ellis IO, Elston CW. Histological features useful in the distinction of phyllodes tumour and fibroadenoma on needle core biopsy of the breast. Histopathology. 2007;51(3):336–44.

25. Van Osdol AD, Landercasper J, Andersen JJ, Ellis RL, Gensch EM, Johnson JM, et al. Determining whether excision of all fibroepithelial lesions of the breast is needed to exclude phyllodes tumor: upgrade rate of fibroepithelial lesions of the breast to phyllodes tumor. JAMA Surg. 2014;149(10):1081–5.

26. Lacroix-Triki M, Geyer FC, Lambros MB, Savage K, Ellis IO, Lee AH, et al. β-catenin/Wnt signalling pathway in fibromatosis, metaplastic carcinomas and phyllodes tumours of the breast. Mod Pathol. 2010;23(11):1438–48.

27. Burga AM, Tavassoli FA. Periductal stromal tumor: a rare lesion with low-grade sarcomatous behavior. Am J Surg Pathol. 2003;27(3):343–8.

28. Zhang Y, Kleer CG. Phyllodes tumor of the breast: histopathologic features, differential diagnosis, and molecular/genetic updates. Arch Pathol Lab Med. 2016;140(7):665–71.

29. Liu H. Application of immunohistochemistry in breast pathology: a review and update. Arch Pathol Lab Med. 2014;138(12):1629–42.

30. Tse GM, Lee CS, Kung FY, Scolyer RA, Law BK, Lau TS, et al. Hormonal receptors expression in epithelial cells of mammary phyllodes tumors correlates with pathologic grade of the tumor: a multicenter study of 143 cases. Am J Clin Pathol. 2002;118(4):522–6.

Anna Biernacka and Melinda F. Lerwill

Ductal hyperplasia of the breast is an intraductal proliferation of epithelial cells that is subdivided into two diagnostic categories: usual ductal hyperplasia and atypical ductal hyperplasia. Usual ductal hyperplasia represents a non-neoplastic proliferation that is commonly encountered as a component of fibrocystic changes. Atypical ductal hyperplasia, on the other hand, represents a neoplastic proliferation that shares cytologic and architectural features with ductal carcinoma in situ. Accurate differentiation between these two forms of ductal hyperplasia is important for patient management and breast cancer risk assessment.

10.1 Usual Ductal Hyperplasia

Usual ductal hyperplasia is a form of benign proliferative change in the breast. It is part of the spectrum of fibrocystic changes, and the amount of proliferation can range from slight to florid. It is not a direct precursor to carcinoma but is an indicator of breast tissue at a slightly increased risk for subsequent carcinoma.

10.1.1 Clinical Features

Usual ductal hyperplasia occurs over a broad age range, with a mean age of diagnosis of 54 years [1]. It is not associated with specific clinical findings. It does not usually represent the targeted lesion in stereotactic- or ultrasound-guided breast biopsies, although it may be a component of an underlying lesion (such as a radial scar or papilloma) that is targeted. In the setting of breast magnetic resonance imaging, usual ductal hyperplasia may contribute to abnormal enhancement as a component of proliferative fibrocystic changes [2].

A. Biernacka, MD, PhD
Department of Pathology, The University of Chicago Medicine and Biological Sciences, Chicago, IL, USA
e-mail: abiernacka@bsd.uchicago.edu

M. F. Lerwill, MD (⊠)
Department of Pathology, Massachusetts General Hospital and Harvard Medical School, Boston, MA, USA
e-mail: mlerwill@mgh.harvard.edu

© Springer International Publishing AG, part of Springer Nature 2018
S. Stolnicu, I. Alvarado-Cabrero (eds.), *Practical Atlas of Breast Pathology*, https://doi.org/10.1007/978-3-319-93257-6_10

10.1.2 Cytologic Features

Usual ductal hyperplasia is characterized by cells with relatively small nuclei that show mild variation in their sizes and shapes, lending a polymorphic appearance to the proliferation (Figs. 10.1, 10.2, 10.3, 10.4, 10.5, 10.6, 10.7, 10.8, and 10.9, Table 10.1). Some nuclei are plump while others are narrow; some are larger and others smaller. The nuclei are typically oval in contour, and they frequently have longitudinal grooves (imparting a "coffee bean"-like appearance) or simple folds in their nuclear membranes (Fig. 10.6). Some nuclei show asymmetrically tapered ends that result in teardrop-like shapes (Fig. 10.6). This variability in size and shape is a hallmark of usual ductal hyperplasia, but it should be noted that the degree of variation is relatively mild and overt pleomorphism or highly convoluted nuclei are not features of usual ductal hyperplasia.

The chromatin of the proliferative cells is euchromatic and lightly speckled, and small nucleoli are present (Fig. 10.5). Smaller, shrunken nuclei located in the center of the proliferation may demonstrate darker chromatin with loss of chromatinic detail (Figs. 10.4, 10.8, and 10.9). Eosinophilic intranuclear pseudoinclusions are common but are not present in every example of usual ductal hyperplasia (Figs. 10.2 and 10.6). The cytoplasm is eosinophilic and is not abundant, and the cell borders are typically indistinct.

Cellular maturation is seen in many examples of usual ductal hyperplasia: as the cells progress from a basal location toward the center of the proliferation, they progressively become smaller (Figs. 10.4, 10.8, and 10.9). The central mature cells have scant cytoplasm and small, almost pyknotic nuclei. While maturation is not seen in every case, it can be a useful diagnostic feature when present.

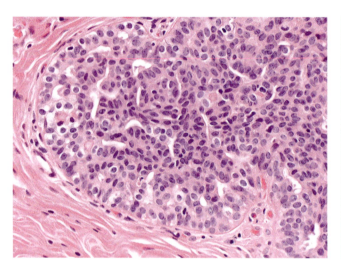

Fig. 10.1 Usual ductal hyperplasia is composed of a population of cells showing mild variation in nuclear size and shape and a streaming growth pattern

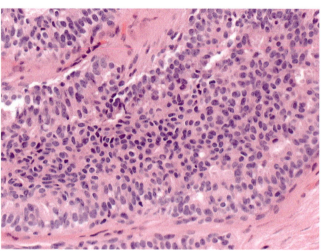

Fig. 10.3 Haphazardly arrayed nuclei in usual ductal hyperplasia

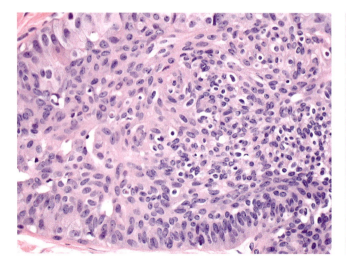

Fig. 10.2 The cells of usual ductal hyperplasia show a mild degree of cytologic variability and an uneven distribution of nuclei. Several intranuclear pseudoinclusions are also present (upper left)

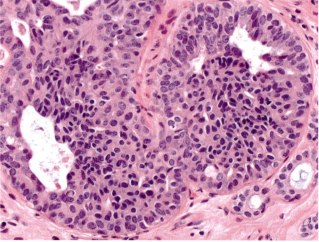

Fig. 10.4 Usual ductal hyperplasia showing overlapping, jumbled nuclei with variation in their sizes and shapes. Cells in the center of the proliferation are smaller with less cytoplasm and shrunken dark nuclei, a phenomenon known as maturation

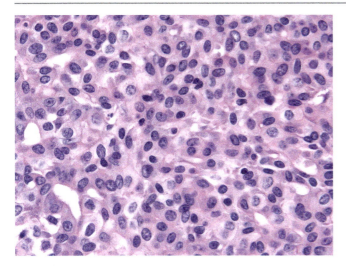

Fig. 10.5 Nuclei in usual ductal hyperplasia are oval with euchromatic chromatin and small nucleoli. They show a mild degree of variability in their size, shape, and distribution

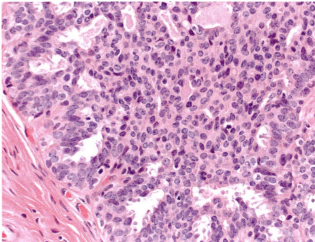

Fig. 10.7 Characteristic haphazard distribution of cells in usual ductal hyperplasia. Nuclei are euchromatic with mild variability and frequent nuclear grooves. Cellular polarity seen at the periphery is not an abnormal architectural feature if the polarized ductal cells rest upon the basement membrane

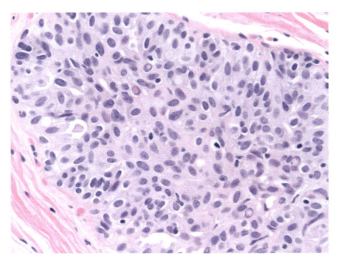

Fig. 10.6 Nuclei in usual ductal hyperplasia frequently show simple longitudinal grooves, tapered ends, and eosinophilic intranuclear pseudoinclusions

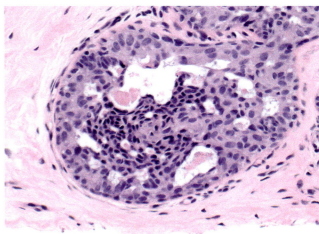

Fig. 10.8 The transition from plumper cells at the base to smaller cells with shrunken dark nuclei in the center is referred to as maturation. Maturation is seen in many examples of usual ductal hyperplasia

10.1.3 Architectural Features

The cells of usual ductal hyperplasia form a cohesive mass that displays an uneven distribution of nuclei, with some areas showing greater nuclear overlap than others. The oval nuclei are haphazardly arrayed along intersecting axes, imparting a jumbled appearance to the overall proliferation (Figs. 10.10, 10.11, and 10.12 and Table 10.1). The overall growth pattern has a streaming quality.

As the proliferative cells traverse the duct lumen, they often do so incompletely with the resulting formation of fenestrated gaps (Figs. 10.10, 10.11, 10.12, 10.13, and 10.14). These fenestrated spaces represent residual portions of the native duct lumen. The spaces classically have crescentic, slit-like shapes, and they are often prominent around the periphery of the proliferation but may also be found within the central mass of cells. The cells that border the fenestrations stream along the edge of the spaces, with the long axes of their nuclei running in parallel with the space. The cells do not demonstrate any regular apical-basal polarity relative to the luminal space (Figs. 10.10, 10.11, 10.12, 10.13, 10.14, and 10.15), which is in contrast to the polarized architectural features of atypical ductal hyperplasia (see Sect. 10.2.3). Thin strands of hyperplastic cells that connect proliferative aggregates often show conspicuous streaming growth.

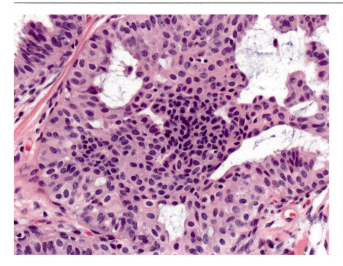

Fig. 10.9 Central mature nuclei often show a tight, overlapping distribution

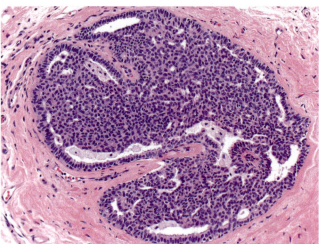

Fig. 10.10 Characteristic peripheral fenestrations of usual ductal hyperplasia

Table 10.1 Criteria for distinguishing usual ductal hyperplasia from low-grade ductal neoplasia

Cytologic features	Usual ductal hyperplasia	Atypical ductal hyperplasia and low-grade ductal carcinoma in situ
Cell population	Polymorphic	Monomorphic
Nuclear shape	Oval, elongated to tapered	Round or oval
Nuclear contours	Simple grooves	Smooth
Chromatin	Granular, slightly open, euchromatic	Homogeneous, fine, hyperchromatic
Nucleoli	Small nucleoli present	Usually inconspicuous
Nuclear pseudoinclusions	Often present	Rare
Cytoplasm – amount	Modest	Increased
Cytoplasm – staining quality	Eosinophilic	Eosinophilic or amphophilic, pale
Cell borders	Inconspicuous	Often conspicuous
Cellular maturation	Often present	Absent
Architectural features	**Usual ductal hyperplasia**	**Atypical ductal hyperplasia and low-grade ductal carcinoma in situ**
Cell distribution	Jumbled, overlapping nuclei	Uniformly spaced nuclei
Polarization around luminal spaces	Absent	Present
Architectural patterns	Fenestrations, solid growth with overlapping nuclei, uncommonly micropapillae	Cribriform spaces, Roman arches, trabecular bars, micropapillae, solid growth with regular nuclear spacing

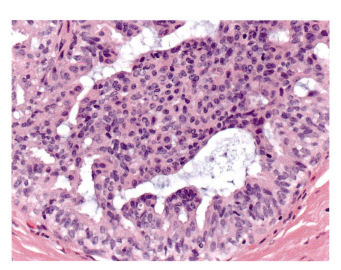

Fig. 10.11 The hyperplastic cells stream along the edges of the spaces, with the long axes of their nuclei in parallel with the edge of the space

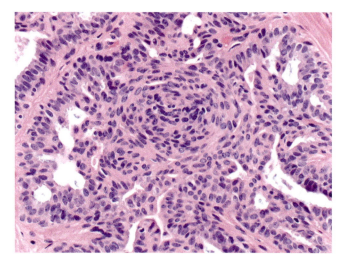

Fig. 10.12 Swirling growth pattern that is common in usual ductal hyperplasia

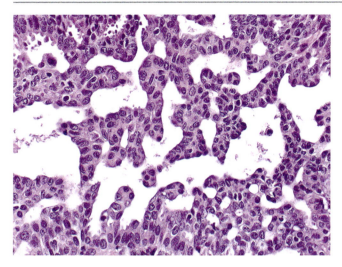

Fig. 10.13 Complex fenestrated spaces in usual ductal hyperplasia. The spaces have irregular shapes, and the cells are randomly arrayed relative to the space and do not show evidence of polarity

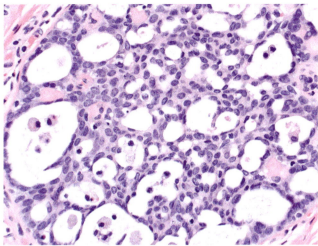

Fig. 10.15 Although the spaces in this example of usual ductal hyperplasia are round and superficially mimic cribriform spaces, the cells that border the spaces stream along the edges and lack polarity. The arrangement of the cells relative to the space is more important diagnostically than the shape of the space

10.1.4 Variant Features

Occasional variant features may be encountered that can lead to diagnostic consideration of atypical ductal hyperplasia or ductal carcinoma in situ.

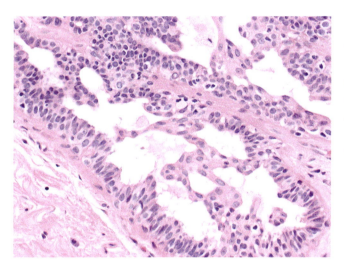

Fig. 10.14 Thin strands of hyperplastic cells traversing the duct lumen show a streaming pattern of growth

- **Necrosis**. Central necrosis is typically a sign of carcinoma. However, rare cases of usual ductal hyperplasia may demonstrate central necrosis (Fig. 10.18). This occurs in the setting of florid usual ductal hyperplasia that is associated with a background proliferative lesion, such as a radial scar, nipple adenoma, or juvenile papillomatosis. The cytologic and architectural features are otherwise those of conventional usual ductal hyperplasia.
- **Mild Nuclear Enlargement in Radial Scars**. Florid usual ductal hyperplasia within radial scars can occasionally have active-appearing nuclei with mild nuclear enlargement (Figs. 10.19 and 10.20). The nuclear size may give an initial impression of atypia. However, the mild increase in size is the only anomalous feature, and the remaining cytologic characteristics (such as mild nuclear variability, nuclear grooves and folds, euchromatic chromatin, and small nucleoli) and lack of architectural atypia will together support a diagnosis of usual ductal hyperplasia.
- **Immature Usual Ductal Hyperplasia**. An uncommon variant of usual ductal hyperplasia occurs when the immature hyperplastic cells near the basement membrane are increased beyond their usual one or two cell layers and are instead several cell layers thick (Figs. 10.21 and 10.22). Because basally-located

Occasional examples of usual ductal hyperplasia demonstrate micropapillary tufting (Figs. 10.16 and 10.17). In women, this is most often a focal pattern in a background of otherwise conventional usual ductal hyperplasia. It is only rarely the dominant pattern, and is usually confined in such cases to a proliferative lesion such as a nipple adenoma (Fig. 10.17). In men with gynecomastia, however, micropapillary usual ductal hyperplasia is typically diffuse. The micropapillary tufts in all these scenarios are short and stubby and are of similar height and appearance. The tips of the micropapillae are formed by small knots of mature cells with shrunken, hyperchromatic nuclei and scant cytoplasm. The cells swirl together and lack evidence of polarization. Elongated, bulbous, broad, or architecturally complex micropapillae are not seen.

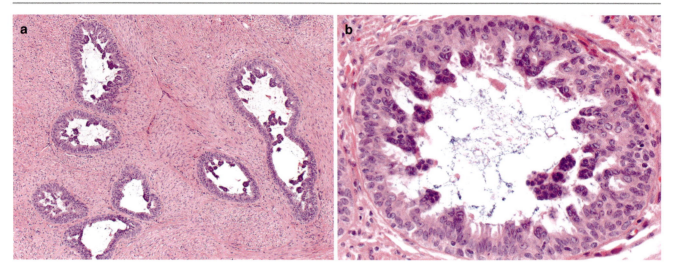

Fig. 10.16 Micropapillary usual ductal hyperplasia in a myoid hamartoma from an 11-year-old girl. (**a**) Short micropapillae of even height are present within mildly dilated glands. (**b**) The micropapillary tufts are composed of small knots of hyperchromatic cells that show matura-tion relative to the larger basal cells. The proliferation demonstrates the haphazard cellular distribution, a mild degree of cytologic variability, and nuclear morphology that characterize usual ductal hyperplasia

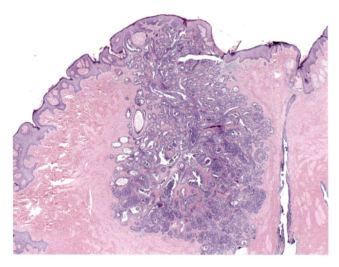

Fig. 10.17 Nipple adenoma with florid micropapillary usual ductal hyperplasia. Micropapillary usual ductal hyperplasia in women is typically focal within a background of otherwise conventional usual ductal hyperplasia. It may be more extensive, however, when it involves a background lesion such as a nipple adenoma. This example was initially misinterpreted as ductal carcinoma in situ due to the florid nature of the micropapillary proliferation

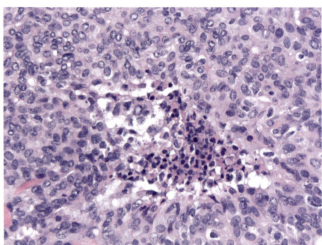

Fig. 10.18 Necrosis can be seen in rare examples of florid usual ductal hyperplasia when it is present within a proliferative lesion such as a radial scar. The cytologic and architectural features are otherwise those of usual ductal hyperplasia

hyperplastic cells contain larger nuclei with more prominent nucleoli than centrally-located hyperplastic cells, their prominence can lead to concern for atypia. The immature hyperplastic cells show a striking transition to smaller mature cells, which is a diagnostically helpful feature. The immature hyperplastic cells usually do not exceed four or five cell layers before they begin to mature. The involved ducts show only mild-to-moderate expansion, and the amount of proliferation tends to be conspicuously uniform across a single involved duct as well as from duct to duct. This pattern of usual ductal hyperplasia with a predominance of immature cells is most often encountered within cellular fibroepithelial lesions; it is not a common pattern in background breast parenchyma with fibrocystic changes.

10.1.5 Immunohistochemistry

Because the proliferative cells in usual ductal hyperplasia are not fully luminal in their phenotype, they retain positivity for basal-type high molecular weight cytokeratins (HMWCK), such as CK5, CK14, and K903 (Figs. 10.23 and 10.24, Table 10.2) [3, 4]. The pattern of reactivity tends to be heterogeneous with intermixed positive and negative cells (mosaic pattern). Some examples show diffuse positivity. Positivity is greatest in the central areas of the proliferation, while peripheral immature hyperplastic cells are often negative.

Usual ductal hyperplasia also shows a heterogeneous pattern of positivity for estrogen receptor (ER) (Fig. 10.24). Many but not all cells stain for ER, and they demonstrate variation in their staining intensity.

10.1.6 Clinical Management

Usual ductal hyperplasia is associated with an approximately 1.5–2× relative risk for subsequent breast cancer [1, 5, 6]. It is not a pre-neoplastic alteration itself but instead an indicator of breast tissue at mild increased risk. A diagnosis of usual ductal hyperplasia does not necessitate additional surgical or medical therapy, and patients are followed under standard screening protocols. In the core biopsy setting, usual ductal hyperplasia in and of itself is not an indication for follow-up excision, but it can be a component of a lesion (such as a radial scar or papilloma) that may be considered for excision.

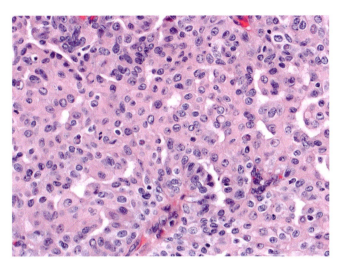

Fig. 10.19 Florid usual ductal hyperplasia in radial scars can occasionally have cells with increased cytoplasm and distinct cell borders, which can mimic the appearance of an atypical proliferation. However, the nuclear features are those of usual ductal hyperplasia

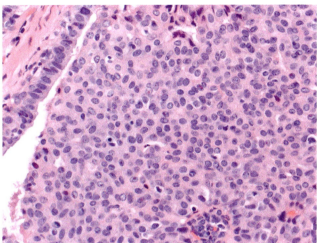

Fig. 10.20 Usual ductal hyperplasia in radial scars sometimes demonstrates a slightly uniform appearance with plump oval nuclei, which can raise concern for atypia. Other features, however, such as euchromatic chromatin, nuclear grooves, intranuclear pseduoinclusions, and haphazard cellular distribution, support a diagnosis of usual ductal hyperplasia

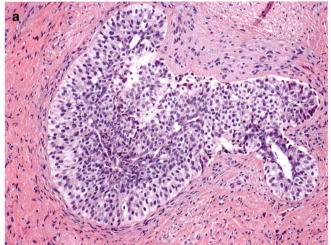

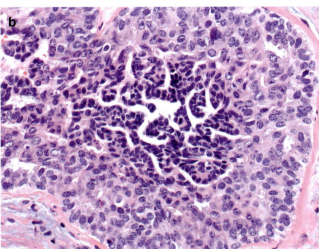

Fig. 10.21 Immature usual ductal hyperplasia. An increase in the number of immature basal hyperplastic cells may lead to concern for atypia because the nuclei can appear more monotonous (**a**) or larger (**b**) than those in the average example of usual ductal hyperplasia. The immature hyperplastic cells form a layer of uniform thickness that typically does not exceed four or five cells, and they merge into smaller cells showing conventional features of usual ductal hyperplasia and often striking maturation

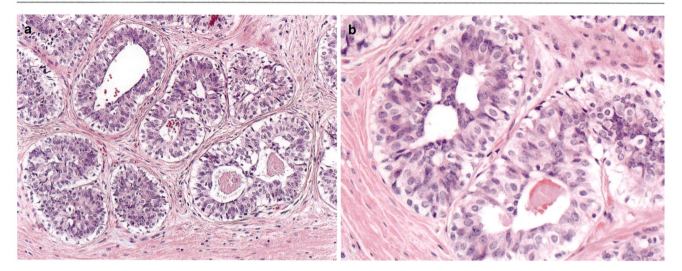

Fig. 10.22 Early immature usual ductal hyperplasia in a hamartoma. (**a**) Plump, active-appearing basal hyperplastic cells predominate. They show a similar thickness of 2–3 cells across multiple ducts. (**b**) The larger immature cells transition into central smaller cells showing architectural and cytologic features of usual ductal hyperplasia

Fig. 10.23 Cytokeratin 5/6 showing a mosaic pattern of staining in usual ductal hyperplasia. Staining is best evaluated in the central proliferative mass of cells, as the peripheral basal hyperplastic cells are often negative. Myoepithelial cells around the ducts are also immunoreactive

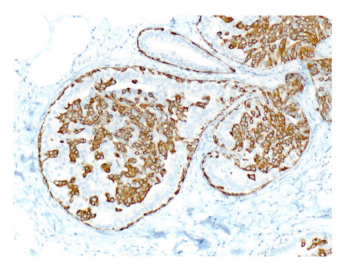

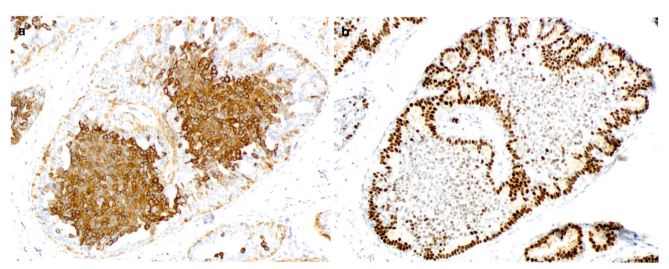

Fig. 10.24 High molecular weight cytokeratin and estrogen receptor profile of usual ductal hyperplasia. (**a**) In this example, cytokeratin 5/6 shows diffuse reactivity within the central mass of proliferative cells. (**b**) Estrogen receptor shows a heterogeneous pattern of reactivity, with intermixed positive and negative cells and variable staining intensity

Table 10.2 High molecular weight cytokeratin and estrogen receptor expression

	Usual ductal hyperplasia	Atypical ductal hyperplasia and low-grade ductal carcinoma in situ
High molecular weight cytokeratin (e.g., CK5/6, CK14, K903)	Positive	Negative
Estrogen receptor	Positive, heterogeneous	Positive, diffuse and strong

10.2 Atypical Ductal Hyperplasia

Atypical ductal hyperplasia is part of the spectrum of low-grade ductal neoplasia in the breast. It shares morphologic, immunohistochemical, and molecular findings with low-grade ductal carcinoma in situ [7]. These observations support a role as a non-obligate precursor to carcinoma. It arises from differentiated glandular cells and does not appear to represent a neoplastic transformation of usual ductal hyperplasia [3, 7].

10.2.1 Clinical Features

Atypical ductal hyperplasia occurs over a wide age range and is diagnosed at a mean age of 49 years [6]. It is seen in approximately 10% of biopsies with benign findings [8]. It is often associated with mammographically-detected microcalcifications but can be an incidental finding in biopsies performed for other indications.

10.2.2 Cytologic Features

Atypical ductal hyperplasia is characterized by a monomorphic, low-grade cytologic atypia that is identical to that seen in low-grade ductal carcinoma in situ (Figs. 10.25, 10.26, and 10.27, Table 10.1). The atypical cells have mildly enlarged nuclei that have round or oval shapes. The chromatin is hyperchromatic, fine and powdery, and evenly distributed. Nucleoli are generally inconspicuous. Nuclear membranes are typically smoothly contoured. Occasional cases may show variant nuclear characteristics, with slightly granular hyperchromatic chromatin and distinct but small nucleoli. The cytoplasm is increased in amount in comparison to normal cells and has a pale quality. Cell borders are frequently more distinct than in usual ductal hyperplasia. The atypical cells have a uniform appearance throughout the proliferation, and genuine cellular maturation is absent.

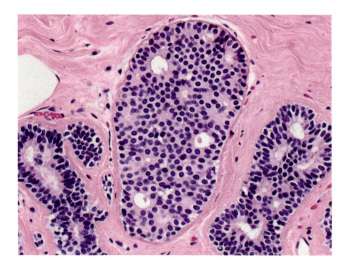

Fig. 10.25 Atypical ductal hyperplasia. Limited intraductal proliferation showing monomorphic cells with round, hyperchromatic nuclei and early cribriform space formation

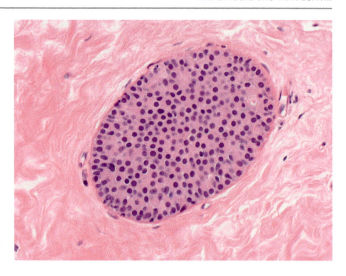

Fig. 10.26 Atypical ductal hyperplasia. Classic low-grade ductal atypia comprised of a monomorphic population of cells showing uniform, round-to-plump oval nuclei, with fine, evenly dispersed, hyperchromatic chromatin. Nucleoli are relatively inconspicuous and nuclear membranes are smooth. The cells have an increased amount of cytoplasm, and cell borders are distinct

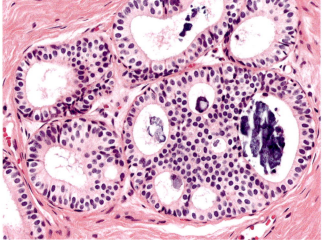

Fig. 10.27 Atypical ductal hyperplasia. These nuclei show a variant morphology with slightly granular chromatin and small nucleoli, but the uniformity and hyperchromasia permit recognition of the cells as atypical. Calcifications are commonly associated with atypical ductal hyperplasia

10.2.3 Architectural Features

Atypical ductal hyperplasia shows the same forms of architectural atypia as ductal carcinoma in situ, albeit on a more limited scale. Cribriform spaces, trabecular bars, Roman arches, micropapillae, and uniform solid growth are the main patterns that are encountered (Figs. 10.25, 10.26, 10.27, 10.28, 10.29, 10.30, and 10.31, Table 10.1). With the exception of solid growth, these architectural formations are characterized by the presence of cellular polarity. The atypical cells radially orient their apical cytoplasmic compartments toward the abutting luminal space, thus recapitulating the apical-basal polarity of normal ductal cells. In the classical

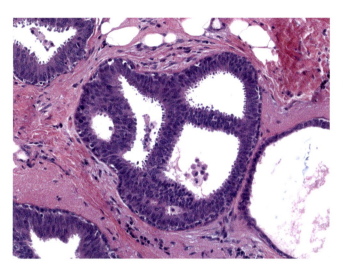

Fig. 10.28 Architectural atypia. In trabecular bars, the cells are arrayed with their apical cytoplasmic compartments radially oriented toward the luminal space. In this case, the apical cytoplasmic snouts provide a clear indication of apical polarity

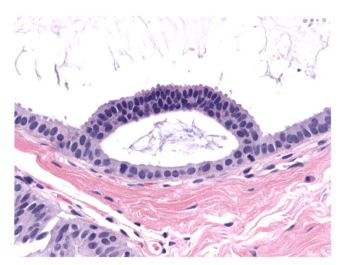

Fig. 10.29 Architectural atypia. Roman arches are so-named for their palisaded arrangement of cells across the arch, mimicking the pattern in a Roman stone arch. The cells are radially oriented with their apical compartments facing the luminal space

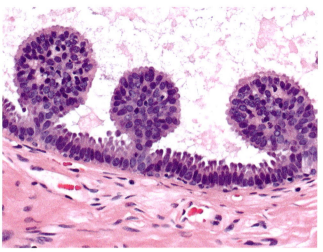

Fig. 10.30 Architectural atypia. Micropapillae in atypical proliferations show a polarized orientation of the outer layer of cells toward the luminal space. The apices of the cells, identified by a zone of cytoplasm and, in this case, apical snouts, point outward toward the lumen. Bulbous micropapillae such as these are not a feature of micropapillary usual ductal hyperplasia

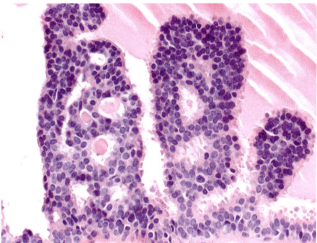

Fig. 10.31 Architectural atypia. Complex micropapillae of variable length and with bulbous shapes are indicative of an atypical proliferation, although evidence of polarization is the key defining feature of architectural atypia. In this example, polarity can be seen at the epithelial-luminal interface as well as within the papillae themselves with the formation of cribriform spaces

cribriform space, the polarized cells form a *de novo* neoplastic lumen within the proliferative aggregate. Trabecular bars, Roman arches, and micropapillae show cellular polarization relative to the existing luminal space. When the proliferation is solid, cellular polarity is not discernable; however, the atypical cells tend to be evenly distributed with less nuclear overlap than in usual ductal hyperplasia.

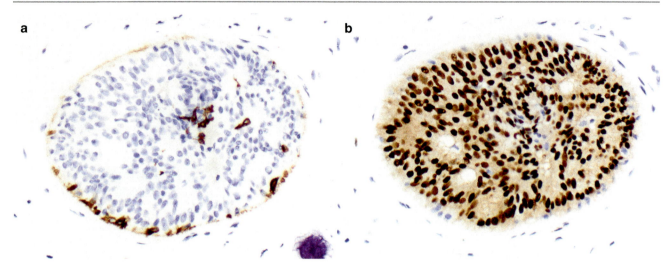

Fig. 10.32 High molecular weight cytokeratin and estrogen receptor profile of atypical ductal hyperplasia. (**a**) Atypical ductal hyperplasia is negative for high molecular weight cytokeratins, as is seen in this cyto- keratin 5/6 immunostain. Residual entrapped normal luminal cells and peripheral myoepithelial cells account for the positive cells. (**b**) The atypical cells show diffuse strong positivity for estrogen receptor

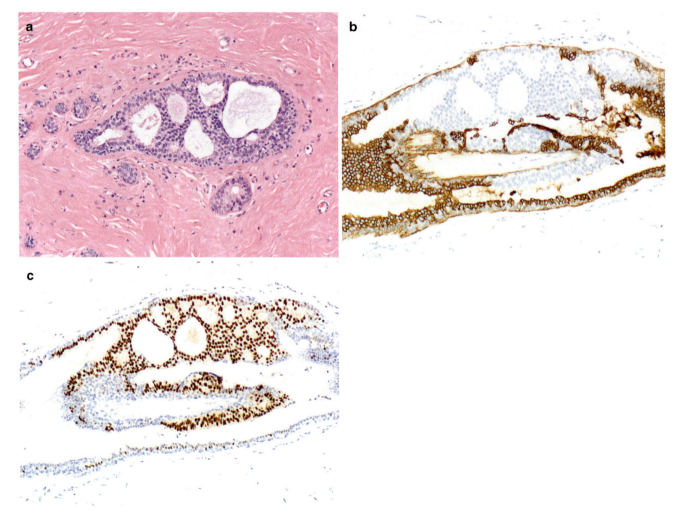

Fig. 10.33 Atypical ductal hyperplasia. (**a**) A limited proliferation of small but monotonous ductal cells expands a single duct profile. (**b**) The proliferative cells are negative for cytokeratin 5/6. Normal luminal cells and myoepithelial cells account for immunopositive regions. (**c**) The proliferative area shows strong diffuse positivity for estrogen receptor. Together the morphological and immunohistochemical findings support a diagnosis of atypical ductal hyperplasia

10.2.4 Immunohistochemistry

Atypical ductal hyperplasia is negative for HMWCK (Figs. 10.32 and 10.33, Table 10.2) [3, 4]. Residual normal luminal cells may be a source of positivity within the proliferation, however, and should not be mistaken for staining of the proliferative cells. Residual normal cells usually appear as a thin, flat layer appliqued along the luminal edge or as small discrete groups, and thus can be distinguished from the proliferative cells by their size and location. The cells of atypical ductal hyperplasia show diffuse strong staining for ER (Figs. 10.32 and 10.33). The HMWCK/ER immunoprofile is identical to that of low-grade ductal carcinoma in situ.

10.2.5 Clinical Management

Atypical ductal hyperplasia is associated with an approximately 4× increased risk for subsequent breast cancer [1, 5, 6]. Its management depends on the context in which it is diagnosed.

When identified in a core biopsy specimen, atypical ductal hyperplasia is associated with a 23% mean upgrade rate to ductal carcinoma in situ or invasive carcinoma on follow-up excision, although results from individual studies vary widely (0% to >50%) [9]. Its presence in a core biopsy is generally considered an indication for surgical excision. The goal of surgery is not to treat the atypical ductal hyperplasia *per se*, but to rule out the presence of carcinoma in the adjacent parenchyma. Parameters to identify patients who can be managed with active surveillance instead of excision have yet to be determined.

Atypical ductal hyperplasia is frequently associated with biopsy-targeted calcifications and therefore represents a correlative finding in such cases. It is not, however, an adequate explanation for a mass lesion or architectural distortion. In cases with radiographic-pathologic discordance, upgrade rates may be higher.

Atypical ductal hyperplasia that is diagnosed in a surgical excision specimen is managed primarily as a risk factor and does not require further surgical therapy, assuming there is correlation with the clinical and radiographic findings. As such, margins are not reported for atypical ductal hyperplasia. An exception is made at our institution if there is severely atypical ductal hyperplasia bordering on ductal carcinoma in situ (see below). We report the margins to these borderline lesions because re-excision may be considered if the severely atypical ductal hyperplasia is present at or <0.1 cm from the margin.

Patients with atypical ductal hyperplasia have an approximately fourfold increased risk for subsequent breast cancer [1, 5, 6]. The increased risk affects both breasts and persists over decades. Data from the Mayo Clinic indicate a cumulative incidence of carcinoma of 29% at 25 years for patients with atypical hyperplasia (ductal or lobular) [10]. Screening recommendations include annual mammogram and clinical breast exam. Chemoprevention with hormonal agents such as tamoxifen, raloxifene, or exemestane can reduce the relative risk of breast cancer by 41–79% [11, 12]. Overall chemoprevention usage in high-risk patients, however, remains relatively low at approximately 16% [13].

10.3 Differential Diagnosis

The classification of ductal proliferations is a recurrent source of diagnostic difficulty [14]. Problems center on two main issues: (1) determining whether a proliferation is atypical or not; and (2) if it is atypical, whether it is best classified as atypical ductal hyperplasia or ductal carcinoma in situ.

10.3.1 Atypical vs. Non-atypical Intraductal Proliferations

Most diagnostic difficulties occur at the low-grade end of the spectrum in differentiating low-grade ductal neoplasia (atypical ductal hyperplasia and low-grade ductal carcinoma in situ) from usual ductal hyperplasia. Intermediate-grade ductal carcinoma in situ can also occasionally have some features that mimic those of usual ductal hyperplasia and thus raise its own set of diagnostic issues.

- **Low-Grade Ductal Neoplasia vs. Usual Ductal Hyperplasia**

The presence of cytologic atypia distinguishes both atypical ductal hyperplasia and low-grade ductal carcinoma in situ from usual ductal hyperplasia. The monomorphic nuclei of low-grade atypia show a set of morphologic features that are distinct from the polymorphic nuclei of usual ductal hyperplasia (Table 10.1). While no individual feature is 100% sensitive or specific, the combined evaluation of multiple features will enable one to determine which diagnosis has greater evidence to support it. Of the cytologic criteria listed in Table 10.1, the characteristics of the cell population, nuclear shape, and chromatin are the most consistent and therefore the most reliable. Awareness of the occasional variant features of usual ductal hyperplasia (see above) will aid in the prevention of an overdiagnosis of atypia.

Architectural features are less reliable than cytologic ones. Proliferations with unusual architecture but benign cytologic features are not atypical ductal hyperplasia; the architecture can usually be explained by tangential sectioning or involvement of a pre-existing lesion (Figs. 10.34 and 10.35).

Micropapillary proliferations can be a source of diagnostic difficulty. While cytologic atypia and polarized architecture are the keys to recognizing an atypical micropapillary proliferation, the presence of long, complex, or bulbous micropapillae should also alert one to the possibility of atypia (Figs. 10.30 and 10.31).

Secondary findings, while not present in every case, can provide helpful clues. Merging of apocrine cells with a ductal proliferation is suggestive of a diagnosis of usual ductal hyperplasia (Fig. 10.36). Atypical ductal hyperplasia and ductal carcinoma in situ may collide with apocrine metaplasia, but an intimate admixture of the ductal and apocrine cell types is generally not seen. Abundant calcifications within a ductal proliferation are more common in atypical proliferations. It is relatively uncommon to see prominent calcifications within the proliferative mass of cells in usual ductal hyperplasia, although calcifications are frequent within the other associated elements of fibrocystic change.

In difficult cases, use of immunohistochemistry for HMWCK and ER can be helpful, as usual ductal hyperplasia and low-grade ductal neoplasia demonstrate differing profiles (Figs. 10.23, 10.24, 10.32, and 10.33, Table 10.2). In usual ductal hyperplasia, the proliferative cells are positive for HMWCK and show heterogeneous reactivity for ER. In atypical ductal hyperplasia and low-grade ductal carcinoma in situ, the proliferative cells are negative for HMWCK and show diffuse strong reactivity for ER.

- **Intermediate-Grade Ductal Carcinoma In Situ vs. Usual Ductal Hyperplasia**

The cytologic features of intermediate-grade ductal carcinoma in situ are more variable than those of low-grade ductal

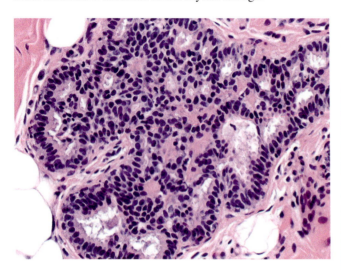

Fig. 10.34 Tangential sectioning through a duct profile can mimic atypical ductal hyperplasia. Polarized spaces are present; however, examination reveals strands of waxy eosinophilic basement membrane material traversing between them. Ductal cells sitting on basement membrane are polarized regardless of whether they are atypical or not. There is no evidence of true architectural atypia or even significant epithelial proliferation

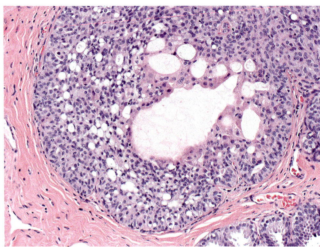

Fig. 10.36 Intimate merging of a ductal proliferation with apocrine cells is a finding associated with usual ductal hyperplasia

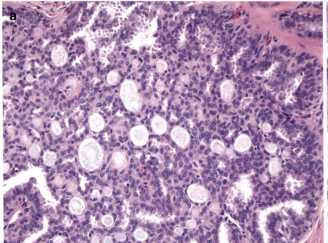
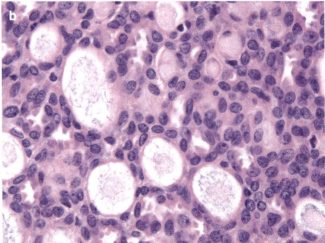

Fig. 10.35 Usual ductal hyperplasia involving collagenous spherulosis. (a) The round spaces mimic a cribriform architecture. (b) The spaces, however, are lined by small flattened myoepithelial cells with an associated waxy rim of basement membrane. The spaces contain eosin-ophilic to basophilic basement membrane material rather than intraluminal secretions. The surrounding cells demonstrate the typical cytologic features of usual ductal hyperplasia

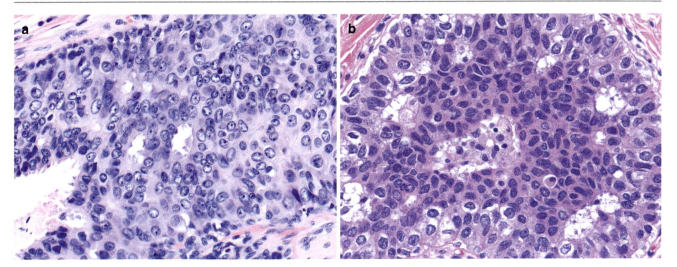

Fig. 10.37 Intermediate-grade ductal carcinoma in situ. (**a**) The oval nuclei show open chromatin, distinct nuclei, and occasional nuclear grooves, features that descriptively overlap with those of usual ductal hyperplasia. However, the nuclei are uniformly enlarged, the chromatin is abnormally cleared, and there is polarized cribriform space forma-

tion. Early cellular necrosis is also present (bottom left). The overall features are indicative of intermediate-grade atypia. (**b**) In this example, the nuclei are larger, more hyperchromatic, and show greater nuclear irregularity than would be expected for usual ductal hyperplasia

neoplasia. The nuclei show moderate enlargement in size and can have variable shapes. The chromatin may be hyperchromatic, open, coarse, or clumped and cleared, and nucleoli are usually conspicuous. Nuclear membrane irregularities can be seen. The presence of polymorphism, open chromatin, nucleoli, and/or nuclear membrane irregularities may raise consideration of usual ductal hyperplasia (Fig. 10.37). However, the nuclei in intermediate-grade ductal carcinoma in situ are larger than those of usual ductal hyperplasia, and this moderate nuclear enlargement is maintained throughout the proliferation. While cells of comparable size may sometimes be found in usual ductal hyperplasia, they are restricted to the basal layers and do not persist into the central zones of the proliferation, instead maturing into smaller cells.

The cytologic features of intermediate-grade ductal atypia vary from case to case, and thus they do not lend themselves to a generally applicable set of diagnostic criteria as for low-grade atypia. However, the moderate nuclear size enlargement is a consistent feature. The presence of hyperchromasia, red nucleoli, or marked nuclear irregularity point toward a neoplastic process, as does the presence of polarized architectural atypia. Comedonecrosis is a concerning feature, although it may be seen in rare examples of usual ductal hyperplasia. Although individual features of intermediate-grade atypia may descriptively overlap with those of usual ductal hyperplasia, the diagnosis usually becomes clear when the entirety of the cytologic and architectural findings is considered.

In difficult cases, immunohistochemistry for HMWCK and ER can be helpful. Most examples of intermediate-grade ductal carcinoma in situ are negative for HMWCK, although there can be rare exceptions. ER is helpful if it is diffusely strongly positive or completely negative, findings that are

indicative of a neoplastic process rather than usual ductal hyperplasia. However, heterogeneous ER expression akin to that of usual ductal hyperplasia can be also seen in intermediate-grade ductal carcinoma in situ, and the immunohistochemical findings must be weighed in combination with the morphologic ones.

10.3.2 Atypical Ductal Hyperplasia vs. Ductal Carcinoma In Situ

After establishment of a ductal proliferation as atypical, one must decide whether it is best classified as atypical ductal hyperplasia or ductal carcinoma in situ. The distinction bears important clinical consequences, as atypical ductal hyperplasia is managed as a risk factor but ductal carcinoma in situ is treated as a malignancy. Despite the clinical dichotomy, the pathology is not binary. Atypical ductal hyperplasia and ductal carcinoma in situ are composed of the same type of neoplastic cells and demonstrate the same forms of architectural atypia. They represent points along a biologic continuum rather than discrete entities. The lack of clear qualitative differences between the two has led to the development of quantitative criteria for diagnostic purposes. Such quantitative criteria are arbitrary but have become established within clinical practice.

• **Quantitative Criteria**

Fundamentally, atypical ductal hyperplasia is a proliferation with low-grade cytologic atypia and limited architectural atypia, whereas low-grade ductal carcinoma in situ is a proliferation with low-grade cytologic atypia and well-developed architectural atypia. The distinction between

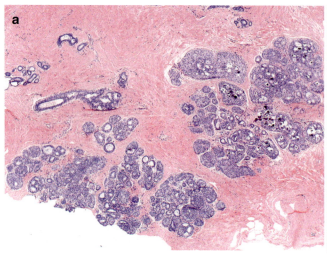
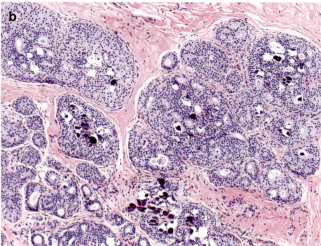

Fig. 10.38 Small focus of low-grade ductal carcinoma in situ. (**a**) This 3.5 mm focus shows a well-developed proliferation that (**b**) demonstrates both cytologic and architectural atypia. There is a robust prolif-

eration within individual glands, and the proliferation is greater than 2 mm in size. It therefore meets the criteria for low-grade ductal carcinoma in situ

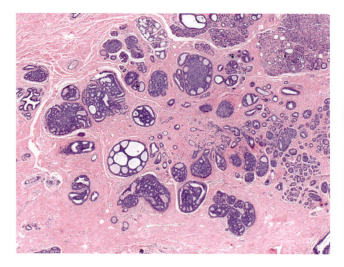
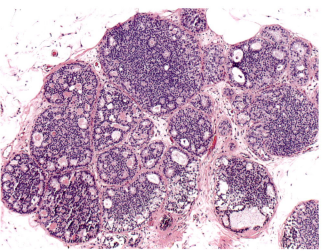

Fig. 10.39 Small focus of low-grade ductal carcinoma in situ. The proliferation shows notable duct distension compared to the background glands and spans 3 mm in size, thus meeting the minimal criteria for low-grade ductal carcinoma in situ

Fig. 10.40 The atypical intraductal proliferation shows prominent duct expansion and spans 2 mm, thus meeting the minimal criteria for low-grade ductal carcinoma in situ. In practice, however, classification of proliferations right around the size cutoff can be controversial

"limited" and "well-developed" architectural features rests on both the overall extent of the atypical proliferation and the degree of proliferation within individual ducts.

Extent can be determined by measuring the size of the atypical proliferation, which can then provide a quantitative threshold for diagnosis. One commonly used cutoff point is 2 mm: atypical proliferations 2 mm or greater in size meet minimum criteria for low-grade ductal carcinoma in situ, whereas smaller proliferations are regarded as atypical ductal hyperplasia (Figs. 10.38, 10.39, 10.40, 10.41, 10.42, 10.43, and 10.44) [15]. An alternative approach is to use complete involvement of two separate duct profiles by the atypical proliferation as a minimum criterion for ductal car-

cinoma in situ [5]. Quantitative size criteria such as these are inherently subject to the limitations of evaluating a complex three-dimensional structure in a two-dimensional plane, as well as those based on the random nature of tissue sampling. Both criteria are arbitrary and do not indicate known biological differences between proliferations immediately above or below the size thresholds. Nevertheless, they represent accepted guideposts that pathologists can use to gain greater diagnostic concordance in the classification of small atypical ductal proliferations.

While the 2 mm size criterion was initially proposed by Tavassoli and Norris [15] as an "aggregate diameter," in current practice it is usually applied to a continuous focus. A

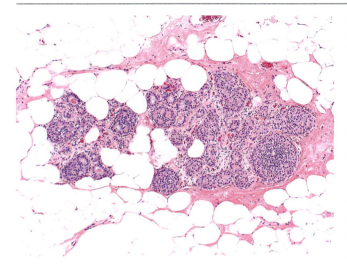

Fig. 10.41 Atypical ductal hyperplasia. The atypical proliferation shows only mild-to-moderate duct expansion and is less than 2 mm in size

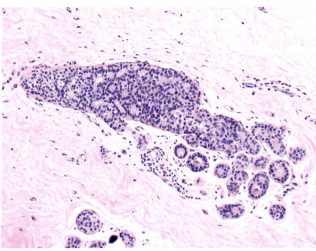

Fig. 10.43 Atypical ductal hyperplasia. Moderate expansion of a terminal duct by a cytologically atypical proliferation with cribriform space formation. The focus is limited in both the amount of proliferation and in size (less than 2 mm), and it is thus best classified as atypical ductal hyperplasia

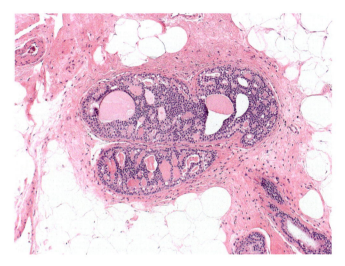

Fig. 10.42 Atypical ductal hyperplasia. The degree of atypical proliferation is fairly robust, but the focus spans only 1 mm in size. While two duct profiles are involved, these likely represent a single contiguous duct and thus do not clearly fulfill the alternative minimal criterion for ductal carcinoma in situ of complete involvement of two separate duct profiles

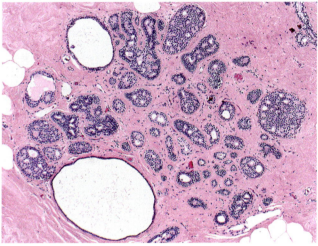

Fig. 10.44 Atypical ductal hyperplasia. Mild-to-moderate expansion of multiple glands by an atypical ductal proliferation that spans less than 2 mm in size

common question is whether several foci of atypia should be spanned or individually measured to determine the size. It is hard to make a diagnostic rule that applies in all examples, given that individual cases differ in their appearance and distribution of atypical foci. In general, if the foci seem likely to be contiguous in three dimensions, then using a span seems reasonable. However, if they are separated by moderate amounts of normal breast tissue, then considering them as separate foci seems most appropriate.

The robustness of the proliferation within individual ducts also influences whether the architectural changes are considered limited or well-developed. Because atypical ductal

hyperplasia represents an early stage of neoplasia, it shows a relatively limited amount of proliferation within the lumen (Figs. 10.45 and 10.46). It is not usually associated with marked ductal distortion and expansion. If there is marked duct expansion by a florid atypical proliferation but the focus is less than 2 mm in size, the possibility of an under-sampled ductal carcinoma in situ should be considered. Conversely, one should be cautious about diagnosing low-grade ductal carcinoma in situ even in a focus larger than 2 mm if the ducts show only a minimal amount of proliferation.

Pathologists also typically require complete involvement of the ducts to render a diagnosis of a low-grade ductal carcinoma in situ [5]. The phrase "complete involvement"

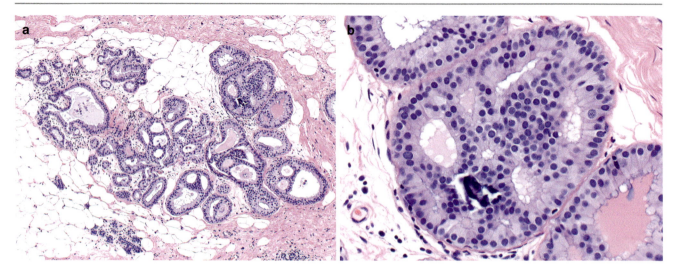

Fig. 10.45 Atypical ductal hyperplasia. (**a**) The amount of proliferation within individual glands is relatively limited. (**b**) The proliferation demonstrates monomorphic low-grade cytologic atypia and limited architectural atypia (early cribriform space formation)

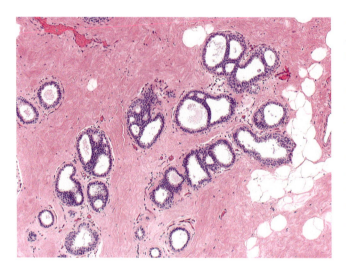

Fig. 10.46 Although the atypical proliferation spans 2 mm, the amount of proliferation within the individual glands is limited; the proliferation is therefore best classified as atypical ductal hyperplasia

sometimes leads to the expectation that the ducts should be entirely filled by the atypical proliferation. Bear in mind, however, that some growth patterns of ductal carcinoma in situ can show complete and circumferential replacement of the duct lining by neoplastic cells but never solidly fill the duct lumen. Micropapillary ductal carcinoma in situ is one such example. Small lesions that just meet minimal criteria for ductal carcinoma in situ around the 2 mm size threshold may still be controversial in practice (Fig. 10.40). A second opinion from colleagues or a consultant is helpful in providing a consistent approach to classification within one's practice. Communication to the clinician that a proliferation is of a borderline nature is also of value.

- **Severely Atypical Ductal Hyperplasia**

Occasional cases of atypical ductal hyperplasia may closely approach a diagnosis of low-grade ductal carcinoma in situ, either based on size criteria and/or the presence of marked duct expansion. In such instances, we may render a

diagnosis of severely atypical ductal hyperplasia bordering on low-grade ductal carcinoma in situ (Figs. 10.47 and 10.48). Such findings on core biopsy warrant follow-up excision. In an excision specimen, a borderline lesion at or < 0.1 cm from the margin may raise consideration of re-excision.

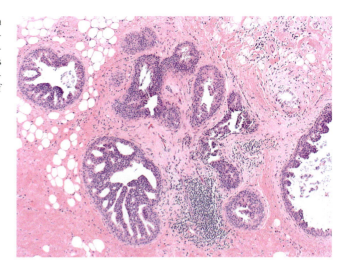

Fig. 10.47 Core biopsy demonstrating an atypical ductal proliferation that is robust within individual glands and 2 mm in overall size. A diagnosis of severely atypical ductal hyperplasia bordering on ductal carcinoma in situ was rendered. Others might diagnose it as a limited focus of low-grade ductal carcinoma in situ. The robustness of the proliferation does raise the possibility of under-sampling of a broader area of ductal carcinoma in situ

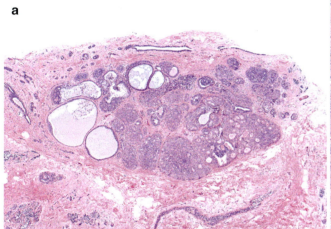
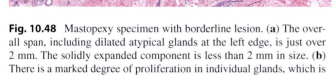
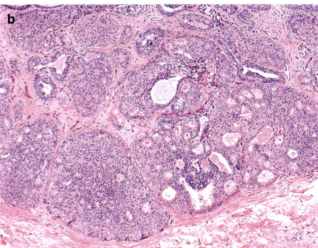

Fig. 10.48 Mastopexy specimen with borderline lesion. (**a**) The overall span, including dilated atypical glands at the left edge, is just over 2 mm. The solidly expanded component is less than 2 mm in size. (**b**) There is a marked degree of proliferation in individual glands, which is

concerning for ductal carcinoma in situ. Some pathologists may diagnose such a lesion as a limited focus of low-grade ductal carcinoma in situ, whereas others may classify it as severely atypical ductal hyperplasia bordering on ductal carcinoma in situ

- **High- or Intermediate-Grade Cytologic Atypia**

The above quantitative considerations apply to ductal proliferations showing low-grade cytologic atypia. The presence of high-grade cytologic atypia warrants a diagnosis of high-grade ductal carcinoma in situ regardless of size (Fig. 10.49). Pathologists are variable in their approach to proliferations with intermediate-grade cytologic atypia. Many apply the same quantitative criteria as in low-grade proliferations to determine if there are sufficiently well-developed architectural features to warrant a diagnosis of ductal carcinoma in situ. The threshold may be lowered if concerning features such as necrosis are present (Fig. 10.50). Others take the approach that a proliferation with intermediate-grade atypia is indicative of ductal carcinoma in situ regardless of size [16].

Conclusion

The evaluation of ductal hyperplasia is one of the most common diagnostic scenarios in breast pathology. Attention to a combined set of cytologic and architectural features permits distinction of usual ductal hyperplasia from atypical ductal hyperplasia. Diagnostic separation of atypical ductal hyperplasia from low-grade ductal carcinoma in situ can be difficult because the two represent points along a biologic continuum rather than unique entities. Accepted quantitative criteria provide a practical means of making the distinction.

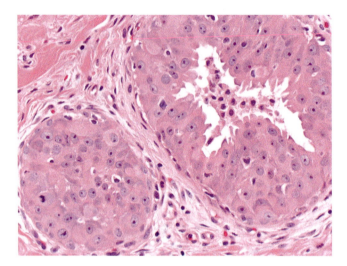

Fig. 10.49 High-grade cytologic atypia warrants a diagnosis of high-grade ductal carcinoma in situ regardless of size

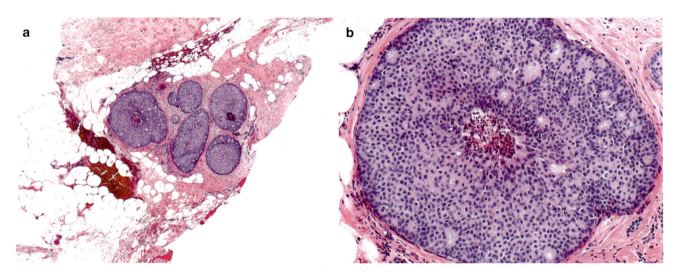

Fig. 10.50 Small focus of intermediate grade ductal carcinoma in situ. (**a**) Core biopsy with a 1.5 mm focus of a robust intraductal proliferation with (**b**) intermediate-grade nuclear atypia and central necrosis

References

1. Hartmann LC, Sellers TA, Frost MH, Lingle WL, Degnim AC, Ghosh K, et al. Benign breast disease and the risk of breast cancer. N Engl J Med. 2005;353:229–37.
2. Jabbar SB, Lynch B, Seiler S, Hwang H, Sahoo S. Pathologic findings of breast lesions detected on magnetic resonance imaging. Arch Pathol Lab Med. 2017;141:1513–22.
3. Boecker W, Moll R, Dervan P, Buerger H, Poremba C, Diallo RI, et al. Usual ductal hyperplasia of the breast is a committed stem (progenitor) cell lesion distinct from atypical ductal hyperplasia and ductal carcinoma in-situ. J Pathol. 2002;198:458–67.
4. Otterbach F, Bànkfalvi A, Bergner S, Decker T, Krech R, Boecker W. Cytokeratin 5/6 immunohistochemistry assists the differential diagnosis of atypical proliferations of the breast. Histopathology. 2000;37:232–40.
5. Page DL, Dupont WD, Rogers LW, Rados MS. Atypical hyperplastic lesions of the female breast. A long-term follow-up study. Cancer. 1985;55:2698–708.
6. Collins LC, Baer HJ, Tamimi RM, Connolly JL, Colditz GA, Schnitt SJ. The influence of family history on breast cancer risk in women with biopsy-confirmed benign breast disease: results from the nurses' health study. Cancer. 2006;107:1240–7.
7. Lopez-Garcia MA, Geyer FC, Lacroix-Triki M, Marchió C, Reis-Filho JS. Breast cancer precursors revisited: molecular features and progression pathways. Histopathology. 2010;57:171–92.
8. Simpson JF. Update on atypical epithelial hyperplasia and ductal carcinoma in situ. Pathology. 2009;41:36–9.
9. Mooney KL, Bassett LW, Apple SK. Upgrade rates of high-risk breast lesions diagnosed on core needle biopsy: a single-institution experience and literature review. Mod Pathol. 2016;29:1471–84.
10. Hartmann LC, Radisky DC, Frost MH, Santen RJ, Vierkant RA, Benetti LL, et al. Understanding the premalignant potential of atypical hyperplasia through its natural history: a longitudinal cohort study. Cancer Prev Res (Phila). 2014;7:211–7.
11. Hartmann LC, Degnim AC, Santen RJ, Dupont WD, Ghosh K. Atypical hyperplasia of the breast – risk assessment and management options. N Engl J Med. 2015;372:78–89.
12. Coopey SB, Mazzola E, Buckley JM, Sharko J, Belli AK, Kim EM, et al. The role of chemoprevention in modifying the risk of breast cancer in women with atypical breast lesions. Breast Cancer Res Treat. 2012;136:627–33.
13. Smith SG, Sestak I, Forster A, Partridge A, Side L, Wolf MS, et al. Factors affecting uptake and adherence to breast cancer chemoprevention: a systematic review and meta-analysis. Ann Oncol. 2016;27:575–90.
14. Elmore JG, Longton GM, Carney PA, Geller BM, Onega T, Tosteson AN, et al. Diagnostic concordance among pathologists interpreting breast biopsy specimens. JAMA. 2015;313:1122–32.
15. Tavassoli FA, Norris HJ. A comparison of the results of long-term follow-up for atypical intraductal hyperplasia and intraductal hyperplasia of the breast. Cancer. 1990;65:518–29.
16. Schnitt SJ, Collins LC. Intraductal proliferative lesions: usual ductal hyperplasia, atypical ductal hyperplasia, and ductal carcinoma in situ. In: Biopsy Interpretation of the Breast. 2nd ed. Philadelphia, PA: Lippincott Williams & Wilkins; 2013. p. 78.

Ductal Carcinoma In Situ

11

Isabel Alvarado-Cabrero

Ductal carcinoma in situ (DCIS) is a malignant, clonal proliferation of cells growing within the basement membrane-bound structures of the breast, with no evidence of invasion into the surrounding stroma [1]. The increased use of screening mammography has led to a significant increase in the diagnosis of earlier stage breast cancers, including DCIS.

Specifically, DCIS is detected as mammographic microcalcifications in more than three quarters (75%) of cases, as a non-palpable mass in 11%, and as a combination of the above in 13%. Furthermore, DCIS constitutes 30–40% of breast cases diagnosed mammographically, with one case of DCIS detected in every 1300 screening mammograms. Ten to 20% of DCIS cases are seen bilaterally [2]. In some cases, DCIS presents clinically as nipple discharge, usually hemorrhagic, and is often seen in association with Paget disease of the nipple [3].

Risk factors for the development of DCIS are similar to those for invasive breast cancer, suggesting that these diseases are etiologically related and include increasing age (mean age at diagnosis for DCIS, 50–59 years), family history of a first-degree relative with breast cancer, nulliparity or late age of first birth, late age of menopause, long-term use of postmenopausal hormonal therapy, elevated body-mass index in postmenopausal women, BRCA mutational status, and high mammographic breast density [4, 5]. DCIS is considered a precursor lesion with a relative risk of 8–11 for the subsequent development of invasive carcinoma [1, 2].

11.1 Histologic Parameters

Ductal carcinoma in situ is a heterogeneous group of neoplastic intraductal lesions characterized by increased epithelial proliferation of different architectural patterns and various degrees of cytological atypia, ranging from mild to severe. The microscopic heterogeneity of DCIS has led to the development of several systems for classification. Historically, DCIS has been classified based on architectural patterns of proliferation, including comedo, cribriform, micropapillary, solid, or mixed subtypes [1, 6].

I. Alvarado-Cabrero, MD, PhD
Department of Pathology, Hospital de Oncologia, Centro Medico Nacional Siglo XXI, Instituto Mexicano del Seguro Social, Mexico City, Mexico

© Springer International Publishing AG, part of Springer Nature 2018
S. Stolnicu, I. Alvarado-Cabrero (eds.), *Practical Atlas of Breast Pathology*, https://doi.org/10.1007/978-3-319-93257-6_11

11.2 Low-Grade Ductal Carcinoma In Situ

Low-grade DCIS is characterized by a proliferation of small cells with well-defined cell membranes that exhibit uniform size, shape, and placement. Cells are 1.5–2 times the size of a red blood cell, or similar in size to the adjacent ductal epithelial cells. In the solid growth pattern, cells completely fill ductal spaces (Figs. 11.1 and 11.2). The nuclei are small, with relatively homogeneous chromatin distribution and inconspicuous nucleoli (Fig. 11.3). Because of their polarized nature, these carcinomas cells consistently display better-developed glandular characteristics than hyperplastic cells. Cribriform and micropapillary architecture are more common than a solid growth pattern.

The cribriform pattern features extracellular lumens within the proliferation (Figs. 11.4 and 11.5). These are typically round and rigid with a punched-out appearance (Fig. 11.6).

Micropapillary DCIS consists of ducts lined by a layer of neoplastic cells giving rise to papillary/micropapillary fronds or arcuate formations protruding into the duct lumen (Fig. 11.7). Micropapillary DCIS is recognized to more often be multiquadrant (71%) than comedo-type disease (8%) [7]. Rare cases of low-grade DCIS may have comedo type necrosis (Fig. 11.8).

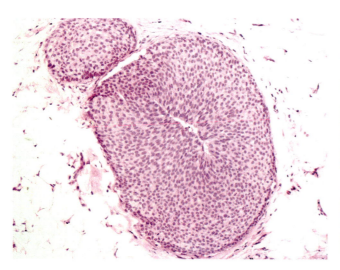

Fig. 11.1 Low-grade ductal carcinoma in situ, solid pattern. Involved ductal spaces are filled with solid sheets of cohesive cells; numerous microacini are present

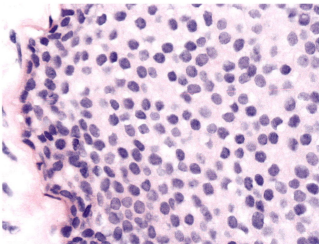

Fig. 11.3 Low-grade ductal carcinoma in situ. The nuclei are small, with small, relatively homogeneous chromatin distribution and inconspicuous nucleoli. The cells show a subtle increase in N:C ratio

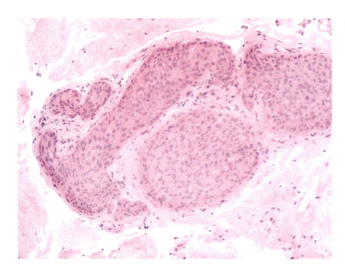

Fig. 11.2 Low-grade ductal carcinoma in situ, solid pattern

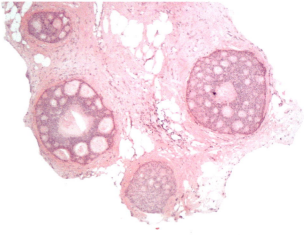

Fig. 11.4 Low-grade ductal carcinoma in situ, with cribriform pattern. Round lumens within the proliferation

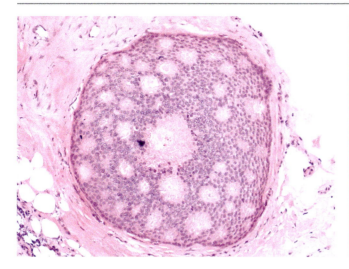

Fig. 11.5 Low-grade ductal carcinoma in situ with a cribriform pattern

Fig. 11.6 Low-grade ductal carcinoma in situ with a cribriform pattern. The neoplastic cells show polarization around these lumens

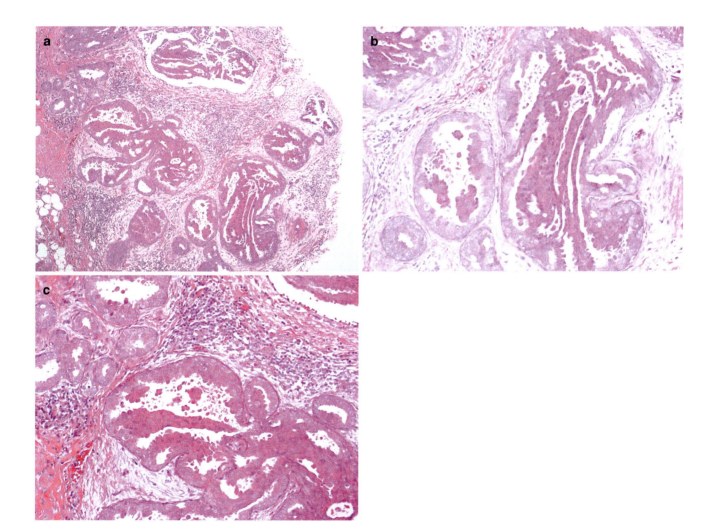

Fig. 11.7 Micropapillary carcinoma. (**a**, **b**) Slender fronds of micropapillary ductal carcinoma in situ form an irregular network of arches at the periphery. (**c**) Tufts of proliferating cells project into the lumen of the ducts

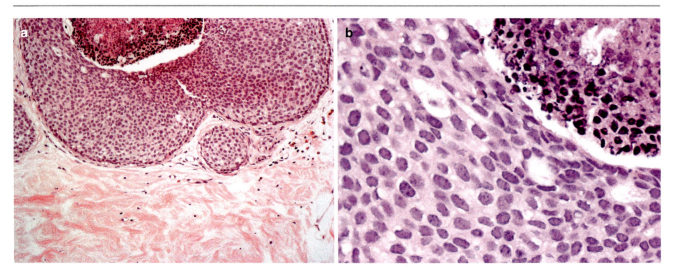

Fig. 11.8 (**a**, **b**) Low-grade ductal carcinoma in situ with comedo necrosis

11.3   High-Grade Ductal Carcinoma In Situ

High-grade DCIS consists of cells showing the archetypical characteristics of malignancy. The cells appear greatly enlarged and pleomorphic, and the nuclei and nucleoli usually look large, irregular, and pleomorphic (Fig. 11.9). Assessment of the size of the nuclei compared with adjacent normal cells (epithelial or red blood cells) provides particular assistance in classification. The nuclei of high-grade DCIS are typically more than 2.5 red-blood cells in diameter (Fig. 11.10) [8].

This grade of DCIS is often solid architecture, tends not to show polarization of cells, and frequently bears central (comedo-type) necrosis with or without associated microcalcifications (Fig. 11.11). Necrosis may be so extensive that only one layer or a few cell layers are present at the periphery of the involved space. Fibroblastic proliferation with collagen deposition (Fig. 11.12), chronic inflammation, and vascular proliferation are often seen in the stroma surrounding the involved spaces (Fig. 11.13).

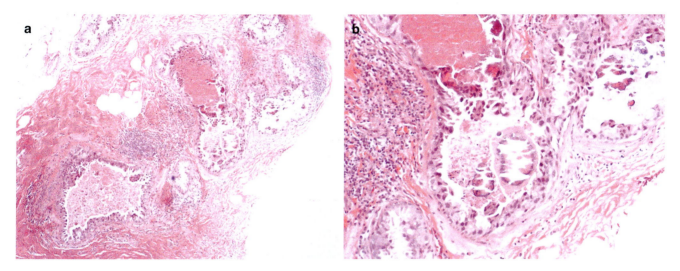

Fig. 11.9   High-grade ductal carcinoma in situ. (**a**, **b**) High-grade ductal carcinoma in situ with comedo necrosis and amorphous calcification

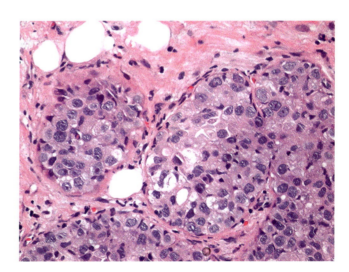

Fig. 11.10   High-grade ductal carcinoma in situ. Cells with large, pleomorphic nuclei that have vesicular or coarse chromatin and prominent nucleoli

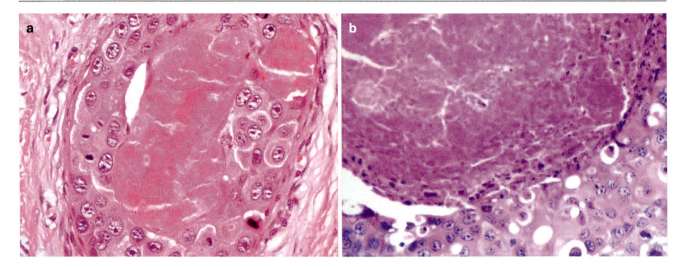

Fig. 11.11 High-grade ductal carcinoma in situ. (**a, b**) Ductal carcinoma in situ with comedo necrosis

Fig. 11.12 High-grade ductal carcinoma in situ. Marked periductal fibrosis can be associated with extensive obliteration of ducts, a process referred to as healing

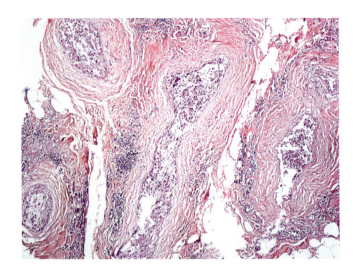

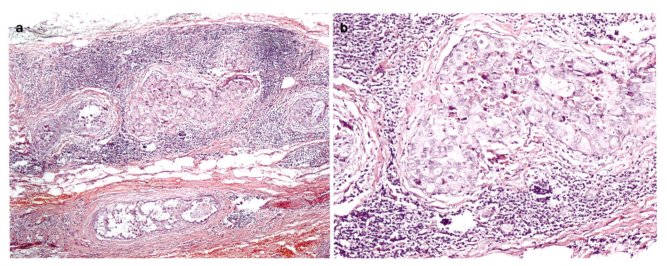

Fig. 11.13 (**a, b**) High-grade ductal carcinoma in situ with prominent chronic inflammation in the surrounding stroma

11.4 Intermediate-Grade Ductal Carcinoma In Situ

Intermediate-grade DCIS is diagnosed when the lesion cannot be assigned to high- or low-nuclear-grade categories. The cells may also grow in a cribriform pattern but without prominent cell polarization (Fig. 11.14). The nuclear–cytoplasmic (N:C) ratio is often high, and one or two small nucleoli may be present but are not prominent. The difference in ipsilateral recurrence rates between low- and intermediate-grade DCIS is not significant [9].

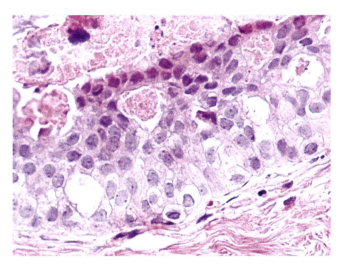

Fig. 11.14 Intermediate-grade cribriform DCIS. This duct is filled by cribriform DCIS without prominent cell polarization. N:C ratio is often high, and one or two small nucleoli may be present but are not prominent

11.5 Rare Variants of Ductal Carcinoma In Situ

A range of cell types is found in DCIS. Certain distinct variants have been identified and described by specific names. Signet ring cells, usually associated with lobular carcinoma, also occur in DCIS, most often in papillary and cribriform types [10]. Clear cell DCIS [11] is a poorly defined variant typically encountered with solid and "comedo" patterns (Fig. 11.15). The presence of a monomorphic clear cell population in a ductal proliferative lesion is highly suggestive of intraductal carcinoma.

Apocrine DCIS is characterized by cells that have abundant, eosinophilic cytoplasm (Fig. 11.16) [12]. The growth pattern may be solid, cribriform, or micropapillary, and necrosis can be present (either punctate or comedo).

Less commonly, DCIS may exhibit spindle cells (Fig. 11.17) [13], small cell, or adenoid cystic differentiation.

Cystic hypersecretory carcinoma is an uncommon variant of ductal carcinoma in situ that is recognized by its cystic appearance and characteristic luminal secretion. The cysts are lined by atypical epithelial cells, most often with a micropapillary pattern, but clinging, cribriform, and solid patterns may also be seen (Fig. 11.18) [14].

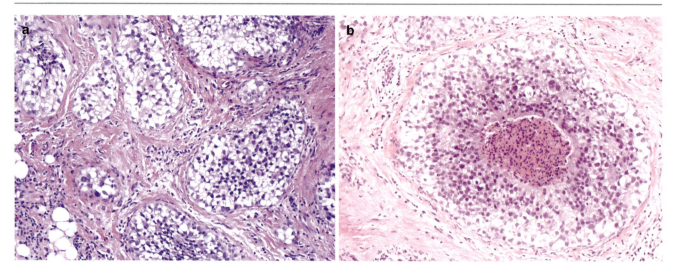

Fig. 11.15 (**a**, **b**) Ductal carcinoma in situ with clear cell features, the cells show prominent cytoplasmic clearing

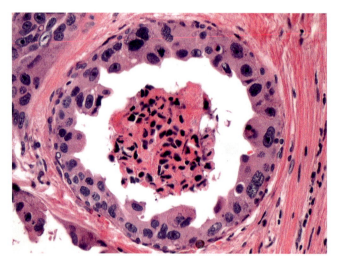

Fig. 11.16 High-grade ductal carcinoma in situ with enlarged nuclei and abundant eosinophilic cytoplasm

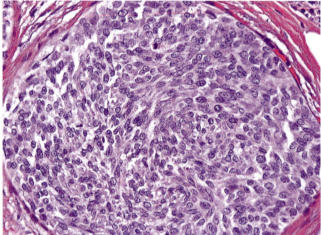

Fig. 11.17 Ductal carcinoma in situ with spindle cell features. The proliferation is composed of spindle-shaped cells with elongated nuclei that fill the involved space

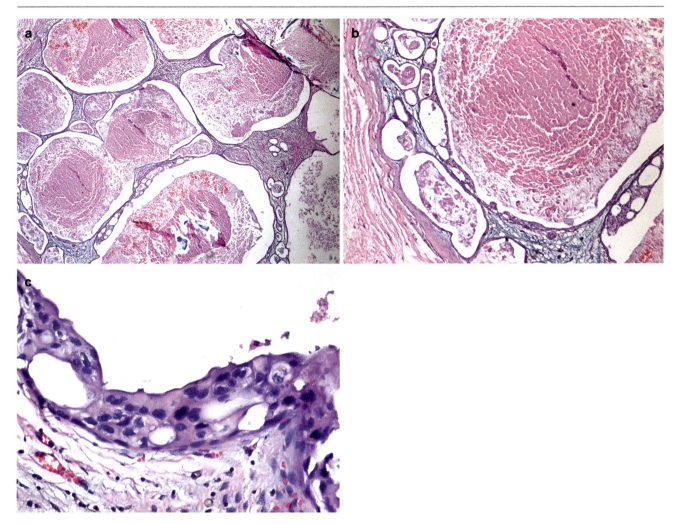

Fig. 11.18 Cystic hypersecretory ductal carcinoma in situ. (**a**) Low-power multiple cyst-like structures containing eosinophilic material and comedo necrosis. (**b**) The spaces are lined by epithelium with a cribriform pattern. (**c**) Epithelium with atypical cells

11.6   Immunohistochemistry

The distribution of receptor expression in DCIS is similar to that seen in invasive breast cancer. About 75–80% show positive nuclear staining for estrogen receptor (ER) (range, <1–100% of cells) (Fig. 11.19) [15]. The frequency of progesterone receptor (PR) expression in DCIS is somewhat lower.

Low-grade DCIS lesions typically show diffuse and strong ER and PR expression (Fig. 11.17). In contrast, high-grade DCIS lesions may be ER and PR positive or negative, have a high proliferative rate, and frequently show HER2 (human epidermal growth factor receptor 2) protein overexpression (Fig. 11.20) [16].

Fig. 11.19 Low-grade ductal carcinoma in situ and estrogen receptor immunostain. The neoplastic cells show intense strong nuclear staining

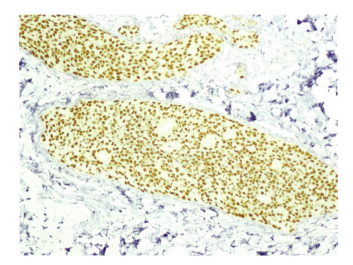

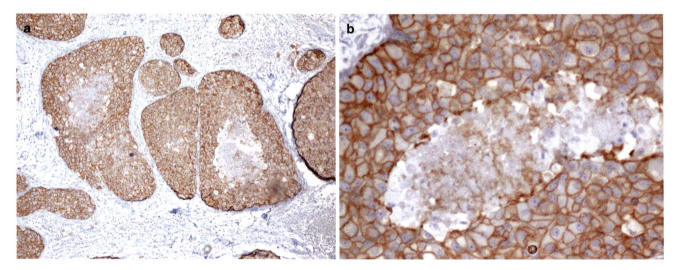

Fig. 11.20 High-grade ductal carcinoma in situ with comedo necrosis and HER2 immunostain. (**a**, **b**) The neoplastic cells show intense membrane staining (HER2 protein overexpression)

References

1. Pinder SE. Ductal carcinoma in situ (DCIS): pathological features, differential diagnosis, prognostic factors and specimen evaluation. Mod Pathol. 2010;23(suppl 2):S8–13.
2. Sizioprkou KP. Ductal carcinoma in situ of the breast. Current concepts and future directions. Arch Pathol Lab Med. 2013;137:462–6.
3. Kerlikowske K, Walker R, Miglioretti DL, Desai A, Ballard-Barbash R, Buist DSM. Obesity, mammography use and accuracy, and advanced breast cancer risk. J Natl Cancer Inst. 2008;23:1724–33.
4. Kerlikowske K, Miglioretti DL, Ballard-Barbash R, Weaver DL, Buist DS, Barlow WE, et al. Prognostic characteristics of breast cancer among postmenopausal hormone users in a screened population. J Clin Oncol. 2003;21:4314–21.
5. Sakorafas GH, Farley DR. Optimal management of ductal carcinoma in situ of the breast. Surg Oncol. 2003;12:221–40.
6. Mardekian SK, Bombonati A, Palazzo JO. Ductal carcinoma in situ of the breast: the importance of morphologic and molecular interactions. Hum Pathol. 2016;49:114–23.
7. Bellamy CO, McDonald C, Salter DM, Chetty U, Anderson TJ. Noninvasive ductal carcinoma of the breast: the relevance of histologic categorization. Hum Pathol. 1993;24:16–23.
8. Lester SC, Bose S, Chen YY, Connolly JL, de Baca ME, Fitzgibbons PL, et al. Protocol for the examination of specimens from patients with ductal carcinoma in situ of the breast. Arch Pathol Lab Med. 2009;133:15–25.
9. Pinder SE, Duggan C, Ellis IO, Cuzick J, Forbes JF, Bishop H, et al. A new pathological system for grading DCIS with improved prediction of local recurrence: results from the UKCCCR/ANZ DCIS trial. Br J Cancer. 2010;103:94–100.
10. Fisher ER, Brown R. Intraductal signet ring cell carcinoma. A hitherto undescribed form of intraductal carcinoma of the breast. Cancer. 1985;55:2533–7.
11. Terada T. Clear cell variant of ductal carcinoma in situ of the breast. Breast J. 2012;18:279–80.
12. Vranic S, Schmitt F, Sapino A, Costa JL, Reddy S, Castro M, et al. Apocrine carcinoma of the breast: a comprehensive review. Histol Histopathol. 2013;28:1393–409.
13. Tan PH, Lui GG, Chiang G, Yap WM, Poh WT, Bay BH. Ductal carcinoma in situ with spindle cells: a potential diagnostic pitfall in the evaluation of breast lesions. Histopathology. 2004;45:343–51.
14. D'Alfonso TM, Ginters PS, Liu YF, Shin SJ. Cystic hypersecretory (in situ) carcinoma of the breast: a clinicopathologic and immunohistochemical characterization of 10 cases with clinical follow-up. Am J Surg Pathol. 2014;32:45–53.
15. Lari SA, Kuerer HM. Biological markers in DCIS and risk of breast recurrence: a systematic review. J Cancer. 2011;2:232–61.
16. Han K, Nofech-Mozes S, Narod S, Hanna W, Vesprini D, Saskin R, et al. Expression of HER2neu in ductal carcinoma in situ is associated with local recurrence. Clin Oncol (R Coll Radiol). 2012;24:183–9.

Microinvasive Carcinoma

12

Simona Stolnicu

Microinvasive breast carcinoma is a rare lesion, in which foci of intralobular or intraductal carcinoma are associated with one or more microscopic foci of atypical cells located outside the basement membrane, in the adjacent intralobular or interlobular stroma [1]. In rare cases, microinvasive carcinoma can be identified without an adjacent in situ lesion (Fig. 12.1). Frequently, microinvasive carcinomas have a multifocal character. There is no international consensus regarding this lesion and its definition and all definitions are arbitrary. Some authors consider that the maximum size of the invasive focus should be 1 mm for the diagnosis of microinvasive carcinoma [1]. Other authors define microinvasive carcinoma as having a single focus with a maximum size less than 2 mm, while others consider 2–3 foci, none exceeding 1 mm in diameter [2]. However, the presence of microinvasive breast carcinoma and distinction from in situ carcinoma may have therapeutic and prognostic implications, consequently recognizing it is of paramount importance. During microscopic examination, the pathologist establishes microinvasion on the basis of several morphological criteria. Sometimes, these criteria may be difficult to assess and may not be perfectly reproducible among pathologists.

Microinvasive breast carcinoma does not display clinical signs and can only be identified on mammography and macroscopic examination due to its association with intraductal or, rarely, intralobular carcinoma. As a consequence, microinvasion is only detected when examining the microscopic slides, making the role of the pathologist essential in the diagnosis of this lesion.

Microscopically, invasive tumor cells usually invade the stroma by forming small nests or tubular structures, while in other cases the cells are isolated (Fig. 12.2). Sometimes we can only detect tongue-like projections of cohesive cells that have not lost continuity with the in situ component through a minor disruption of the basement membrane. Most of the time, however, the invasive cells are found dissociated from the in situ component, infiltrating the stroma. Neither the microscopic type nor the grade of malignancy can be established due to its small size, but mostly, the morphological appearance suggests an infiltrating carcinoma of no special type (NST). A desmoplastic stroma and an inflammatory infiltrate can be noticed around microinvasive foci (especially if the in situ component is of high grade) (Fig. 12.3). Consistency in the recognition of microinvasion significantly improves with the use of additional stains. Immunohistochemically, the absence of myoepithelial cells around the clusters of invasive tumor cells can be demonstrated using stains for Calponin, smooth muscle myosin heavy chain (SMMHC), p63 (these markers being reported with excellent sensitivity and specificity) and more recently, p40, D2–40. Ideally, the three markers should be used in association. However, it is important to keep in mind that myoepithelial cells surrounding spaces involved by ductal carcinoma in situ may show phenotypic differences from normal myoepithelial cells [3, 4]. Ductal carcinoma in situ-associated myoepithelial cells show decreased expression of one or more myoepithelial markers (such as SMMHC, CD10, CK5/6, calponin, p63, p75, smooth muscle actin) when compared with normal myoepithelial cells. As such, for practical implications, it is always advisable to use a panel of markers. Also, the absence of the basement membrane around the nests of microinvasive cells can be demonstrated using Laminin or Collagen IV. However, careful consideration should be given to rare situations in which invasive carcinomas may produce basement membrane components. It is always advisable to combine myoepithelial markers and basement membrane markers with a keratin stain, which can also better determine the extent of the invasive component, especially in cases in which the tumor cells are isolated.

In routine practice, the evaluation of ER, PR, Ki-67, and HER2 is recommended in microinvasive foci as for any other

S. Stolnicu, MD, PhD
Department of Pathology, University of Medicine and Pharmacy, Tîrgu Mureș, Romania

© Springer International Publishing AG, part of Springer Nature 2018
S. Stolnicu, I. Alvarado-Cabrero (eds.), *Practical Atlas of Breast Pathology*, https://doi.org/10.1007/978-3-319-93257-6_12

foci of certain invasive tumors. In some cases, however, this is not possible due to the small size of the foci. In these particular cases, these four markers can be reported in the adjacent in situ lesion since the molecular profile of the two lesions (in situ and microinvasive) is identical in most of the cases.

The pathology report of a microinvasive carcinoma must necessarily include the number of the microinvasive foci, their size (in case there are multiple foci, the size of the largest one must be mentioned), as well as any special test that was performed for the diagnosis. It is essential that multiple sections should be performed in any intraductal carcinoma (especially if it is extensive) in order to exclude the presence of microinvasive foci. Similarly, it is recommended that multiple sections should be performed in a microinvasive lesion to exclude the presence of an invasive carcinoma of larger size.

Differential diagnosis is performed with intraductal carcinoma. Of interest, the features of ductal in situ carcinoma associated with microinvasion are the following: more extensive in situ component, high-grade, central necrosis, and periductal inflammatory infiltrate. In intraductal carcinoma, the branching layout of the duct on a small cross section can sometimes mimic adjacent invasive foci (Fig. 12.4). In most of these cases, the myoepithelial cells can be detected on hematoxylin-eosin slides (Fig. 12.5). In difficult cases, however, laminin or collagen IV allows the identification of a continuous basal membrane around these foci. If around such a duct with in situ carcinoma there are small portions where laminin is negative and the microscopic appearance suggests a microinvasion, the microinvasion focus being directly connected to the duct, the lesion should be reported as possibly microinvasive. It is noteworthy, however, that some intraductal carcinoma lesions may sometimes have a discontinuous basement membrane, and some microinvasive

foci may sometimes have areas of basement membrane around them, so that the diagnosis remains a morphological one. Also, problems in distinguishing ductal in situ carcinoma from microinvasion occur when the in situ component may involve the lobules, sometimes with distortion of involved spaces, tangential sectioning, crushed artifact, cautery effect, and artifactual displacement of cells in ductal in situ lesions. In all these situations, the lesion can be overdiagnosed, but there are also situations in which the microinvasive carcinoma can be under-diagnosed (when the microinvasive foci can be overlooked or may not be sampled). Also, because differential diagnosis includes frank invasive foci with a diameter greater than 1 mm, invasive foci should be carefully measured under the microscope.

Cases of previous biopsy in which the area is associated with architectural distortion, inflammation, hemorrhage, and fibrosis may pose difficulty in diagnosing. Microinvasive diagnosis is difficult especially if intralobular or intraductal carcinoma foci are associated with radial scars, sclerosing adenosis, or complex sclerosing lesions [3]. In these situations, it is important to remember that myoepithelial cells associated with benign sclerosing lesions of the breast may show immunophenotypic differences from normal myoepithelial cells. In one published study, myoepithelial cells associated with benign sclerosing lesions showed reduced expression of SMMHC, CD10, p63 and calponin [3]. This needs to be taken into consideration when selecting myoepithelial markers to help distinguish benign sclerosing lesions from invasive breast cancer.

Microinvasive carcinoma is rarely associated with lymph node metastases. Lack of consensus regarding the definition of the lesion makes the predictability of its evolution difficult, although it is usually favorable.

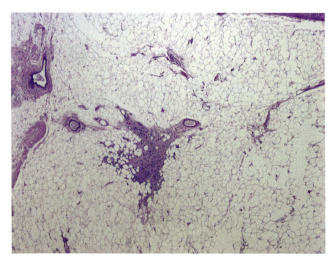

Fig. 12.1 Focus of microinvasive carcinoma (size <1 mm diameter) identified at microscopic examination lacking an adjacent in situ lesion

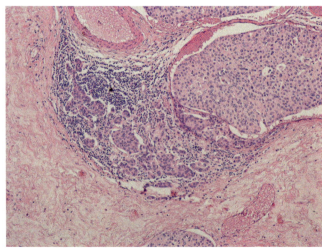

Fig. 12.2 Microinvasive carcinoma: invasive tumor cells invade the stroma in the vicinity of DCIS

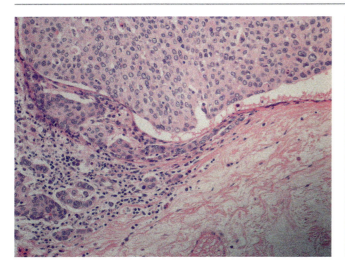

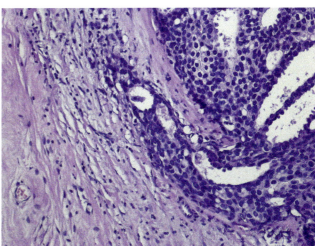

Fig. 12.3 Microinvasive carcinoma: the invasive tumor cells are forming small nests or have a trabecular arrangement while others are isolated into the stroma; an inflammatory infiltrate can be appreciated surrounding the invasive foci

Fig. 12.5 Intraductal carcinoma mimicking a microinvasive focus by the branching layout of the duct; however, the myoepithelial cells can be detected on the hematoxylin-eosin slide

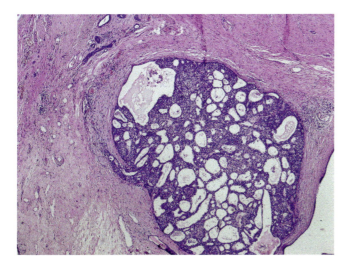

Fig. 12.4 Intraductal carcinoma: the branching layout of the duct on a small cross section can mimic adjacent invasive foci

References

1. Lakhani SR, Schnitt SJ, Tan PH, van deVijver MJ. WHO classification of tumors of the breast. Lyon: IARC; 2012.
2. Tavassoli FA. Pathology of the breast. 2nd ed. Stamford, CT: Appleton and Lange; 1999. p. 410.
3. Hilson JB, Schnitt SJ, Collins LC. Phenotypic alterations in myoepithelial cells associated with benign sclerosing lesions of the breast. Am J Surg Pathol. 2010;34(6):896–900.
4. Hilson JB, Schnitt SJ, Collins LC. Phenotypic alterations in ductal carcinoma in situ-associated myoepithelial cells: biologic and diagnostic implications. Am J Surg Pathol. 2009;33(2):227–32.

Atypical Lobular Hyperplasia and Lobular Carcinoma In Situ

13

Isabel Alvarado-Cabrero

Despite the earlier description by Ewing [1], the term lobular carcinoma is largely credited to Foote and Stewart [2] who, in 1941, published their seminal paper describing a detailed morphologic analysis of a distinctive subgroup of in situ carcinoma of the breast. Almost 40 years after the first description of lobular carcinoma in situ (LCIS), Haagensen et al. [3] published their own experience with this disease and concluded that "lobular neoplasia" was a more appropriate term for this lesion, as few cases appeared to progress to invasive carcinoma. With increasing recognition of LCIS, it became apparent that less well-developed forms were more frequently seen in the breast. Page et al. [4] used the term atypical lobular hyperplasia for these lesions.

Lobular neoplasia has also been termed lobular intraepithelial neoplasia (LIN), which divides these lesions using a 3-tiered grading scale based on extent and degree of lobular involvement and/or nuclear atypia (LIN1, LIN2, LIN3) [5]. Lobular neoplasia and LIN nomenclatures have not been widely adopted, and use of the terms ALH and LCIS is still prevalent in the literature as well as in patients' diagnostic reports today.

The incidence of both in situ and invasive forms of lobular carcinoma has increased over the last decades [6]. Between 1978 and 1988, the incidence of LCIS increased from 0.90/100,000 person-per-years to 3.19/100,000 person-per-year in the North American population [7]. Lobular neoplastic lesions (ALH and LCIS) are often multi-centric and bilateral. They occur predominantly in premenopausal women, with most cases being diagnosed in women between 40 and 50 years of age [8].

They are clinically occult, and although they are often also mammographically silent, a significant minority of lobular neoplasia cases diagnosed on core biopsy have associated microcalcifications [9]. Epidemiologic studies have clearly shown lobular neoplasia as a marker of increased risk [10]. In recent years, however, there is increasing evidence that LCIS may also act as a non-obligate precursor in the progression to invasive carcinoma [11].

Atypical lobular hyperplasia (ALH) and lobular carcinoma in situ (LCIS) are not associated with any grossly recognizable features.

Lobular carcinoma in situ is composed of acini filled with a monomorphic population of small, round, polygonal, or cuboidal cells, with a thin rim of clear cytoplasm and a high nuclear-to-cytoplasmic rate. The nuclei are round-to-oval. The nuclei have homogeneous chromatin and nucleoli that are inconspicuous to absent, and mitoses are infrequent (Fig. 13.1).

The distinction between ALH and LCIS is quantitative. More than half of the acini of a lobular unit needs to be distended (not just filled) and distorted by the neoplastic cells for a diagnosis of LCIS; anything less than that is ALH. In objective terms, criterion to distinguish LCIS from ALH is based on extent; at least 50–75% of acini in a lobular unit must be filled and distended with no residual lumina (Fig. 13.2). Involved lobules may be compared to uninvolved lobules to estimate degree of distension.

In classical LCIS, two types of cells may be seen: (1) type A cells with small-to-slightly enlarged nuclei (1.5× size of lymphocyte), with uniform round nuclei and inconspicuous nucleoli (Fig. 13.3); and (2) type B cells with larger nuclei (2× size of lymphocyte), more abundant cytoplasm, and more prominent nucleoli (Fig. 13.4). Type A and B cells can coexist in the same lesion (Fig. 13.5). Regardless of cell nuclear size, the cytoplasm of LCIS cells is typically pale-to-lightly eosinophilic.

Most cases of LCIS have a discohesive growth pattern and the presence of intracytoplasmic vacuoles (Fig. 13.6). These vacuoles may be so subtle that special histochemical stains for mucin are required for their demonstration. At the other end of the spectrum, the vacuoles may be large enough to produce signet ring cell forms. Signet ring cells can have low, intermediate, or high-grade nuclei (Fig. 13.7).

I. Alvarado-Cabrero, MD, PhD
Department of Pathology, Hospital de Oncologia, Centro Medico Nacional Siglo XXI, Instituto Mexicano del Seguro Social, Mexico City, Mexico

© Springer International Publishing AG, part of Springer Nature 2018
S. Stolnicu, I. Alvarado-Cabrero (eds.), *Practical Atlas of Breast Pathology*, https://doi.org/10.1007/978-3-319-93257-6_13

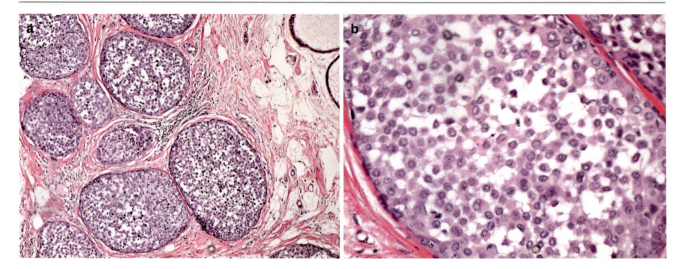

Fig. 13.1 Lobular carcinoma in situ. (**a**) A low-power view illustrating several enlarged terminal duct. (**b**) Lobular units in which the acini are filled with and distended by a population of uniform cells

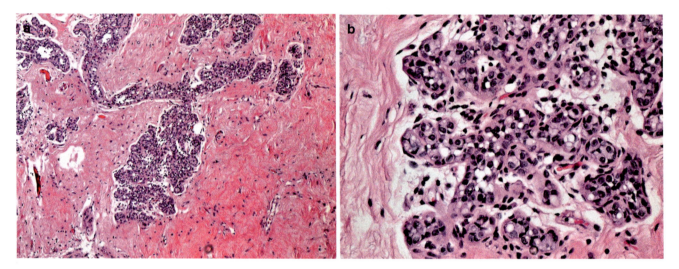

Fig. 13.2 Atypical lobular hyperplasia. (**a**) Involved terminal duct-lobular units are not completely distended by neoplastic cells. (**b**) Duct lobular unit contains a cellular proliferation that only minimally distends the involved acini

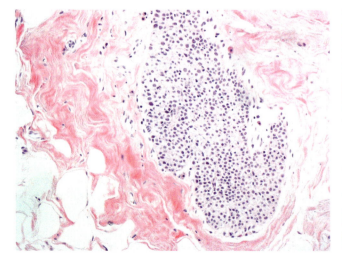

Fig. 13.3 Lobular carcinoma in situ with small cells with uniform nuclei often referred as type A

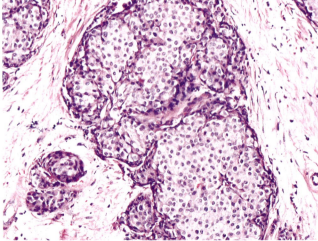

Fig. 13.4 Lobular carcinoma in situ with cells that show more abundant cytoplasm and slightly more variation in cell and nuclei size and shape, and by the presence of nucleoli. These have been referred as type B

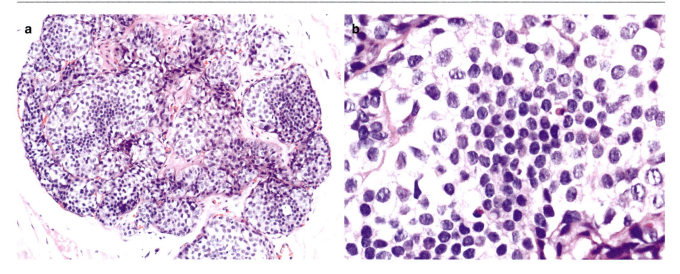

Fig. 13.5 Lobular carcinoma in situ with a mixture of two cell types. (**a**) Small cells with small uniform nuclei or smaller, central type A cells and larger, peripheral type B cells (**b**)

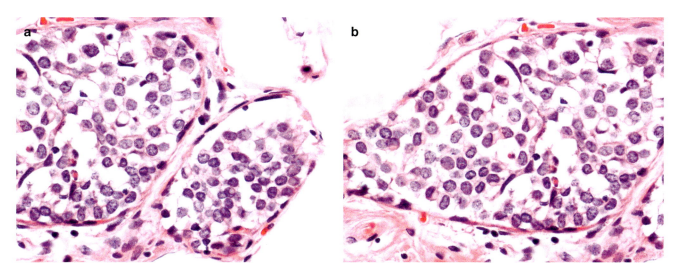

Fig. 13.6 (**a**, **b**) Most cases of LCIS are readily distinguished from low-grade DCIS with hematoxylin-eosin stain. Dyscohesive growth pattern and the presence of prominent intracytoplasmic vacuoles favor the diagnosis of LCIS

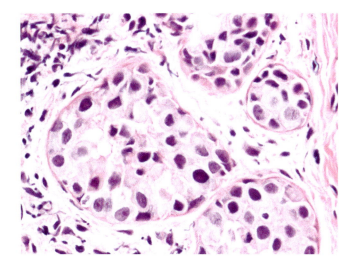

Fig. 13.7 Lobular carcinoma in situ with signet ring cells. Spaces expanded by a discohesive population of cells. Intracytoplasmic vacuoles are evident

Lobular carcinoma in situ typically involves intralobular and extralobular or terminal ductules as well as acinar units within the lobule. The irregular configuration of ductules affected by LCIS has been described as "saw-toothed" or as resembling a cloverleaf (Fig. 13.8). Pagetoid LCIS growing beneath the non-neoplastic ductal epithelium may be distributed continuously or discontinuously along the ductal system, undermining, and ultimately displacing, the normal ductal epithelium (Fig. 13.9). LCIS can also involve lactiferous ducts, but usually does not extend to epidermis. On the other hand, LCIS may colonize preexisting breast lesions such as fibroadenomas (Fig. 13.10), sclerosing adenosis, radial sclerosing lesions, collagenous spherulosis, and papillomas.

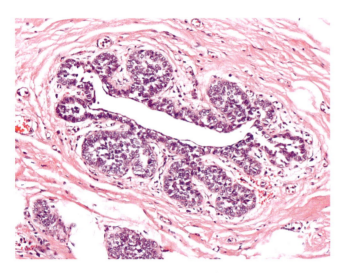

Fig. 13.8 Lobular carcinoma in situ with duct involvement in a cloverleaf pattern

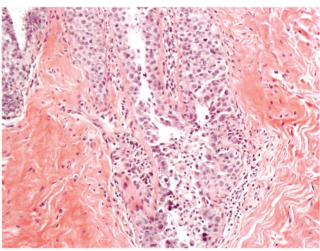

Fig. 13.10 LCIS involving an area of lobular units in a fibroadenoma

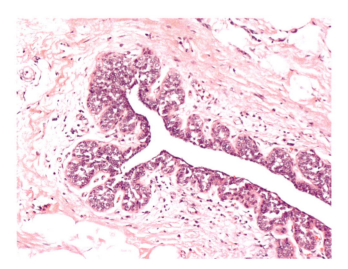

Fig. 13.9 Lobular carcinoma in situ. Pagetoid spread in ducts may be present. The neoplastic cells extend along ducts between intact overlying epithelium and underlying basement membrane

13.1 Variants of Lobular Carcinoma In Situ

Several variants of LCIS have been recognized. These include florid LCIS with comedo necrosis, Florid LCIS with signet ring cells, central necrosis and calcifications, and pleomorphic LCIS.

- **Lobular Carcinoma In Situ with Comedonecrosis**

LCIS with comedonecrosis has recently been described. Before the widespread use of E-cadherin, such cases were categorized as mixed ductal and lobular carcinoma or carcinoma in situ with indeterminate features. These lesions are comprised of cells identical to those of classic LCIS; namely, small, uniform cells and a discohesive growth pattern, but which also contain central areas of comedonecrosis (Fig. 13.11). An associated invasive carcinoma was present in 12 (67%) of 18 cases described by Fadare et al. (seven classic lobular, one pleomorphic lobular, one ductal, one mixed lobular and ductal, one tubular, and one case with ductal and lobular carcinomas as separate foci) [12]. Because LCIS with comedonecrosis is rare in its pure form, re-excision is recommended when this lesion is detected in isolation in a core biopsy or at the margin of an excision specimen.

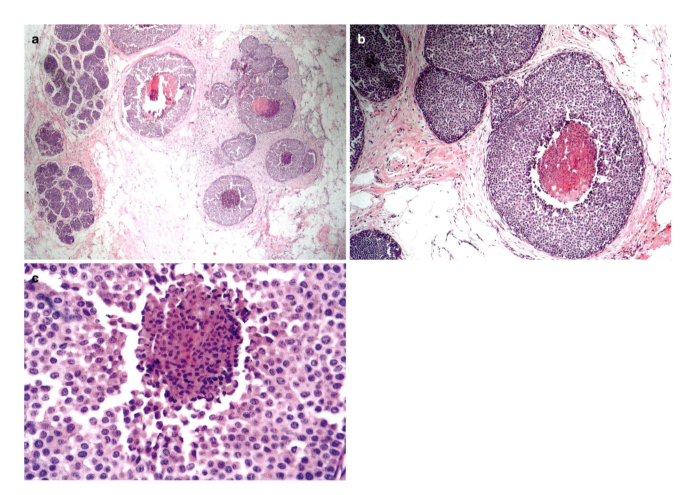

Fig. 13.11 Lobular carcinoma in situ with necrosis. (**a**) Low-power showing LCIS with necrosis in a background of classical LCIS. (**b, c**) Same lesion showing typical cytologic features of classical lobular carcinoma in situ

- **Lobular Carcinoma In Situ (Lobular Intraepithelial Neoplasia) with Signet Ring Cells, Central Necrosis, and Calcifications**

Alvarado-Cabrero et al. [13] described ten cases of LCIS (lobular intraepithelial neoplasia), composed of signet ring cells with central necrosis and calcifications. In this series, eight patients had associated invasive carcinoma (six lobular carcinomas and one mixed lobular and ductal) (Fig. 13.12).

- **Pleomorphic Lobular Carcinoma In Situ**

Pleomorphic lobular carcinoma in situ was first identified as a distinct entity by Eusebi et al. [14] in 1992. The cytological appearances of these cells are quite different to those of classic LCIS. Although the cells appear discohesive, as in classic LCIS, they exhibit a greater degree of nuclear pleomorphism and usually contain abundant cytoplasm. Occasionally, the cytoplasm can appear eosinophilic and finely granular (Fig. 13.13).

Regarding the immunohistochemical (IHC) profile, almost all cases of LCIS express estrogen receptors (ER) and progesterone receptors (PR) and lack for membranous E-cadherin (Fig. 13.14) and p120 expression by IHC. Classic LCIS is usually negative for HER2 protein overexpression/gene amplification, lack p53 mutations, and has a low ki-67 labeling index. In contrast, PLCIS may show HER2 protein overexpression/gene amplification, p53 expression, and moderate-to-high Ki-67 labeling index [15].

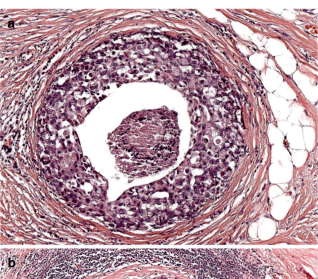

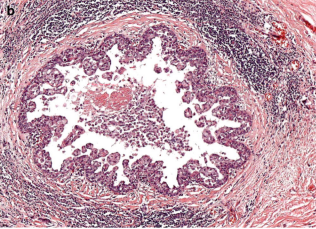

Fig. 13.12 Lobular carcinoma in situ. (**a**) Low-power microscopic examination of this case reveal distention of a duct by a population of signet ring cells. Foci of comedo type necrosis (central). (**b**) Duct involvement in a cloverleaf pattern (same case)

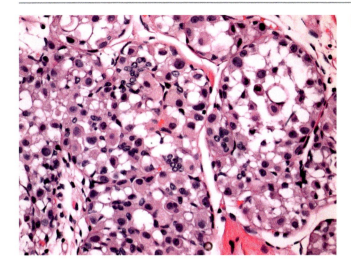

Fig. 13.13 Pleomorphic lobular carcinoma in situ (PLCIS). The neoplastic cells in PLCIS show marked pleomorphism and are larger with abundant eosinophilic cytoplasm. Signet-ring cells may be found in some cases

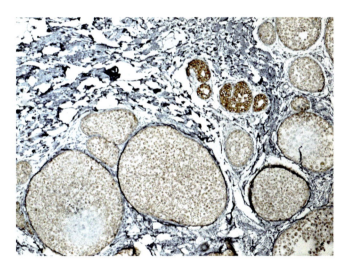

Fig. 13.14 Lobular carcinoma in situ (LCIS). The lack of membranous E-cadherin expression characterizes LCIS and is useful for distinction from ductal proliferations

References

1. Ewing J. Neoplastic diseases: a textbook on tumors. 1st ed. Philadelphia, PA: WB Saunders; 1919.
2. Foote F, Stewart F. Lobular carcinoma in situ: a rare form of mammary cancer. Am J Pathol. 1941;17:491–6.
3. Haagensen CD, Lane N, Lattes R, Bodian C. Lobular neoplasia (so-called lobular carcinoma in situ) of the breast. Cancer. 1978;42:737–69.
4. Page DL, Dupont WD, Rogers LW, Rados MS. Atypical hyperplastic lesions of the female breast. A long-term follow-up study. Cancer. 1985;55:2698–708.
5. Bratthauer GL, Tavassoli FA. Lobular intraepithelial neoplasia: previously unexplored aspects assessed in 775 cases and their clinical implications. Virchows Arch. 2002;440:134–8.
6. Chickman B, Lavy R, Davidson T, Wassermann I, Sandbank J, Siegelmann-Danieli N, et al. Factors affecting rise in the incidence of infiltrating lobular carcinoma of the breast. Isr Med Assoc J. 2010;12:697–700.
7. Li CI, Anderson BO, Daling JR, Moe RE. Changing incidence of lobular carcinoma in situ of the breast. Breast Cancer Res Treat. 2002;75:259–68.
8. Malley FO. Lobular neoplasia: morphology, biological potential and management in core biopsies. Mod Pathol. 2010;23(Suppl 2):S14–25.
9. Middleton LP, Grant S, Stephens T, Stelling CB, Sneige N, Sahin AA. Lobular carcinoma in situ diagnosed by core needle biopsy: when should it be excised? Mod Pathol. 2003;16:120–9.
10. Bodian CA, Perzin KH, Lattes R. Lobular neoplasia. Long term risk of breast cancer and relation to other factors. Cancer. 1996;78:1024–34.
11. Lakhani SR. In situ lobular neoplasia: time for an awakening. Lancet. 2003;361:96.
12. Fadare O, Dadmanesh F, Alvarado-Cabrero I, Snyder R, Stephen Mitchell J, Tot T, et al. Lobular Intraepithelial (lobular carcinoma in situ) with comedo-type necrosis: a clinico-pathologic study of 18 cases. Am J Surg Pathol. 2006;30:1445–53.
13. Alvarado-Cabrero I, Picón Coronel G, Valencia Cedillo R, Canedo N, Tavassoli FA. Florid lobular intraepithelial neoplasia with signet ring cells, central necrosis and calcifications: a clinicopathological and immunohistochemical analysis of ten cases associated with invasive lobular carcinoma. Arch Med Res. 2010;41:436–41.
14. Bentz JS, Yassa N, Clayton F. Pleomorphic lobular carcinoma of the breast: clinicopathologic features of 12 cases. Mod Pathol. 1998;11:814–22.
15. Dabbs DJ, Kaplai M, Chivukula M, Kanbour A, Kanbour-Shakir A, Carter GJ. The spectrum of morphomolecular abnormalities of the E-cadherin/catenin complex in pleomorphic lobular carcinoma of the breast. Appl Immunohistochem Mol Morphol. 2007;15:260–6.

Infiltrating Carcinoma of No Special Type

14

Simona Stolnicu

Infiltrating breast carcinoma is a category of malignant epithelial tumors characterized by adjacent tissue invasion and distance metastasis. This category includes several microscopic types that differ from one another from morphological, immunohistochemical, molecular, and prognostic points of view. It is currently known that all these microscopic types have their origin in the terminal duct/lobular unit. The WHO 2012 classification categorized both invasive carcinomas of no special type (NST), previously termed as ductal carcinomas, and lobular and other special and rare subtypes of carcinomas, as infiltrating epithelial tumors, only distinguishing between these types in terms of morphological appearance, but disregarding the origin of proliferation [1].

14.1   NST Infiltrating Carcinoma

The NST infiltrating carcinoma, also called ductal, classic, or not otherwise specified (NOS), is the most common form, accounting for 40–75% of invasive breast carcinomas [1]. Its origin is in the epithelium of ducts and acini. By definition, it describes a heterogeneous group in which the microscopic appearance is uncharacteristic of any of the specific microscopic variants of breast carcinoma (like tubular, medullary carcinoma, etc.). Grossly, the tumor size is highly variable, from a few millimeters (Fig. 14.1) to more than 10 cm (Fig. 14.2) with infiltrating edges, while its shape may be stellate or nodular (Figs. 14.3, 14.4, and 14.5) but usually solid, and rarely with cystic changes determined by tumor necrosis (Fig. 14.6). Tumor consistency is high and sometimes the tumor is so hard that its hardness is comparable to that of wood. It is rare, however, due to the minor stromal component, that the tumor consistency is soft. The color varies between white and gray with yellow striations (confirming the presence of elastosis in the tumor) but sometimes has

a yellow color (Fig. 14.7) or red color due to intratumor hemorrhage (Figs. 14.8 and 14.9). When the tumor is high-stage, it invades the skin and can produce skin ulceration (Figs. 14.10, 14.11, and 14.12).

The microscopic diagnosis of NST type is based on the growth pattern of the tumor. Microscopic appearance is highly variable and can be challenging for an inexperienced pathologist because the tumor cells may be present in clusters, nests, cords, tubules (with evident central lumen), or isolated in a more or less abundant stroma (Figs. 14.13, 14.14, 14.15, 14.16, and 14.17). These structures are comprised of only epithelial tumor cells and are not accompanied by myoepithelial cells or basement membrane (Fig. 14.18). Tumor cells are sometimes arranged in a "single file" or a targetoid pattern, as in infiltrating lobular carcinoma, but they have a completely different morphologic appearance and they are cohesive (Fig. 14.19). Some pathologists, however, indicate that the presence of the lumina itself is in favor of NST (ductal) differentiation, because lobular in situ carcinomas or invasive carcinomas lack lumina [2]. Tumor cells are typically round or polygonal, with abundant and eosinophilic cytoplasm, and sometimes with vacuolated cytoplasm or signet-ring appearance, and have nuclei with variable pleomorphism and with one or more evident nucleoli (Figs. 14.20, 14.21, and 14.22). Mitotic activity varies from one tumor to another or from one microscopic field to another within the same tumor (Fig. 14.23). Tumor stroma is highly variable in quantity, and in some tumors, it is cellular and fibroblastic, while in others it may be hypocellular with extensive hyalinization. The stroma may have stromal elastosis (periductal and perivascular), necrosis, as well as inflammatory lymphoplasmacytic infiltrate, sometimes with a granulomatous character and microcalcifications (Figs. 14.24, 14.25, 14.26, and 14.27). Rarely, the tumor may present minor or sometimes extensive hemorrhage, which may obstruct the tumor cells and may lead to difficulty in microscopic interpretation (Fig. 14.28). Some tumors may be associated with perineural invasion. The presence of

S. Stolnicu, MD, PhD
Department of Pathology, University of Medicine and Pharmacy, Tîrgu Mureş, Romania

© Springer International Publishing AG, part of Springer Nature 2018
S. Stolnicu, I. Alvarado-Cabrero (eds.), *Practical Atlas of Breast Pathology*, https://doi.org/10.1007/978-3-319-93257-6_14

vascular tumor emboli can be better appreciated at the periphery of the tumor. The tumor cells, however, must be detected within vascular channels lined by endothelial cells and not within artifactual spaces that have been caused by tissue shrinkage occurring during the processing of the tissue (Fig. 14.29).

Also, areas of in situ carcinoma (ductal or lobular or both, with identical microscopic grade as in the infiltrating component) can be detected at the periphery of the tumor in more than 80% of cases (Figs. 14.30 and 14.31). Immunohistochemically, the tumor cells have a variable positivity for the ER, PR, HER2. E-cadherin is typically positive, but positivity may be low in some cases (Fig. 14.32). Also, E-cadherin-positivity does not equal ductal differentiation in the context of appropriate histologic features, and one should be aware of the limitation in the use of E-cadherin immunostaining. The Ki67 index is highly variable and it correlates with the tumor microscopic grade.

Regarding differential diagnosis, it should be emphasized that the diagnosis of NST infiltrating ductal carcinoma is a diagnosis of exclusion. It is a form of carcinoma that does not meet classic criteria for other microscopic types. As a rule, it is advisable that in difficult situations, a diagnosis of NST infiltrating ductal carcinoma be preferred, especially when the tumor reveals tubular structures, because most authors consider that NST infiltrating ductal carcinoma is the most common form of breast cancer. The most important differential diagnosis is with infiltrating lobular carcinoma. The appearance of the latter carcinoma is characterized by the presence of small and uniform dyscohesive cells arranged in "single file" in its classic form. Sometimes, NST infiltrating carcinoma may also present a linear "single file" arrangement, where the abundant fibrous stroma compresses the trabeculae of tumor cells (Fig. 14.33). NST infiltrating ductal carcinoma cells are more uneven and more pleomorphic, but especially more cohesive than, those of infiltrating lobular carcinoma. Immunohistochemical stains (with E-cadherin and p120 catenin) can help differentiate between the two lesions, but with some limitations

(Fig. 14.34). The solid subtype of infiltrating lobular carcinoma must be distinguished from poorly differentiated NST infiltrating ductal carcinoma in which the tumor cells are arranged in large nests and glandular lumen formation is rarely seen (Fig. 14.35). In this case, however, differential diagnosis is favored by the fact that tumor cells of NST infiltrating ductal carcinoma are more pleomorphic. If the cells are small, uniform, and arranged predominantly in nests, the question of alveolar subtype of infiltrating lobular carcinoma arises (in the alveolar subtype of infiltrating lobular carcinoma, however, cells have more eosinophilic cytoplasm and lack cohesiveness). A clue in recognizing the lobular infiltrating carcinoma is the presence of intracytoplasmic lumina with eosinophilic material, but one must be aware of the fact that rare NST carcinomas can display similar features (Figs. 14.36 and 14.37). The increased amount of intracytoplasmic mucin must be differentiated by using special stains for the presence of glycogen (PAS-positive) or lipids (Sudan III-positive), characteristic of breast carcinoma variants containing abundant lipids and of clear cell carcinoma abundant in glycogen. If the cells appear uniform with low and elongated cytoplasm arranged in nests, NST carcinoma must be differentiated by a carcinoma with neuroendocrine differentiation (the latter is positive for neuroendocrine markers such as chromogranin, synaptophysin, etc.) (Fig. 14.38). The occasional presence of extracellular mucin must be differentiated from a mucinous carcinoma, and the presence of an abundant inflammatory infiltrate of lymphoplasmacytic type in the stroma should not be confused with the similar appearance of medullary carcinoma, especially when the tumor has "pushing" margins. Finally, NST infiltrating carcinoma should not be confused with adenosis, a benign lesion that can sometimes mimic an infiltrating carcinoma (but in which epithelial cells do not have atypia and myoepithelial cells can be distinguished in most of the cases).

The prognosis of NST invasive carcinoma of the breast is variable and depends on several prognostic parameters, which will be discussed in detail in another chapter.

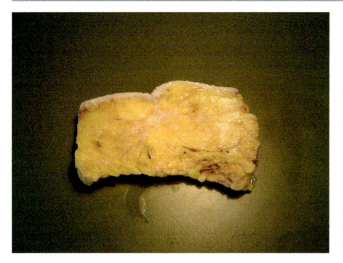

Fig. 14.1 Invasive carcinoma of NST subtype with small size (10 mm of diameter)

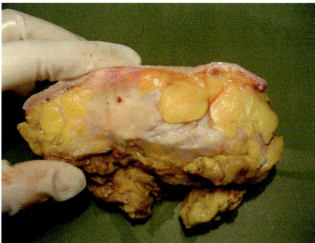

Fig. 14.4 Invasive carcinoma of NST subtype with infiltrating margins

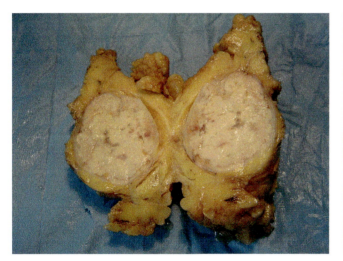

Fig. 14.2 Invasive carcinoma of NST subtype with large size (locally advanced tumor)

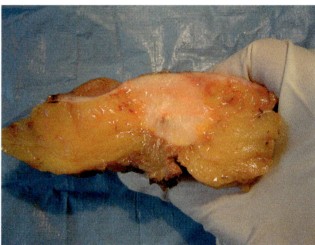

Fig. 14.5 Invasive carcinoma of NST subtype with partially infiltrating margins

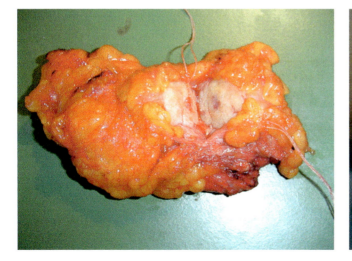

Fig. 14.3 Invasive carcinoma of NST subtype with lobulated margins

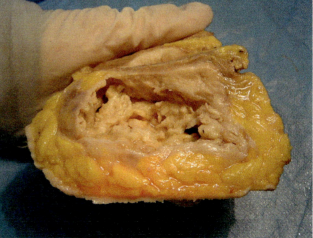

Fig. 14.6 Invasive carcinoma of NST subtype with cystic changes determined by central tumor necrosis

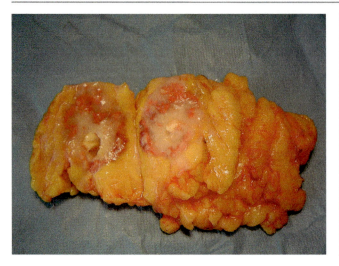

Fig. 14.7 Invasive carcinoma of NST subtype with cystic changes and yellow color on the section surface

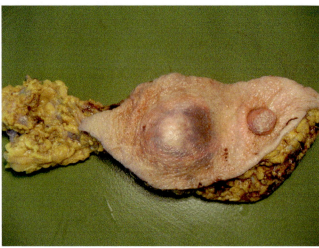

Fig. 14.10 High stage Invasive carcinoma of NST subtype infiltrating the skin

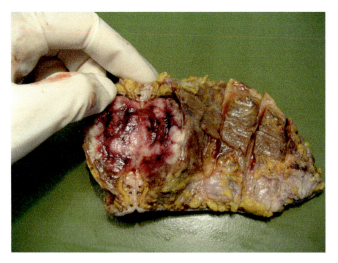

Fig. 14.8 Invasive carcinoma of NST subtype with red color due to intratumor focus of hemorrhage

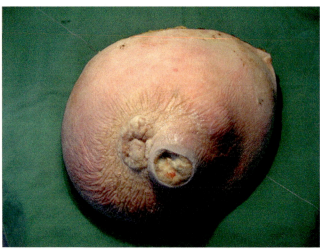

Fig. 14.11 Invasive carcinoma of NST subtype infiltrating the skin and the nipple

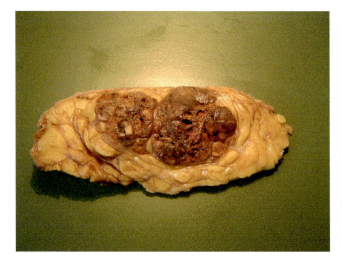

Fig. 14.9 Invasive carcinoma of NST subtype with red color and cystic spaces due to intratumor hemorrhage

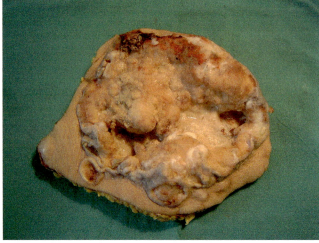

Fig. 14.12 Invasive carcinoma of NST subtype with massive skin ulceration

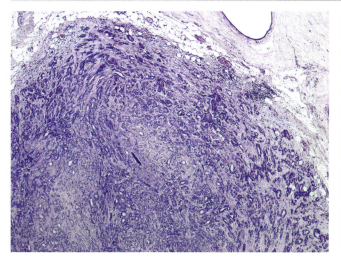

Fig. 14.13 Invasive carcinoma of NST subtype: microscopic architectural and cellular appearance is highly variable

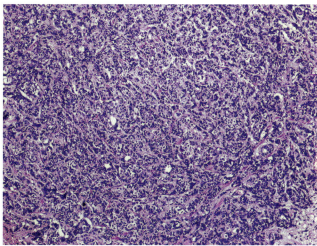

Fig. 14.16 Invasive carcinoma of NST subtype: trabecular and alveolar arrangement

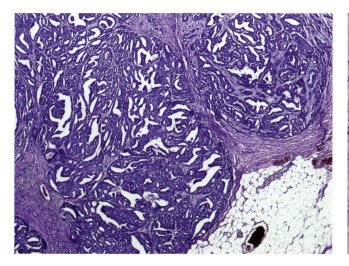

Fig. 14.14 Invasive carcinoma of NST subtype: in this case, the tumor cells are mostly arranged in tubules

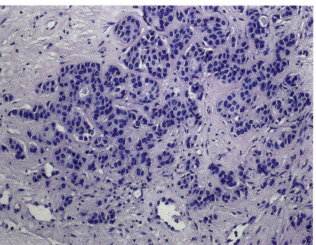

Fig. 14.17 Invasive carcinoma of NST subtype: alveolar arrangement of the tumor cells

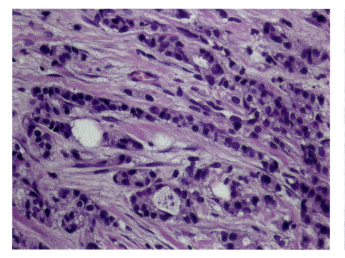

Fig. 14.15 Invasive carcinoma of NST subtype: in this case, the tumor cells are mostly arranged in cords

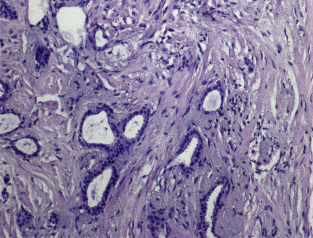

Fig. 14.18 Invasive carcinoma of NST subtype: tubular structures are composed of only epithelial tumor cells, which are not accompanied by myoepithelial cells or basement membrane

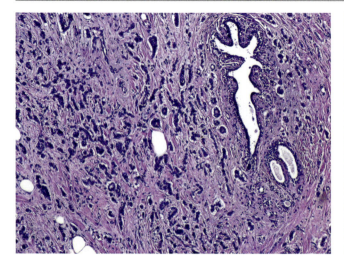

Fig. 14.19 Invasive carcinoma of NST subtype: in this case, the tumor cells are arranged in a targetoid pattern around a normal duct, mimicking an infiltrating lobular carcinoma; however, they have a completely different morphologic appearance and are associated with tubular formation

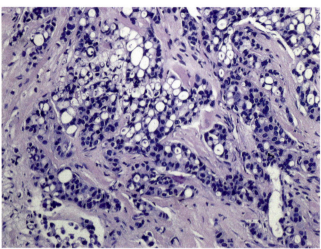

Fig. 14.22 Invasive carcinoma of NST subtype: most of the tumor cells have a signet-ring appearance; in this case, however, E-cadherin was positive, differentiating from an invasive lobular carcinoma with signet-ring cells (not shown here)

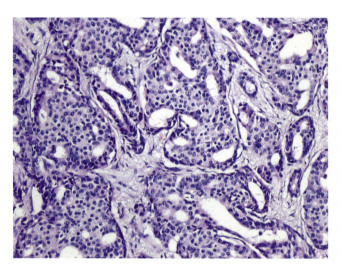

Fig. 14.20 Invasive carcinoma of NST subtype: the tumor cells are typically round or polygonal, with abundant and eosinophilic cytoplasm

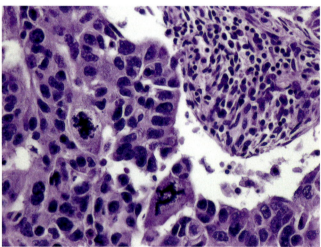

Fig. 14.23 Invasive carcinoma of NST subtype: high-grade tumor with numerous atypical mitotic figures

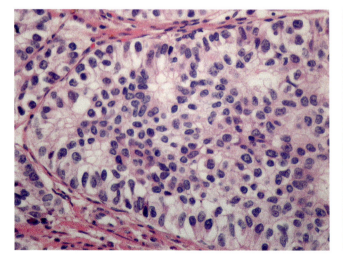

Fig. 14.21 Invasive carcinoma of NST subtype: sometimes the tumor cells have a vacuolated cytoplasm

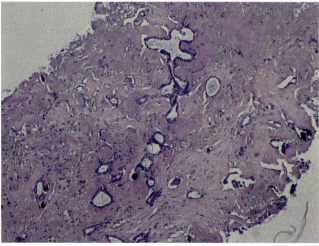

Fig. 14.24 Invasive carcinoma of NST subtype: the stroma displays abundant stromal elastosis

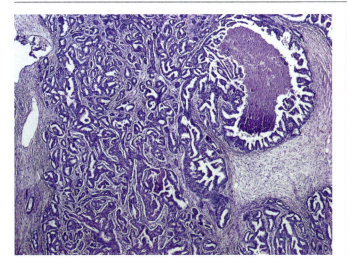

Fig. 14.25 Invasive carcinoma of NST subtype with focal necrosis

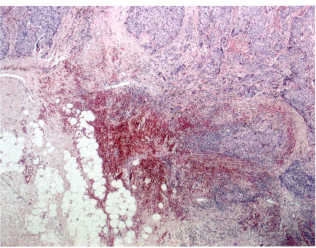

Fig. 14.28 Invasive carcinoma of NST subtype: the tumor presents minor hemorrhagic area

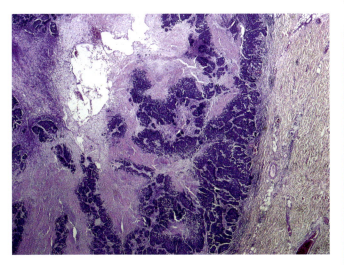

Fig. 14.26 Invasive carcinoma of NST subtype with extensive geographic-type necrosis (typically associated with basal-like invasive carcinomas)

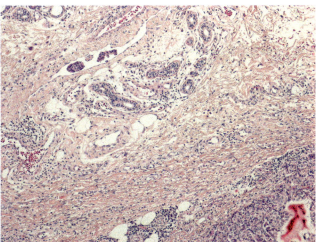

Fig. 14.29 Invasive carcinoma of NST subtype: at the periphery and outside of the tumor border, the presence of vascular tumor emboli can be better appreciated

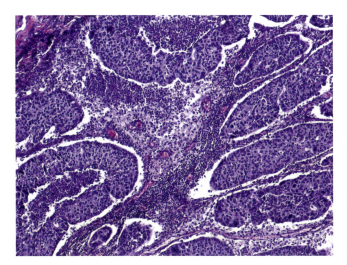

Fig. 14.27 Invasive carcinoma of NST subtype presenting an inflammatory lymphoplasmacytic infiltrate, with numerous macrophages within the tumor stroma

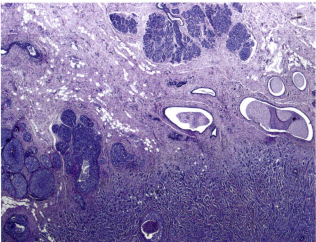

Fig. 14.30 Invasive carcinoma of NST subtype: areas of both in situ ductal and lobular carcinoma are detected at the periphery of this tumor

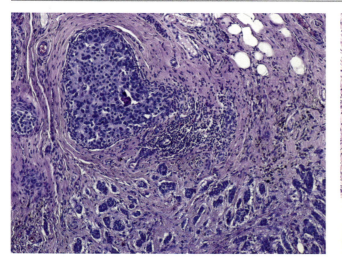

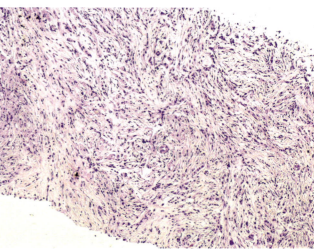

Fig. 14.31 Invasive carcinoma of NST subtype: identical morphological appearance of the tumor cells is present in both in situ and infiltrating component

Fig. 14.33 Invasive carcinoma of NST subtype: tumor cells are arranged predominantly in trabeculae, mimicking an invasive lobular carcinoma

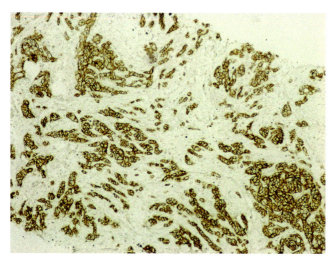

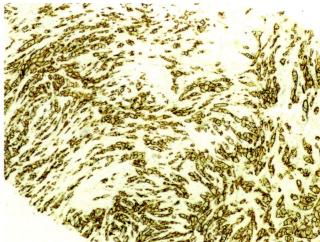

Fig. 14.32 Invasive carcinoma of NST subtype: the tumor cells are positive for E-cadherin

Fig. 14.34 Invasive carcinoma of NST subtype with tumor cells are arranged in trabeculae, mimicking invasive lobular carcinoma; however, the E-cadherin is positive helping in differentiating the two entities

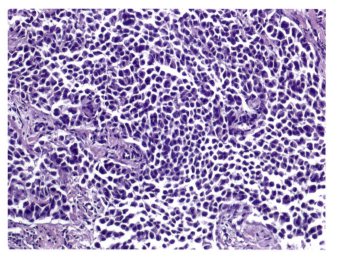

Fig. 14.35 The solid subtype of infiltrating lobular carcinoma must be distinguished from poorly differentiated NST infiltrating ductal carcinoma; however, in the lobular invasive carcinoma the cells are dyscohesive (as shown in this picture)

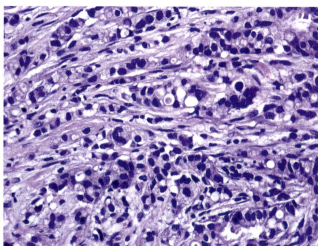

Fig. 14.37 Invasive carcinoma of NST subtype: some tumor cells may also display intracitoplasmic lumina with eosinophilic content, similar to lobular invasive carcinoma. But the cells are more cohesive

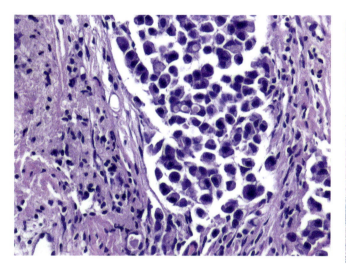

Fig. 14.36 Invasive lobular carcinoma: high-power examination reveals the presence of intracytoplasmatic lumina with eosinophilic material, a very characteristic feature of this tumor, besides the fact that the tumor cells are dyscohesive

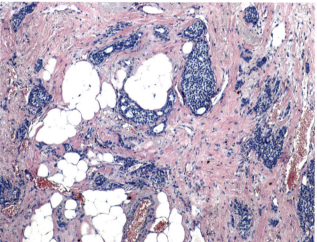

Fig. 14.38 Invasive carcinoma with neuroendocrine differentiation: of note, the cells are uniform and arranged in nests, a finding that can also occur in the infiltrating NSY subtype

14.2 Mixed Carcinoma

To qualify as NST type, this pattern must be present in more than 90% of the tumor. Mixed carcinoma is a microscopic variant in which NST infiltrating carcinoma features should represent 10–49% of the tumor, while other microscopic subtypes represent the rest. Both components should be reported and microscopically graded (Figs. 14.39 and 14.40).

The 2012 WHO classification distinguishes four subtypes of NST infiltrating ductal carcinoma: pleomorphic carcinoma, carcinoma with osteoclast-like stromal giant cells, carcinoma with choriocarcinomatous features, and carcinoma with melanotic features [1].

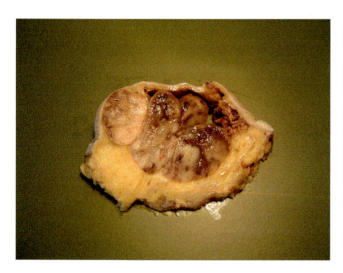

Fig. 14.39 Mixed infiltrating carcinoma: macroscopic examination of the tumor cut surface demonstrates a solid infiltrating NST component with hard consistency (left side) associated with a larger, more gelatinous and softer mucinous component (right side)

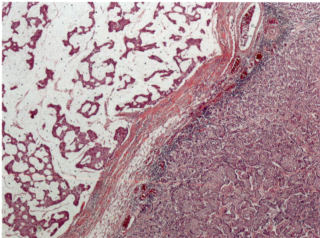

Fig. 14.40 Mixed infiltrating carcinoma with a mucinous hypercellular component (left side) and a second component of NST subtype (right side)

14.3   Pleomorphic Carcinoma

Pleomorphic carcinoma is a rare variant, characterized by a proliferation of large, pleomorphic, and bizarre tumor cells, which comprise over 50% of the tumor. The remaining tumor is usually represented by an NST infiltrating carcinoma (rarely by a metaplastic, squamous cell or spindle-cell carcinoma, in which case the lesion should be diagnosed as metaplastic carcinoma). Macroscopically, the tumor resembles an NST infiltrating carcinoma often accompanied by central necrosis. Microscopically, tumor cells are large, bizarre, with abundant eosinophilic cytoplasm, have a nucleus with marked pleomorphism, and the cells are frequently multinucleated and have numerous mitotic figures (this tumor is always of high-grade of malignancy). Sometimes the cells are spindle, resembling a sarcomatous component (Figs. 14.41 and 14.42). An intraductal carcinoma can be noticed at the margin of the tumor, as well as numerous vascular tumor emboli. Most of these tumors are either triple negative or ER and PR-negative, while the HER2 is positive. Tumor cells are diffusely positive for pan-Cytokeratin. Differential diagnosis should be done with various forms of sarcoma

(immunohistochemical tests are useful for this purpose). It is important to bear in mind that primary breast sarcomas are very rare, and by combining a good sample of the tumor with ancillary stains (it is advisable to use a panel of markers for the epithelial differentiation as well as for the exclusion of the mesenchymal differentiation), one can almost always recognize a pleomorphic carcinoma [3]. Of note, some sarcomas can be pan-CK positive, while other carcinomas can show positivity for Vimentin. Also, a differential diagnosis with metaplastic (also called sarcomatous carcinoma or myoepithelial carcinoma, as the two lesions represent the same entity) needs to be considered in cases in which a malignant mesenchymal-looking carcinoma is present. In metaplastic carcinoma, however, the NST component is not identified. Of interest, several publications demonstrated positivity for myoepithelial markers in metaplastic (sarcomatoid) carcinomas (such as p63, CD 10, SMA, S100), as well as for basal cell markers (CK5/6, CK14, CK34betaE12) [4].

This pleomorphic carcinoma has a very aggressive behavior and is very rarely associated with axillary lymph node metastases, being characterized by a behavior more like that of a sarcoma.

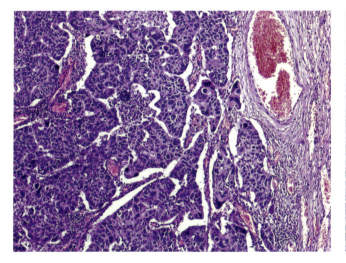

Fig. 14.41 Pleomorphic carcinoma with solid architecture and composed of very pleomorphic tumor cells, some of them with large and bizarre nuclei

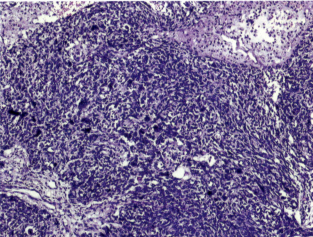

Fig. 14.42 Pleomorphic carcinoma: another example of tumor composed of spindle- shaped tumor cells, resembling a sarcomatous component

14.4   Carcinoma with Osteoclast-Like Stromal Giant Cells

This microscopic subtype is a rare form of infiltrating carcinoma. Macroscopically, it has a soft consistency, brownish color due to bleeding foci, and may have clearly defined or infiltrating margins. Microscopically, the tumor is characterized by the presence of giant multinucleated stromal cells that are similar to osteoclasts [5]. Inflammatory infiltrate can be found in the stroma, as well as numerous blood vessels, extravasated erythrocytes, and histiocytes with intracytoplasmic hemosiderin. Giant stromal cells vary in shape and are located in the stroma, arranged around nests of tumor cells (usually of NST type, well or moderately differentiated), or even inside the lumens formed by the tumor cells. They have an abundant eosinophilic cytoplasm and numerous nonatypical round nuclei, usually arranged in the center of the cell, resembling osteoclasts. Immunohistochemically, multinucleated giant stromal cells are positive for CD-68, acid phosphatase, non-specific esterase, and lysozyme, and are negative for alkaline phosphatase, S-100 protein, actin, Cytokeratin, EMA, ER, and PR. Immunohistochemical and ultrastructural studies have confirmed the histiocytic origin of these cells. The invasive carcinoma component is represented by an NST infiltrating ductal carcinoma. Prognosis depends on the characteristics of the invasive NST carcinoma component and is not influenced by the presence of multinucleated giant stromal cells. The prognosis is driven by the NST component and does not appear to be influenced by the presence of the giant stromal cells.

14.5   Carcinoma with Choriocarcinomatous Features

An extremely rare variant of infiltrating breast carcinoma, this type is associated with increased ß-HCG (β-Human chorionic gonadotropin) serum [6–8]. The microscopic appearance of NST infiltrating ductal carcinoma is associated with choriocarcinomatous areas of differentiation, formed by multinucleated giant cells with eosinophilic cytoplasm and syncytial appearance (syncytiotrophoblast-type of differentiation), together with groups of small, uniform, mononuclear cells, with cytotrophoblastic differentiation. The tumor must be differentiated from metastatic choriocarcinoma originating in the uterus (associated with evidence of primary uterine tumor). A large number of NST cases may have HCG-positive cells without morphological identification of these cells as having trophoblast appearance. Prognosis is difficult to establish because there are very few cases of this microscopic subtype reported in the literature.

14.6   Carcinoma with Melanotic Features

This is a very rare breast carcinoma, which likely appears as the result of a process of metaplasia to a melanocytic component of an infiltrating breast carcinoma. Grossly, the tumor has a brownish color, while microscopically it is composed of areas with an NST infiltrating ductal carcinoma appearance and areas of malignant melanoma (with spindle cell or epithelioid tumor cells). Immunohistochemically, areas of NST infiltrating carcinoma type are positive for Cytokeratin and negative for HMB-45, Melan A, and S-100 protein. The melanocytic-appearing differentiations are negative for Cytokeratin and positive for HMB-45, Melan A, and S-100 protein. Differential diagnosis must include infiltrating breast carcinomas that may have melanin pigment (due to its phagocytosis by tumor cells), and breast carcinomas infiltrating the skin (without areas with melanocytic differentiation). Also, the tumor must be distinguished from infiltrating breast tumors, which sometimes may contain lipofuscin deposits (special stains differentiate the two pigments). Another differential diagnosis is made with metastasis of malignant melanoma with an extramammary origin (clinical evidence of another primary tumor) and intramammary metastasis of malignant cutaneous melanoma, which starts in the skin of the mammary gland or another location (without areas appearing as NST infiltrating ductal carcinoma). Sometimes an NST carcinoma may have Melan A positive cells lacking an association with a component with melanocytic features. This tumor usually has an aggressive behavior.

References

1. Lakhani SR, Schnitt SJ, Tan PH, van deVijver MJ. WHO classification of tumors of the breast. Lyon: IARC; 2012.
2. Tavassoli FA. Pathology of the breast. 2nd ed. New York, NY: McGraw-Hill; 1999.
3. Moinfar F. Essentials of diagnostic breast pathology. Berlin: Springer; 2007. p. 236.
4. Leibl S, Gogg-Kammerer M, Sommersacher A, Denk H, Moinfar F. Metaplastic breast carcinoma: are they of myoepithelial differentiation? Immunohistochemical profile of the sarcomatoid subtype using novel myoepithelial markers. Am J Surg Pathol. 2005;29:347–53.
5. Pettinato G, Petrella G, Manco A, di Prisco B, Salvatore G, Angrisani P. Carcinoma of the breast with osteoclast-like giant cells. Fine-needle aspiration cytology, histology and electron microscopy of 5 cases. Appl Pathol. 1984;2(3):168–78.
6. Saigo PE, Rosen PP. Mammary carcinoma with choriocarcinomatous features. Am J Surg Pathol. 1981;5(8):773–8.
7. Resetkova E, Sahin A, Ayala AG, Sneige N. Breast carcinoma with choriocarcinomatous features. Ann Diagn Pathol. 2004;8(2):74–9.
8. Zhu Y, Liu M, Li J, Jung F, Linghu R, Guo X, et al. Breast carcinoma with choriocarcinomatous features: a case report and review of the literature. World J Surg Oncol. 2014;12:239.

Special Types of Invasive Breast Carcinoma

15

Javier A. Arias-Stella III, Isabel Alvarado-Cabrero, and Fresia Pareja

Breast carcinoma is a vastly heterogeneous disease encompassing a wide array of entities with different morphology, biology, clinical behavior, and prognosis. Special types of breast carcinoma include tumors with morphologies that deviate from invasive carcinoma of no special type (NST). As a group, special types comprise up to 25% of all breast cancers, and encompass entities ranging from low to high-grade, and with different hormone receptor and HER2 status. The recognition of the different special types of breast cancer is of paramount importance, as their proper classification is relevant not only for taxonomic purposes, but has also therapeutic implications.

15.1 Invasive Lobular Carcinoma

Invasive lobular carcinoma (ILC) is the most common special type of breast cancer and accounts for approximately 15% of breast invasive carcinomas [1]. While the incidence of invasive carcinoma of no special type (NST) has been stable, incidence of ILC appears to have increased [2].

Patients with ILC usually present with an ill-defined palpable mass or diffuse breast nodularity, at an older age, and with larger tumors than patients with invasive carcinoma, NST [3]. ILC has a tendency to occur bilaterally and multicentrically [4]. The most frequent mammographic finding of ILC is a mass with irregular borders, while microcalcifications are rarely seen [5–7]. However, mammography has a relatively low sensitivity for the detection of ILC, with up to 30% of false negative cases [7]. On ultrasonogram, ILC is

J. A. Arias-Stella III, MD · F. Pareja, MD, PhD (✉)
Department of Pathology, Memorial Sloan Kettering Cancer Center, New York, NY, USA
e-mail: ariasstj@mskcc.org; parejaf@mskcc.org

I. Alvarado-Cabrero, MD, PhD
Department of Pathology, Hospital de Oncologia, Centro Medico Nacional Siglo XXI, Instituto Mexicano del Seguro Social, Mexico City, Mexico

commonly detected as an irregular hypoechoic mass with spiculated borders; posterior acoustic shadowing is observed more frequently than in invasive carcinoma, NST [5]. While the tumor size of ILC is frequently underestimated by mammography and ultrasonogram [8], magnetic resonance imaging (MRI) findings correlate better with the histologic size of the tumor [9].

Classic ILC is composed of discohesive tumor cells arranged in a linear pattern or as single cells. Classic ILC is associated with negligible desmoplasia or host lymphocytic reaction and does not disrupt the normal breast architecture (Fig. 15.1), displaying a targetoid concentric distribution around ducts and lobules (Fig. 15.2). The tumor cells resemble those of lobular carcinoma in situ (LCIS), and are small and uniform with occasional intracellular lumina, round and uniform nuclei, inconspicuous nucleoli, and infrequent mitotic figures (Fig.15.3).

A wide array of ILC variants can be recognized, which differ from classical ILC in their morphology and behavior, including the solid, alveolar, trabecular, tubulolobular, signet ring cell, and pleomorphic variants. ILC histologic variants are found occasionally admixed with classic ILC or with other ILC variants. The solid variant of ILC is characterized by discohesive tumor cells growing in solid nests, and may show pleomorphism or increased mitotic activity (Fig. 15.4) [10]. The alveolar variant of ILC is composed of tumor cells arranged in discrete clusters or aggregates of 20 or more cells, separated by thin fibrous septa (Fig. 15.5) [11]. The trabecular variant of ILC is characterized by tumor cells growing in bands thicker than two cells. The tubulolobular variant of ILC is composed of small cords and tubules of tumor cells arranged in a linear fashion, with a hybrid tubular and lobular morphology [12]. Pleomorphic ILC has the same growth pattern as classic ILC, but the tumor cells show greater cytological atypia and pleomorphism and display a higher mitotic rate (Figs. 15.6 and 15.7) [13].

Cytologic smears of ILC show small tumor cells in poorly cohesive clusters or as isolated cells, with occasional single-cell linear alignments (Fig. 15.8) [14]. Despite the challenges associated with the diagnosis ILC on cytology, fine-needle aspiration (FNA) remains a useful diagnostic tool. Nonetheless, caution should be exerted to distinguish ILC from its mimickers, such as inflammatory cells in mastitis, which may result in a false positive interpretation.

The differential diagnosis of ILC includes lymphoma, metastatic carcinoma, tubulolobular carcinoma, and invasive carcinoma NST with lobular features. Classic ILC, and in particular its histologic variants, must sometimes be distinguished from invasive carcinoma NST, and E-cadherin is widely used for this purpose. *CDH1* mutations cause loss of expression of E-cadherin, a molecule involved in cell-to-cell adhesion, which results in the facilitation of epithelial to mesenchymal transition and tumorigenesis [15]. The expression of E-cadherin is reduced or completely absent in ILC (Fig. 15.9) [16], although some cases may express E-cadherin aberrantly [17]. Notably, the cadherin-catenin complex appears to be non-functional in ILC with aberrant E-cadherin expression, and the latter should not preclude the diagnosis of ILC in cases with a typical lobular morphology [17].

Immunohistochemical stains for β-catenin, which is reduced in ILC, and p120, which shows a diffuse cytoplasmic expression, are also helpful to define a lobular phenotype. ILCs are generally positive for estrogen receptor (ER) and progesterone receptor (PR), while negative for the human epidermal growth factor receptor 2 (HER2), although ILC variants, such as pleomorphic ILC, may more frequently display a HER2-positive or triple negative phenotype [18]. ILCs are enriched for mutations in *CDH1*, *PTEN*, *TBX3*, and *FOXA1* [19], and the majority of them are of luminal A molecular subtype [20].

ILC has a favorable clinical outcome and has a significantly better 5-year disease-free survival than invasive carcinoma NST. Nonetheless, ILC is associated with late recurrences and metastasis in atypical locations [21], and with a higher frequency of positive or close surgical margins than invasive carcinoma NST [22]. Moreover, some histologic variants of ILC, such as pleomorphic ILC, have more aggressive clinicopathologic features. Older age and triple negative phenotype have been shown to significantly correlate with a worse clinical outcome in pleomorphic ILC [23].

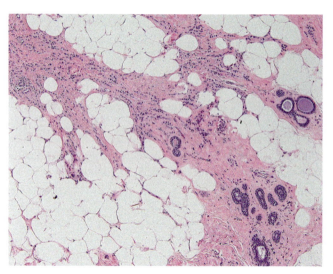

Fig. 15.1 Classic invasive lobular carcinoma: the carcinoma is composed of discohesive cells growing in a linear pattern without disrupting the normal breast architecture

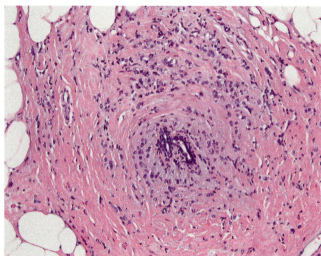

Fig. 15.2 Classic invasive lobular carcinoma: the tumor cells show a targetoid growth around normal ducts

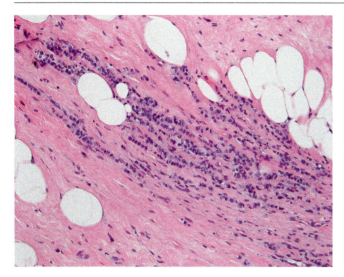

Fig. 15.3 Classic invasive lobular carcinoma: the carcinoma is composed of small monotonous bland cells

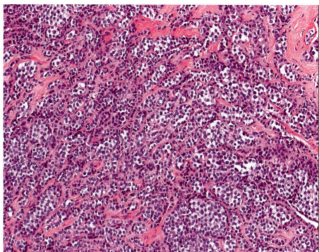

Fig. 15.5 Alveolar variant of invasive lobular carcinoma: the carcinoma cells are arranged in small clusters of cells separated by fibrous septae

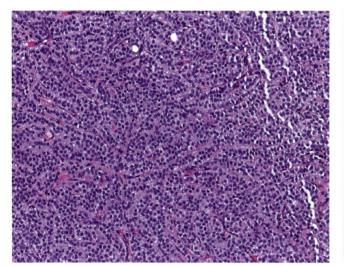

Fig. 15.4 Solid variant of invasive lobular carcinoma: the carcinoma cells are arranged in sheets

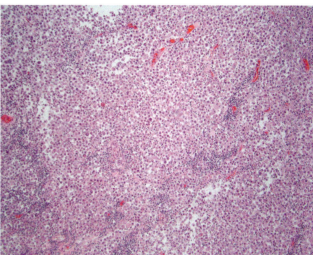

Fig. 15.6 Pleomorphic lobular carcinoma: the carcinoma is arranged in solid sheets and is composed of discohesive large atypical cells with marked pleomorphism

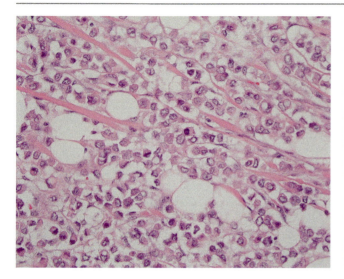

Fig. 15.7 Pleomorphic lobular carcinoma: the tumor cells show a high nuclear/cytoplasmic ratio and frequent mitoses

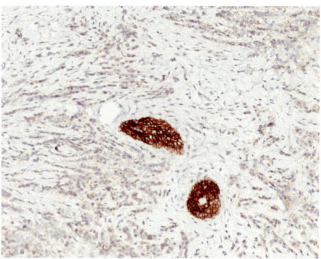

Fig. 15.9 Invasive lobular carcinoma, immunohistochemical stain for E-cadherin: the carcinoma cells show markedly decreased E-cadherin expression compared to the normal breast epithelium which exhibits strong E-cadherin membranous expression

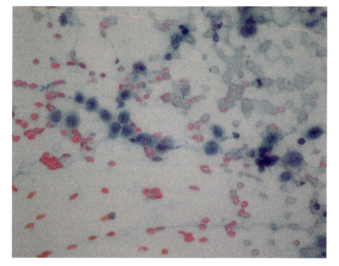

Fig. 15.8 Invasive lobular carcinoma, cytology: FNA smear shows discohesive tumor cells arranged in a linear pattern

15.2 Tubular Carcinoma

Tubular carcinoma is an uncommon histologic subtype, accounting for approximately 1–4% of breast invasive carcinomas [24]. Tubular carcinoma is not commonly associated with a palpable mass and is usually detected as an incidental finding on screening mammography [25]. On mammogram, tubular carcinomas appear as irregularly shaped masses with central densities and spiculated margins, and as hypoechoic masses with irregular margins and posterior acoustic shadowing on ultrasonogram [26].

Tubular carcinomas are composed of tubules with open lumina and oval or angulated contours in a haphazard arrangement. The tubules are lined by a single layer of epithelium with cuboidal or columnar cells with minimal pleomorphism and basally located round-to-oval nuclei (Fig. 15.10) [27]. More than 90% of the tumor should have the aforementioned morphologic features for it to be classified as a pure tubular carcinoma, whereas tumors with >50–75% of tubular component are best categorized as mixed tubular carcinomas.

The diagnosis of tubular carcinoma on FNA smears is challenging. Cytologic features of tubular carcinoma include moderate-to-high cellularity, angular epithelial clusters of oval cells, and dispersed single epithelial cells with minimal atypia in the background [28].

Tubular carcinomas are classically ER-positive and HER2-negative, and have a luminal A phenotype (Fig. 15.11) [29]. Tubular carcinomas belong to the "low-grade breast neoplasia family" and are frequently seen in association with columnar cell lesions, atypical ductal hyperplasia, low-grade ductal carcinoma in situ, and lobular neoplasia [20]. In a way akin to low-grade IDC-NST, ILC, cribriform, and tubulolobular carcinomas, tubular carcinomas are characterized by 16q losses coupled to 1q gains [20].

Benign sclerosing lesions, such as radial scars or sclerosing adenosis, may show a pseudoinvasive morphology and mimic tubular carcinoma, and myoepithelial markers such as p63 and CD10 have been proven useful to discriminate between these lesions [30]. Microglandular adenosis is another mimicker of tubular carcinoma. However, tubular carcinoma lacks the characteristic eosinophilic secretions and strong S100 positivity characteristic of microglandular adenosis [31].

Tubular carcinoma of the breast is associated with a low rate of nodal metastasis and recurrences, and a life expectancy that is close to normal [24].

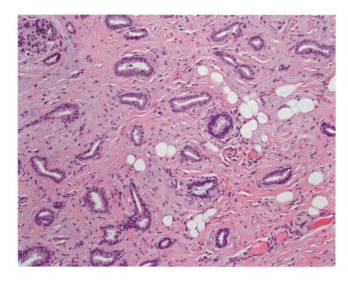

Fig. 15.10 Tubular carcinoma: neoplastic oval and angular glands with open lumens invading fibroadipose tissue

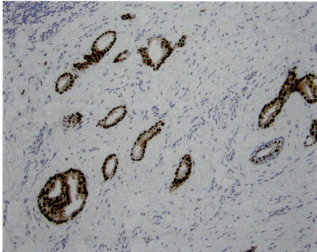

Fig. 15.11 Tubular carcinoma: the tumor cells display strong and diffuse expression of estrogen receptor

15.3   Mucinous Carcinoma

Mucinous carcinomas represent approximately 1.5% of all breast carcinomas [32]. Patients present at a significantly older age than those with IDC-NST [33]. The diagnosis of pure mucinous carcinoma requires >90% of tumor to be admixed with mucin, whereas tumors in which the mucinous component is less than 90% should be classified as mixed mucinous carcinomas (Figs. 15.12 and 15.13) [34].

On mammography, pure mucinous carcinomas appear as well-circumscribed oval masses, whereas mixed mucinous carcinomas show more aggressive imaging features [35]. On ultrasound, pure and mixed mucinous carcinomas are isoechogenic and hypoechogenic to subcutaneous fat, respectively [35, 36]. Pure mucinous carcinomas show MRI features which may be observed in benign lesions, such as a circumscribed shape, and a very high signal intensity of fat-saturated T2-weighted images, whereas mixed lesions display more suspicious imaging findings [35, 37].

Mucinous carcinoma is characterized by an invasive component admixed with varying amounts of extracellular mucin. The tumor cells are arranged in architectural patterns, such as nests, trabeculae, sheets, and cell clusters with glandular lumen formation. According to criteria put forward by Capella et al., two morphologic subtypes may be distinguished: type A and B [38]. Type A mucinous carcinomas are characterized by abundant extracellular mucin, whereas type B tumors have less extracellular mucin and show neuroendo-crine differentiation (Figs. 15.14 and 15.15). Tumors with an intermediate morphology are classified as of type AB [38].

Typically, mucinous carcinomas display strong and diffuse positivity for ER and PR (Fig. 15.16), have a low Ki67 index, and express WT1 more frequently than ER-matched invasive carcinoma NST [39]. Expression of neuroendocrine markers is more frequent in type B mucinous carcinomas [39].

The features of breast mucinous carcinomas in FNA smears include a mucinous background, branching capillaries, and tumor cells in clusters or as single cells (Figs. 15.17 and 15.18) Nevertheless, these findings may be present in other malignant or benign breast lesions, making the identification of mucinous carcinoma on cytology specimens challenging [40].

The main differential diagnoses of stromal mucin in a core-needle biopsy specimen are mucinous carcinomas and mucocele-like lesions, which may be associated with benign, atypical, or malignant epithelium [41, 42].

Pure mucinous carcinomas show more favorable clinico-pathologic features than invasive carcinoma NST, such as smaller tumor sizes, lower rates of lymph node positivity, and higher rates of ER and PR positivity [43]. Patients with pure breast mucinous carcinomas have better relapse-free survival than those with invasive carcinoma NST [43]. Even though type A mucinous carcinomas occur in older patients, have a lower nuclear grade, and lower rates of HER2 positivity and nodal involvement than type B tumors [44], the prognostic significance of this morphologic classification is uncertain and warrants further study.

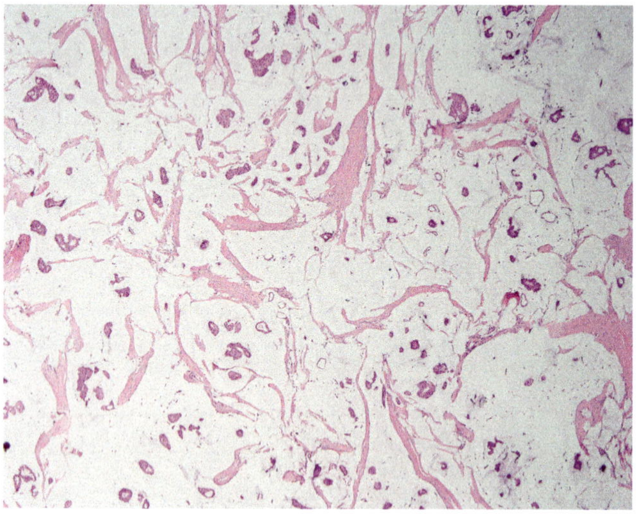

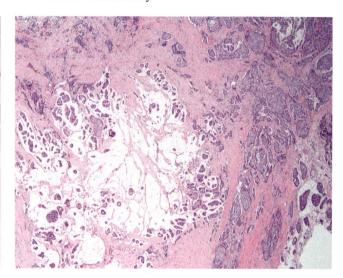

Fig. 15.12 Pure mucinous carcinoma: the tumor is entirely composed of nests of carcinoma cells floating in pools of mucin

Fig. 15.13 Mixed mucinous carcinoma: the tumor has a predominant mucinous component admixed with a ductal component

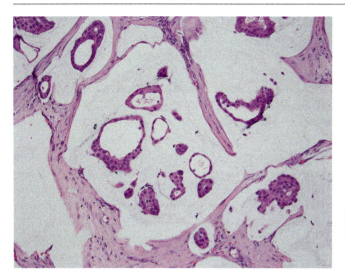

Fig. 15.14 Mucinous carcinoma, type A: the tumor is hypocellular and has abundant extracellular mucin

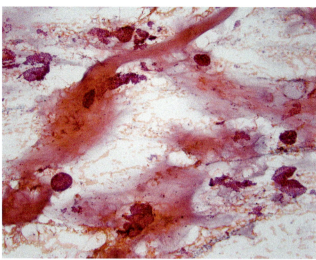

Fig. 15.17 Mucinous carcinoma, cytology: FNA smear showing cohesive clusters of carcinoma cells in a background of abundant mucin

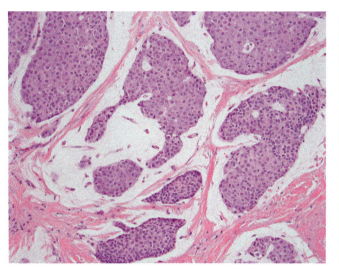

Fig. 15.15 Mucinous carcinoma, type B: the carcinoma is hypercellular

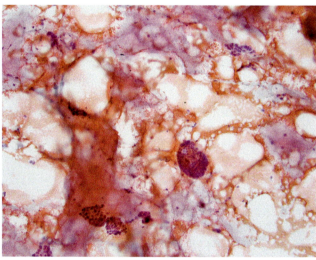

Fig. 15.18 Mucinous carcinoma, cytology: FNA smear shows tumor cells with a bland appearance admixed with mucin

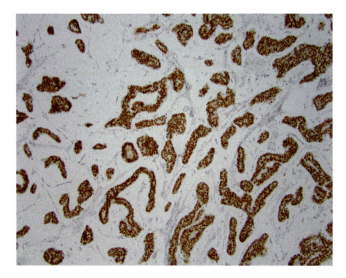

Fig. 15.16 Mucinous carcinoma: the carcinoma cells are strongly and diffusely positive for estrogen receptor

15.4 Micropapillary Carcinoma

Micropapillary carcinoma is rare and accounts for <2% of breast carcinomas [45]. Patients usually present with a palpable mass.

On mammogram, micropapillary carcinomas appear as masses with irregular shape and spiculated margins, frequently associated with microcalcifications [46]. Sonographically, these masses are hypoechoic and lack posterior acoustic enhancement or shadowing [46, 47]. MRI demonstrates masses with irregular or spiculated margins, with initial rapid enhancement and washout [46, 47].

Histologically, breast micropapillary carcinomas are composed of small morule-like clusters of tumor cells lacking fibrovascular cores within empty spaces, which may resemble lymphovascular invasion (Fig. 15.19) [48]. The tumor clusters show reverse polarity (inside-out growth pattern), with the apical aspect of the cells facing the stroma [48]. Pleomorphism and atypia are usually moderate, and mitotic activity is variable. Associated psammomatous calcifications are not infrequent (Fig. 15.20) [49, 50]. Invasive carcinoma NST and other histologic subtypes of breast cancer may be associated with a minor micropapillary component [49].

FNA smears of micropapillary carcinomas have a moderate-to-high cellularity and show tightly cohesive angular cell clusters of mildly to moderately pleomorphic tumor cells with high nuclear/cytoplasmic ratio and an inside-out pattern, admixed with single discohesive cells [51].

Micropapillary carcinomas are usually positive for ER and PR, and have variable rates of HER2 expression [52]. Expression of HER2 is restricted to the basolateral membranes of the tumor cells, as it is absent in the membrane aspect facing the stroma [53], posing challenges to its accurate interpretation. Notably, almost half of micropapillary carcinomas with a HER2 score of 1+ by immunohistochemistry (IHC) were found to be HER2 amplified by FISH [54]. Indeed, the American Society of Clinical Oncology (ASCO) and the College of American Pathologists (CAP) guidelines recommend the use of an alternative method for evaluation of HER2 expression in micropapillary carcinomas that show intense but incomplete HER2 expression by IHC [55].

The reverse polarization of the tumor cells in micropapillary carcinomas can be highlighted by MUC1 and EMA, which are positive in the apical, stroma-facing aspect of the tumor cell membranes [56, 57], and by E-cadherin and p120, which have a "cup-shaped" staining pattern, present in the lateral cell borders, and absent in the apical membrane facing the stroma [57, 58]. Vascular markers such as CD31, CD34, factor VIII, and D2-40 may be useful for the discrimination of true lymphovascular invasion from the clear stromal spaces of micropapillary carcinoma [59]. Micropapillary carcinomas are mostly of luminal B molecular subtype [60], and harbor recurrent mutations in *NBPF10* and in genes of the mitogen-activated protein kinase (MAPK) family [61].

Micropapillary carcinoma should be distinguished from invasive carcinoma NST with marked retraction artifact, which lacks inside-out morphology. Importantly, in the absence of clear *in situ* carcinoma, or in the metastatic setting, a panel of immunohistochemical stains including uroplakin, CK20, TTF-1, ER, WT1, PAX8, and mammaglobin might be useful to discriminate breast micropapillary carcinoma from micropapillary carcinoma of other anatomic origins, such as ovary, bladder, lung, salivary glands, and the gastrointestinal tract [62].

Micropapillary carcinoma is associated with more aggressive clinicopathologic features than invasive carcinoma NST, such as larger tumor size, increased incidence of lymphovascular invasion, and a higher rate of lymph node metastasis [63, 64]. Indeed, the majority of patients present with nodal metastasis at diagnosis, and nodal positivity is the most important independent prognostic predictor of recurrence-free survival [64]. Nonetheless, the disease-specific and overall survival of patients with micropapillary carcinoma does not appear to differ from that of patients with invasive carcinoma NST of similar stage [65].

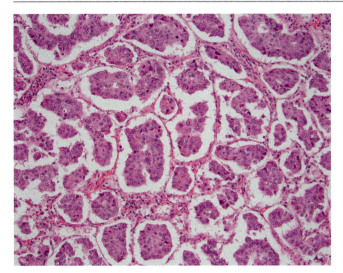

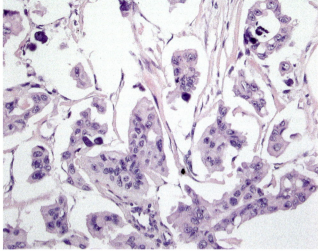

Fig. 15.19 Micropapillary carcinoma: the tumor is arranged in morule-like clusters, with no fibrovascular cores, in empty spaces separating them from the stroma

Fig. 15.20 Micropapillary carcinoma: the carcinoma cells have high nuclear grade. Psammomatous calcifications are seen

15.5 Mucinous Micropapillary Carcinoma

Mucinous micropapillary carcinoma, also known as micropapillary variant of mucinous carcinoma, is an unusual form of invasive breast cancer that exhibits dual mucinous and micropapillary morphology [66].

Mucinous micropapillary carcinomas display a hybrid histology, characterized by floret-like or pseudoacinar structures of hobnail cells in stromal spaces filled with mucin (Figs. 15.21 and 15.22) [67]. Psammomatous calcifications can be readily identified.

Akin to micropapillary carcinomas and pure mucinous carcinomas, mucinous micropapillary carcinomas display reverse polarity, which may be highlighted by IHC stains for EMA and MUC1 [67]. These tumors are diffusely positive for ER and PR [67], and show a higher rate of HER2 overexpression/amplification than mucinous carcinomas, which ranges between 10% and 20% [44, 66].

Cytologic preparations have a moderate cellularity, and show micropapillary clusters of tumor cells with nuclear hobnailing in pools of mucin. Single cells in the background are present to a lesser degree than in micropapillary carcinoma, and psammomatous calcifications are not uncommon [68, 69].

Mucinous micropapillary carcinoma displays clinicopathologic features intermediate between mucinous and micropapillary carcinoma, such as an intermediate rate of lymphovascular invasion, nodal metastasis, and HER2 overexpression/amplification. The rate of regional recurrence and distant metastasis of mucinous micropapillary carcinoma is also intermediate, between the rates of recurrence and distant metastasis of mucinous and micropapillary carcinomas [44, 66, 67].

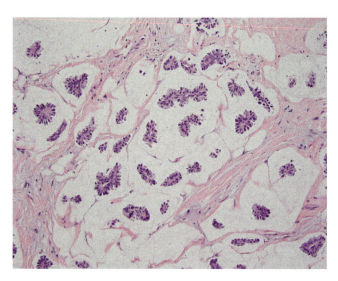

Fig. 15.21 Mucinous micropapillary carcinoma: tumor cells are arranged in morule-like clusters with hobnail cells floating in pools of mucin

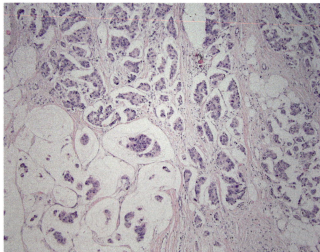

Fig. 15.22 Mucinous micropapillary carcinoma: mucinous micropapillary carcinoma (left) with tumor clusters floating in mucin transitions to an area with micropapillary morphology in which the carcinoma cells are present in empty spaces (right)

15.6   Carcinoma with Medullary Features

Carcinoma with medullary features is a category encompassing tumors previously designated as medullary carcinoma and atypical medullary carcinoma. Grouping of these entities under this category is recommended due to their overlapping morphology associated with diagnostic challenges and a poor inter-observer reproducibility. Carcinomas with medullary features are rare, and represent <5% of breast invasive carcinomas [70]. Patients with carcinomas with medullary features present at a younger age than those with invasive carcinoma NST [71].

Carcinomas with medullary features present as well-circumscribed masses on mammography and ultrasound. Posterior acoustic enhancement on sonogram is more frequent in typical than in atypical medullary carcinomas [72]. On MRI, carcinomas with medullary features show an oval shape, well-circumscribed borders, and frequent rim enhancement with or without enhancing internal septations [73].

The classic morphologic criteria used to define typical medullary carcinomas include predominant syncytial growth (>75% of the tumor), circumscribed and pushing borders, lack of tubule formation, diffuse prominent stromal lympho-plasmacytic infiltrate, and high nuclear grade (Figs. 15.23 and 15.24) [74]. Tumors that don't display all these features were called atypical medullary carcinomas.

On FNA specimens, carcinomas with medullary features are highly cellular and show distinctive characteristics, such as syncytial sheets of cells with bizarre nuclei and prominent nucleoli, and marked chronic lymphoplasmacytic infiltrate [75].

Carcinomas with medullary features are usually triple negative [76], and display a basal immunophenotype (ER−, PR−, HER2−, CK5/6+ and/or EGFR+) more frequently than does high-grade invasive carcinoma NST [77].

Despite their aggressive morphologic features, carcinomas with medullary features are associated with a favorable prognosis [78], and the outcome of typical and atypical medullary carcinomas does not seem to differ [79]. Notably, the prognosis of carcinoma with medullary features is similar to the one of high-grade ductal carcinoma with prominent inflammatory infiltrate [80], and the excellent outcome of these tumors appears to be related to their associated host inflammatory response, a favorable prognostic and predictive marker of triple negative breast cancer (TNBC) treated with chemotherapy [81].

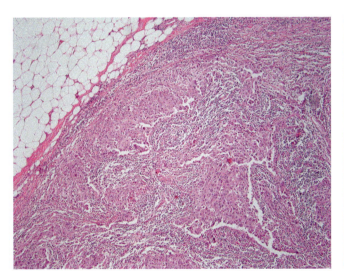

Fig. 15.23 Carcinoma with medullary features: the tumor has a circumscribed pushing border. The tumor cells grow in a syncytial pattern and are intermixed with marked host lymphoplasmacytic infiltrate

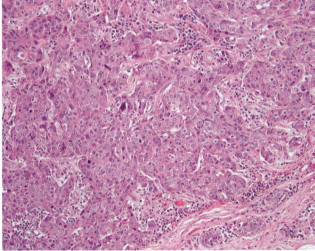

Fig. 15.24 Carcinoma with medullary features: the tumor cells show marked atypia and frequent mitoses

15.7 Apocrine Carcinoma

Apocrine carcinomas are composed of tumor cells with abundant densely eosinophilic cytoplasm with large nuclei and prominent nucleoli, and represent up to 4% of all breast carcinomas [82, 83]. Apocrine morphology may be present in different breast cancer histologic subtypes, and there is currently a lack of uniformity in the diagnostic criteria for apocrine carcinoma. Some authors advocate to restrict this diagnosis to tumors composed of more than 90% of apocrine cells [84].

A large SEER database study showed that patients present with apocrine carcinoma at an older age and with larger tumors than patients with invasive carcinoma NST [85]. Sonographic, mammographic, and MRI findings of apocrine carcinomas do not differ from those of invasive carcinoma NST [86–88].

Apocrine carcinomas may be composed of type A cells, which have an abundant eosinophilic granular cytoplasm, type B cells, which have a foamy and vacuolated cytoplasm, or a combination of both. The tumor cells exhibit large centrally to eccentrically located nuclei, prominent nucleoli, and distinctive cell borders (Figs. 15.25, 15.26, and 15.27).

Apocrine carcinomas are mostly negative for ER and PR [83, 84], although it has been shown that they frequently express ER-α36, an isoform of ER [89]. Approximately half of apocrine carcinomas display HER2 overexpression/ampli-fication [90], and most of them are positive for androgen receptor (AR) [90]. Indeed, some authors consider tumors that display apocrine morphology, are negative for ER and PR, and positive for AR as "pure apocrine" carcinomas, while those that exhibit ER or PR positivity, and are negative for AR are considered "apocrine-like carcinomas" [91]. Apocrine carcinomas belong to the luminal androgen receptor transcriptomic subtype of TNBC [92], and harbor a higher rate of mutations in *PIK3CA* and other genes of the Phosphoinositide 3-kinase (PI3K) pathway, and a lower frequency of *TP53* mutations and *MYC* gains compared to other TNBCs [93, 94].

The diagnosis of apocrine carcinoma in cytology specimens is challenging due to their morphologic overlap with benign apocrine lesions [95, 96]. FNA smears of apocrine carcinomas are usually highly cellular and show tumor cells arranged in sheets, clusters, and singly scattered. The tumor cells show moderate-to-marked pleomorphism, a dense granular cytoplasm, large nuclei with coarse chromatin, prominent nucleoli, and occasional intranuclear inclusions (Fig. 15.28) [95, 96].

The recurrence-free survival of patients with apocrine carcinomas appears to be similar to that of patients with non-apocrine ductal carcinomas when matched for stage [97]. Nonetheless, a study indicated that patients with "pure apocrine" carcinoma have a worse outcome that those with invasive carcinoma NST [91].

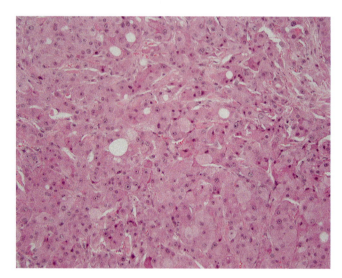

Fig. 15.25 Apocrine carcinoma: the tumor is composed of cells with abundant eosinophilic cytoplasm and cells with foamy cytoplasm. Scattered intracytoplasmic vacuoles can be seen

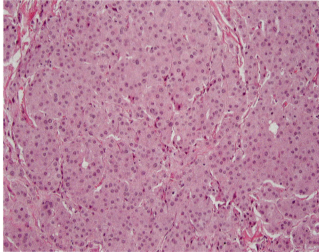

Fig. 15.26 Apocrine carcinoma: the tumor has a nested architecture with focal glandular formation. The tumor cells have an intermediate nuclear grade

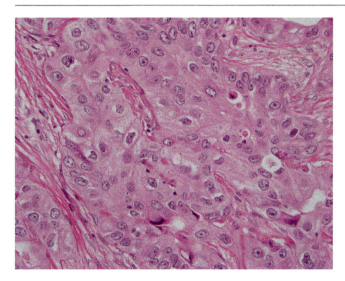

Fig. 15.27 Apocrine carcinoma: the tumor cells show marked pleomorphism and prominent nucleoli

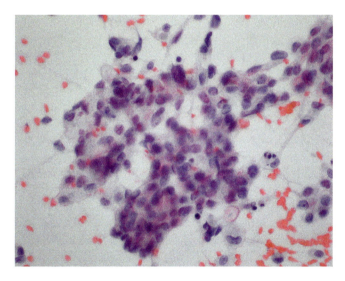

Fig. 15.28 Apocrine carcinoma: FNA smear shows tumor cells with moderate pleomorphism, dense granular cytoplasm and large nuclei with prominent nucleoli

15.8   Metaplastic Breast Carcinoma

Metaplastic carcinomas encompass a heterogenous group of carcinomas characterized by non-glandular morphology, including squamous or mesenchymal differentiation, such as spindle, chondroid, and osseous features [98]. There is currently no consensus regarding the extent of metaplastic elements required for the diagnosis of metaplastic carcinoma, and a wide range of cutoffs have been used [99, 100]. Although most metaplastic carcinomas are high-grade tumors, low-grade variants are also recognized. Metaplastic carcinomas are rare and account for 0.2–5% of breast carcinomas [98].

Patients with metaplastic carcinoma present usually with a palpable mass, and at an older age and with larger tumors than patients with invasive carcinoma NST [101, 102]. Most metaplastic carcinomas are identified as masses on mammogram and ultrasound, and show enhancing, and not uncommonly central necrosis on MRI [103]. Areas of calcification in metaplastic carcinomas with osseous or chondroid differentiation are occasionally detected by imaging [104]. Although the imaging features of metaplastic carcinomas show overlap with those of invasive carcinoma NST [105, 106], features of malignancy, such as irregular shape, spiculated margins, pleomorphic calcifications in a segmental distribution, and posterior acoustic shadowing have been reported to be less frequent in metaplastic carcinomas than in invasive carcinomas NST [107].

Morphologically, metaplastic carcinomas are a heterogeneous group of tumors with marked inter- and intra-tumor heterogeneity. Several subtypes are recognized, including squamous cell carcinoma, metaplastic carcinoma with mesenchymal differentiation, spindle cell carcinoma, including intermediate- and high-grade spindle cell carcinomas, as well as the low-grade fibromatosis-like spindle cell carcinoma and low-grade adenosquamous carcinoma.

Confirmation of epithelial differentiation, such as focal epithelial morphology, presence of ductal carcinoma in situ (DCIS), or positivity for epithelial or myoepithelial markers is required for the diagnosis of metaplastic carcinoma.

The diagnosis of squamous cell carcinoma is reserved for tumors composed of least 90% of squamous elements. Squamous cell carcinomas are frequently associated with cysts (Fig. 15.29) and are composed of polygonal cells with abundant eosinophilic and occasionally clear cytoplasm infiltrating the stroma, frequently associated with marked host lymphocytic reaction (Figs. 15.30 and 15.31). A spindle cell component may be present. Breast squamous cell carcinomas are morphologically similar to squamous cell carcinomas arising in other locations [108, 109].

Metaplastic carcinomas with mesenchymal differentiation are tumors with an overt carcinoma component associated with a mesenchymal component with chondroid or osseous differentiation (Figs. 15.32 and 15.33), or less frequently with rhabdomyosarcomatous, liposarcomatous, or angiosarcomatous differentiation. Matrix-producing carcinomas were classically defined as those in which the carcinoma component directly transitions to chondroid or osseous matrix, without the presence of intervening spindle cells or osteoclastic giant cells (Fig.15.34). The matrix-producing component may occasionally display a mucoid appearance and mimic mucinous carcinoma (Fig. 15.35) [110].

Metaplastic spindle cell carcinomas may arise in association with fibrosclerotic lesions of the breast, like papillomas, complex sclerosing lesions and nipple adenomas [111]. Metaplastic spindle cell carcinomas have infiltrative margins and are composed of spindle cells with moderate-to-marked atypia, arranged haphazardly, or in fascicular, herringbone, and storiform architectural patterns, and frequently show associated inflammatory infiltrate (Fig. 15.36) [112]. Necrosis and numerous mitoses and are common (Fig. 15.37). Focal clusters of cells with more epithelioid morphology or squamous differentiation or focal areas of conventional invasive carcinoma, usually poorly differentiated, and ductal carcinoma in situ (DCIS) may be present (Figs. 15.38 and 15.39) [112].

Low-grade fibromatosis-like metaplastic spindle cell carcinoma (LG-FLMC) is a low-grade form of spindle cell carcinoma with morphologic resemblance to fibromatosis. LG-FLMCs have irregular infiltrative margins with finger-like projections (Figs. 15.40 and 15.41), and are composed of bland spindle cells with absent-to-minimal atypia, arranged in wavy fascicles in more than 95% of the tumor (Fig. 15.42). LG-FLMCs range from hypocellular to hypercellular and are intermixed with collagenous areas [113]. The spindle cells are frequently admixed with few clusters of glandular or squamous epithelial cells [113].

Low-grade adenosquamous carcinomas (LGASC) have a stellate configuration with poorly defined borders, and are composed of elongated or ovoid infiltrating glands with tumor cells of low nuclear grade and various degrees of squamous differentiation (Fig. 15.43). The LGASC glands appear to blend with the surrounding stroma, which ranges from hyalinized to cellular (Fig. 15.44). Lymphocytic aggregates are frequently seen in the periphery of the lesions [114, 115].

FNA smears of metaplastic carcinomas are usually highly cellular and frequently show necrosis. Clues for the diagnosis of metaplastic carcinoma on cytology material include squamous carcinoma cells, atypical spindle cells, and heterologous elements fragments (Fig. 15.45) [116–118]. Nonetheless, identification of both epithelial and heterologous elements in cytology specimens is uncommon, and the

diagnosis of metaplastic carcinoma on cytology material is challenging (Fig. 15.46).

Metaplastic carcinomas are usually triple negative, have a basal immunophenotype [119, 120], and are of basal-like molecular subtype [112, 121, 122]. The identification of epithelial differentiation in metaplastic carcinomas requires a broad panel of epithelial and myoepithelial markers, as the immunoreactivity of metaplastic carcinomas to cytokeratins or myoepithelial markers is highly variable and may be focal, and no individual marker has been found to be uniformly positive. The majority (70–80%) of metaplastic carcinomas are positive for broad spectrum cytokeratins (AE1/AE3 and MNF116) and for high molecular weight cytokeratins (34βE12, CK5/6, CK14 and CK17), whereas low molecular weight cytokeratins (CK8/18, CK7 and CK19) are less frequently positive in metaplastic carcinomas (30–60%) (Fig. 15.47) [120]. Myoepithelial markers, such as p63, are frequently positive [112]. Metaplastic breast carcinomas share the complex genetic abnormalities and high frequency of TP53 mutations with conventional TNBCs, and are associated with mutations in PIK3CA, PIK3R1, PTEN, FAT1 and AXIN1 resulting in an increased activation of the PI3K and Wnt pathways [123, 124].

The differential diagnosis of metaplastic carcinoma is broad. Therefore, metastatic squamous cell carcinoma from a distant anatomical site or direct extension from a squamous cell carcinoma arising in the overlying skin should be excluded before rendering the diagnosis of breast squamous cell carcinoma. Phyllodes tumor with stromal overgrowth should be considered in the differential diagnosis of spindle cell metaplastic carcinomas, and cytokeratins and p63 are useful IHC markers in this scenario. Nevertheless, caution should be exerted, as a subset of phyllodes tumors may be focally positive for p63 and cytokeratins [125]. CD34 is consistently negative in metaplastic carcinomas and may help differentiate metaplastic carcinomas from phyllodes tumors [120]. Discrimination of LG-FLMC from fibromatosis might be particularly challenging due to their marked morphologic overlap. While fibromatosis is negative for cytokeratins and shows nuclear β-catenin expression [126], β-catenin may also be expressed in metaplastic carcinomas, and should not be used as the sole marker for the distinction between these entities [123]. LGASCs may show morphologic overlap with tubular carcinoma, adenomyoepithelioma, and syringomatous tumor of the nipple [127]. A study using lineage-tracing analysis suggested that LGASCs and syringomatous tumors of the nipple are identical or nearly identical lesions [127].

Metaplastic carcinomas show a lower rate of nodal metastasis than invasive carcinoma NST [101, 102, 128]. Like other TNBCs, metaplastic carcinomas may develop distant metastasis in the absence of nodal metastasis [106]. These tumors show a lower response rate to neoadjuvant and adjuvant chemotherapy [129–131]. Several studies indicate that metaplastic carcinomas have a worse prognosis than invasive carcinoma NST [122, 129, 132–134], although a multi-institutional study that included over 400 cases showed that when matched for grade, nodal status, and ER/HER2 receptor status, metaplastic carcinomas have an outcome similar to invasive carcinoma NST. In the aforementioned study, spindle cell carcinoma had a worse outcome than other subtypes of metaplastic carcinoma [119]. Unlike other types of metaplastic carcinomas, LGASCs and LG-FLMCs have an indolent clinical behavior and a good prognosis [135, 136].

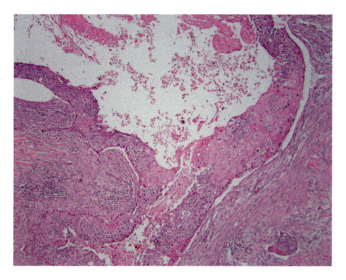

Fig. 15.29 Squamous cell carcinoma: the carcinoma is associated with cystic areas

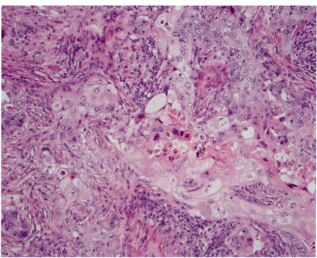

Fig. 15.31 Squamous cell carcinoma: tumor cells show abundant eosinophilic cytoplasm, focal clearing, and marked pleomorphism

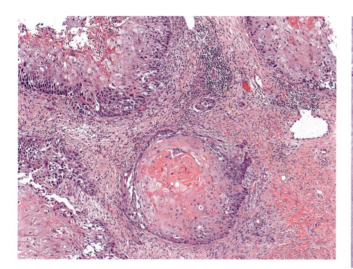

Fig. 15.30 Squamous cell carcinoma: nests of tumor cells with marked keratinization associated with host inflammatory infiltrate

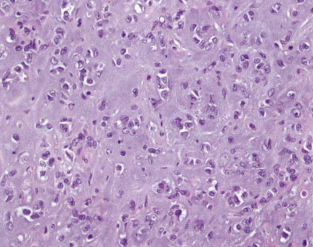

Fig. 15.32 Metaplastic carcinoma with chondroid differentiation: the carcinoma shows chondroid morphology

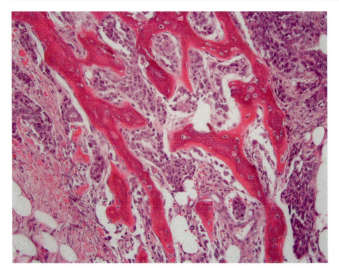

Fig. 15.33 Metaplastic carcinoma with osseous differentiation: the carcinoma shows osteoid production

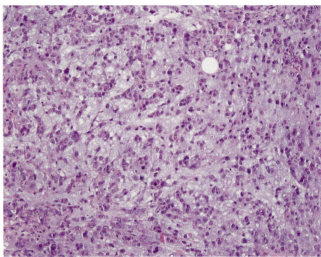

Fig. 15.35 Metaplastic carcinoma, matrix-producing: poorly differentiated carcinoma admixed with matrix material with a mucin-like morphology

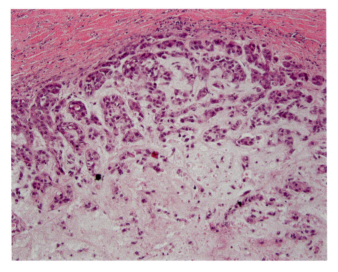

Fig. 15.34 Metaplastic carcinoma, matrix-producing: poorly differentiated carcinoma transitioning to a hypocellular matrix area with focal necrosis

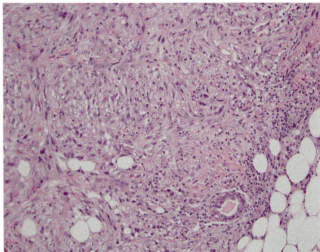

Fig. 15.36 Metaplastic carcinoma, spindle cell: the spindle cells are arranged haphazardly and are associated with peritumoral lymphocytic infiltrate

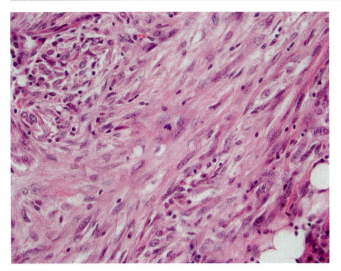

Fig. 15.37 Metaplastic carcinoma, spindle cell: the tumor cells display marked atypia and frequent mitoses

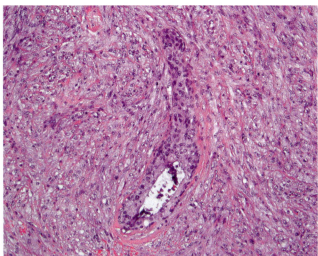

Fig. 15.39 Metaplastic carcinoma, spindle cell: focal high-grade DCIS is identified admixed with the spindle cell carcinoma

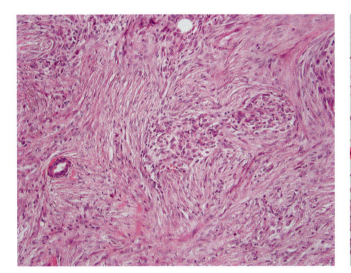

Fig. 15.38 Metaplastic carcinoma, spindle cell: the spindle carcinoma cells are admixed with clusters of cells with epithelioid morphology

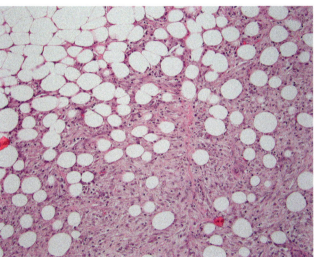

Fig. 15.40 Low-grade fibromatosis-like metaplastic spindle cell carcinoma: bland-appearing spindle cells infiltrate adipose tissue

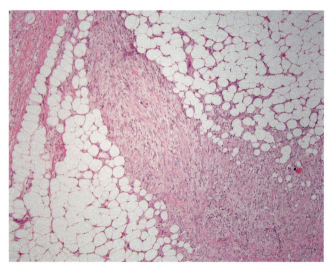

Fig. 15.41 Low-grade fibromatosis-like metaplastic spindle cell carcinoma: the carcinoma has an infiltrative growth with finger-like projections

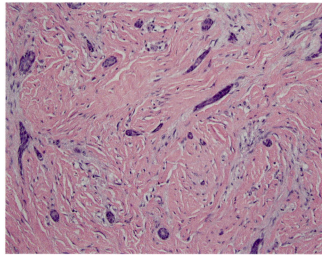

Fig. 15.43 Low-grade adenosquamous carcinoma: neoplastic cells are arranged in nests and glands with an infiltrative pattern

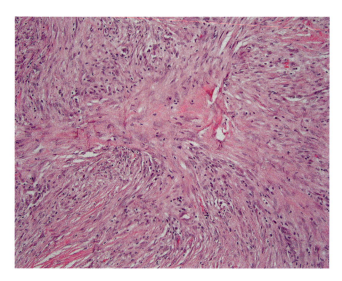

Fig. 15.42 Low-grade fibromatosis-like metaplastic spindle cell carcinoma: the tumor cells are arranged in wavy fascicles surrounded by collagenous stroma

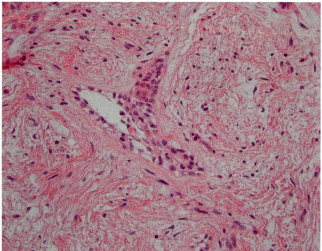

Fig. 15.44 Low-grade adenosquamous carcinoma: angulated gland with tumor cells with low nuclear grade and squamous differentiation, surrounded by a hypocellular stroma

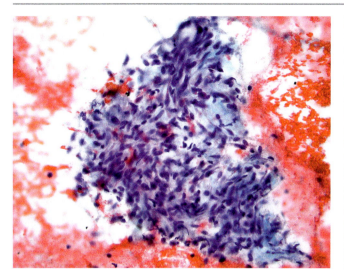

Fig. 15.45 Metaplastic carcinoma, spindle cell, cytology: FNA smear shows large clusters of spindle tumor cells in a background of red blood cells

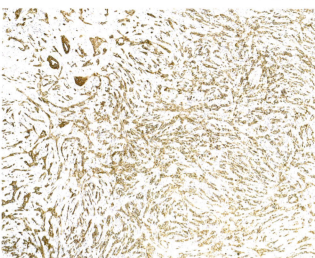

Fig. 15.47 Metaplastic carcinoma, spindle cell: the spindle cell metaplastic carcinoma shows diffuse positivity for 34βE12

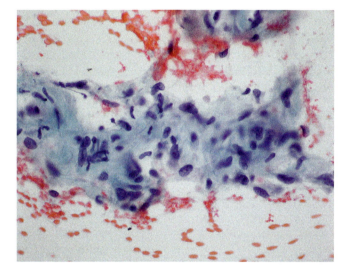

Fig. 15.46 Metaplastic carcinoma, matrix-producing, cytology: FNA smear shows tumor cells admixed with matrix

15.9   Adenoid Cystic Carcinoma

Adenoid cystic carcinoma (AdCC) typically arises in the salivary glands, but may also originate at other anatomic locations, such as the respiratory and gastrointestinal tracts, skin, and breast [137]. Breast AdCCs account for approximately 0.1% of breast carcinomas [138]. The usual clinical presentation of AdCC is a palpable mass, frequently located in the subareolar region.

On mammography, AdCCs appear as irregular or lobulated masses [139], and are usually heterogenous or hypoechoic on sonogram [140]. On MRI they display suspicious enhancement kinetics [140].

AdCCs are biphasic tumors, composed of epithelial and myoepithelial cells arranged in different patterns, histologically indistinguishable from their counterparts arising in other anatomic locations [141]. The most characteristic growth pattern of AdCC is the cribriform one. Cribriform AdCCs are composed of islands of tumor cells with smooth contours and a sieve-like appearance with pseudolumina formed by the invagination of the stroma, containing eosinophilic PAS-positive hyaline and/or alcian blue-positive myxoid material, and less frequent true glandular spaces surrounded by epithelial cells (Figs. 15.48 and 15.49) [142]. Other AdCC morphologies include the tubular/glandular, trabecular/reticular, and solid patterns (Fig. 15.50 and 15.51) [141]. A solid variant of AdCC with basaloid features has been described, and is characterized by large infiltrative solid nests of basaloid cells with marked nuclear atypia within hyalinized, myxoid, or desmoplastic stroma [143].

The luminal epithelial component of AdCC is positive for low molecular weight cytokeratins, such as CK7, CK8/18, and for EMA and CD117, whereas the myoepithelial cells are positive for basal cytokeratins, like CK5/6, CK14, and for myoepithelial markers such as smooth muscle actin and p63 [144–146]. Breast AdCCs generally have a triple negative phenotype and are of basal-like molecular subtype [20, 147]. Akin to their salivary gland counterparts, breast AdCCs are underpinned by the t(6;9)(q22–23;p23–24) translocation, which results in the *MYB-NFIB* fusion gene and subsequent overexpression of the MYB oncogene [148], a sensitive and specific finding for AdCC [149]. Recently, breast *MYB-NFIB* fusion gene-negative AdCCs have been shown to be driven by alternative genetic alterations, such as *MYBL1* rearrangements and *MYB* amplification [150].

Cytologic preparations of breast AdCCs show cellular smears with three-dimensional clusters of basaloid and epithelial cells surrounding extracellular metachromatic spherules (Figs. 15.52 and 15.53) [151, 152].

The differential diagnosis of breast AdCC includes invasive cribriform carcinoma, cribriform DCIS, and collagenous spherulosis. The distinction of AdCC from collagenous spherulosis might be particularly challenging in core-needle biopsies. CD117, which is positive in AdCC and negative in collagenous spherulosis, and calponin and smooth muscle myosin heavy chain, which is negative in AdCC but strongly positive in collagenous spherulosis, may be useful for such diagnostic distinction [153].

Breast AdCCs show a low rate of nodal metastasis [154], and unlike their salivary gland counterparts and conventional TNBC, they have a favorable clinical course [155]. Nevertheless, transformation to high-grade TNBC has been described [156].

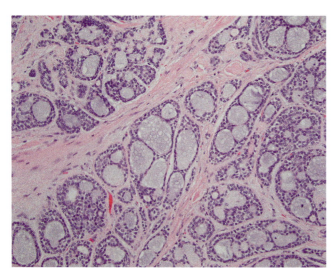

Fig. 15.48 Adenoid cystic carcinoma: the carcinoma shows a cribriform growth pattern with basophilic secretions within pseudolumina

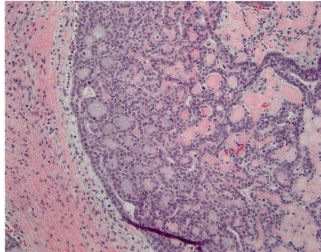

Fig. 15.49 Adenoid cystic carcinoma: the pseudolumina contained myxoid material or invaginated collagenous stroma

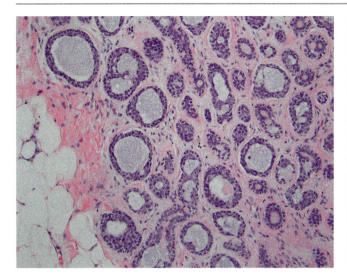

Fig. 15.50 Adenoid cystic carcinoma: the tumor shows a tubular/glandular growth pattern

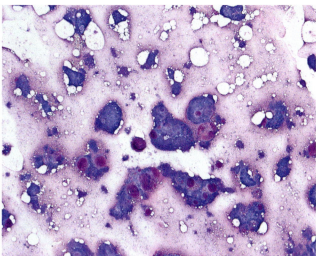

Fig. 15.52 Adenoid cystic carcinoma, cytology: FNA smear shows cohesive clusters of basaloid cells surrounding spheres of basement metachromatic material. Numerous bare nuclei are present in the background

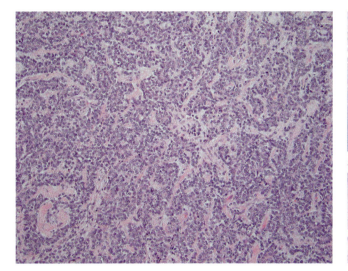

Fig. 15.51 Adenoid cystic carcinoma: the carcinoma displays a trabecular growth pattern

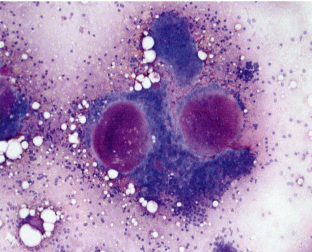

Fig. 15.53 Adenoid cystic carcinoma, cytology: FNA smear show small uniform cells with scant cytoplasm and round-to-oval nuclei surrounding amorphous acellular material

15.10 Secretory Carcinoma

Secretory carcinoma was originally described in children and initially named juvenile carcinoma [157]. However, it occurs at a later age than initially recognized, with the median age at diagnosis of 53 years [158]. Secretory carcinomas are extremely rare and represent less than 0.1% of breast carcinomas [158].

The imaging features of secretory carcinomas are variable and nonspecific. Mammographic findings range from well-circumscribed isodense masses to suspicious lesions with spiculated margins [159]. On sonography, they appear as well-circumscribed or partially microlobulated iso- or hypoechoic nodules [159, 160].

Secretory carcinomas grow in different architectural patterns (microcystic, tubular, solid, and papillary), which often coexist (Figs. 15.54 and 15.55) [161, 162]. Tumor cells have a granular eosinophilic-to-clear cytoplasm with low-grade nuclei, inconspicuous nucleoli, and minimal mitotic activity. The hallmark of secretory carcinomas is abundant intra- and extracellular dense PAS-positive eosinophilic secretions, which may resemble thyroid colloid when found in association with microcystic regions (Fig. 15.56) [162].

Although few cases have been reported to weakly express hormone receptors, most secretory carcinomas are triple negative and show a basal-like immunoprofile [161]. Secretory carcinomas are positive for S-100, mammaglobin, alpha-lactalbumin, EMA, MUC4, and SOX10 [162–165].

Akin to mammary analog secretory carcinomas (MASCs) in salivary glands or skin, breast secretory carcinomas are underpinned by the t(12;15)(p13;q25) translocation, which results in the *ETV6-NTRK3* fusion gene [165]. In contrast to high-grade TNBC, secretory carcinomas show a low mutational burden, no pathogenic mutations in genes frequently altered in breast cancer, and few copy number alterations [165].

Cytologic preparations of breast secretory carcinomas are of low cellularity and show bland tumor cells with cytoplasmic vacuoles admixed with colloid material [166, 167].

The differential diagnosis of secretory carcinoma includes entities with cystic architecture and prominent secretions, such as acinic cell carcinoma and cystic hypersecretory carcinoma [168]. Cystic hypersecretory carcinomas are mostly *in situ* lesions, composed by large cysts and abundant secretions, and are generally ER-positive, whereas secretory carcinomas frequently display a microcystic pattern and are triple negative [169]. Unlike secretory carcinomas, acinic cell carcinomas are positive for amylase, lysozyme and α1-antytripsin [170]. Importantly, the *ETV6-NTRK3* fusion gene is pathognomonic for secretory carcinoma in a breast-specific context [171].

Secretory carcinomas have an excellent outcome, even in the presence of nodal involvement [158].

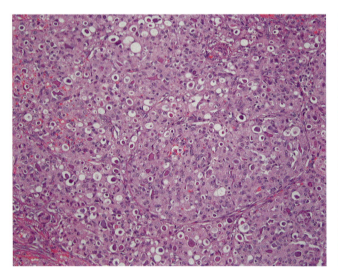

Fig. 15.54 Secretory carcinoma: the carcinoma shows a microcystic growth pattern.

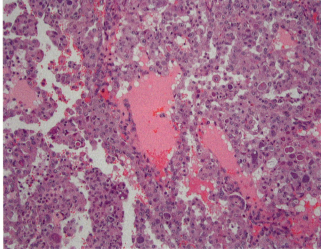

Fig. 15.55 Secretory carcinoma: the carcinoma shows a papillary growth pattern with a focal microcystic component

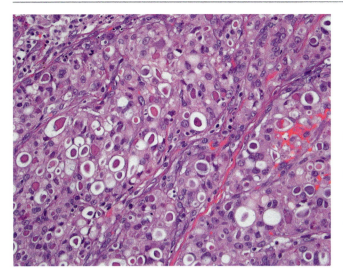

Fig. 15.56 Secretory carcinoma: the carcinoma displays abundant intra and extracellular secretions

15.11 Solid Papillary Breast Carcinoma Resembling the Tall Cell Variant of Papillary Thyroid Neoplasms/Solid Papillary Carcinoma with Reverse Polarity

These tumors have been described by different names, including solid papillary carcinoma resembling the tall cell variant of papillary thyroid neoplasms (BPTC), and solid papillary carcinoma with reverse polarity (SPCRP). They constitute a vanishingly rare histologic type of breast carcinoma, with less than 50 cases reported in the literature to date [172–177]. They have a benign appearance with regular margins on mammography or ultrasound [177].

BPTCs/SPCRPs have a very distinctive morphology, reminiscent of the morphology of the tall cell variant of papillary thyroid carcinoma. They are composed of circumscribed tumor nodules with solid, papillary, and follicular architectural patterns, and often coexist in the same case. The follicular structures contain a colloid-like eosinophilic material (Fig. 15.57). The tumor cells are cuboidal-to-columnar with eosinophilic granular cytoplasm and apically polarized nuclei, simulating reverse polarization (Fig. 15.58), although MUC1 is expressed in the apical cellular border [175]. Akin to papillary thyroid carcinomas, SPCRPs have nuclei with clear chromatin, grooves, and pseudoinclusions (Fig. 15.59 and 15.60) [172].

Despite their resemblance to papillary thyroid neoplasms, BPTCs/SPCRPs are negative for thyroid markers, such as thyroglobulin and TTF-1 [172, 175, 178], and show focal positivity for GCDFP-15 and GATA-3 [172, 177]. These tumors are HER2-negative, and two-thirds of cases are also negative for ER and PR [172, 175, 177].

BPTCs/SPCRPs are underpinned by highly recurrent *IDH2* R172 hotspot mutations or *TET2* mutations, with frequent concurrent mutations targeting genes of the PI3K pathway [175, 176]. Despite their morphological overlap with the tall cell variant of papillary thyroid carcinoma, no *RET/PTC* and *BRAF* genetic alterations have been described in these tumors [172, 173, 179].

Due to their remarkably similar morphology, metastasis from a tall cell variant of papillary thyroid carcinoma should be considered in the differential diagnosis of BPTCs/SPCRPs. IHC stains for thyroglobulin and TTF-1 are useful for this distinction. BPTCs/SPCRPs may show morphologic overlap with secretory carcinomas, another low-grade TNBC, and assessment of the *IDH2* mutational status and of the presence of *ETV6-NTRK3* fusion gene might be useful in this scenario.

BTPCs/SPCRPs have an indolent behavior and a favorable course, and there have been only occasional reports of regional or distant metastasis [173, 175, 177, 178, 180].

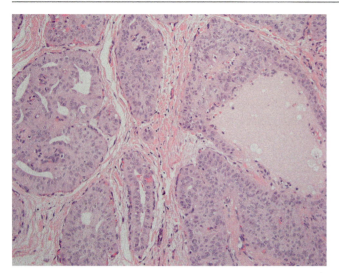

Fig. 15.57 Solid papillary breast carcinoma resembling the tall cell variant of papillary thyroid neoplasms/solid papillary carcinoma with reverse polarity: tumor nodules with solid papillary and follicular patterns. Thick eosinophilic material is identified within the follicles

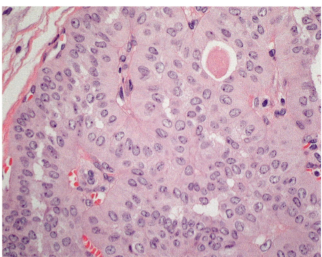

Fig. 15.59 Solid papillary breast carcinoma resembling the tall cell variant of papillary thyroid neoplasms/solid papillary carcinoma with reverse polarity: the carcinoma cells show nuclear clearing and nuclear grooves

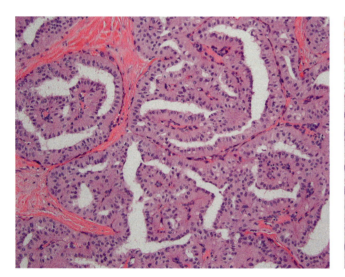

Fig. 15.58 Solid papillary breast carcinoma resembling the tall cell variant of papillary thyroid neoplasms/solid papillary carcinoma with reverse polarity: the tumor cells appear to have a reverse polarization with nuclei located in the apical aspect of the cells

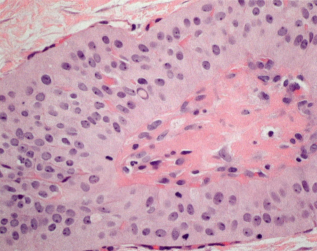

Fig. 15.60 Solid papillary breast carcinoma resembling the tall cell variant of papillary thyroid neoplasms/solid papillary carcinoma with reverse polarity: the carcinoma cells show occasional nuclear pseudoinclusions

15.12 Inflammatory Breast Cancer

Inflammatory breast cancer (IBC) is a rare and aggressive form of breast cancer. This phenotype is characterized clinically by acute inflammatory changes of the breast presenting, within ≤3 months, diffuse erythema and edema, with or without palpable mass.

IBC accounts for 1–2% of all invasive breast cancer [181]. It is characterized by a higher risk of early recurrence, distant metastases, and metastases to the central nervous system compared with non-inflammatory locally advanced cancer.

The classic histologic finding in IBC on biopsy of affected skin is dermal lymphatic invasion by tumor cells (Fig. 15.61). These malignant cells form tumor emboli which are responsible for both the local signs and symptoms and for the development of metastatic disease [182].

Inflammatory breast cancer includes basal (20–40%), HER2 (20–40%) and luminal A and B subtypes. Loss of heterozygosity is detected in approximately one-half of IBC, and the most frequently loss alleles are at 3p, 6p, 8p, 11q, 13q, and 17q [183].

The differential diagnosis includes:

- Infection (mastitis, cellulitis, abscess). Mammary infection should be distinguished from IBC clinically. Mastitis typically develops rapidly over a few days; erythema is associated with tenderness and typically occupies a wedge-shaped quadrant of breast. However, symptomatic women improvement should occur within 24–48 h of initiation of antibiotics.
- Locally advanced carcinoma with skin invasion. Large carcinomas may directly invade into skin and cause skin ulceration. Focal dermal lymph vascular invasion may be present adjacent to the area of skin invasion. This type of cancer should not be classified as IBC.

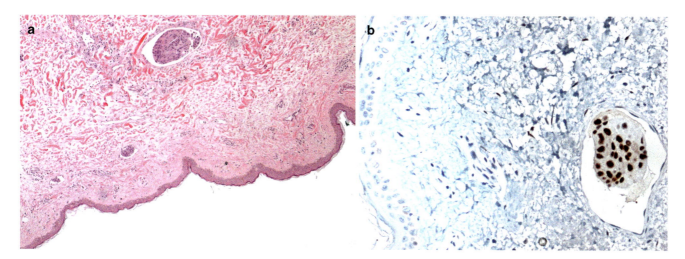

Fig. 15.61 Inflammatory breast carcinoma. (**a**) Dermal lymphovascular invasion is present. (**b**) Tumor cells showing staining with estrogen receptor

References

1. McCart Reed AE, Kutasovic JR, Lakhani SR, Simpson PT. Invasive lobular carcinoma of the breast: morphology, biomarkers and omics. Breast Cancer Res. 2015;17:12.
2. Li CI, Anderson BO, Daling JR, Moe RE. Trends in incidence rates of invasive lobular and ductal breast carcinoma. JAMA. 2003;289(11):1421–4.
3. Chen Z, Yang J, Li S, Lv M, Shen Y, Wang B, et al. Invasive lobular carcinoma of the breast: a special histological type compared with invasive ductal carcinoma. PLoS One. 2017;12(9):e0182397.
4. Lewis TR, Casey J, Buerk CA, Cammack KV. Incidence of lobular carcinoma in bilateral breast cancer. Am J Surg. 1982;144(6):635–8.
5. Kim SH, Cha ES, Park CS, Kang BJ, Whang IY, Lee AW, et al. Imaging features of invasive lobular carcinoma: comparison with invasive ductal carcinoma. Jpn J Radiol. 2011;29(7):475–82.
6. Le Gal M, Ollivier L, Asselain B, Meunier M, Laurent M, Vielh P, et al. Mammographic features of 455 invasive lobular carcinomas. Radiology. 1992;185(3):705–8.
7. Porter AJ, Evans EB, Foxcroft LM, Simpson PT, Lakhani SR. Mammographic and ultrasound features of invasive lobular carcinoma of the breast. J Med Imaging Radiat Oncol. 2014;58(1):1–10.
8. Gruber IV, Rueckert M, Kagan KO, Staebler A, Siegmann KC, Hartkopf A, et al. Measurement of tumour size with mammography, sonography and magnetic resonance imaging as compared to histological tumour size in primary breast cancer. BMC Cancer. 2013;13:328.
9. Parvaiz MA, Yang P, Razia E, Mascarenhas M, Deacon C, Matey P, et al. Breast MRI in invasive lobular carcinoma: a useful investigation in surgical planning? Breast J. 2016;22(2):143–50.
10. Fechner RE. Histologic variants of infiltrating lobular carcinoma of the breast. Hum Pathol. 1975;6(3):373–8.
11. Shousha S, Backhous CM, Alaghband-Zadeh J, Burn I. Alveolar variant of invasive lobular carcinoma of the breast. A tumor rich in estrogen receptors. Am J Clin Pathol. 1986;85(1):1–5.
12. Esposito NN, Chivukula M, Dabbs DJ. The ductal phenotypic expression of the E-cadherin/catenin complex in tubulolobular carcinoma of the breast: an immunohistochemical and clinicopathologic study. Mod Pathol. 2007;20(1):130–8.
13. Butler D, Rosa M. Pleomorphic lobular carcinoma of the breast: a morphologically and clinically distinct variant of lobular carcinoma. Arch Pathol Lab Med. 2013;137(11):1688–92.
14. Menet E, Becette V, Briffod M. Cytologic diagnosis of lobular carcinoma of the breast: experience with 555 patients in the Rene Huguenin Cancer Center. Cancer. 2008;114(2):111–7.
15. Derksen PW, Liu X, Saridin F, van der Gulden H, Zevenhoven J, Evers B, et al. Somatic inactivation of E-cadherin and p53 in mice leads to metastatic lobular mammary carcinoma through induction of anoikis resistance and angiogenesis. Cancer Cell. 2006;10(5):437–49.
16. Moriya T, Kozuka Y, Kanomata N, Tse GM, Tan PH. The role of immunohistochemistry in the differential diagnosis of breast lesions. Pathology. 2009;41(1):68–76.
17. Da Silva L, Parry S, Reid L, Keith P, Waddell N, Kossai M, et al. Aberrant expression of E-cadherin in lobular carcinomas of the breast. Am J Surg Pathol. 2008;32(5):773–83.
18. Sahin S, Karatas F, Erdem GU, Hacioglu B, Altundag K. Invasive pleomorphic lobular histology is an adverse prognostic factor on survival in patients with breast cancer. Am Surg. 2017;83(4):359–64.
19. Ciriello G, Gatza ML, Beck AH, Wilkerson MD, Rhie SK, Pastore A, et al. Comprehensive molecular portraits of invasive lobular breast cancer. Cell. 2015;163(2):506–19.
20. Weigelt B, Geyer FC, Reis-Filho JS. Histological types of breast cancer: how special are they? Mol Oncol. 2010;4(3):192–208.
21. Mamtani A, King TA. Lobular breast cancer: different disease, different algorithms? Surg Oncol Clin N Am. 2018;27(1):81–94.
22. Sakr RA, Poulet B, Kaufman GJ, Nos C, Clough KB. Clear margins for invasive lobular carcinoma: a surgical challenge. Eur J Surg Oncol. 2011;37(4):350–6.
23. Monhollen L, Morrison C, Ademuyiwa FO, Chandrasekhar R, Khoury T. Pleomorphic lobular carcinoma: a distinctive clinical and molecular breast cancer type. Histopathology. 2012;61(3):365–77.
24. Rakha EA, Lee AH, Evans AJ, Menon S, Assad NY, Hodi Z, et al. Tubular carcinoma of the breast: further evidence to support its excellent prognosis. J Clin Oncol. 2010;28(1):99–104.
25. Leibman AJ, Lewis M, Kruse B. Tubular carcinoma of the breast: mammographic appearance. AJR Am J Roentgenol. 1993;160(2):263–5.
26. Sheppard DG, Whitman GJ, Huynh PT, Sahin AA, Fornage BD, Stelling CB. Tubular carcinoma of the breast: mammographic and sonographic features. AJR Am J Roentgenol. 2000;174(1):253–7.
27. Rakha E, Pinder SE, Shin SJ, Tsuda H. Tubular carcioma and cribriform carcinoma. In: Lakhani SR, Ellis IO, Schnitt SJ, Tan PH, MJvd V, editors. WHO classification of tumours of the breast. Lyon: IARC; 2012.
28. Cangiarella J, Waisman J, Shapiro RL, Simsir A. Cytologic features of tubular adenocarcinoma of the breast by aspiration biopsy. Diagn Cytopathol. 2001;25(5):311–5.
29. Dieci MV, Orvieto E, Dominici M, Conte P, Guarneri V. Rare breast cancer subtypes: histological, molecular, and clinical peculiarities. Oncologist. 2014;19(8):805–13.
30. de Moraes Schenka NG, Schenka AA, de Souza Queiroz L, de Almeida Matsura M, Alvarenga M, Vassallo J. p63 and CD10: reliable markers in discriminating benign sclerosing lesions from tubular carcinoma of the breast? Appl Immunohistochem Mol Morphol. 2006;14(1):71–7.
31. Spruill L. Benign mimickers of malignant breast lesions. Semin Diagn Pathol. 2016;33(1):2–12.
32. Albrektsen G, Heuch I, Thoresen SO. Histological type and grade of breast cancer tumors by parity, age at birth, and time since birth: a register-based study in Norway. BMC Cancer. 2010;10:226.
33. Di Saverio S, Gutierrez J, Avisar E. A retrospective review with long term follow up of 11,400 cases of pure mucinous breast carcinoma. Breast Cancer Res Treat. 2008;111(3):541–7.
34. Tan PH, Tse GM, Bay BH. Mucinous breast lesions: diagnostic challenges. J Clin Pathol. 2008;61(1):11–9.
35. Bitencourt AG, Graziano L, Osório CA, Guatelli CS, Souza JA, Mendonça MH, et al. MRI features of mucinous cancer of the breast: correlation with pathologic findings and other imaging methods. AJR Am J Roentgenol. 2016;206(2):238–46.
36. Lam WW, Chu WC, Tse GM, Ma TK. Sonographic appearance of mucinous carcinoma of the breast. AJR Am J Roentgenol. 2004;182(4):1069–74.
37. Linda A, Zuiani C, Girometti R, Londero V, Machin P, Brondani G, et al. Unusual malignant tumors of the breast: MRI features and pathologic correlation. Eur J Radiol. 2010;75(2):178–84.
38. Capella C, Eusebi V, Mann B, Azzopardi JG. Endocrine differentiation in mucoid carcinoma of the breast. Histopathology. 1980;4(6):613–30.
39. Lacroix-Triki M, Suarez PH, MacKay A, Lambros MB, Natrajan R, Savage K, et al. Mucinous carcinoma of the breast is genomically distinct from invasive ductal carcinomas of no special type. J Pathol. 2010;222(3):282–98.
40. Laucirica R, Bentz JS, Khalbuss WE, Clayton AC, Souers RJ, Moriarty AT. Performance characteristics of mucinous (colloid) carcinoma of the breast in fine-needle aspirates: observations from the College of American Pathologists Interlaboratory Comparison

Program in Nongynecologic Cytopathology. Arch Pathol Lab Med. 2011;135(12):1533–8.

41. Tang SL, Yang JQ, Du ZG, Tan QW, Zhou YT, Zhang D, et al. Clinicopathologic study of invasive micropapillary carcinoma of the breast. Oncotarget. 2017;8(26):42455–65.

42. Edelweiss M, Corben AD, Liberman L, Kaplan J, Nehhozina T, Catalano JP, et al. Focal extravasated mucin in breast core needle biopsies: is surgical excision always necessary? Breast J. 2013;19(3):302–9.

43. Cao AY, He M, Liu ZB, Di GH, Wu J, Lu JS, et al. Outcome of pure mucinous breast carcinoma compared to infiltrating ductal carcinoma: a population-based study from China. Ann Surg Oncol. 2012;19(9):3019–27.

44. Ranade A, Batra R, Sandhu G, Chitale RA, Balderacchi J. Clinicopathological evaluation of 100 cases of mucinous carcinoma of breast with emphasis on axillary staging and special reference to a micropapillary pattern. J Clin Pathol. 2010;63(12):1043–7.

45. Paterakos M, Watkin WG, Edgerton SM, Moore DH 2nd, Thor AD. Invasive micropapillary carcinoma of the breast: a prognostic study. Hum Pathol. 1999;30(12):1459–63.

46. Alsharif S, Daghistani R, Kamberoğlu EA, Omeroglu A, Meterissian S, Mesurolle B. Mammographic, sonographic and MR imaging features of invasive micropapillary breast cancer. Eur J Radiol. 2014;83(8):1375–80.

47. Adrada B, Arribas E, Gilcrease M, Yang WT. Invasive micropapillary carcinoma of the breast: mammographic, sonographic, and MRI features. AJR Am J Roentgenol. 2009;193(1):W58–63.

48. Yang YL, Liu BB, Zhang X, Fu L. Invasive micropapillary carcinoma of the breast: an update. Arch Pathol Lab Med. 2016;140(8):799–805.

49. Nassar H. Carcinomas with micropapillary morphology: clinical significance and current concepts. Adv Anat Pathol. 2004;11(6):297–303.

50. Siriaunkgul S, Tavassoli FA. Invasive micropapillary carcinoma of the breast. Mod Pathol. 1993;6(6):660–2.

51. Kelten EC, Akbulut M, Duzcan SE. Diagnostic dilemma in cytologic features of micropapillary carcinoma of the breast: a report of 2 cases. Acta Cytol. 2009;53(4):463–6.

52. Vingiani A, Maisonneuve P, Dell'orto P, Farante G, Rotmensz N, Lissidini G, et al. The clinical relevance of micropapillary carcinoma of the breast: a case-control study. Histopathology. 2013;63(2):217–24.

53. Yang W, Wei B, Chen M, Bu H. Evaluation of immunohistochemistry HER2 results interpretation in invasive micropapillary carcinoma of the breast. Zhonghua Bing Li Xue Za Zhi. 2015;44(1):48–52.

54. Stewart RL, Caron JE, Gulbahce EH, Factor RE, Geiersbach KB, Downs-Kelly E. HER2 immunohistochemical and fluorescence in situ hybridization discordances in invasive breast carcinoma with micropapillary features. Mod Pathol. 2017;30(11):1561–6.

55. Wolff AC, Hammond ME, Hicks DG, Dowsett M, McShane LM, Allison KH, et al. Recommendations for human epidermal growth factor receptor 2 testing in breast cancer: American Society of Clinical Oncology/College of American Pathologists clinical practice guideline update. J Clin Oncol. 2013;31(31):3997–4013.

56. Nassar H, Pansare V, Zhang H, Che M, Sakr W, Ali-Fehmi R, et al. Pathogenesis of invasive micropapillary carcinoma: role of MUC1 glycoprotein. Mod Pathol. 2004;17(9):1045–50.

57. Pettinato G, Manivel CJ, Panico L, Sparano L, Petrella G. Invasive micropapillary carcinoma of the breast: clinicopathologic study of 62 cases of a poorly recognized variant with highly aggressive behavior. Am J Clin Pathol. 2004;121(6):857–66.

58. Lepe M, Kalife ET, Ou J, Quddus MR, Singh K. 'Inside-out' p120 immunostaining pattern in invasive micropapillary carcinoma of the breast; additional unequivocal evidence of reversed polarity. Histopathology. 2017;70(5):832–4.

59. Ueng SH, Mezzetti T, Tavassoli FA. Papillary neoplasms of the breast: a review. Arch Pathol Lab Med. 2009;133(6):893–907.

60. Marchiò C, Iravani M, Natrajan R, Lambros MB, Savage K, Tamber N, et al. Genomic and immunophenotypical characterization of pure micropapillary carcinomas of the breast. J Pathol. 2008;215(4):398–410.

61. Natrajan R, Wilkerson PM, Marchiò C, Piscuoglio S, Ng CK, Wai P, et al. Characterization of the genomic features and expressed fusion genes in micropapillary carcinomas of the breast. J Pathol. 2014;232(5):553–65.

62. Lotan TL, Ye H, Melamed J, Wu XR, Shih IM, Epstein JI. Immunohistochemical panel to identify the primary site of invasive micropapillary carcinoma. Am J Surg Pathol. 2009;33(7):1037–41.

63. Guo X, Chen L, Lang R, Fan Y, Zhang X, Fu L. Invasive micropapillary carcinoma of the breast: association of pathologic features with lymph node metastasis. Am J Clin Pathol. 2006;126(5):740–6.

64. Chen HL, Ding A. Comparison of invasive micropapillary and triple negative invasive ductal carcinoma of the breast. Breast. 2015;24(6):723–31.

65. Chen AC, Paulino AC, Schwartz MR, Rodriguez AA, Bass BL, Chang JC, et al. Population-based comparison of prognostic factors in invasive micropapillary and invasive ductal carcinoma of the breast. Br J Cancer. 2014;111(3):619–22.

66. Liu F, Yang M, Li Z, Guo X, Lin Y, Lang R, et al. Invasive micropapillary mucinous carcinoma of the breast is associated with poor prognosis. Breast Cancer Res Treat. 2015;151(2):443–51.

67. Barbashina V, Corben AD, Akram M, Vallejo C, Tan LK. Mucinous micropapillary carcinoma of the breast: an aggressive counterpart to conventional pure mucinous tumors. Hum Pathol. 2013;44(8):1577–85.

68. Madur B, Shet T, Chinoy R. Cytologic findings in infiltrating micropapillary carcinoma and mucinous carcinomas with micropapillary pattern. Acta Cytol. 2007;51(1):25–32.

69. Jain S, Khurana N, Rao S, Garg A, Kaza R. Psammomatous colloid carcinoma of the breast with micropapillary pattern. Breast J. 2012;18(2):178–80.

70. Pedersen L, Zedeler K, Holck S, Schiødt T, Mouridsen HT. Medullary carcinoma of the breast. Prevalence and prognostic importance of classical risk factors in breast cancer. Eur J Cancer. 1995;31A(13–14):2289–95.

71. Wang XX, Jiang YZ, Liu XY, Li JJ, Song CG, Shao ZM. Difference in characteristics and outcomes between medullary breast carcinoma and invasive ductal carcinoma: a population based study from SEER 18 database. Oncotarget. 2016;7(16):22665–73.

72. Yilmaz E, Lebe B, Balci P, Sal S, Canda T. Comparison of mammographic and sonographic findings in typical and atypical medullary carcinomas of the breast. Clin Radiol. 2002;57(7):640–5.

73. Jeong SJ, Lim HS, Lee JS, Park MH, Yoon JH, Park JG, et al. Medullary carcinoma of the breast: MRI findings. AJR Am J Roentgenol. 2012;198(5):W482–7.

74. Ridolfi RL, Rosen PP, Port A, Kinne D, Mike V. Medullary carcinoma of the breast: a clinicopathologic study with 10 year follow-up. Cancer. 1977;40(4):1365–85.

75. Racz MM, Pommier RF, Troxell ML. Fine-needle aspiration cytology of medullary breast carcinoma: report of two cases and review of the literature with emphasis on differential diagnosis. Diagn Cytopathol. 2007;35(6):313–8.

76. Xu R, Feiner H, Li P, Yee H, Inghirami G, Delgado Y, et al. Differential amplification and overexpression of HER-2/neu, p53, MIB1, and estrogen receptor/progesterone receptor among medullary carcinoma, atypical medullary carcinoma, and high-grade

invasive ductal carcinoma of breast. Arch Pathol Lab Med. 2003;127(11):1458–64.

77. Rodriguez-Pinilla SM, Rodríguez-Gil Y, Moreno-Bueno G, Sarrió D, Martin-Guijarro Mdel C, Hernandez L, et al. Sporadic invasive breast carcinomas with medullary features display a basal-like phenotype: an immunohistochemical and gene amplification study. Am J Surg Pathol 2007;31(4):501–8.

78. Huober J, Gelber S, Goldhirsch A, Coates AS, Viale G, Öhlschlegel C, et al. Prognosis of medullary breast cancer: analysis of 13 International Breast Cancer Study Group (IBCSG) trials. Ann Oncol. 2012;23(11):2843–51.

79. Mateo AM, Pezzi TA, Sundermeyer M, Kelley CA, Klimberg VS, Pezzi CM. Atypical medullary carcinoma of the breast has similar prognostic factors and survival to typical medullary breast carcinoma: 3,976 cases from the National Cancer Data Base. J Surg Oncol. 2016;114(5):533–6.

80. Rakha EA, Aleskandarany M, El-Sayed ME, Blamey RW, Elston CW, Ellis IO, et al. The prognostic significance of inflammation and medullary histological type in invasive carcinoma of the breast. Eur J Cancer. 2009;45(10):1780–7.

81. Loi S, Sirtaine N, Piette F, Salgado R, Viale G, Van Eenoo F, et al. Prognostic and predictive value of tumor-infiltrating lymphocytes in a phase III randomized adjuvant breast cancer trial in node-positive breast cancer comparing the addition of docetaxel to doxorubicin with doxorubicin-based chemotherapy: BIG 02-98. J Clin Oncol. 2013;31(7):860–7.

82. O'Malley FP, Bane A. An update on apocrine lesions of the breast. Histopathology. 2008;52(1):3–10.

83. Tanaka K, Imoto S, Wada N, Sakemura N, Hasebe K. Invasive apocrine carcinoma of the breast: clinicopathologic features of 57 patients. Breast J. 2008;14(2):164–8.

84. Vranic S, Schmitt F, Sapino A, Costa JL, Reddy S, Castro M, et al. Apocrine carcinoma of the breast: a comprehensive review. Histol Histopathol. 2013;28(11):1393–409.

85. Zhang N, Zhang H, Chen T, Yang Q. Dose invasive apocrine adenocarcinoma has worse prognosis than invasive ductal carcinoma of breast: evidence from SEER database. Oncotarget. 2017;8(15):24579–92.

86. Gilles R, Lesnik A, Guinebretière JM, Tardivon A, Masselot J, Contesso G, et al. Apocrine carcinoma: clinical and mammographic features. Radiology. 1994;190(2):495–7.

87. Yuen S, Uematsu T, Kasami M, Tanaka K, Kimura K, Sanuki J, et al. Breast carcinomas with strong high-signal intensity on T2-weighted MR images: pathological characteristics and differential diagnosis. J Magn Reson Imaging. 2007;25(3):502–10.

88. Seo KJ, An YY, Whang IY, Chang ED, Kang BJ, Kim SH, et al. Sonography of invasive apocrine carcinoma of the breast in five cases. Korean J Radiol. 2015;16(5):1006–11.

89. Vranic S, Gatalica Z, Deng H, Frkovic-Grazio S, Lee LM, Gurjeva O, et al. ER-alpha36, a novel isoform of ER-alpha66, is commonly over-expressed in apocrine and adenoid cystic carcinomas of the breast. J Clin Pathol. 2011;64(1):54–7.

90. Vranic S, Marchiò C, Castellano I, Botta C, Scalzo MS, Bender RP, et al. Immunohistochemical and molecular profiling of histologically defined apocrine carcinomas of the breast. Hum Pathol. 2015;46(9):1350–9.

91. Dellapasqua S, Maisonneuve P, Viale G, Pruneri G, Mazzarol G, Ghisini R, et al. Immunohistochemically defined subtypes and outcome of apocrine breast cancer. Clin Breast Cancer. 2013;13(2):95–102.

92. Turner NC, Reis-Filho JS. Tackling the diversity of triple-negative breast cancer. Clin Cancer Res. 2013;19(23):6380–8.

93. Weisman PS, Ng CK, Brogi E, Eisenberg RE, Won HH, Piscuoglio S, et al. Genetic alterations of triple negative breast cancer by targeted next-generation sequencing and correlation with tumor morphology. Mod Pathol. 2016;29(5):476–88.

94. Lehmann BD, Bauer JA, Schafer JM, Pendleton CS, Tang L, Johnson KC, et al. PIK3CA mutations in androgen receptor-positive triple negative breast cancer confer sensitivity to the combination of PI3K and androgen receptor inhibitors. Breast Cancer Res. 2014;16(4):406.

95. Agarwal C, Pujani M, Sharma N, Rana D, Prajapati D. Apocrine carcinoma of breast: a rare entity posing cytological challenge. Diagn Cytopathol. 2017;45(12):1156–8.

96. Ng WK. Fine needle aspiration cytology of apocrine carcinoma of the breast. Review of cases in a three-year period. Acta Cytol. 2002;46(3):507–12.

97. Abati AD, Kimmel M, Rosen PP. Apocrine mammary carcinoma. A clinicopathologic study of 72 cases. Am J Clin Pathol. 1990;94(4):371–7.

98. Weigelt B, Eberle C, Cowell CF, Ng CK, Reis-Filho JS. Metaplastic breast carcinoma: more than a special type. Nat Rev Cancer. 2014;14(3):147–8.

99. Downs-Kelly E, Nayeemuddin KM, Albarracin C, Wu Y, Hunt KK, Gilcrease MZ. Matrix-producing carcinoma of the breast: an aggressive subtype of metaplastic carcinoma. Am J Surg Pathol. 2009;33(4):534–41.

100. Yamaguchi R, Horii R, Maeda I, Suga S, Makita M, Iwase T, et al. Clinicopathologic study of 53 metaplastic breast carcinomas: their elements and prognostic implications. Hum Pathol. 2010;41(5):679–85.

101. Pezzi CM, Patel-Parekh L, Cole K, Franko J, Klimberg VS, Bland K. Characteristics and treatment of metaplastic breast cancer: analysis of 892 cases from the National Cancer Data Base. Ann Surg Oncol. 2007;14(1):166–73.

102. Nelson RA, Guye ML, Luu T, Lai LL. Survival outcomes of metaplastic breast cancer patients: results from a US population-based analysis. Ann Surg Oncol. 2015;22(1):24–31.

103. Langlands F, Cornford E, Rakha E, Dall B, Gutteridge E, Dodwell D, et al. Imaging overview of metaplastic carcinomas of the breast: a large study of 71 cases. Br J Radiol. 2016:20140644.

104. Lang R, Fan Y, Fu X, Fu L. Metaplastic breast carcinoma with extensive osseous differentiation: a report of two cases and review of the literature. Tumori. 2011;97(4):e1–5.

105. Leddy R, Irshad A, Rumboldt T, Cluver A, Campbell A, Ackerman S. Review of metaplastic carcinoma of the breast: imaging findings and pathologic features. J Clin Imaging Sci. 2012;2:21.

106. McKinnon E, Xiao P. Metaplastic carcinoma of the breast. Arch Pathol Lab Med. 2015;139(6):819–22.

107. Yang WT, Hennessy B, Broglio K, Mills C, Sneige N, Davis WG, et al. Imaging differences in metaplastic and invasive ductal carcinomas of the breast. AJR Am J Roentgenol. 2007;189(6):1288–93.

108. Nayak A, Wu Y, Gilcrease MZ. Primary squamous cell carcinoma of the breast: predictors of locoregional recurrence and overall survival. Am J Surg Pathol. 2013;37(6):867–73.

109. DeLair DF, Corben AD, Catalano JP, Vallejo CE, Brogi E, Tan LK. Non-mammary metastases to the breast and axilla: a study of 85 cases. Mod Pathol. 2013;26(3):343–9.

110. Wargotz ES, Norris HJ. Metaplastic carcinomas of the breast. I. Matrix-producing carcinoma. Hum Pathol. 1989;20(7):628–35.

111. Gobbi H, Simpson JF, Jensen RA, Olson SJ, Page DL. Metaplastic spindle cell breast tumors arising within papillomas, complex sclerosing lesions, and nipple adenomas. Mod Pathol. 2003;16(9):893–901.

112. Carter MR, Hornick JL, Lester S, Fletcher CD. Spindle cell (sarcomatoid) carcinoma of the breast: a clinicopathologic and immunohistochemical analysis of 29 cases. Am J Surg Pathol. 2006;30(3):300–9.

113. Dwyer JB, Clark BZ. Low-grade fibromatosis-like spindle cell carcinoma of the breast. Arch Pathol Lab Med. 2015;139(4):552–7.

114. Kawaguchi K, Shin SJ. Immunohistochemical staining characteristics of low-grade adenosquamous carcinoma of the breast. Am J Surg Pathol. 2012;36(7):1009–20.

115. Geyer FC, Lambros MB, Natrajan R, Mehta R, Mackay A, Savage K, et al. Genomic and immunohistochemical analysis of adenosquamous carcinoma of the breast. Mod Pathol. 2010;23(7):951–60.

116. Lui PC, Tse GM, Tan PH, Jayaram G, Putti TC, Chaiwun B, et al. Fine-needle aspiration cytology of metaplastic carcinoma of the breast. J Clin Pathol. 2007;60(5):529–33.

117. Murata T, Ihara S, Kato H, Tanigawa K, Higashiguchi T, Imai T, et al. Matrix-producing carcinoma of the breast: case report with radiographical and cytopathological features. Pathol Int. 1998;48(10):824–8.

118. Joshi D, Singh P, Zonunfawni Y, Gangane N. Metaplastic carcinoma of the breast: cytological diagnosis and diagnostic pitfalls. Acta Cytol. 2011;55(4):313–8.

119. Rakha EA, Tan PH, Varga Z, Tse GM, Shaaban AM, Climent F, et al. Prognostic factors in metaplastic carcinoma of the breast: a multi-institutional study. Br J Cancer. 2015;112(2):283–9.

120. Rakha EA, Coimbra ND, Hodi Z, Juneinah E, Ellis IO, Lee AH. Immunoprofile of metaplastic carcinomas of the breast. Histopathology. 2017;70(6):975–85.

121. Davis WG, Hennessy B, Babiera G, Hunt K, Valero V, Buchholz TA, et al. Metaplastic sarcomatoid carcinoma of the breast with absent or minimal overt invasive carcinomatous component: a misnomer. Am J Surg Pathol. 2005;29(11):1456–63.

122. Lester TR, Hunt KK, Nayeemuddin KM, Bassett RL Jr, Gonzalez-Angulo AM, Feig BW, et al. Metaplastic sarcomatoid carcinoma of the breast appears more aggressive than other triple receptor-negative breast cancers. Breast Cancer Res Treat 2012;131(1):41–48.

123. Lacroix-Triki M, Geyer FC, Lambros MB, Savage K, Ellis IO, Lee AH, et al. Beta-catenin/Wnt signalling pathway in fibromatosis, metaplastic carcinomas and phyllodes tumours of the breast. Mod Pathol. 2010;23(11):1438–48.

124. Ng CKY, Piscuoglio S, Geyer FC, Burke KA, Pareja F, Eberle CA, et al. The landscape of somatic genetic alterations in metaplastic breast carcinomas. Clin Cancer Res. 2017;23(14):3859–70.

125. Cimino-Mathews A, Sharma R, Illei PB, Vang R, Argani P. A subset of malignant phyllodes tumors express p63 and p40: a diagnostic pitfall in breast core needle biopsies. Am J Surg Pathol. 2014;38(12):1689–96.

126. Rungta S, Kleer CG. Metaplastic carcinomas of the breast: diagnostic challenges and new translational insights. Arch Pathol Lab Med. 2012;136(8):896–900.

127. Boecker W, Stenman G, Loening T, Andersson MK, Sinn HP, Barth P, et al. Differentiation and histogenesis of syringomatous tumour of the nipple and low-grade adenosquamous carcinoma: evidence for a common origin. Histopathology. 2014;65(1):9–23.

128. Cimino-Mathews A, Verma S, Figueroa-Magalhaes MC, Jeter SC, Zhang Z, Argani P, et al. A clinicopathologic analysis of 45 patients with metaplastic breast carcinoma. Am J Clin Pathol. 2016;145(3):365–72.

129. Hennessy BT, Giordano S, Broglio K, Duan Z, Trent J, Buchholz TA, et al. Biphasic metaplastic sarcomatoid carcinoma of the breast. Ann Oncol. 2006;17(4):605–13.

130. Jung SY, Kim HY, Nam BH, Min SY, Lee SJ, Park C, et al. Worse prognosis of metaplastic breast cancer patients than other patients with triple-negative breast cancer. Breast Cancer Res Treat. 2010;120(3):627–37.

131. Nagao T, Kinoshita T, Hojo T, Tsuda H, Tamura K, Fujiwara Y. The differences in the histological types of breast cancer and the response to neoadjuvant chemotherapy: the relationship between the outcome and the clinicopathological characteristics. Breast. 2012;21(3):289–95.

132. El Zein D, Hughes M, Kumar S, Peng X, Oyasiji T, Jabbour H, et al. Metaplastic carcinoma of the breast is more aggressive than triple-negative breast cancer: a study from a single institution and review of literature. Clin Breast Cancer. 2017;17(5):382–91.

133. Zhang Y, Lv F, Yang Y, Qian X, Lang R, Fan Y, et al. Clinicopathological features and prognosis of metaplastic breast carcinoma: experience of a major Chinese cancer center. PLoS One. 2015;10(6):e0131409.

134. Lai HW, Tseng LM, Chang TW, Kuo YL, Hsieh CM, Chen ST, et al. The prognostic significance of metaplastic carcinoma of the breast (MCB)—a case controlled comparison study with infiltrating ductal carcinoma. Breast. 2013;22(5):968–73.

135. Tan QT, Chuwa EW, Chew SH, Lim-Tan SK, Lim SH. Low-grade adenosquamous carcinoma of the breast: a diagnostic and clinical challenge. Int J Surg. 2015;19:22–6.

136. Gobbi H, Simpson JF, Borowsky A, Jensen RA, Page DL. Metaplastic breast tumors with a dominant fibromatosis-like phenotype have a high risk of local recurrence. Cancer. 1999;85(10):2170–82.

137. Jaso J, Malhotra R. Adenoid cystic carcinoma. Arch Pathol Lab Med. 2011;135(4):511–5.

138. Treitl D, Radkani P, Rizer M, El Hussein S, Paramo JC, Mesko TW. Adenoid cystic carcinoma of the breast, 20 years of experience in a single center with review of literature. Breast Cancer. 2017. https://doi.org/10.1007/s12282-017-0780-1.

139. Boujelbene N, Khabir A, Boujelbene N, Jeanneret Sozzi W, Mirimanoff RO, Khanfir K. Clinical review—breast adenoid cystic carcinoma. Breast. 2012;21(2):124–7.

140. Glazebrook KN, Reynolds C, Smith RL, Gimenez EI, Boughey JC. Adenoid cystic carcinoma of the breast. AJR Am J Roentgenol. 2010;194(5):1391–6.

141. Foschini MP, Morandi L, Asioli S, Giove G, Corradini AG, Eusebi V. The morphological spectrum of salivary gland type tumours of the breast. Pathology. 2017;49(2):215–27.

142. Marchiò C, Weigelt B, Reis-Filho JS. Adenoid cystic carcinomas of the breast and salivary glands (or 'The strange case of Dr Jekyll and Mr Hyde' of exocrine gland carcinomas). J Clin Pathol. 2010;63(3):220–8.

143. Shin SJ, Rosen PP. Solid variant of mammary adenoid cystic carcinoma with basaloid features: a study of nine cases. Am J Surg Pathol. 2002;26(4):413–20.

144. Mastropasqua MG, Maiorano E, Pruneri G, Orvieto E, Mazzarol G, Vento AR, et al. Immunoreactivity for c-kit and p63 as an adjunct in the diagnosis of adenoid cystic carcinoma of the breast. Mod Pathol. 2005;18(10):1277–82.

145. Azoulay S, Laé M, Fréneaux P, Merle S, Al Ghuzlan A, Chnecker C, et al. KIT is highly expressed in adenoid cystic carcinoma of the breast, a basal-like carcinoma associated with a favorable outcome. Mod Pathol. 2005;18(12):1623–31.

146. Nakai T, Ichihara S, Kada A, Ito N, Moritani S, Kawasaki T, et al. The unique luminal staining pattern of cytokeratin 5/6 in adenoid cystic carcinoma of the breast may aid in differentiating it from its mimickers. Virchows Arch. 2016;469(2):213–22.

147. Wetterskog D, Lopez-Garcia MA, Lambros MB, A'Hern R, Geyer FC, Milanezi F, et al. Adenoid cystic carcinomas constitute a genomically distinct subgroup of triple-negative and basal-like breast cancers. J Pathol. 2012;226(1):84–96.

148. Persson M, Andrén Y, Mark J, Horlings HM, Persson F, Stenman G. Recurrent fusion of MYB and NFIB transcription factor genes in carcinomas of the breast and head and neck. Proc Natl Acad Sci U S A. 2009;106(44):18740–4.

149. Poling JS, Yonescu R, Subhawong AP, Sharma R, Argani P, Ning Y, et al. MYB labeling by immunohistochemistry is more sensitive and specific for breast adenoid cystic carcinoma than MYB labeling by FISH. Am J Surg Pathol. 2017;41(7):973–9.

150. Kim J, Geyer FC, Martelotto LG, Ng CKY, Lim RS, Selenica P, et al. MYBL1 rearrangements and MYB amplification in breast adenoid cystic carcinomas lacking the MYB-NFIB fusion gene. J Pathol. 2017. https://doi.org/10.1002/path.5006.

151. Saqi A, Mercado CL, Hamele-Bena D. Adenoid cystic carcinoma of the breast diagnosed by fine-needle aspiration. Diagn Cytopathol. 2004;30(4):271–4.

152. Ilkay TM, Gozde K, Ozgur S, Dilaver D. Diagnosis of adenoid cystic carcinoma of the breast using fine-needle aspiration cytology: a case report and review of the literature. Diagn Cytopathol. 2015;43(9):722–6.

153. Rabban JT, Swain RS, Zaloudek CJ, Chase DR, Chen YY. Immunophenotypic overlap between adenoid cystic carcinoma and collagenous spherulosis of the breast: potential diagnostic pitfalls using myoepithelial markers. Mod Pathol. 2006;19(10):1351–7.

154. Welsh JL, Keeney MG, Hoskin TL, Glazebrook KN, Boughey JC, Shah SS, et al. Is axillary surgery beneficial for patients with adenoid cystic carcinoma of the breast? J Surg Oncol. 2017;116(6):690–5.

155. Ghabach B, Anderson WF, Curtis RE, Huycke MM, Lavigne JA, Dores GM. Adenoid cystic carcinoma of the breast in the United States (1977 to 2006): a population-based cohort study. Breast Cancer Res. 2010;12(4):R54.

156. Fusco N, Geyer FC, De Filippo MR, Martelotto LG, Ng CK, Piscuoglio S, et al. Genetic events in the progression of adenoid cystic carcinoma of the breast to high-grade triple-negative breast cancer. Mod Pathol. 2016;29(11):1292–305.

157. McDivitt RW, Stewart FW. Breast carcinoma in children. JAMA. 1966;195(5):388–90.

158. Horowitz DP, Sharma CS, Connolly E, Gidea-Addeo D, Deutsch I. Secretory carcinoma of the breast: results from the survival, epidemiology and end results database. Breast. 2012;21(3):350–3.

159. Mun SH, Ko EY, Han BK, Shin JH, Kim SJ, Cho EY. Secretory carcinoma of the breast: sonographic features. J Ultrasound Med. 2008;27(6):947–54.

160. Paeng MH, Choi HY, Sung SH, Moon BI, Shim SS. Secretory carcinoma of the breast. J Clin Ultrasound. 2003;31(8):425–9.

161. Del Castillo M, Chibon F, Arnould L, Croce S, Ribeiro A, Perot G, et al. Secretory breast carcinoma: a histopathologic and genomic spectrum characterized by a joint specific ETV6-NTRK3 gene fusion. Am J Surg Pathol. 2015;39(11):1458–67.

162. Li D, Xiao X, Yang W, Shui R, Tu X, Lu H, et al. Secretory breast carcinoma: a clinicopathological and immunophenotypic study of 15 cases with a review of the literature. Mod Pathol. 2012;25(4):567–75.

163. Lamovec J, Bracko M. Secretory carcinoma of the breast: light microscopical, immunohistochemical and flow cytometric study. Mod Pathol. 1994;7(4):475–9.

164. Lae M, Fréneaux P, Sastre-Garau X, Chouchane O, Sigal-Zafrani B, Vincent-Salomon A. Secretory breast carcinomas with ETV6-NTRK3 fusion gene belong to the basal-like carcinoma spectrum. Mod Pathol. 2009;22(2):291–8.

165. Krings G, Joseph NM, Bean GR, Solomon D, Onodera C, Talevich E, et al. Genomic profiling of breast secretory carcinomas reveals distinct genetics from other breast cancers and similarity to mammary analog secretory carcinomas. Mod Pathol. 2017;30(8):1086–99.

166. Shanthi V, Rama Krishna BA, Rao NM, Sujatha C. Cytodiagnosis of secretory carcinoma of the breast. J Cytol. 2012;29(1):63–5.

167. Jayaram G, Looi LM, Yip CH. Fine needle aspiration cytology of secretory carcinoma of breast: a case report. Malays J Pathol. 1997;19(1):69–73.

168. Osako T, Takeuchi K, Horii R, Iwase T, Akiyama F. Secretory carcinoma of the breast and its histopathological mimics: value of markers for differential diagnosis. Histopathology. 2013;63(4):509–19.

169. D'Alfonso TM, Ginter PS, Liu YF, Shin SJ. Cystic hypersecretory (in situ) carcinoma of the breast: a clinicopathologic and immuno-histochemical characterization of 10 cases with clinical follow-up. Am J Surg Pathol. 2014;38(1):45–53.

170. Peintinger F, Leibl S, Reitsamer R, Moinfar F. Primary acinic cell carcinoma of the breast: a case report with long-term follow-up and review of the literature. Histopathology. 2004;45(6):645–8.

171. Geyer FC, Pareja F, Weigelt B, Rakha E, Ellis IO, Schnitt SJ, et al. The spectrum of triple-negative breast disease: high- and low-grade lesions. Am J Pathol. 2017;187(10):2139–51.

172. Eusebi V, Damiani S, Ellis IO, Azzopardi JG, Rosai J. Breast tumor resembling the tall cell variant of papillary thyroid carcinoma: report of 5 cases. Am J Surg Pathol. 2003;27(8):1114–8.

173. Cameselle-Teijeiro J, Abdulkader I, Barreiro-Morandeira F, Ruiz-Ponte C, Reyes-Santias R, Chavez E, et al. Breast tumor resembling the tall cell variant of papillary thyroid carcinoma: a case report. Int J Surg Pathol. 2006;14(1):79–84.

174. Masood S, Davis C, Kubik MJ. Changing the term "breast tumor resembling the tall cell variant of papillary thyroid carcinoma" to "tall cell variant of papillary breast carcinoma". Adv Anat Pathol. 2012;19(2):108–10.

175. Chiang S, Weigelt B, Wen HC, Pareja F, Raghavendra A, Martelotto LG, et al. IDH2 mutations define a unique subtype of breast cancer with altered nuclear polarity. Cancer Res. 2016;76(24):7118–29.

176. Bhargava R, Florea AV, Pelmus M, Jones MW, Bonaventura M, Wald A, et al. Breast tumor resembling tall cell variant of papillary thyroid carcinoma: a solid papillary neoplasm with characteristic immunohistochemical profile and few recurrent mutations. Am J Clin Pathol. 2017;147(4):399–410.

177. Foschini MP, Asioli S, Foreid S, Cserni G, Ellis IO, Eusebi V, et al. Solid papillary breast carcinomas resembling the tall cell variant of papillary thyroid neoplasms: a unique invasive tumor with indolent behavior. Am J Surg Pathol. 2017;41(7):887–95.

178. Tosi AL, Ragazzi M, Asioli S, Del Vecchio M, Cavalieri M, Eusebi LH, et al. Breast tumor resembling the tall cell variant of papillary thyroid carcinoma: report of 4 cases with evidence of malignant potential. Int J Surg Pathol. 2007;15(1):14–9.

179. Hameed O, Perry A, Banerjee R, Zhu X, Pfeifer JD. Papillary carcinoma of the breast lacks evidence of RET rearrangements despite morphological similarities to papillary thyroid carcinoma. Mod Pathol. 2009;22(9):1236–42.

180. Colella R, Guerriero A, Giansanti M, Sidoni A, Bellezza G. An additional case of breast tumor resembling the tall cell variant of papillary thyroid carcinoma. Int J Surg Pathol. 2015;23(3):217–20.

181. Robertson FM, Bondy M, Yang W, Yamauchi H, Wiggins S, Kamrudin S, et al. Inflammatory breast cancer: the disease, the biology, the treatment. CA Cancer J Clin. 2010;60(6):351–75.

182. Cristofanilli M, Valero V, Buzdar AV, Kau SW, Broglio KR, Gonzalez-Angulo AM, et al. Inflammatory breast cancer (IBC) and patterns of recurrence: understanding the biology of a unique disease. Cancer. 2007;110(7):1436–44.

183. Raghav K, French JT, Ueno NT, Lei X, Krishnamurthy S, Reuben JM, et al. Inflammatory Breast Cancer: a distinct clinicopathologic entity transcending histological distinction. PLoS One. 2016;11(1):e0145534.

Isabel Alvarado-Cabrero

The diagnosis of primary breast lymphoma (PBL) is limited to patients without evidence of systemic lymphoma or leukemia at the time that the breast lesion is detected. Clinically, the disease should involve only the breast or the breast and ipsilateral lymph nodes. PBL is a rare clinical entity that accounts for less than 1% of all patients with non-Hodgkin lymphoma (NHL) and approximately 1.7% of all patients with extra lymph node NHL.

Among patients with malignant breast neoplasms, patients with PBL reportedly represent between 0.04% and 1%. Clinically, it is presented as a palpable mass, unpainful, without clear radiologic differences from carcinomas. More than 95% of the cases correspond to B-type non-Hodgkin lymphoma, of which 60–80% are diffuse large B-cell lymphoma.

16.1 Introduction

Primary breast lymphoma (PBL) is a rare form of presentation of extranodal lymphoid neoplasm. It represents approximately 0.5% of all primary malignant neoplasms of the breast and between 1.7% and 2.2% of extranodal lymphomas [1]. Primary breast lymphoma is mainly found in female patients, accounting for 95–100% of all the PBL. It is very rare in men and only a few cases have been reported [2]. Clinically, it presents as a palpable mass, unpainful, without clear radiologic differences from carcinomas (Fig. 16.1) and can be associated with ipsilateral axillary lymph nodes [3]. Approximately 11% of the cases of PBL show bilateral involvement [4].

The median age at diagnosis in Western countries is 62–64 years; however, the age range is broad. In East Asian countries, the median age is lower (45–53 years), a finding which (as with breast carcinoma) likely reflects differences in demographics rather than biology [2, 4].

Once a diagnosis of lymphoma of the breast has been made, it is important to realize that it can represent primary or secondary disease. The distinction between primary breast lymphoma and secondary breast lymphoma (SBL) is based on several criteria first defined by Wiseman et al. [5]. Studying a group of 31 patients diagnosed between 1951 and 1970, they defined the distinction as the infiltration of the breast tissue by lymphoma, with or without regional lymph node, in patients with no history of prior nodal or extranodal lymphoma or systemic disease at the time of diagnosis. These criteria were reviewed in 1990 by Hugh et al. [6].

The origins of PBL are not completely understood. It has been postulated that the breast can act as a mucosal immune system site with development of lymphoid tissue associated with autoimmune mechanism or other inciting events, or in general terms, the breast behaves as a mucosal-associated lymphoid tissue [7, 8].

I. Alvarado-Cabrero, MD, PhD
Department of Pathology, Hospital de Oncologia, Centro Medico Nacional Siglo XXI, Instituto Mexicano del Seguro Social, Mexico City, Mexico

© Springer International Publishing AG, part of Springer Nature 2018
S. Stolnicu, I. Alvarado-Cabrero (eds.), *Practical Atlas of Breast Pathology*, https://doi.org/10.1007/978-3-319-93257-6_16

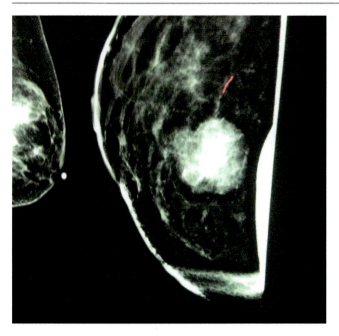

Fig. 16.1 Mammographic appearance of diffuse large B-cell lymphoma. Mammogram shows a high density circumscribed mass with partially irregular margins

16.2 Diffuse Large B-Cell Lymphoma (DLBCL)

Diffuse large B-cell lymphoma typically occurs in the fifth or sixth decade with a unilateral, solitary, palpable mass that is indistinguishable from a breast cancer [9]. Therefore, diagnosis is usually only obtained after a breast biopsy. Lesions range from 1 to 20 cm in greatest dimension, with a median size of 4–5 cm. A few patients have diffuse breast enlargement. Grossly, primary breast lymphoma can have a lobulated, well-circumscribed appearance (Fig. 16.2a). The tumor is composed of a proliferation of large lymphoid cells, with frequent infiltration of normal breast epithelium and occasional lymphoepithelial lesions (Figs. 16.2b and 16.3) [1, 10].

Immunophenotypic features overlap with those seen in other sites. The lymphomas are CD45+ and CD20+ (Fig. 16.4), with rare CD5+ cases; in addition, they have a relatively high proliferation index (60–90%) [11].

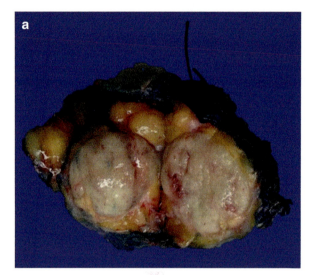

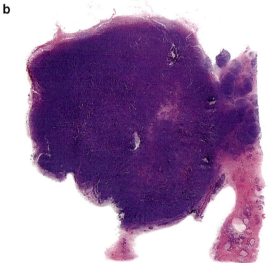

Fig. 16.2 Diffuse large B-cell lymphoma. (**a**) Gross appearance: well-circumscribed solid mass. (**b**) Microscopic appearance: solid proliferation of malignant lymphoid cells within breast tissue

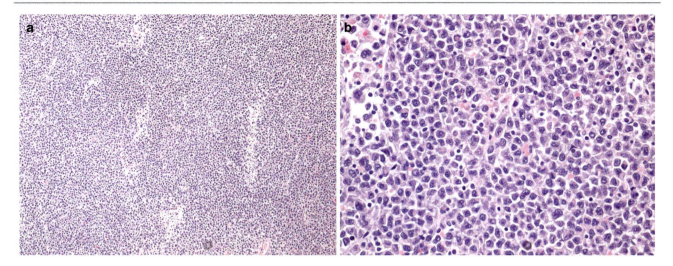

Fig. 16.3 Diffuse large B-cell lymphoma. (**a**) This needle core biopsy shows a dense, diffuse infiltrate of lymphoid cells. (**b**) High power shows closely packed large atypical lymphoid cells

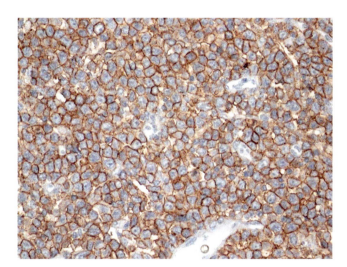

Fig. 16.4 Diffuse large B-cell lymphoma. The tumor is typically positive for the B-cell markers such as CD20

16.3 Extranodal Marginal Zone B-Cell Lymphoma (MALT Lymphoma)

The breast is suggested to be one component of mucosal immunity and may acquire lymphoid tissue from which lymphoma can develop [12]. MALT Lymphoma represents approximately 9% of all primary breast lymphomas [13]. Despite being the second most common variant of primary breast lymphoma, it occurs exceedingly rarely. In the largest multicenter retrospective study (1980–2003), only 24 cases of MALT lymphoma were reported [14].

The most common presentation of MALT lymphoma is an enlarging painless breast mass in an elderly patient. Bilateral presentation is not uncommon. The median age at presentation is 68 years (47–92 years), with a higher female predilection. The lymphomas range from <1 to 20 cm, with a median size of approximately 3 cm. Their histologic features are similar to those of MALT lymphomas in other sites [12–14]. The lymphomas have a vaguely nodular-to-diffuse appearance on low-power microscopic examination (Fig. 16.5a). They are composed of small-to-medium-sized cells with slightly irregular nuclei and a scan-to-abundant quantity of pale cytoplasm (Fig. 16.5b). Bands of sclerosis can also be seen (Fig. 16.5c). Mitotic activity is low, except in residual reactive follicles [15].

Well-formed lymphoepithelial lesions are found less often than in MALT lymphomas involving some other sites. The neoplastic cells are typically CD45+, CD20+, CD5−, CD10−, CD23−, CD43+/−, Bcl2+/−, cyclin D-1− (Fig. 16.6), and cytokeratin cocktail AE1&AE3 negative (Fig. 16.7). The proliferation index is low. The translocation, t(11;18) (q21; q21), is found in most anatomical sites and is seen in nearly 50% of the cases [16].

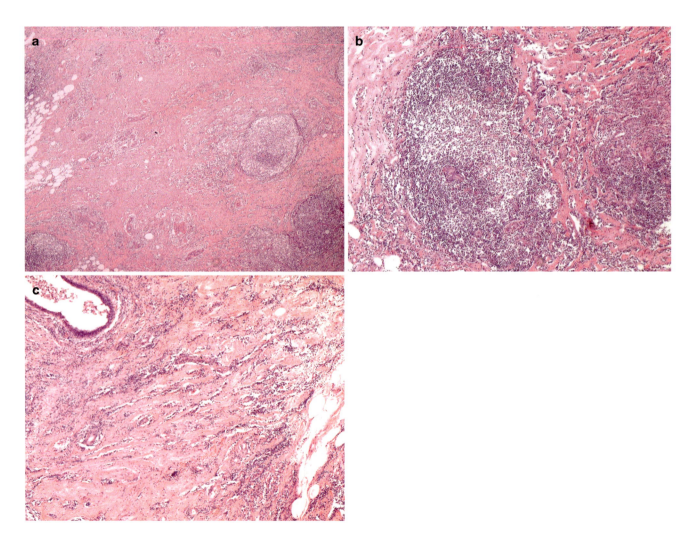

Fig. 16.5 MALT lymphoma. (**a**) On low-power microscopic examination the lymphoma has a vaguely nodular to diffuse appearance. (**b**) Neoplasm has a nodular pattern, cytologically, predominant cell type is small. (**c**) Lymphoid infiltrate and bands of sclerosis

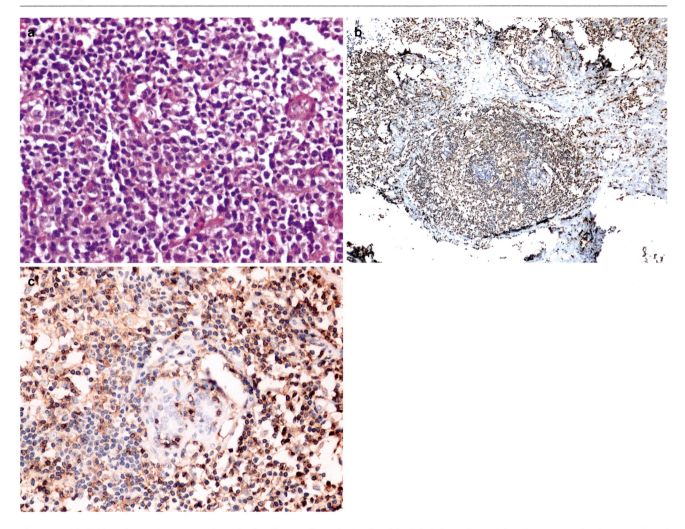

Fig. 16.6 MALT lymphoma. Immunomarkers. (**a**) Small-to medium-sized cells with slightly irregular nuclei and a scant-to-abundant quantity of pale cytoplasm. (**b**) The tumor cells are reactive for CD43. (**c**) Small cells with clear cytoplasm are reactive for CD20

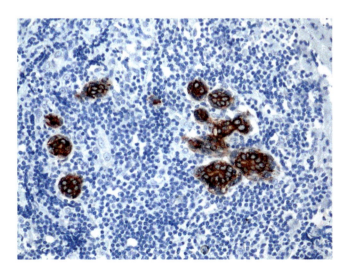

Fig. 16.7 MALT lymphoma. The lymphoma cells are negative for cytokeratin cocktail AE1&AE3. Keratins are preferred markers for identifying carcinomas

16.4 Follicular Lymphoma

Primary follicular lymphoma of the breast (PFLB) is the third most prevalent primary breast lymphoma, preceded by diffuse large B-cell lymphoma and marginal zone lymphoma. Martinelli et al. [14] reported on a multicentered study, 36 cases of PFLB over a period of 23 years. On the other hand, Talwalkar et al. [7] described 106 cases of lymphomas involving the breast; of the 106 lymphomas, 15 were documented as follicular lymphomas.

Patients present with lesions that are unilateral in approximately 95% of the cases, typically unaccompanied by constitutional symptoms. The tumors appear to range from <1 to 9 cm, with a median size of 2–3 cm. Grossly, they can be unifocal or multifocal (Fig. 16.8). Histologic and immunophenotypic features are similar to those of nodal follicular lymphomas, and they might have a nodular or diffuse pattern or growth (Figs. 16.9 and 16.10). Tumors are composed by back-to back neoplastic follicles comprised of centrocytes (small cleaved cells without nucleoli) and centroblast (large noncleaved cells with multiple nucleoli), and lymphoepithelial lesions are generally not seen. Infiltration in collagenous tissue in single-file pattern can mimic invasive lobular carcinoma. Neoplastic follicles are typically CD45+, CD20+,CD10+, CD5−, CD43− and cyclin D1− [17].

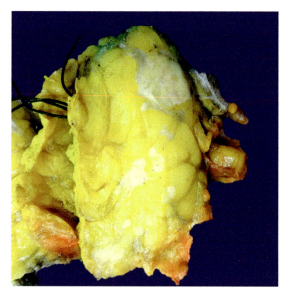

Fig. 16.8 Follicular lymphoma. Gross specimen: this specimen contains multiple lesions. There are several adjacent, but separate irregular masses

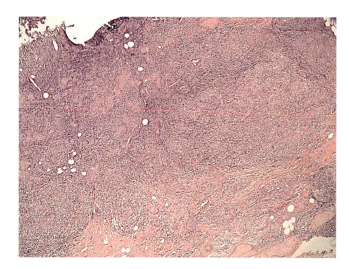

Fig. 16.9 Follicular lymphoma, follicular pattern. A nodular lymphoid infiltrate is present and involves the interlobular and intralobular stroma

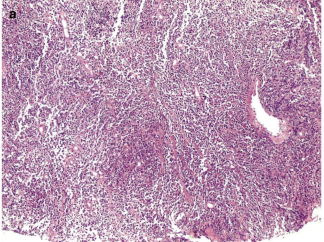
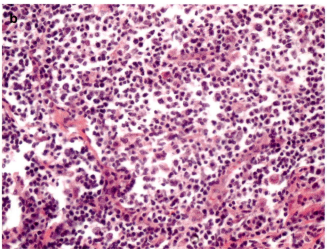

Fig. 16.10 Follicular lymphoma. (**a**) Diffuse pattern. (**b**) High magnification shows lymphomatous infiltrate composed of centrocytes and occasional centroblast in a background of small lymphocytes

16.5 Burkitt Lymphoma

Burkitt lymphoma (BL) of the breast occurs most commonly in endemic BL areas such as malaria-endemic areas including equatorial Africa, Brazil, and Papua New Guinea. Epstein-Barr virus infection is present in almost all patients (>95%). Burkitt lymphoma mainly affects young-to-middle-aged females, some have been pregnant or postpartum at the time of diagnosis, but presentation during puberty is also seen [2, 3, 7]. Patients present with massive bilateral breast swelling, rather than discrete tumor masses, as more often seen in diffuse large B-cell lymphoma (Fig. 16.11). The tumor is composed of sheets of medium-sized cells with basophilic cytoplasm, round, noncleaved nuclei with multiple nucleoli. Numerous tangible-body macrophages produce a "starry-sky" pattern (Fig. 16.12). Pattern-surrounding epithelial elements can closely mimic lymphocytic (diabetic) mastopathy [18].

Burkitt lymphoma also has a characteristic immunophenotype: The neoplastic cells are uniformly CD20+, CD10+, BCl6+, BCL-2−, monotypic surface immunoglobulin (IgM) +, with virtually all cells positive for Ki-67 (Fig. 16.13) [19].

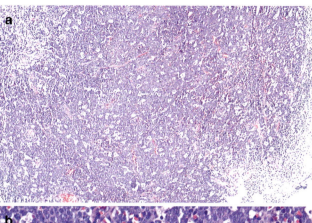
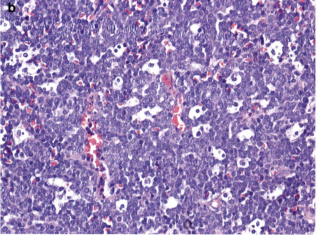

Fig. 16.12 Burkitt Lymphoma. Microscopic features. (**a**, and **b**) The tumor shows starry-sky appearance due to scattered histiocytes among the monotonous proliferation of intermediate-sized transformed lymphoid cells

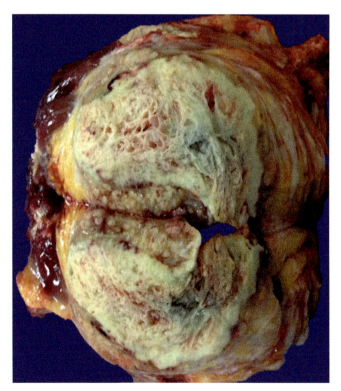

Fig. 16.11 Burkitt lymphoma. Gross appearance: cut section through the breast mass reveals a fleshy solid yellow-colored tumor with necrotic areas

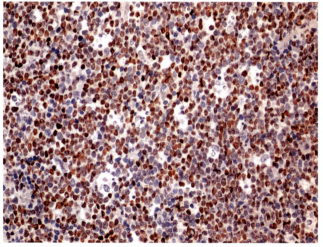

Fig. 16.13 Burkitt lymphoma. Ki-67 immunostain highlights an extremely high proliferation index

16.6 Hodgkin Lymphoma

According to the literature, primary Hodgkin lymphomas of the breast represent one of the rarer entities in the primary breast lymphoma scenario. In 1981 Schouten et al. [20, 21] reported a retrospective review of 13 patients over a 10-year period; two of those patients had primary HL of breast. In 1995 Ariad et al. [22] published a 10-year retrospective review in which they found 16 patients affected by breast lymphoma. Seven patients out of the sixteen fulfilled the criteria for primary breast lymphoma. In this group, one case of primary HL of the breast was found.

Typically, Hodgkin lymphoma involves the breast in the setting of concurrent lymph node involvement, and sometimes widespread disease [23]. Breast involvement is usually unilateral, but occasionally bilateral. As in other sites, Hodgkin lymphoma in the breast shows malignant multinucleated giant Reed-Sternberg (RS) cells within the characteristic reactive cellular background (lymphocytes, histiocytes, eosinophils, plasma cells, and/or neutrophils) (Fig. 16.14a, b). The RS cells are CD30+, CD15+ (Fig. 16.14c), PAX5 dim+, CD20−, CD3−, and ALK1−.

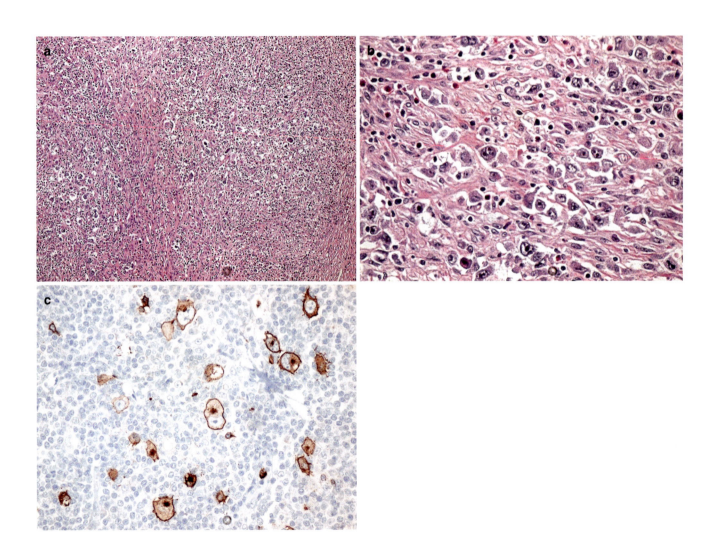

Fig. 16.14 Hodgkin lymphoma. Microscopic examination. (**a**, **b**) Large atypical cells are present in a background of sclerosis with scattered reactive cells. (**c**) Reed-Sternberg cells show intense membranous positivity for CD15

16.7 T-Cell Lymphoma

T-cell lymphomas rarely involve the breast as a primary site, but can secondarily involve the breast as part of disseminated disease. T-cell lymphomas account for only about 2–3% of the cases [24]. In one study the most common types of T-cell lymphoma to involve the breast were anaplastic large cell lymphomas (ALCL), either positive or negative for ALK, in patients with a history of systemic or cutaneous ALCL [12].

16.8 Breast Implant-Associated Anaplastic Large T-Cell Lymphoma

Lymphoma has rarely arisen adjacent to both silicone and saline implants, with cases diagnosed 1–32 years after placement of implant (median: 9 years). Most patients present symptoms usually though to be related to implant, seroma, or infection. Other common presentations include a mass in the fibrous capsule or severe contracture of the fibrous capsule surrounding the implant. The vast majority of lymphomas arising in patients with implants have almost all been ALK-negative anaplastic large cell lymphomas [25].

16.9 Differential Diagnosis of Mammary Lymphoma

Mastitis, such as granulomatous mastitis (Fig. 16.15) can present with clinical and morphologic features that mimic carcinoma or lymphoma. It may have an infectious etiology, reflect a localized manifestation of a systemic disease, or be idiopathic [26].

Lymphocytic mastitis is generally lobulocentric lymphocytic infiltrate associated with a poorly defined area of stromal fibrosis. It is referred to by a variety of designations, including diabetic mastopathy (Fig. 16.16) and fibrous mastopathy [27].

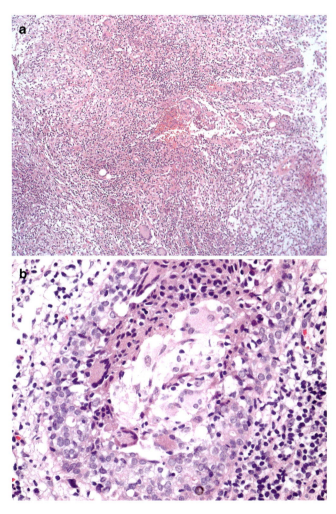

Fig. 16.15 Granulomatous mastitis. (**a**) There is a total granulomatous inflammatory destruction of the ducts. (**b**) A granuloma surrounding a mammary duct

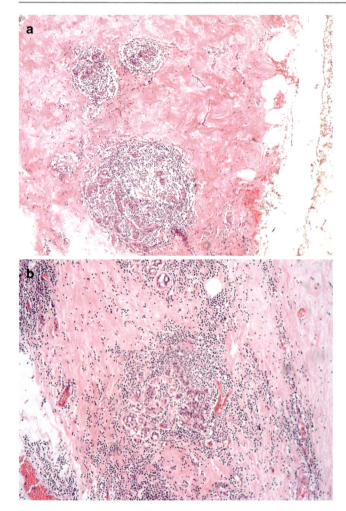

Fig. 16.16 Diabetic mastopathy. (**a**) A lymphocytic infiltrate is noted in the lobules. (**b**) Mature lymphocytes are clustered around a lobule and small blood vessels

16.10 Other Hematopoietic Lesions

Infrequently, the breast is involved by leukemia of either lymphoid or myeloid types. Involvement by chronic lymphocytic leukemia/small lymphocytic lymphoma (Fig. 16.17) may be mistaken for chronic inflammatory cell infiltrates [28].

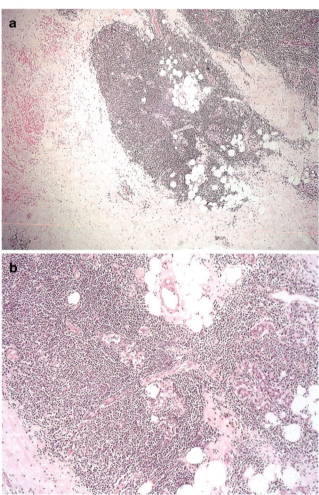

Fig. 16.17 Chronic lymphocytic leukemia involving the breast. (**a**) The tumor shows stromal aggregates of lymphocytes. (**b**) The neoplasia consists of small lymphocytes characteristic of chronic lymphocytic leukemia

16.11   Histiocytic Proliferations

Rosai-Dorfman Disease (RDD), also known as sinus histio-cytosis with massive lymphadenopathy, was characterized as a distinct clinicopathological disorder in 1969 by Rosai and Dorfman [29]. Although the disease has a predilection for the lymph nodes in the head and neck, RDD can also present in any extranodal site. Most patients with RD disease involv-ing the breast are adults, with rare occurrence during adoles-cence. Patients range in age from 15 to 84 years. Histologically, the lesions are multinodular and the pale his-tiocytes are located in the stroma, including in the special-ized stroma of the lobules (Fig. 16.18) [30]. Histiocytes have intracytoplasmic lymphocytes and are positive for S-100 protein (Fig. 16.19).

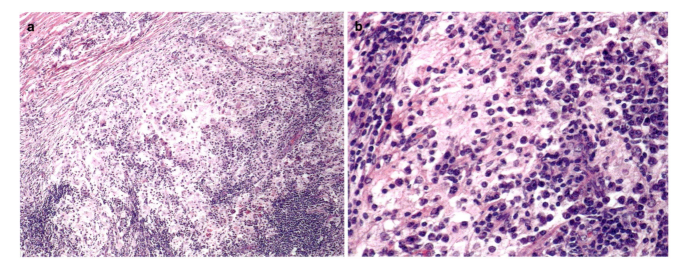

Fig. 16.18   Extranodal Rosai-Dorfman disease. (**a**) Proliferation of histiocytes. (**b**) Plasma cells are sprinkled among the histiocytes

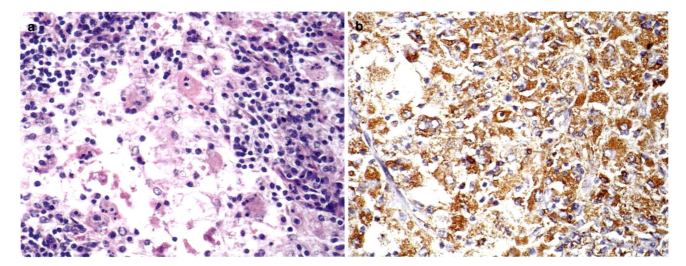

Fig. 16.19   (**a**) Histiocytes with intracytoplasmic lymphocytes. (**b**) Histiocytes showing strong immunoreactivity for the S-100 protein

Hormone receptors, i.e., estrogen receptor (ER) and progesterone receptors (PR), are variably positive in the epithelial cells (approximately 5–25%, moderate-to-strong) of benign breast glands. Myoepithelial cells are invariably ER (−) and PR (−), whereas myofibroblasts are typically ER (+) and PR (+). The proportion and intensity of hormone receptor staining in "normal" breast epithelial cells depend mainly upon the patient's age and menstrual phase. Certain types of breast epithelial cells are relatively more predictable in this regard: columnar cells are almost always strongly and diffusely ER (+) and PR (+),

and apocrine metaplastic cells are almost always ER (−) and PR (−) [8]. Benign and malignant apocrine cells are typically also positive for androgen receptors (AR) [9].

The mammary stroma comprises mainly adipose tissue, myofibroblasts, fibroblasts, and blood vessels. Smooth muscle bundles are present around lactiferous ducts of the nipple and hair follicles of overlying skin. The individual components of the stroma show immunohistochemical reactivities characteristic of each structure (e.g., myofibroblasts are positive for CD34, etc.).

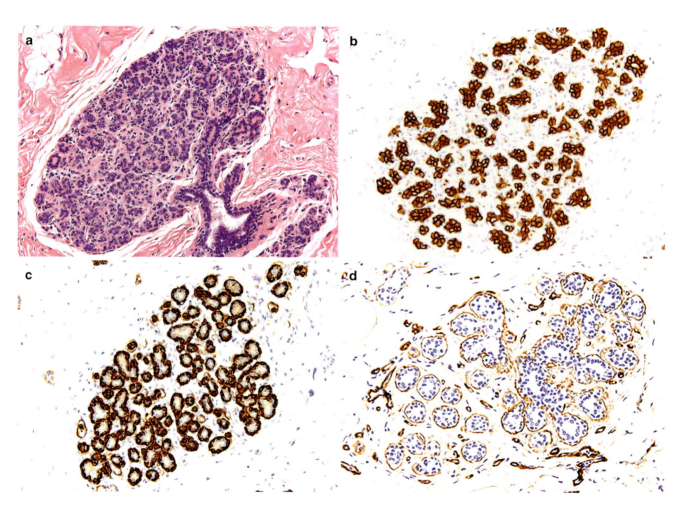

Fig. 17.1 Structure of inactive terminal duct lobular unit (TDLU) of breast. (**a**) This TDLU is from an adult female. Almost all benign glands in the breast have three layers, which may not be evident on routinely stained sections (H&E). (**b**), The luminal layer comprises of a single layer of cytokeratin-positive epithelial cells (CK AE1/AE3). (**c**) The abluminal layer comprises of smooth muscle myosin-positive myoepithelial layer (SMM). (**d**) Below the abluminal myoepithelial layer is the linear basement membrane, which stains for reticulin, collagen IV, and laminin (laminin)

17.1   Usual Ductal Hyperplasia, Atypical Ductal Hyperplasia and Ductal Carcinoma In Situ

The correct interpretation of proliferative epithelial lesions is possibly the most common diagnostic dilemma in everyday pathology practice. Although there are well-established criteria for various degrees of epithelial proliferation (including for usual, florid, and atypical hyperplasia, as well as for low-grade intraductal carcinoma), these criteria can be rather difficult to apply in practice. Immunostains—especially for high molecular weight-cytokeratins (HMW-CK) and estrogen receptors (ER)—can be helpful in this regard. Proliferation marker (i.e., Ki-67) is unhelpful in the differential diagnosis of proliferative epithelial lesions.

HMW-CK (i.e., CK5, CK5/6 and 34BE12/K903), can be regarded as a marker of epithelial "differentiation," and is positive in benign breast epithelium and in UDH. Conversely, atypical ductal hyperplasia (ADH) and ductal carcinoma in situ (DCIS) show "loss of differentiation" and consequently lose reactivity with HMW-CK. HMW-CK positivity is observed in most epithelial cells of florid ductal hyperplasia in a heteroge-neous pattern that is described as "mosaic-like" (Fig. 17.2). Furthermore, florid ductal hyperplasia is usually focally and weakly ER (+). In more than 90% of cases, ADH and low-grade DCIS are strongly and diffusely ER (+) and HMW-CK (−) (Fig. 17.3). ADH and low-grade DCIS cannot be distinguished based on immunoreactivity patterns with HMW-CK and ER—therefore, established histopathological criteria must be used to render the diagnosis [10–12]. High-grade DCIS (including the so-called "basal-like" DCIS) does not usually present a diagnostic problem. HER2 is positive (3+, on a scale of 0–3+) and ER is negative in a large proportion of high-grade DCIS.

HMW-CK immunostaining is *not* helpful in the differential diagnosis of usual ductal hyperplasia (UDH) versus atypical ductal hyperplasia (ADH) in three specific settings: (a) proliferative columnar cell lesions; (b) proliferative apocrine lesions; and (c) some papillary lesions. Furthermore, columnar cell change and columnar cell hyperplasia are almost always strongly ER (+), and nearly all apocrine lesions (including atypical apocrine hyperplasia and apocrine DCIS) are usually ER (−). In these situations, diagnostic evaluation of the lesions on H&E-stained sections must be relied upon.

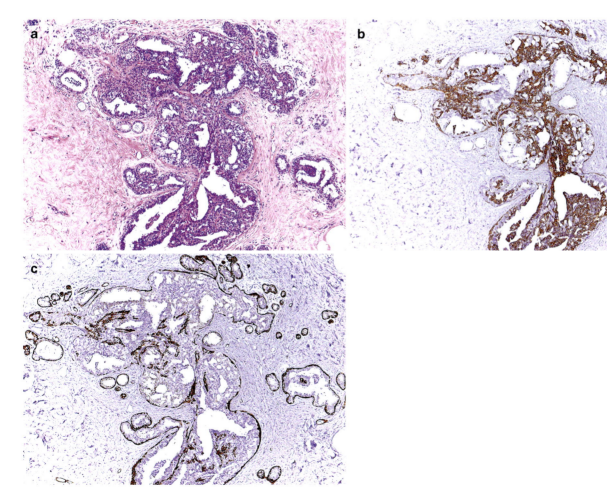

Fig. 17.2 Florid ductal hyperplasia. (**a**) Florid hyperplasia is characterized by exuberant epithelial proliferation (H&E). (**b**) CK 5/6 positivity is observed in some epithelial cells of florid ductal hyperplasia in a heterogeneous pattern that is described as "mosaic-like" (CK 5/6). (**c**) Smooth muscle myosin highlights the presence of myoepithelial cells within and around florid hyperplasia (SMM)

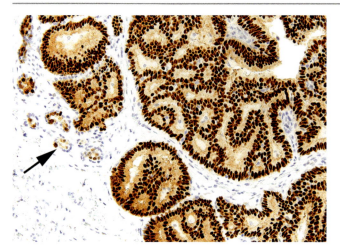

Fig. 17.3 Estrogen receptor (ER) in ductal carcinoma in situ (DCIS). A low-grade DCIS is characterized by strong and diffuse ER-positivity. Note patchy and weaker ER-staining (arrow) in benign glands (ER)

17.2 Lobular Versus Ductal Differentiation of Epithelial Lesions

The distinction between "lobular" and "ductal" carcinomas has clinical implications—especially with regard to differences in anatomical distribution, disease management, risk-stratification, and metastatic pattern. IHC, specifically E-cadherin, can play a vital role in this differential diagnosis. Cadherins (of which E-cadherin is among the best-studied) are a group of transmembrane glycoproteins located in desmosomes, and form complexes with catenins. The latter control several processes including cell migration, differentiation, and proliferation.

E-cadherin is present in benign ductal structures and ductal lesions, and is absent in lobular lesions (Fig. 17.4). Notably, E-cadherin positivity in ductal lesions is present only along the cytoplasmic membrane of the lesional cells. All ductal lesions (including usual ductal hyperplasia, ADH, DCIS, and invasive ductal carcinoma, the latter being called now as invasive carcinoma of NST type) show immunoreactivity with E-cadherin. Lobular lesions (including atypical lobular hyperplasia [ALH], lobular carcinoma in situ [LCIS] and invasive lobular carcinoma) are negative for E-cadherin.

p120 catenin (generally referred to as p120) binds with E-cadherin to form a stable cadherin-catenin complex. This complex is essential for formation of intercellular junctions. Absence of E-cadherin explains the "loss of cohesiveness" in lobular lesions. When E-cadherin is absent, the cytoplasmic pool of p120 increases. It follows that in normal ducts and in ductal lesions, p120 shows cytoplasmic membrane staining, and in lobular lesions with absent or non-functional E-cadherin, p120 localizes within the cytoplasm (Fig. 17.5). Notably, p120 reactivity in ADH and DCIS is similar to that seen with E-cadherin, i.e., positivity is present along the cytoplasmic membrane; and, in lobular lesions, p120 localizes within the cytoplasm—and not along the cytoplasmic membrane. p120 enhances diagnostic accuracy by virtue of being a "positive" stain for lobular carcinoma. Use of E-cadherin and p120 together reduces the rate of equivocal E-cadherin staining [13].

Invasive lobular carcinoma of the classic and pleomorphic types, as well as LCIS of the classic, florid, and pleomorphic types, are all negative for E-cadherin. Rarely, "aberrant" E-cadherin immunoreactivity (i.e., granular "dot-like" cytoplasmic staining) can be encountered in some lobular lesions—particularly in pleomorphic variants of LCIS and invasive lobular carcinoma (Fig. 17.6) [14]. Other immunostains that have been used to distinguish lobular and ductal lesions, with questionable reliability, include beta-catenin (usually negative in lobular lesions) and HMW-CK (usually positive in lobular lesions in a distinctive "perinuclear" pattern). In practice, E-cadherin suffices to establish the diagnosis. p120 immunostain can be additionally evaluated in cases considered equivocal on E-cadherin. Occasionally, invasive ductal carcinoma can display a lobular-like ("single-file") architectural pattern, at least focally. In most such cases, E-cadherin immunostain can unequivocally establish ductal differentiation (Fig. 17.7).

Rarely, LCIS can coexist with collagenous spherulosis; the resultant lesion can simulate cribriform type of intraductal carcinoma. E-cadherin immunostain can be particularly helpful in this regard [15].

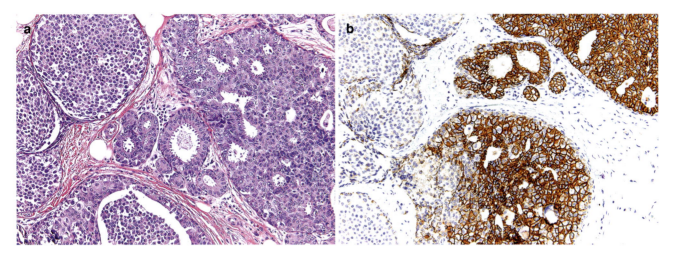

Fig. 17.4 Use of E-cadherin in diagnosing lobular carcinoma in situ (LCIS) and ductal carcinoma in situ (DCIS). (**a**) LCIS is evident on the left, and DCIS is seen on the right (H&E). (**b**) E-cadherin is negative in LCIS and positive in DCIS (E-cadherin)

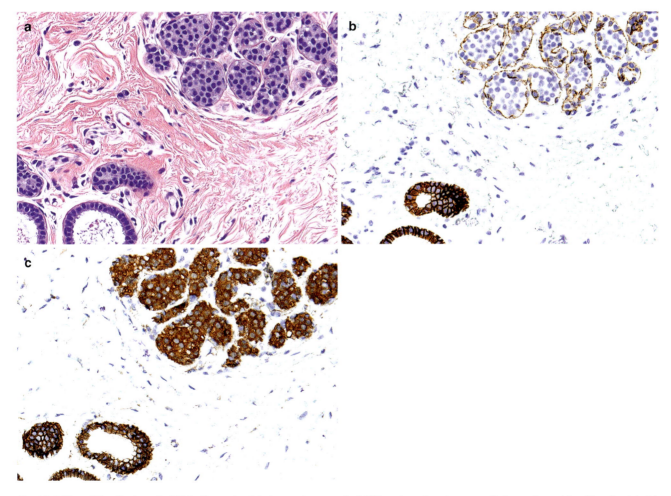

Fig. 17.5 Use of E-cadherin and p120 in diagnosing lobular carcinoma in situ (LCIS). (**a**) LCIS of classic type is seen on upper-right, columnar cell change is present on lower-left (H&E). (**b**) E-cadherin is negative in LCIS, and cystic columnar cell change is positive (E-cadherin). (**c**) p120 is seen to localize within the cytoplasm of LCIS cells, and is positive along the cytoplasmic membrane of columnar cell change (p120)

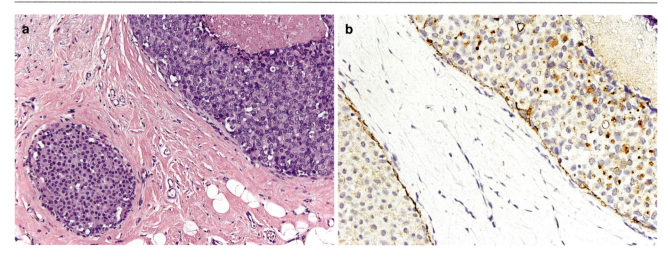

Fig. 17.6 E-cadherin staining in pleomorphic and classic types of lobular carcinoma in situ (LCIS). (**a**) LCIS of pleomorphic type (with "pleomorphic" high-grade nuclei) is seen on upper right, LCIS of classic type is present on lower left (H&E). (**b**) E-cadherin is negative in classic LCIS, and shows "aberrant" E-cadherin immunoreactivity (i.e., granular "dot-like" cytoplasmic staining) in pleomorphic LCIS (E-cadherin)

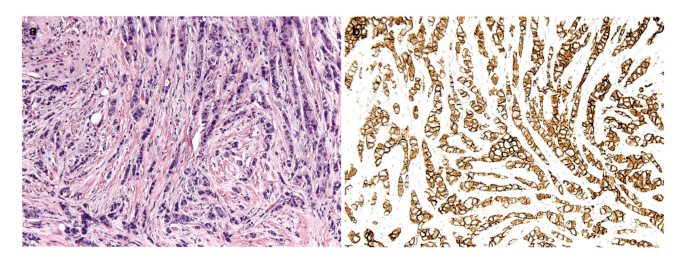

Fig. 17.7 E-cadherin staining in invasive ductal carcinoma. (**a**) Invasive ductal carcinoma with lobular-like ("single-file") architectural pattern (H&E). (**b**) E-cadherin shows positivity in the malignant cells—unequivocally establishing ductal differentiation thereof (E-cadherin)

17.3 Papillary Neoplasms

Immunostains can be helpful in the assessment of some, but not all, papillary lesions of the breast. It must be emphasized that the histological and cytological appearance of papillary lesions on H&E-stained sections is paramount to the diagnosis [16, 17].

Myoepithelial cells typically line fibrovascular stalks (papillae) within benign intraductal papilloma, and also line the perimeter (wall) of an intraductal papilloma. Myoepithelial cells can be diminished or absent in the papillae and/or in the walls of various types of papillary carcinomas. On this premise, IHC for myoepithelial cells (i.e., actin, CD10, calponin, myosin, p40, p63, etc.) are helpful in the evaluation of such lesions. Combination of IHC stains, such as p63 and myosin (in a dual stain, which combines nuclear and cytoplasmic reactivity within the myoepithelial cells) is helpful in demonstrating myoepithelial cells; and the addition of a cytokeratin immunostain to this combination (in a triple stain) can be even more helpful by highlighting the juxtaposition of epithelial and myoepithelial cells within a papillary lesion.

The two fundamental questions to be answered in the assessment of any papillary lesion are (a) Is carcinoma present? and (b) Is invasive carcinoma present?

Myoepithelial cells are uniformly present within the papillae and along the wall of all **benign intraductal papilloma** (Fig. 17.8). In benign papillomas, ER is only sporadically positive. HMW-CK can show a "mosaic-like" staining pattern in the hyperplastic epithelial cells of a benign papilloma.

In an **atypical papilloma**, there is focal ADH within the papilloma. The criteria for diagnosing ADH within a papilloma should be the same within a papilloma as outside it. The myoepithelial cells are usually diminished within the ADH portion of a papilloma, and are present all around the wall of the papilloma.

The criteria for diagnosing **focal DCIS within a papilloma** should be the same within a papilloma as outside of it. The myoepithelial cells are usually absent in the DCIS portion of a papilloma, but are present all around the perimeter (wall) of the papilloma.

Intraductal papillary carcinoma (i.e., papillary DCIS) can be diagnosed when the entire lesion is considered cytologically and histologically malignant, and there is no evidence of invasive carcinoma. The architectural pattern of the DCIS is usually entirely papillary, and sometimes there is a secondary cribriform growth pattern therein. The myoepithelial cells are typically present around the wall of the intraductal papillary carcinoma (Fig. 17.9).

Encysted, encapsulated, intracystic, and solid-papillary carcinomas are all circumscribed papillary carcinomas that usually (but not always) lack myoepithelial cells within the lesion, i.e., in the papillae, and may or may not lack myoepithelial cells in the wall, i.e., at the perimeter. In the absence of frankly invasive carcinoma, these carcinomas behave in an indolent manner. Encysted/encapsulated/intracystic and solid-papillary are terms that essentially imply *non-invasive papillary carcinoma*, and these terms have been used sometimes synonymously and occasionally interchangeably, although some differences have been described between these entities [18, 19]. Cyst formation is prominent in encysted/encapsulated/intracystic papillary lesions, and solid-papillary lesions are characterized by relatively "solid" epithelial proliferation. Often, the only clue to the solid-papillary nature of the lesion is the subtle presence of fibrovascular cores therein. Myoepithelial cells are usually absent within and around the perimeter of these lesions; however, occasionally rare myoepithelial cells can be identified on IHC (in either location). Neuroendocrine differentiation (as evidenced by CD56, chromogranin and synaptophysin immunoreactivity) can be encountered in approximately one-half of solid-papillary carcinomas of the breast.

In sum, myoepithelial cells can be demonstrated to be present around the perimeter of intraductal papilloma, atypical papilloma, papilloma with DCIS, and papillary DCIS. Myoepithelial immunostains show little or no reactivity within and around the perimeter of encysted/encapsulated/intracystic and solid-papillary carcinomas (Fig. 17.10).

The assessment of invasion in papillary carcinomas can be difficult. In general, non-invasive papillary carcinomas have smooth and rounded outer contours, and invasive papillary carcinomas have irregular and jagged outer contours (Fig. 17.11). There may be some degree of stromal reaction around some foci of invasive papillary carcinomas. As outlined above, the absence of myoepithelial cells at the perimeter of papillary carcinomas, as evidenced by IHC, cannot be regarded *per se* as being diagnostic of invasive carcinoma.

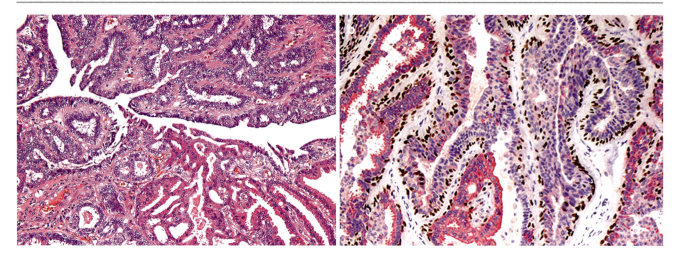

Fig. 17.8 Intraductal papilloma. (**a**) The lesion is characterized by relatively thick fibrovascular cores lined by bland epithelial cells, some of which exhibit apocrine metaplastic cells (H&E). (**b**) Myoepithelial cells are decorated by p63 immunostain (cells with brown staining nuclei) and epithelial cells are stained by cytokeratin immunostain (cells with red-staining cytoplasm); (p63 + CK AE1/AE3 double stain)

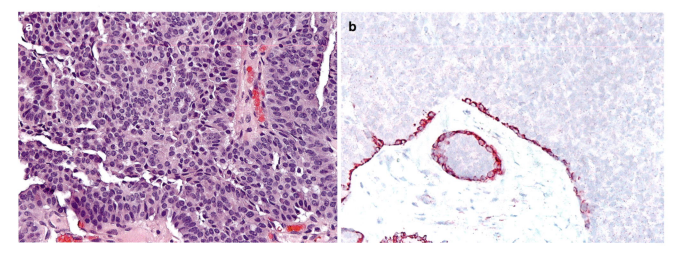

Fig. 17.9 Intraductal papillary carcinoma. (**a**) Intraductal papillary carcinoma (i.e., papillary DCIS) can be diagnosed when the entire lesion is considered cytologically and histologically malignant, and there is no evidence of invasive carcinoma. (**b**) Myoepithelial cells are present around the wall of the intraductal papillary carcinoma (Myosin)

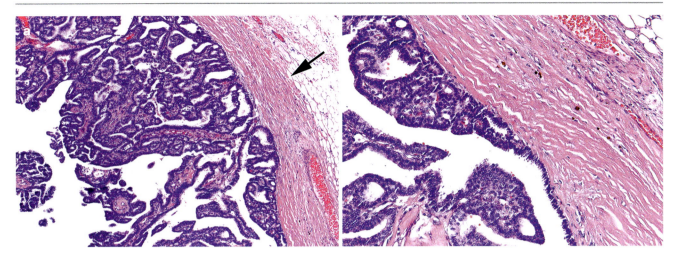

Fig. 17.10 Encapsulated papillary carcinoma. (**a**) The thick "capsule" is present around the papillary carcinoma (arrow). Immunostains for myo-epithelial cells were negative (not shown) within and around the perimeter of these lesions. (**b**) Detail of the "capsule"

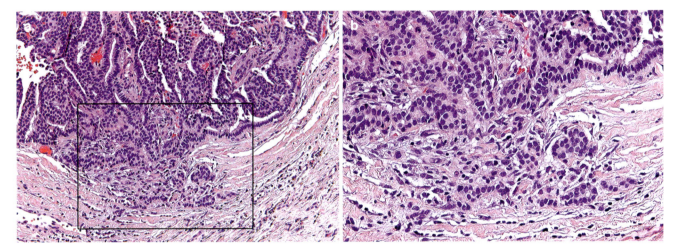

Fig. 17.11 Microinvasive papillary carcinoma. (**a**) The microinvasive papillary carcinoma has irregular and jagged outer contours (box). Non-invasive papillary carcinomas have smooth and rounded outer contours. (**b**) Detail of microinvasive carcinoma

17.4   Sclerosing Lesions

Because of its infiltrative appearance, sclerosing adenosis has a likelihood of being misdiagnosed as invasive carcinoma. The most important diagnostic feature of sclerosing adenosis is that retains a round configuration at low-power magnification. The lesion is more cellular centrally than peripherally, and the glands at the perimeter are dilated relative to those at the center; thus, the lesion has an appearance of a "pinwheel". Histologically, the proliferating glands are lined by two cell types: epithelial and myoepithelial. Occasionally, one component or the other may predominate. Rarely, the myoepithelial cell may show "myoid" or clear change. When the epithelial cells within sclerosing adenosis show apocrine change, the lesion can be referred to as apocrine adenosis. The participation of epithelial cells can be highlighted by cytokeratin immunostains, and that of myoepithelial cells can be demonstrated *via* myoepithelial cells—although the latter may appear to be absent in the center of sclerosing adenosis [20]. Most myoepithelial markers (*except* p63 and p40, both of which are nuclear markers) are immunoreactive in those vascular walls that have smooth muscle and should not be mistaken for myoepithelial cell staining.

Other sclerotic lesions that can display a pseudoinfiltrative appearance include radial scar, sclerosing papilloma, florid papillomatosis of nipple ("nipple adenoma"), and subareolar sclerosing ductal hyperplasia [21]. These lesions can be evaluated by myoepithelial stains if there is any suspicion for invasive carcinoma on H&E-stained slides (Fig. 17.12).

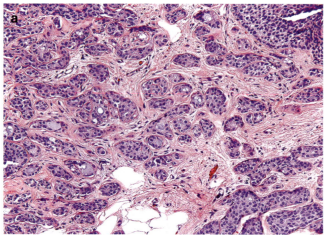
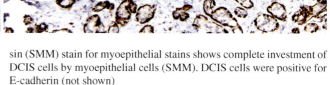

Fig. 17.12 Sclerosing adenosis associated with ductal carcinoma in situ (DCIS). (**a**) Sclerosing adenosis displays a pseudoinfiltrative appearance. Note uniform epithelial cells of DCIS, with intermediate-grade nuclei, inhabiting sclerosing adenosis. (**b**) Smooth muscle myosin (SMM) stain for myoepithelial stains shows complete investment of DCIS cells by myoepithelial cells (SMM). DCIS cells were positive for E-cadherin (not shown)

17.5 Paget Disease of Nipple

The diagnosis of Paget disease of nipple (PDN) may not need immunohistochemical confirmation in cases in which the histopathological features thereof are overt and clinical features (i.e., eczema-like appearance with discolored, oozing, or encrusted nipple or areola) are supportive. However, immunohistochemical confirmation is desirable whenever the diagnosis of PDN is equivocal on routine H&E examination. The majority of PDN cases show the following profile: the neoplastic Paget cells are CK7 (+) and HER2 (+) (Fig. 17.13). Immunoreactivity for ER, PR, GATA3, CEA, and GCDFP15 cannot be relied upon to establish the diagnosis of PDN [22, 23].

Two extremely rare malignancies that involve the nipple may be considered in the differential diagnosis of PDN: Bowen disease (squamous cell carcinoma in situ of skin) and melanoma. Bowen disease is CK7 (−) and p63 (+), and melanomas are CK (−), HMB45 (+), MelanA (+), and MITF1 (+). Toker cells are often included in the differential diagnosis of PDN; however, these cells are cytologically bland, with clear cytoplasm and inconspicuous nucleoli. Toker cells, present in 10% of normal nipples, are typically CK7 (+) and HER2 (−). Rarely, these cells can be relatively large and bear atypical-appearing nuclei [24].

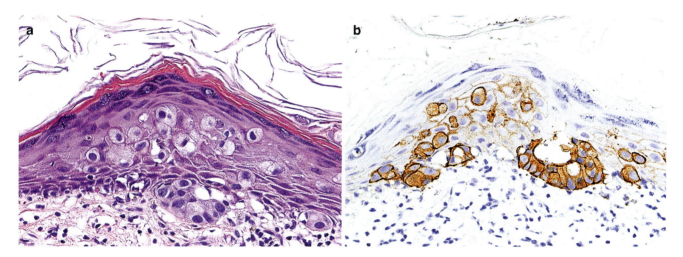

Fig. 17.13 Paget disease of nipple (PDN). (**a**) The intraepidermal carcinoma cells of PDN show marked cytological atypia. (**b**) PDN cells show strong immunoreactivity with HER2 (Hercept)

17.6   Assessment of Invasion

Myoepithelial cells and basement membrane components (i.e., laminin and collagen IV) show a continuously linear pattern of immunoreactivity around benign sclerosing lesions and in non-invasive carcinomas, and are absent around invasive carcinomas (Figs. 17.14, 17.15, and 17.16). Myoepithelial cells can be absent around microglandular adenosis (MGA), and also around some rare apocrine glands. Notably, approximately 5% of DCIS, particularly those of the papillary type, lack myoepithelial cells—at least as these can be demonstrated by immunostains.

Cross-reactivity of SMA and some other myoepithelial markers with myofibroblasts makes identification of myoepithelial cells difficult in some cases of DCIS—especially in cases with marked periductal stromal desmoplasia. Table 17.1 shows the presence and degree of immunohistochemical cross-reactivity of various myoepithelial markers with myofibroblasts and blood vessels.

p63 is a nuclear stain, and it results in apparent "gaps" in myoepithelial cell immunoreactivity. Thus, in the context of DCIS, any nuclear staining around nests of carcinoma should be interpreted as evidence of myoepithelial cell presence. p63 can also be immunoreactive in poorly-differentiated carcinoma.

Microinvasive lobular carcinoma can be particularly difficult to diagnose because often there is minimal stromal reaction (Fig. 17.17). Furthermore, the finding of a few bland microinvasive lobular carcinoma cells amid stromal fibrosis can be particularly subtle, and these cells can be highlighted by cytokeratin immunostain [25].

CK AE1/AE3 immunostain is useful in assessing the *extent* of invasion—particularly in invasive lobular carcinoma (Fig. 17.18). The malignant cells of the latter bear low-grade nuclei that blend imperceptibly amid stromal cells and lymphocytes, and can be difficult to ascertain on H&E-stained histological sections. CK can be especially helpful in detecting invasive carcinoma status-post chemotherapy, and in unequivocal assessment of margins.

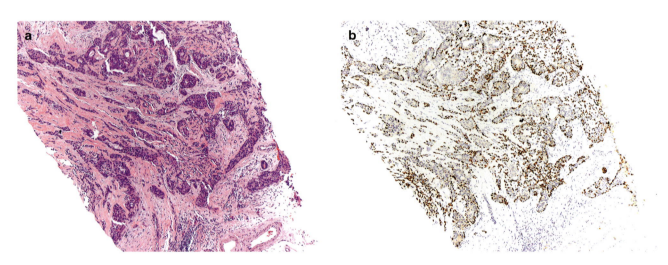

Fig. 17.14 Complex sclerosing papillary lesion. (**a**) Complex sclerosing lesion displays a pseudoinfiltrative appearance. (**b**) Myoepithelial cells show a continuously linear pattern of immunoreactivity with smooth muscle myosin around the sclerosing lesions (SMM)

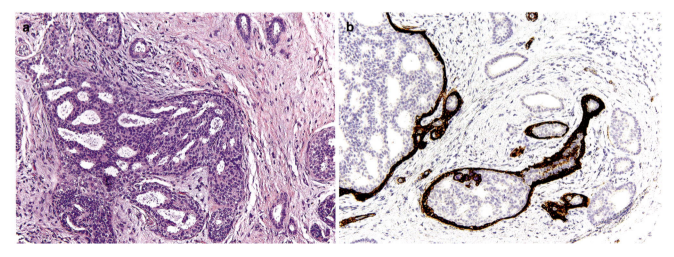

Fig. 17.15 Ductal carcinoma in situ (DCIS) and invasive ductal carcinoma. (**a**) DCIS of cribriform type is associated with invasive ductal carcinoma. (**b**) DCIS shows smooth muscle myosin-positive myoepithelial cells, and absence thereof around invasive carcinoma (SMM)

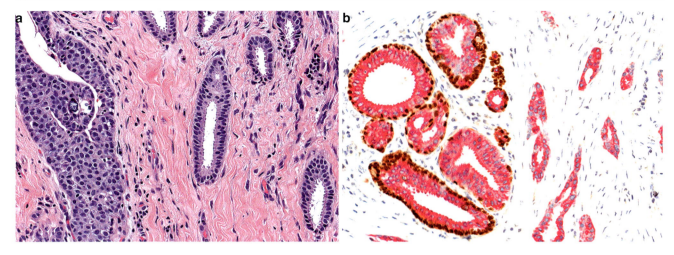

Fig. 17.16 Ductal carcinoma in situ and invasive ductal carcinoma. (**a**) DCIS of cribriform type is associated with invasive ductal carcinoma. (**b**) DCIS shows positivity of myoepithelial cells on combined smooth muscle myosin (SMM) and p63 stain. The malignant epithelial cells show red cytokeratin-positivity, SMM stain shows brown cytoplasmic staining, and p63 shows brown nuclear staining, of myoepithelial cells. No staining of myoepithelial cells is observed around invasive carcinoma (combined cytokeratin+SMM + p63 stain)

Table 17.1 Myoepithelial immunohistochemical stains and cross-reactivity thereof with various other types of cells

	Reactivity in myoepithelial cells	Localization in myoepithelial cells	Reactivity in myofibroblasts	Reactivity in blood vessel walls	Reactivity in epithelial cells
Calponin	++	Cytoplasmic	Uncommon	+	−
CD10	++	Cytoplasmic	Uncommon	+	−
S100p	+	Cytoplasmic	Variable	−	+/−
SMA	++	Cytoplasmic	++	++	−
SMM-HC	++	Cytoplasmic	Uncommon	+	−
p40	++	Nuclear	−	−	−[a]
p63	++	Nuclear	−	−	−[a]

SMA smooth muscle actin, *SMM-HC* smooth muscle myosin-heavy chain
[a]May be positive in rare high-grade carcinoma cells

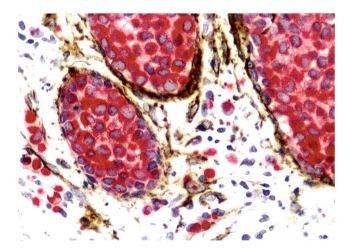

Fig. 17.17 Microinvasive lobular carcinoma. Myoepithelial cells around the in situ carcinoma are decorated by smooth muscle actin (SMA, brown) immunostain, and the malignant epithelial cells are stained by cytokeratin (CK AE1/AE3, red). (SMA + AE1/AE3 double stain). The microinvasive and in situ carcinoma cells were not negative for E-cadherin (not shown)

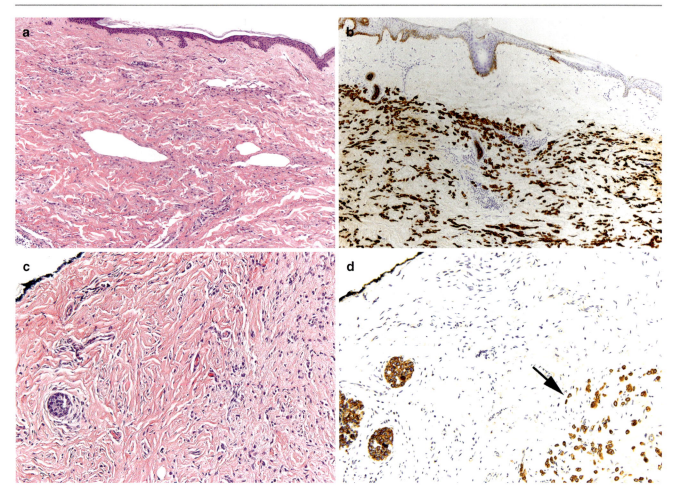

Fig. 17.18 Cytokeratin highlights invasive lobular carcinoma. (**a**, **b**) Dermal invasion by invasive lobular carcinoma (**a**) is highlighted by CK AE1/AE3 immunostain (**b**, CK AE1/AE3). (**c**, **d**) Subtle invasive lobu- lar carcinoma in breast tissue (**c**) is highlighted by CK AE1/AE3 immu- nostain (arrow). Margin-negativity is confirmed by CK AE1/AE3 stain in this case (**d**, CK AE1/AE3)

17.7   Spindle Cell Lesions

Spindle cell lesions of the breast include a wide variety of benign, borderline, and malignant lesions. The benign lesions include scars, pseudoangiomatous stromal hyperplasia (PASH), myofibroblastoma, and benign phyllodes tumor. The malignant lesions include metaplastic spindle cell sarcoma and malignant phyllodes tumor. Borderline malignant spindle cell lesions include borderline phyllodes tumors and fibromatosis. Immunostains can be helpful in the differential diagnosis; however, the key to diagnosis is the correct interpretation of H&E-stained sections [26].

Spindle cell metaplastic carcinoma is almost always immunoreactive (at least focally) with p63, p40, and one of various cytokeratins—especially HMW-CK (Fig. 17.19). A panel of cytokeratins (e.g., CK-K903, Cam 5.2, MNF116, AE1/AE3) should be used, as the tumor can be focally reactive with all or any one of these. Rarely, p63 and cytokeratin can be immunoreactive in some phyllodes tumors and mammary sarcomas. Spindle cell metaplastic carcinoma can also be immunoreactive for SMA, and are negative for CD34, BCL-2, ER, PR, and HER2. It should be remembered that approximately 30% of metaplastic spindle cell carcinomas are positive for beta-catenin; and that spindle cell metaplastic carcinoma can appear to be cytologically as well as architecturally bland, and appear to be "fibromatosis-like."

The stromal cells of phyllodes tumors are variably positive for CD34, BCL-2, actin, and desmin. Immunostain for proliferation marker Ki-67 is unhelpful in grading of fibroepithelial tumors—owing to tumoral

heterogeneity. BCL-2 reactivity is typical of low-grade phyllodes tumor. Malignant phyllodes tumors can be negative for CD34, and can be rarely positive for p40, p63 and HMW-CK [27, 28]. Rarely malignant phyllodes tumors can show focal nuclear staining with beta-catenin—a point worth remembering in the differential diagnosis of fibromatosis. Most cases of mammary fibromatosis are immunoreactive for *nuclear* localization of beta-catenin and for *cytoplasmic* localization of SMA; and are non-reactive for cytokeratins, p63, S100p, CD31, CD34 and ER (Fig. 17.20). Myofibroblastomas and PASH (both being myofibroblastic) are reactive for CD34, desmin, actin, BCL-2, CD99, ER, and PR (Fig. 17.21). The H&E appearance and ER-immunoreactivity of myofibroblastoma can lead to the mistaken diagnosis of invasive lobular carcinoma [29].

p63, a homologue of the tumor suppressor protein p53, is a popular immunostain used in the breast (and in other organs) for the detection of myoepithelial cells. p63 is also useful to detect "myoepithelial" differentiation in metaplastic spindle carcinoma and as a marker of squamous differentiation in low-grade adenosquamous carcinoma. p63 shows nuclear reactivity in the constituent peripheral squamous epithelial cells of cell clusters in low-grade adenosquamous carcinoma (LGASC)—and can possibly lead to its erroneous interpretation as a benign sclerotic lesion with squamous metaplasia (Fig. 17.22). A p40 antibody directed against an N-terminal truncated form of the p63 protein is essentially similar to p63 in its immunoreactivity pattern. Rarely, p63 and p40 may focally stain rare high-grade carcinoma cells.

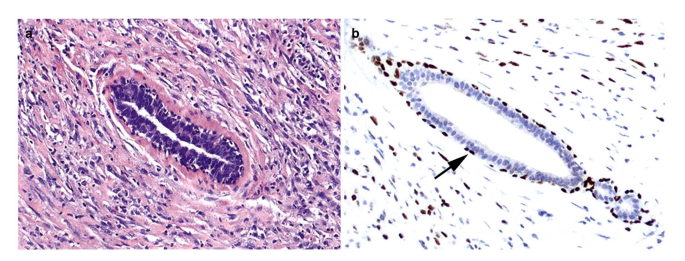

Fig. 17.19 Spindle cell metaplastic carcinoma. (**a**) Spindle cell metaplastic carcinoma infiltrating around a benign duct. (**b**) The metaplastic carcinoma cells are immunoreactive with p63. Note staining of normal myoepithelial cell nuclei of the normal duct by p63 (arrow) (p63)

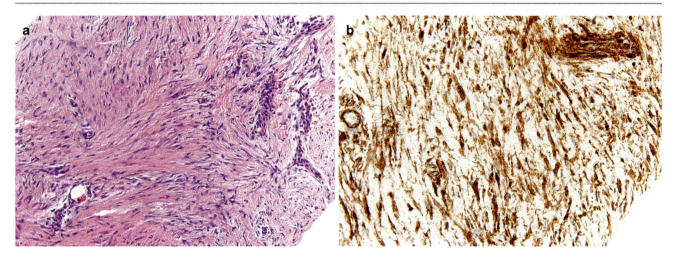

Fig. 17.20 Mammary fibromatosis. (**a**) The typical broad fascicles of "wavy" spindle cells characterize mammary fibromatosis. (**b**) The lesional cells of fibromatosis show nuclear and cytoplasmic staining with beta-catenin (Beta-catenin)

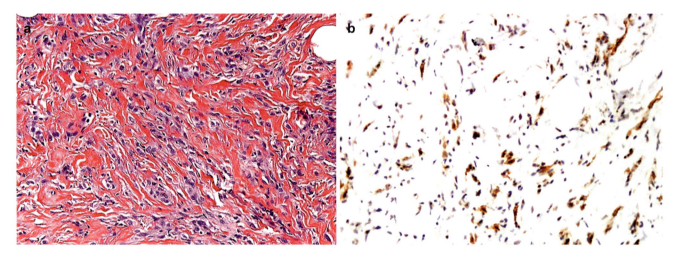

Fig. 17.21 Myofibroblastoma. (**a**) Dense bundles of bland spindle cells lie amid dense collagenous stroma. (**b**) The lesional cells of myofibroblastoma show cytoplasmic staining with CD34 (CD34)

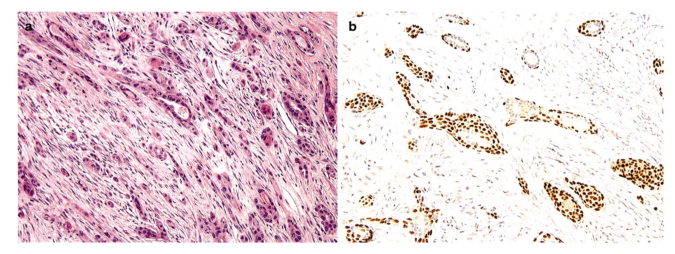

Fig. 17.22 Low-grade adenosquamous carcinoma (LGASC). (**a**) The typical combined "adeno" and "squamous" components of LGASC are evident. (**b**) The neoplastic cells of LGASC show p63-reactivity in the neoplastic squamous cells as well as in some of neoplastic stromal cells. This pattern of p63 staining can lead to erroneous interpretation of LGASC as a benign sclerotic lesion with squamous metaplasia (p63)

17.8   Lymphovascular Channel Involvement

The finding of lymphovascular invasion (LVI) by tumor cells has prognostic significance; however, this important finding can be simulated by tissue retraction. The latter can occur around clusters of in situ or invasive carcinoma in formalin-fixed paraffin-embedded sections [30].

The finding of LVI can be confirmed by adhering to the following criteria: (a) the focus of LVI should be outside the edge of the carcinoma; (b) the tumor emboli should not exactly conform to the space in which they lie; (c) the space should be lined by endothelial cells; and (d) the space is usually accompanied by an artery and vein in its immediate vicinity [31]. The presence of endothelial cells can be confirmed by the use a panel of endothelial markers (e.g., CD31 and D2–40). Lymphovascular endothelia are immunoreactive for CD31, D2–40, ERG, FL1, WT1, and Factor VIII (Fig. 17.23). D2–40 is thought to be specific and sensitive for lymphatic endothelia, and CD31 for vascular endothelia [32]. Notably, D2–40 can be faintly immunoreactive (in a "smudged" pattern) in myoepithelial cells [33].

LVI by tumor cells can also be simulated by artefactual displacement of cells following a needling procedure. In these cases, the artefactual displacement of tumor cell clusters usually appears to be displaced in a linear manner amid granulation tissue along the healing biopsy tract—often accompanied by myoepithelial cells.

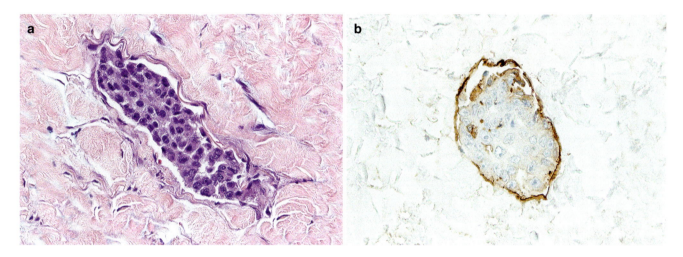

Fig. 17.23 Lymphovascular involvement (LVI) by tumor cells. (**a**) This focus is suspicious for LVI. (**b**) The presence of endothelial cells around the carcinoma cells can be confirmed by the use of CD31 (shown here), D2–40, ERG, FL1, WT1 and Factor VIII (CD31)

17.9   Sentinel Lymph Node

The pathological evaluation of sentinel lymph nodes (SLN) in almost all cases of invasive carcinomas is the standard of care [34, 35]. The SLN should be serially sectioned at 2 mm intervals, and entirely submitted for histopathologial evaluation. H&E-stained sections should be carefully evaluated, and any "suspicious" finding should be further assessed *via* a cytokeratin AE1/3 immunostain (Fig. 17.24). Low molecular weight-cytokeratin (i.e., Cam 5.2) can stain dendritic reticular cells within the lymph node.

Although immunohistochemical staining by cytokeratin is not recommended in the routine processing of SLN examination, a cytokeratin immunostain can be employed in cases of invasive *lobular* carcinoma as even relatively large metastatic tumor aggregates may be missed on H&E examination alone. Furthermore, certain histological findings (e.g., histiocytes, endosalpingiosis, megakaryocytes, etc.) can simulate metastatic carcinoma in SLNs [36–39]. In particular, nevus cell aggregates (positive for S-100 protein and A103/MART1) can be mistaken for micrometastatic carcinoma (Fig. 17.25). In such cases, immunohistochemical confirmation with an *appropriate* immunostain (e.g., CD68 for histocytes) is desirable [40, 41].

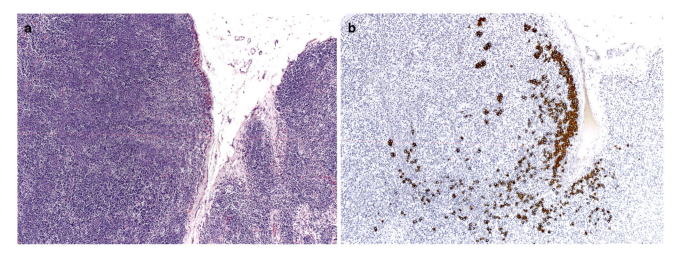

Fig. 17.24 Sentinel lymph node (SLN) with metastatic lobular carcinoma. (**a**) This SLN appears "negative" on H&E. (**b**) CK AE1/AE3 staining of SLN shows more than 200 immunoreactive cells—confirmatory of micrometastasis (CK AE1/AE3)

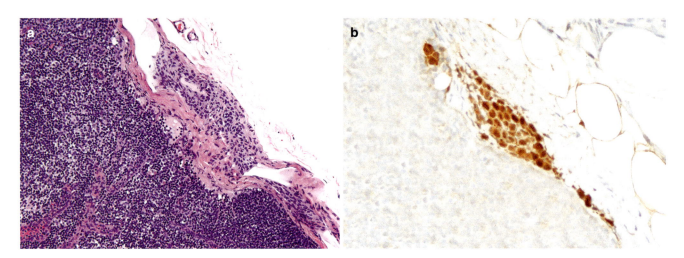

Fig. 17.25 Nevus cell aggregate (NCA) in sentinel lymph node. (**a**) This example of NCA simulates metastatic carcinoma cells. (**b**) S100 protein immunostain can be diagnostic in this regard (S100)

17.10 Metastatic Malignancies

Metastatic neoplasms to the breast can be mistaken, clinically and pathologically, for primary neoplasms [42, 43]. Unless there is a clinical history of another primary neoplasm, the pathologist may not even consider metastatic malignancy in the differential diagnosis.

Most primary breast carcinomas display the following immunoprofile: CK7 (+), GATA3 (+), GCDFP15 (+), mammoglabin (+), ER (+), CK20 (−), TTF1 (−). PAX8 (−), Wilms' tumor protein 1, and WT1 (−). GCDFP-15 is the most specific marker of breast carcinoma, and mammoglobin is a more sensitive marker of breast carcinoma than GCDFP-15; however, GCDFP15 and mammoglobin can be non-reactive in approximately one-quarter of breast carcinomas. Hormone receptors can be present in endometrial, ovarian, and lung primaries. Mammoglobin can also be positive in endometrial carcinomas. GATA3 is reactive in most breast carcinomas (except in about one-third of "triple-negative" carcinomas) [44].

The most common metastatic neoplasms to the breast include lung and melanoma. In most cases, TTF-1 can confirm a primary lung carcinoma. Melanoma markers are negative in breast carcinoma; however, S100 protein can be positive.

Occasionally breast carcinomas need to be distinguished from Mullerian carcinomas (Fig. 17.26). Both groups of carcinomas are CK7 (+) and CK20 (−). However, breast carcinomas are characteristically GATA3 (+), PAX8 (−), and WT-1 (−), and most Mullerian carcinomas are GATA3 (−), PAX8 (+), and WT-1 (+). WT1 can be immunoreactive in some forms of invasive mucinous carcinoma of the breast.

In a metastatic setting, it may be difficult to differentiate between breast, skin, and salivary gland primaries. It is noteworthy that these tumors can show rather similar immunohistochemical results. GCDFP-15 is generally negative in sweat gland carcinomas, CEA is negative in breast carcinomas, and ER is usually negative in salivary gland carcinoma.

In general, a panel of antibodies ought to be used in the workup of metastatic tumors to the breast. Immunohistochemistry can play a role in establishing a non-mammary primary. Reliance on a single antibody to establish any diagnoses (e.g., ER to establish a breast primary) can be misleading.

Malignant lymphoma can involve the breast, usually as part of systemic involvement, and rarely primary—either *de novo* or in association with an implant [45].

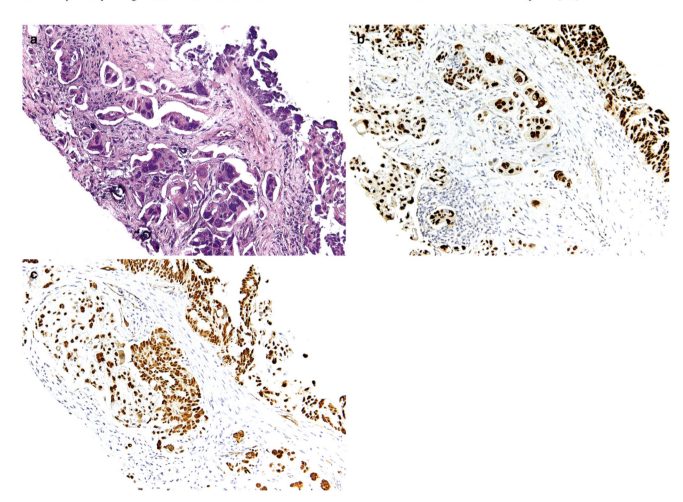

Fig. 17.26 Metastatic Mullerian carcinoma to the breast. (**a**) Note micropapillary architecture of the tumor, "hobnail" appearance of the individual tumor cells, and presence of psammomatous-type calcification. (**b**) This Mullerian carcinoma was positive for both WT1 and PAX8, and negative for GATA3 (PAX8)

17.11 Hormone Receptors and HER2

In the context of oncological pathology, prognostic factors must be differentiated from predictive factors. A prognostic factor is a measure that correlates with disease-free or overall survival in the absence of systemic therapy and is, thus, able to correlate with the natural history of a particular malignancy (e.g., size of invasive carcinoma). A predictive factor is a measure that is associated with response to a given therapy (e.g., HER2). Some factors, such as ER and HER2, should be regarded as both prognostic and predictive (Fig. 17.27). Only the most significant aspects of hormone receptor and HER2 testing via immunostaining are discussed in this section.

Approximately 80% of invasive breast carcinomas are ER (+), and an ER (−) rate of more than 30% in a particular laboratory may be indicative of a technical problem with the assay. In general, PR-positivity parallels ER-positivity. Adequate tissue fixation, appropriate selection of tissue block, and optimal use of control are necessary to obtain excellent results of these tests.

The two parameters that should be evaluated in IHC preparations of ER and PR are the proportion of the tumor cell nuclei stained and the intensity of the staining [46]. These parameters (proportion and intensity) should be reported separately, or the two can be combined using the composite Allred, Quick-score, or H-score systems. Image analysis can be used to assess the results of staining; however, most reporting is being done visually (by "eyeballing"). Although a threshold of >1% immunoreactivity in a carcinoma is considered positive for both ER and PR, there is emerging evidence that <9% immunoreactivity should be regarded as weakly positive (since this result indicates suboptimal response to therapy) [47].

HER2 overexpression (3+, on a scale of 0 to 3+) is observed in approximately 25% of invasive breast carcinomas. Most high-grade DCIS (with "comedo" necrosis) show 3+ reactivity for HER2. On the other hand, it is extremely uncommon for low-grade invasive tumors (including tubular and classic lobular carcinomas) to be HER2 (+). 2+ reactivity in a case is regarded as equivocal, and should be confirmed through FISH testing. Cases negative for HER2 stain either 0 or 1+. 3+ HER2 staining is regarded as positive, and this result need not be confirmed by FISH testing [48].

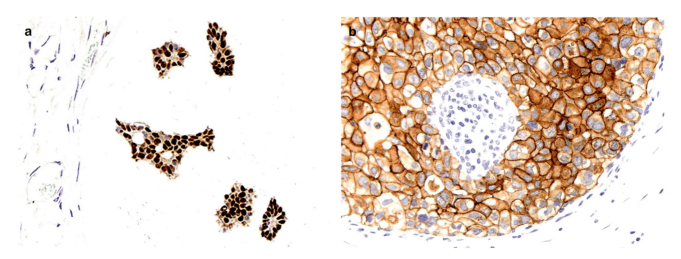

Fig. 17.27 "Biomarkers" in breast carcinoma. (**a**) Estrogen receptor (ER) is strongly and diffusely positive in this invasive mucinous carcinoma (ER). (**b**) HER2 shows 3+ reactivity (on a scale of 0 to 3+) in high-grade ductal carcinoma in situ (Hercept)

17.12   Surrogate Markers for Molecular Classification

Efforts to divide breast carcinomas into distinct groups based on similarities in gene expression profiles using microarray platforms has rapidly evolved into molecular classification thereof. This classification basically divides breast carcinoma into four groups:

- **Luminal A** (with high expression of hormone receptors as well as associated genes, and with the best prognosis)
- **Luminal B** (moderate expression of hormone receptors as well as associated genes, and relatively higher expression of proliferation genes)
- **HER2** (high expression of *HER2* and other genes in amplicon on 17q12)
- **Basal-like** (with low expression of hormone receptors and *HER2* genes, and with the worst prognosis)

Since resources limitations preclude the application of molecular classification of breast carcinomas in each case, efforts have been made to devise a surrogate classification utilizing IHC markers [49, 50].

Although there are limitations to applying IHC markers to molecular classification (e.g., non-standard approach to the assessment of proliferation rate), the following immunoprofiles correspond best to the four groups:

- Luminal A tumors are ER (+), PR (+), and HER2 (−), with a low proliferation rate (<15%).
- Luminal B tumors are ER (+), PR (+), and HER2 (−/+), and are of higher nuclear grade with high proliferation rate (>15%) than luminal A tumors. "Triple-positive" tumors, i.e., ER (+), PR (+) and HER2 (+), belong to luminal B group.
- HER2 group are, as the name implies, HER2 (+), and are ER (−) and PR (−).
- "Triple-negative" tumors are, as the name implies, ER (−), PR (−), and HER2 (−). Most "basal" carcinomas are triple-negative; and in addition, this group of cases are CK5 (+), EGFR (+), and p63 (+). CK5 (a marker for the basal, i.e., myoepithelial layer of the breast glands) is considered the most sensitive immunostain for the identification of "basal" breast carcinomas.

At the present time, the aforementioned surrogate IHC-based molecular classification of breast carcinoma is being used clinically for management purposes in *selected* cases [51]; however, evolutionary refinement in surrogate molecular classification is surely to be expected.

Conclusions

Immunohistochemistry has become an integral part of breast pathology. This *science* can be used to effectively confirm, refine, or refute various pathological diagnoses; however, the appropriate and cost-effective use of immunostains is an *art* that can be mastered—by way of awareness of its advantages, disadvantages, and pitfalls in interpretation.

References

1. Yeh IT, Mies C. Application of immunohistochemistry to breast lesions. Arch Pathol Lab Med. 2008;132:349–58.
2. Moriya T, Kozuka Y, Kanomata N, Tse GM, Tan PH. The role of immunohistochemistry in the differential diagnosis of breast lesions. Pathology. 2009;41:68–76.
3. Gown AM. Diagnostic immunohistochemistry: what can go wrong and how to prevent it. Arch Pathol Lab Med. 2016;140:893–8.
4. Hoda SA, Rosen PP. Contemporaneous H&E sections should be standard practice in diagnostic immunopathology. Am J Surg Pathol. 2007;31:1627.
5. Cserni G. Lack of myoepithelium in apocrine glands of the breast does not necessarily imply malignancy. Histopathology. 2008;52:253–5.
6. Tramm T, Kim JY, Tavassoli FA. Diminished number or complete loss of myoepithelial cells associated with metaplastic and neoplastic apocrine lesions of the breast. Am J Surg Pathol. 2011;35:202–11.
7. Geyer FC, Berman SH, Marchiò C, Burke KA, Guerini-Rocco E, Piscuoglio S, et al. Genetic analysis of microglandular adenosis and acinic cell carcinomas of the breast provides evidence for the existence of a low-grade triple-negative breast neoplasia family. Mod Pathol. 2017;30:69–84.
8. Gatalica Z. Immunohistochemical analysis of apocrine breast lesions. Consistent over-expression of androgen receptor accompanied by the loss of estrogen and progesterone receptors in apocrine metaplasia and apocrine carcinoma in situ. Pathol Res Pract. 1997;193:753–8.
9. Mills AM, Gottlieb EC, Wendroth MS, Brenin MC, Atkins KA. Pure apocrine carcinomas represent a clinicopathologically distinct androgen receptor-positive subset of triple-negative breast cancers. Am J Surg Pathol. 2016;40:1109–16.
10. Nofech-Mozes S, Holloway C, Hanna W. The role of cytokeratin 5/6 as an adjunct diagnostic tool in breast core needle biopsies. Int J Surg Pathol. 2008;16:399–406.
11. Lee AH. Use of immunohistochemistry in the diagnosis of problematic breast lesions. J Clin Pathol. 2013;66:471–7.
12. Khazai L, Rosa M. Use of Immunohistochemical stains in epithelial lesions of the breast. Cancer Control. 2015;22:220–5.
13. Canas-Marques R, Schnitt SJ. E-cadherin immunohistochemistry in breast pathology: uses and pitfalls. Histopathology. 2016;68:57–69.
14. Butler D, Rosa M. Pleomorphic lobular carcinoma of the breast: a morphologically and clinically distinct variant of lobular carcinoma. Arch Pathol Lab Med. 2013;137:1688–92.
15. Eisenberg RE, Hoda SA. Lobular carcinoma in situ with collagenous spherulosis: clinicopathologic characteristics of 38 cases. Breast J. 2014;20:440–1.

16. Jorns JM. Papillary lesions of the breast: a practical approach to diagnosis. Arch Pathol Lab Med. 2016;140:1052–9.

17. Tse GM, Tan PH, Moriya T. The role of immunohistochemistry in the differential diagnosis of papillary lesions of the breast. J Clin Pathol. 2009;62:407–13.

18. Wynveen CA, Nehhozina T, Akram M, Hassan M, Norton L, Van Zee KJ, et al. Intracystic papillary carcinoma of the breast: an in situ or invasive tumor? Results of immunohistochemical analysis and clinical follow-up. Am J Surg Pathol. 2011;35:1–14.

19. Rakha EA, Tun M, Junainah E, Ellis IO, Green A. Encapsulated papillary carcinoma of the breast: a study of invasion associated markers. J Clin Pathol. 2012;65:710–4.

20. Hilson JB, Schnitt SJ, Collins LC. Phenotypic alterations in myoepithelial cells associated with benign sclerosing lesions of the breast. Am J Surg Pathol. 2010;34:896–900.

21. Cheng E, D'Alfonso TM, Arafah M, Marrero Rolon R, Ginter PS, Hoda SA. Subareolar sclerosing ductal hyperplasia. Int J Surg Pathol. 2017;25:4–11.

22. Ozerdem U, Swistel A, Antonio LB, Hoda SA. Invasive Paget disease of the nipple: a brief review of the literature and report of the first case with axillary nodal metastases. Int J Surg Pathol. 2014;22:566–9.

23. Liegl B, Leibl S, Gogg-Kamerer M, Tessaro B, Horn LC, Moinfar F. Mammary and extramammary Paget's disease: an immunohistochemical study of 83 cases. Histopathology. 2007;50:439–47.

24. Park S, Suh YL. Useful immunohistochemical markers for distinguishing Paget cells from Toker cells. Pathology. 2009;41:640–4.

25. Ross DS, Hoda SA. Microinvasive (T1mic) lobular carcinoma of the breast: clinicopathologic profile of 16 cases. Am J Surg Pathol. 2011;35:750–6.

26. Rakha EA, Aleskandarany MA, Lee AH, Ellis IO. An approach to the diagnosis of spindle cell lesions of the breast. Histopathology. 2016;68:33–44.

27. Chia Y, Thike AA, Cheok PY, Yong-Zheng Chong L, Man-Kit Tse G, Tan PH. Stromal keratin expression in phyllodes tumours of the breast: a comparison with other spindle cell breast lesions. J Clin Pathol. 2012;65:339–47.

28. Cimino-Mathews A, Sharma R, Illei PB, Vang R, Argani P. A subset of malignant phyllodes tumors express p63 and p40: a diagnostic pitfall in breast core needle biopsies. Am J Surg Pathol. 2014;38:1689–96.

29. Arafah MA, Ginter PS, D'Alfonso TM, Hoda SA. Epithelioid mammary myofibroblastoma mimicking invasive lobular carcinoma. Int J Surg Pathol. 2015;23:284–8.

30. Hoda SA, Hoda RS, Merlin S, Shamonki J, Rivera M. Issues relating to lymphovascular invasion in breast carcinoma. Adv Anat Pathol. 2006;13:308–15.

31. Rosen PP. Tumor emboli in intramammary lymphatics in breast carcinoma: pathologic criteria for diagnosis and clinical significance. Pathol Annu. 1983;18(Pt 2):215–32.

32. Patton KT, Deyrup AT, Weiss SW. Atypical vascular lesions after surgery and radiation of the breast: a clinicopathologic study of 32 cases analyzing histologic heterogeneity and association with angiosarcoma. Am J Surg Pathol. 2008;32:943–50.

33. Rabban JT, Chen YY. D2–40 expression by breast myoepithelium: potential pitfalls in distinguishing intralymphatic carcinoma from in situ carcinoma. Hum Pathol. 2008;39:175–83.

34. Rivera M, Merlin S, Hoda RS, Gopalan A, Hoda SA. Controversies in surgical pathology: minimal involvement of sentinel lymph node in breast carcinoma: prevailing concepts and challenging problems. Int J Surg Pathol. 2004;12:301–6.

35. Hoda SA, Chiu A, Resetkova E, Harigopal M, Hoda RS, Osborne MP. Pathological examination of sentinel lymph node in breast cancer: potential problems and possible solutions. Microsc Res Tech. 2002;59:85–91.

36. Ozerdem U, Hoda SA. Endosalpingiosis of axillary sentinel lymph node: a mimic of metastatic breast carcinoma. Breast J. 2015;21:194–5.

37. Robinson BD, Amin BD, Hoda SA. Alternaria simulating metastatic breast carcinoma in cytokeratin-stained axillary sentinel node sections. Breast J. 2008;14:120–1.

38. Scognamiglio T, Hoda RS, Edgar MA, Hoda SA. The need for vigilance in the pathologic evaluation of sentinel lymph nodes: a report of two illustrative cases. Breast J. 2003;9:420–2.

39. Hoda SA, Resetkova E, Yusuf Y, Cahan A, Rosen PP. Megakaryocytes mimicking metastatic breast carcinoma. Arch Pathol Lab Med. 2002;126:618–20.

40. Chiu A, Hoda RS, Hoda SA. Pseudomicrometastasis in sentinel lymph node-multinucleated macrophage mimicking micrometastasis. Breast J. 2001;7:440–1.

41. Chiu A, Hoda SA, Yao DX, Rosen PP. A potential source of false-positive sentinel nodes: immunostain misadventure. Arch Pathol Lab Med. 2001;125:1497–9.

42. DeLair DF, Corben AD, Catalano JP, Vallejo CE, Brogi E, Tan LK. Non-mammary metastases to the breast and axilla: a study of 85 cases. Mod Pathol. 2013;26:343–9.

43. Lee AH. The histological diagnosis of metastases to the breast from extramammary malignancies. J Clin Pathol. 2007;60:1333–41.

44. Miettinen M, McCue PA, Sarlomo-Rikala M, Rys J, Czapiewski P, Wazny K, et al. GATA3: a multispecific but potentially useful marker in surgical pathology: a systematic analysis of 2500 epithelial and nonepithelial tumors. Am J Surg Pathol. 2014;38:13–22.

45. Hoda S, Rao R, Hoda RS. Breast implant-associated anaplastic large cell lymphoma. Int J Surg Pathol. 2015;23:209–10.

46. Fitzgibbons PL, Dillon DA, Alsabeh R, Berman MA, Hayes DF, Hicks DG, et al. Template for reporting results of biomarker testing of specimens from patients with carcinoma of the breast. Arch Pathol Lab Med. 2014;138:595–601.

47. Yi M, Huo L, Koenig KB, Mittendorf EA, Meric-Bernstam F, Kuerer HM, et al. Which threshold for ER positivity? a retrospective study based on 9639 patients. Ann Oncol. 2014;25: 1004–11.

48. Wolff AC, Hammond ME, Hicks DG, Dowsett M, McShane LM, Allison KH, et al. Recommendations for human epidermal growth factor receptor 2 testing in breast cancer: American Society of Clinical Oncology/College of American Pathologists clinical practice guideline update. J Clin Oncol. 2013;31:3997–4013.

49. Prat A, Pineda E, Adamo B, Galván P, Fernández A, Gaba L, et al. Clinical implications of the intrinsic molecular subtypes of breast cancer. Breast. 2015;24(Suppl 2):S26–35.

50. Leidy J, Khan A, Kandil D. Basal-like breast cancer: update on clinicopathologic, immunohistochemical, and molecular features. Arch Pathol Lab Med. 2014;138:37–43.

51. Vasconcelos I, Hussainzada A, Berger S, Fietze E, Linke J, Siedentopf F, et al. The St. Gallen surrogate classification for breast cancer subtypes successfully predicts tumor presenting features, nodal involvement, recurrence patterns and disease free survival. Breast. 2016;29:181–5.

18

Prognostic and Predictive Factors in Breast Carcinoma

Simona Stolnicu

Regarding breast cancer, there are well-known clinical, pathological, and molecular prognostic and predictive factors documented by several studies especially within the last decades. From a pathological point of view, these factors need to be evaluated while examining a breast carcinoma, and it is the pathologist's important role to perform this in each case and to include this information in the final pathology report. Based on these factors, patients with breast cancer are divided into those with good prognosis and those with bad prognosis. Also, based on these factors, management is established in every case and the response to the treatment is estimated. Since the evaluation of these parameters is so important in breast pathology, it is necessary for the pathologist dealing with breast carcinoma cases to have experience in this field. Also, especially regarding the evaluation of the markers performed to classify a tumor from a molecular point of view, every laboratory performing these tests is responsible for providing accurate and reproducible results.

Prognostic factors are those parameters that provide information on tumor progression and outcome independent of systemic therapy, while predictive factors indicate the sensitivity or resistance to a particular type of therapy. Related to breast cancer, there are well-known clinical, pathological, and molecular prognostic and predictive factors documented by several studies especially within recent decades. From a pathological point of view, these factors need to be evaluated while examining a breast carcinoma, and it is the pathologist's important role to perform this in each case and to include this information in the final pathology report. Usually, the value of any of these prognostic and predictive factors is established after multivariate statistical tests.

18.1 Clinical Prognostic Factors

18.1.1 Age

Age is a controversial clinical prognostic factor, as some studies have shown that in younger patients with breast cancer, prognosis is more limited, while other studies have shown that prognosis is more favorable, and still others that there is no correlation between age and prognosis.

18.1.2 Pregnancy

Breast cancer associated with pregnancy is clinically defined as a carcinoma diagnosed during pregnancy or in the first year postpartum, and literature insists on separating these two groups of patients. The incidence of breast cancer associated with pregnancy is 0.2–3.8% and about 15% in women under the age of 40 [1]. Traditionally, it has been thought that pregnancy is a factor that aggravates the prognosis of breast cancer. However, studies failed to demonstrate that pregnancy is an independent prognostic factor in breast cancer. Bad prognosis is, rather, related to the fact that pregnancy usually occurs in younger patients and breast tumors are more difficult to detect during pregnancy or breastfeeding, owing to the breast parenchyma edema (especially if the tumor is small in size), and consequently there is a delay in the diagnosis [2, 3]. A large proportion of patients diagnosed with breast carcinoma during pregnancy have already developed axillary metastases at the time of diagnosis and are at higher stage. Also, according to more recent papers, in a small group of susceptible patients, pregnancy can lead to the development of an aggressive form of breast cancer [4]. The management of such cases is greatly dependent on the patient's choice, together with a multidisciplinary team approach.

S. Stolnicu, MD, PhD
Department of Pathology, University of Medicine and Pharmacy, Tîrgu Mureș, Romania

© Springer International Publishing AG, part of Springer Nature 2018
S. Stolnicu, I. Alvarado-Cabrero (eds.), *Practical Atlas of Breast Pathology*, https://doi.org/10.1007/978-3-319-93257-6_18

18.1.3 Bilaterality

Patients with breast cancer have an increased risk of developing such a tumor in the contralateral breast. The risk of developing a contralateral metachronous breast cancer is approximately 1% in the year after mastectomy, while the risk of bilateral synchronous breast cancer is 0.2–2% [5–9]. Synchronous breast cancer is an identified carcinoma within the first two months of primary tumor detection, whereas metachronous breast cancer is a mammary cancer detected more than 2 months after primary tumor diagnosis. The second tumor may be of *in situ* or infiltrating type. By introducing bilateral mammography and screening, the number of patients found to have synchronous breast cancer increased. Also, the frequency of contralateral carcinoma varies among studies because of the patient selection and diagnostic and grossing method. Parameters associated with primary breast cancer that can predict the risk of developing breast cancer in the contralateral breast are: age, tumor size, location, clinical stage, microscopic type and grade (lobular and infiltrating tubular carcinomas and grade 3 carcinomas in general are more commonly associated with bilateral tumors), multicentricity, family history of breast cancer, and association with Peutz-Jeghers syndrome. Some studies have shown that bilateral breast cancer is associated with a more limited prognosis, while other studies have shown that the presence of bilateral breast tumors does not change prognosis [10]. Some of the patients who develop bilateral breast cancer probably have a genetic predisposition.

18.1.4 Multicentricity

In routine practice, most breast carcinomas are diagnosed as unifocal, while a variable proportion is represented by multiple tumors (Fig. 18.1). Data available in the literature regarding the incidence, definition, morphological and molecular profile, treatment, and prognosis of multiple carcinomas are currently contradictory. The incidence of multiple breast carcinomas varies between 6.1% and 77%, due to differences in definition, inclusion/selection criteria, preoperative diagnostic methods (the incidence is 15% when detected with mammographic examination and 35% when detected with MRI and ultrasound), and differences in sampling methods and their correlation with preoperative radiological examinations used in different oncologic hospitals [11, 12]. More recent studies that histopathologically analyzed consecutive cases using the "wide section" method have revealed the presence of multiple foci in most breast carcinoma patients [13]. Traditionally, multiple carcinomas have been classified in two categories: multifocal and multicentric. These definitions were not applied in a uniform manner and these terms are sometimes used together, which can lead to confusion. Also, the distinction between multifocal and multicentric carcinomas was made using several criteria: topographic, histological pattern, and tumor origin. A delimitation between multifocal and multicentric carcinomas was also attempted by using an arbitrary distance between tumor foci. Other authors [14–17] used both terms together, without making a distinction between the two entities by avoiding "quantitative" delimitations. They considered breast carcinomas to be multiple when multiple invasive foci separated by benign breast tissue are seen, regardless of the distance between foci; topographic criteria and distance between tumor foci are considered by these authors to be parameters of debatable biological significance [13]. This definition suggests that, according to more recent studies, the morphology and molecular profile of multiple tumor foci are more important parameters to determine the prognosis than are the location and the distance between multiple foci within the breast.

The latest editions of AJCC and TNM systems define ipsilateral synchronous multiple breast carcinomas as the presence of at least two invasive tumor foci located within the same breast, macroscopically distinct, and assessable using clinical and pathological methods [18, 19]. The multiple foci should only be assessed in terms of their number, which should be reported between parentheses in the final pathology report. However, reporting the histological type, grade, and molecular profile of each tumor focus is imperative, since multiple studies have demonstrated that there is a morphological and molecular heterogeneity among multiple tumor foci, and this should have an impact on management and prognosis [20, 21]. Although multicentricity does not constitute an independent prognostic factor in multivariate analysis, multiple breast carcinomas have a worse prognosis than unifocal ones, and this should be taken into consideration by members of the multidisciplinary tumor board when establishing the treatment [22].

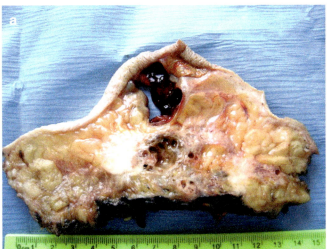
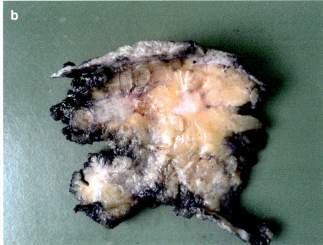

Fig. 18.1 Multiple breast carcinoma: (**a**) Mastectomy specimen with multiple grossly identifiable tumors with infiltrative margins, some of which are of cystic appearance while others are of solid type; (**b**) Quadranectomy specimen with multiple infiltrating breast carcinomas—the number of the tumor foci together with the distance of each focus from the surgical margins must be provided by the pathologist while grossing the specimen

18.1.5 Stage

Stage is an important prognostic factor, but it also serves to determine the type of treatment, and allows for the comparison of outcome results across institutions and national or international clinical trials. This is one of the numerous reasons why it is advisable that all the medical centers involved in diagnosis and treatment of breast cancer should use the same staging system. In 1954, the International Union Against Cancer (UICC) proposed the TNM system, a staging system for breast cancer based on the assessment of the primary tumor (T), regional lymph nodes (N), and distant metastases (M). Within this staging system, regional lymph nodes—axillary, transpectoral, and internal mammary—are taken into account. Therefore, metastases in these lymph node groups (as well as metastases to the intramammary lymph nodes) are considered metastases in N category, while all other metastases are considered distant metastases included in the M category. The TNM system consists of four stages (named I, II, III, IV, in ascending order of severity), and each stage comprises a group of tumors with a similar prognosis. The TNM stage may be clinical (cTNM), based on physical examination and a combination of radiological examinations, or pathological (pTNM), requiring the examination of the primary tumor tissue and regional lymph nodes. Of interest, the clinical and pathological TNM stage do not always correlate. After the UICC proposal in 1954, The American Joint Committee for Cancer Staging and End Results Reporting (AJCC) soon adopted a modified version of the TNM system. The TNM has undergone a number of changes over time, the latest of which was adopted in 2010 and provides more directions related to the specific methods of clinical and pathological tumor size measurement, clarifications of the post-treatment yT and yN classification that are determined after surgical procedure, clarification of the classification of isolated tumor cells and micrometastases in lymph nodes, and definitions of a new category of tumor cells microscopically detectable in bone marrow or circulating blood or found incidentally in other tissues with a size of less than 0.2 mm and without associated symptoms [18]. There are other staging systems for breast carcinoma, but they are not used as often internationally.

18.2 Pathological Prognostic Factors

18.2.1 Tumor Size

Tumor size is an important prognostic factor in that the smaller the size of the tumor, the better the tumor prognosis [23]. The bigger the tumor, the more likely it is to associate with axillary metastases [6]. The way of reporting the size of the tumor is very important, and it varies among pathologists and medical institutions. First of all, the tumor size is reported by the clinicians (through palpation during physical examination) and by the radiologists (using different methods such as ultrasound examination). Of note, all these methods provide information about the tumor; however, the pathological method is best method with which to measure the size. The clinical and pathological size may vary in up to 54% of cases, and a good correlation is needed in all cases.

The clinical and radiological measurements are usually reported in centimeters. The clinical method, utilizing palpation, also takes into account the fat tissue and the skin and using this method, the size may be overestimated. Some pathologists report the macroscopic size (during the grossing of the surgical specimen), others report the microscopic size, the one obtained by measuring the tumor tissue on the glass slide. In terms of macroscopic reporting, the tumor is measured in two dimensions, which is estimated in millimeters (this is done on the breast tissue sections during the grossing process, in the area where the pathologist considers the tumor to have the largest dimensions) (Fig. 18.2). After this assessment, the mammary gland sections are joined, and the third dimension is measured, also given in millimeters. If this dimension is greater than the first two (which is possible because breast carcinomas are not always round and symmetrical), this is the dimension that is reported, along with the next dimension (in descending order). Concerning the microscopic dimension, some pathologists only report the size of the invasive component, but others report the size of both the invasive and the *in situ* component, provided that the latter is situated at a distance of more than 1 mm away from the invasive tumor edge (Fig. 18.3). It has been shown, however, that for the prognosis of the tumor, staging, and management, the size of the invasive component is important; therefore, when there are discrepancies between the macroscopic and microscopic reported size, with regard to the invasive component, the final reporting must include the microscopically detected size. This parameter is considered when staging a malignant breast cancer according to pTNM. Tumor diameter reporting does not take into account vascular invasion foci. This method of measurement applies to unifocal tumors. The international guidelines recommend the use of the maximum diameter of the largest tumor focus in multiple carcinomas, rather than the sum of all diameters when reporting the tumor in the final pathology report [18, 24]. However, the diameter of each tumor focus should be included in the pathology report, since it gives the oncologist an idea about the total volume of the tumor that should be treated; on the other hand, when staging, the largest diameter of the tumor foci should be used [22]. Also, according to the abovementioned international guidelines, these criteria do not apply to tumors with a single macroscopic focus associated with several separate, only microscopically detected, foci, which are called "satellite tumors." If both a macroscopic and a microscopic examination reveals a tumor spread over a variable area in the size of the "spider web" but with no distinct tumor mass, the tumor is called diffuse, and the size of the

entire lesion is measured. Sometimes, especially in invasive lobular carcinoma, diffuse appearance involves the tumor only partially. In this case, if the diffuse aspect concerns less than 50% of the lesion, it is called the mixed tumor type. If a tumor was previously biopsied and preoperatively treated oncologically, the size of the tumor can no longer be determined while grossing or during microscopic examination. In these cases, the tumor diameter established on ultrasound or mammogram is considered in the final staging. As for *in situ* carcinomas, intraductal carcinomas are measured on the microscopic section (and if they form a palpable tumor, they are measured at grossing). The diameter of *in situ* lobular carcinoma is not measured.

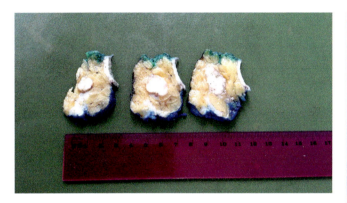

Fig. 18.2 The tumor size is measured during the grossing process and it is estimated in millimeters

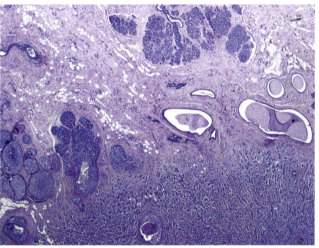

Fig. 18.3 Tumor size: both invasive and *in situ* components can be reported while measuring the size of the tumor, provided that the latter is situated at a distance of more than 1 mm away from the invasive tumor edge, as in this picture

18.2.2 Microscopic Type

Microscopic type is assessed by microscopically examining all the available sections from a tumor and applying the WHO classification [24]. However, establishing the microscopic type is subjective: There is a lack of agreement on diagnostic criteria or lack of good diagnostic criteria, and some pathologists do not recognize the mixed category. For a good assessment of the microscopic type, at least one tissue fragment per 1 cm of tumor is needed to be included in paraffin blocks and then examined under the microscope. Establishing the correct microscopic type is important because in some microscopic types of breast cancer, favorable prognosis has been demonstrated, such as in the following: invasive carcinoma of tubular type, cribriform type, mucinous hypocellular type, and adenoid-cystic type [23, 24]. As for medullary carcinoma, its prognosis is very controversial. Some authors claim that prognosis is better than no special type (NST) infiltrating carcinoma, others claim it is more reserved [24, 25]. In contrast, some microscopic types have an unfavorable prognosis, such as "signet ring" cell carcinoma, inflammatory carcinoma, and metaplastic carcinoma (some but not all of the subtypes of the latter category). Recent guidelines provide information about diverse management of different microscopic types of breast carcinomas (also, in correlation with other prognostic factors). It is advisable that the microscopic type of a breast tumor should be established using the WHO latest edition (2012) [24].

18.2.3 Microscopic Grade

Regardless of the microscopic type, invasive breast cancers are graded, and the microscopic grade is an important prognostic and predictive factor. According to the WHO 2012 criteria, the microscopic grade should be applied to all invasive carcinomas, as it provides important information about tumor prognosis [24, 26]. High-grade invasive carcinomas (grade 3) more frequently exhibit distant metastases and poor prognosis. This also applies to small tumors and even to those without axillary lymph node metastases. Also, the histological grade can provide information on the response to oncological treatment. In this respect, studies have shown that high-grade breast carcinomas respond to chemotherapy treatment better, and most cases with complete pathologic response to neoadjuvant chemotherapy are grade 3 tumors. Also, tumors of different microscopic grades show distinct molecular profiles, and there are studies suggesting that grade 1 and grade 3 tumors are two different diseases with different molecular origins, pathogenesis, and behavior [27, 28]. Currently, histological grade also remains an independent prognostic factor for ER-positive tumors. The grading system established by Patey and Scarff—later modified by Bloom and Richardson and more recently by Elston and Ellis in 1991—is used for grading invasive breast cancers [29]. This microscopic grade is established on microscopic examination by the pathologist and is obtained by adding three numbers representing the estimation of three different parameters: tubular formation (as an expression of glandular differentiation), nuclear pleomorphism, and mitotic activity. Each parameter is scored between 1 and 3 points as follows:

1. Formation of tubules:
   1 point: tubule formation in over 75% of the tumor.
   2 points: tubule formation in 10–75% of the tumor.
   3 points: tubule formation in less than 10% of the tumor.
2. Nuclear pleomorphism:
   1 point: nuclei with minimal variation in size and shape.
   2 points: nuclei with moderate variation in size and shape.
   3 points: nuclei with marked variation in size and shape.
3. Number of mitoses:
   1–3 points depending on the diameter of the microscopic field.

The three numbers are added up and a score is obtained to measure the microscopic grade as follows:

- Grade 1: 3–5 points (well-differentiated).
- Grade 2: 6–7 points (moderately differentiated).
- Grade 3: 8–9 points (poorly differentiated) (Figs. 18.4, 18.5, and 18.6).

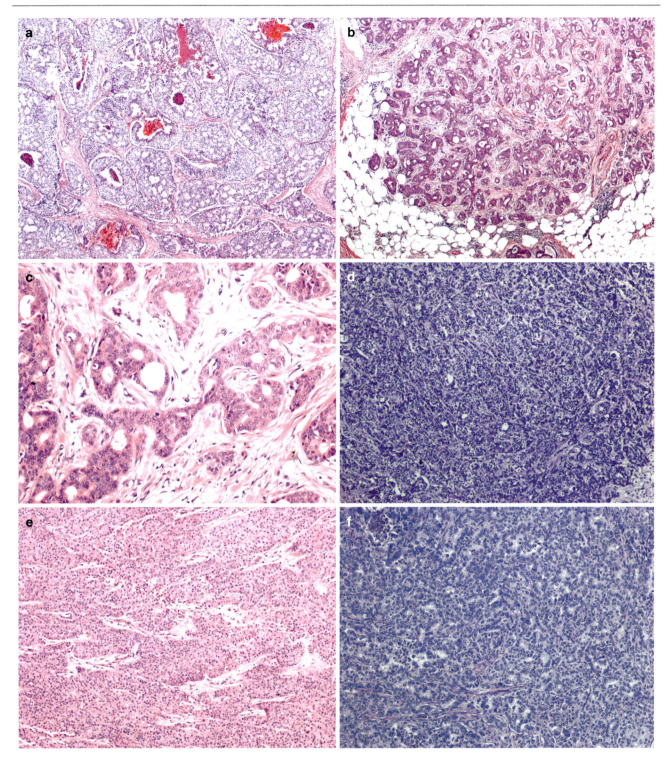

Fig. 18.4 Microscopic grade: (**a**) Tubule formation in over 75% of the tumor; (**b**) another example in which the tubule formation is identified in over 75% of the tumor—1 point; (**c**) same case as (**b**), but at high-power examination with open round lumina surrounded by polarized atypical cells with basal nuclei and apical cytoplasm around the spaces—1 point; (**d**) tubule formation in less than 10% of the tumor (3 points); (**e**) another case with tubules in less than 10% of the tumor (3 points); F, high power examination reveals presence of small round spaces but lacking an open round lumina surrounded by polarized atypical cells (pseudolumina)—3 points

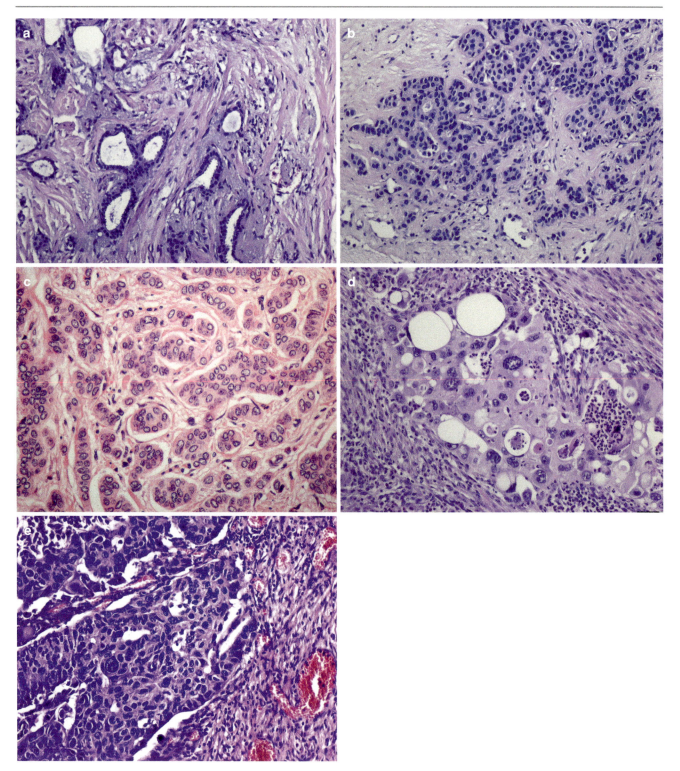

Fig. 18.5 Microscopic grade: (**a**) Nuclei with minimal variation in size and shape—1 point; (**b**, **c**) Nuclei with moderate variation in size and shape—2 points; (**d**, **e**) Nuclei with marked variation in size and shape—3 points

For reporting invasive breast carcinomas, it is advisable to use the term *grade* and specify which grade (1, 2, or 3), instead of *well*, *moderately*, and *poorly differentiated*. Grading is not done on frozen sections or on incorrectly fixed (especially delayed in fixation), cut, or stained sections.

Grading can be done on biopsies, but due to the limited quantity of tissue, the ability to accurately identify the number of mitoses is also limited. This may lead to underestimation of the grade on such specimens, and it is advisable to repeat the grading on the surgical specimen. If for some reason the

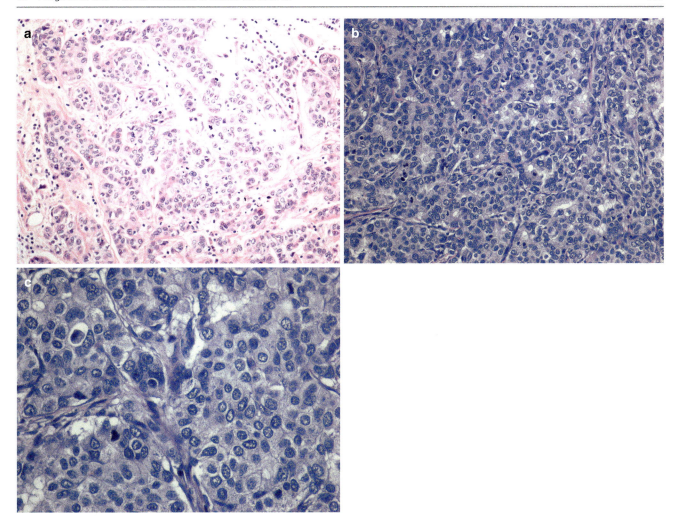

Fig. 18.6 Microscopic grade: number of mitosis will get, depending on the diameter of the microscopic 1 point (**a**) or 3 points (**b** and **c**)

section is not appropriate, it is advisable not to grade the tumor. A good relationship with the surgery department that provides the specimens, as well as training of the staff technicians in the pathology laboratory, are required to properly handle and fix the breast tissue. It is advisable that microscopic grading be done by two pathologists experienced in this field, and in case of inconsistency, grading should be established by consensus. With time and more experience, even one specialized pathologist can grade a breast tumor; however, it is recommended that the pathologist periodically re-check a sample of cases without knowledge of the previous result. Recurrences or tumors treated preoperatively are not graded. If there are multiple tumors present, they must be graded and reported separately. With respect to the formation of tubular structures, only those that have an open and obvious lumen in the center (and surrounded by polarized tumor cells) are considered, and their proportion is appreciated. By tubular formation, one must also take into account the acini, glands, and papillae. Tubular formation is appreciated by examining the entire tumor, including the most undifferenti-

ated areas, on at least three sections from each tumor (it is advisable to examine 4–6 sections, depending on the size of the tumor). Areas of tumor necrosis are avoided. Tubular formation is appreciated on low-power examination. Nuclear pleomorphism is more subjectively appreciated and is done by comparing the appearance of tumor cell nuclei between them and in comparison with normal epithelial cell nuclei in the normal breast tissue adjacent to the tumor. If the normal breast is missing from the slide, then comparison with normal lymphocytes is useful. If one sees only focal pleomorphic nuclei, this should not automatically result in a score 3 for pleomorphism. The pleomorphic nuclei should be found in at least one quarter of the tumor before a score of 3 is allocated for this parameter [29]. Evaluating mitotic figures is even more difficult. Only atypical mitotic figures are considered, and they should not be confused with hyperchromatic nuclei, apoptotic bodies, pycnotic nuclei, or lymphocytes. The total number of mitoses per 10 high-power microscopic fields is calculated. Calculation is done at the periphery of the tumor (the area with the most common mitoses), as well as in the most undifferentiated areas of the tumor, with attempts to assess this parameter also in the central areas within the same tumor (which is less mitotically active). Areas of necrosis are avoided. Of interest, breast carcinomas are heterogeneous, and some degree of variation may occur from one part of the tumor to another concerning the microscopic grade in general, but especially concerning the number of mitoses. To determine the number of mitoses, regardless of the type of the microscope used, it is necessary to determine the field diameter in advance. To obtain this diameter, the following formula is applied:

Field diameter = number of the field / objective magnification
× intermediate magnification.

The number of the field is set for each microscope by the manufacturing company. On each lens, regardless of the type of microscope, both lens and intermediate zooming are indicated. Once the field diameter is determined, the number of mitoses/ten microscopic high-power fields is calculated and then the score is evaluated using the chart provided in the NHS Breast Screening Program (1997) published by the ENHSBSP [23].

This method of appreciating the microscopic grade is applied for each microscopic type of infiltrating breast carcinoma. In mixed type of infiltrating carcinoma (in which two or more microscopic types are identified), each component is graded and reported separately.

Variants of infiltrating breast carcinoma (including the lobular infiltrating carcinoma) are graded according to the same method [29].

Some microscopic subtypes are always grade 1 (like tubular carcinoma) while others are always grade 3 (like medullary carcinoma). Metaplastic carcinoma raises most problems with grading. Squamous carcinoma is graded according to nuclear pleomorphism and cytoplasmic differentiation. In the case of this tumor, the grading system of infiltrating ductal carcinoma is not applied. Adenosquamous carcinoma can be low-grade or high-grade. Regarding adenoid-cystic carcinoma, the same grading system was proposed as in the case of a similar tumor with localization in the salivary gland. The grading system comprises three grades: grade 1 is characterized by the presence of glandular and cystic areas without a solid component; grade 2 contains solids that make up less than 30% of the invasive component; in grade 3, the solid component represents more than 30% of the tumor [30]. Another grading system for mammary adenoid-cystic carcinoma was proposed by Rosen in 1989 [31]. This grading has two categories: low-grade malignancies are characterized by a predominantly glandular or tubular appearance and the solid component is minimal or absent; high-grade malignant tumors are characterized by a predominantly solid appearance.

The microscopic grade set by Ellis and Elston is not perfect, and intraobserver disagreement has been reported by some studies. The subjective criteria are the main reason for reproducibility problems. However, subjectivity can be diminished and reproducibility can be improved with increased experience of the breast pathologist. Grading systems comprising only two grades may be developed in the future.

18.2.4 Vascular Invasion

Vascular invasion is an important prognostic factor. The presence of tumor emboli in vessels is associated with increased risk of metastasis in axillary lymph nodes, with increased frequency of local recurrences and with poor prognosis [32]. Also, the presence of both vascular invasion and lymph node metastases is associated with a worse prognosis than either alone. Of interest, it is important to identify which patients with breast cancer with free regional lymph nodes present vascular invasion, since this group of patients is at higher risk to develop distant metastases. No distinction should be made between the types of vessels (lymphatic or blood), as there is no prognostic significance. Most of the time, however, it cannot be established precisely whether the vessel is of the lymph or blood type, even if immunohistochemical examinations for Factor VIII, CD 31, CD 34, or Ulex europaeus are performed. As a rule, the presence of tumor emboli should be sought around and outside the tumor (at least 1 mm outside) (Figs. 18.7 and 18.8). It should be differentiated from tumor cell nests that are located within empty spaces inside the tumor and represent artefacts produced by stroma retrieval during technical processing (Fig. 18.9). Also, when the tumor cells fill the vascular spaces, it must be differentiated by nests of ductal carcinoma *in situ* (DCIS), which are surrounded by an outer layer of myoepithelial cells (which can be demonstrated with the use of myoepithelial markers). Care must be taken not to over-diagnose foci of micropapillary-infiltrating carcinomas as tumor emboli. To highlight the tumor emboli in the vascular space, it is necessary to visualize a layer of endothelial cells around the space. The presence of erythro-

cytes or thrombi inside the vascular lumen is helpful. Also, the adjacent presence of a venous or arterial lumen is useful. A useful criterion is the shape of the tumor emboli, which in general is not identical to the shape of the space around it. Inflammatory carcinoma demonstrates a particular aspect of this. In this case, the presence of tumor emboli in dermal lymphatic vessels establishes the diagnosis and, as a consequence, the breast skin becomes red, edematous, and warm. Of note, the presence of vascular invasion alone, not associated with residual tumor tissue after neoadjuvant chemotherapy, is resistant to treatment and is associated with a poor prognosis.

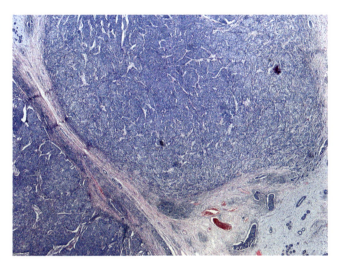

Fig. 18.8 Tumor emboli identified outside the infiltrative tumor margins

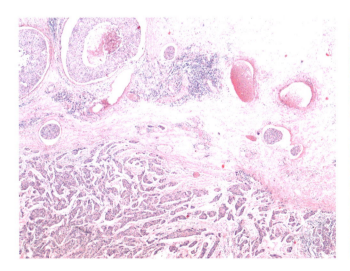

Fig. 18.7 The presence of tumor emboli should be sought around and outside the tumor (at least 1 mm outside)

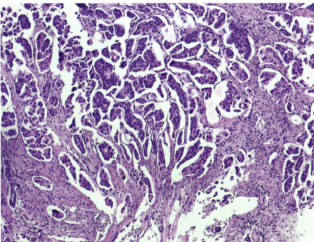

Fig. 18.9 Tumor emboli should be differentiated from tumor cell nests that are located within empty spaces inside the tumor and represent artefacts produced by stroma retrieval during technical processing

18.2.5 Tumor Necrosis

Tumor necrosis is associated with poor prognosis, lack of response to treatment, and early recurrence of the tumor process [33]. The presence of necrosis correlates with tumor size and microscopic grade. In contrast to some invasive mammary carcinomas in which necrosis is focally present, there is a category of such lesions in which necrosis is extensive, located centrally with a geographic-like shape and surrounded by a marginal tissue tumor at the periphery. This latter category is usually basal-like from a molecular point of view and triple negative, and it has a more aggressive prognosis, being frequently associated with pulmonary and cerebral metastases (Fig. 18.10) [34].

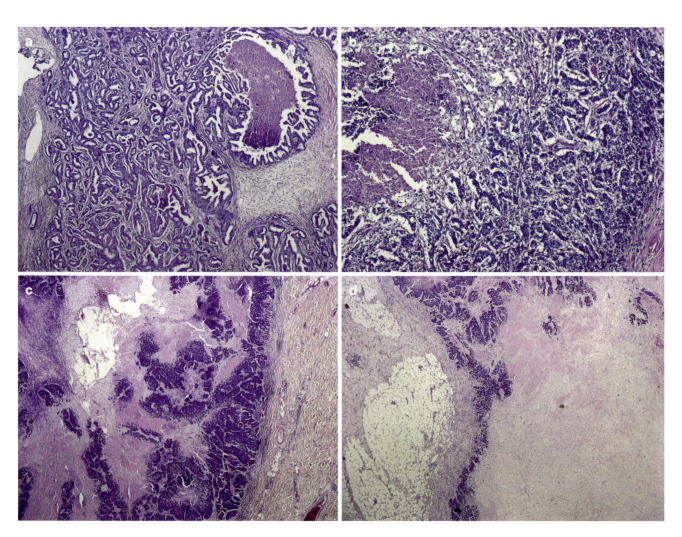

Fig. 18.10 Tumor necrosis: (**a**) Grade 1 invasive mammary carcinomas of NST type in which necrosis is focally present; (**b**) Larger area of necrosis in grade 2 invasive breast carcinoma of NST type; (**c**) Grade 3 infiltrating breast carcinoma of NST type with extensive necrosis; (**d**) Extensive necrosis located centrally with a geographic-like shape and surrounded by a marginal tissue tumor at the periphery in a basal-like triple negative grade 3 infiltrating breast carcinoma

18.2.6 Tumor-Infiltrating Lymphocytes

Several recent papers have evaluated the prognostic and predictive importance of the tumor-infiltrating lymphocytes in breast cancer. In 2013, a consensus meeting sought to provide recommendations for the evaluation of tumor-infiltrating lymphocytes in breast cancer, especially for the clinical routine practice, with a special focus on what area to examine in order to report tumor-infiltrating lymphocytes and how to score the presence of tumor-infiltrating lymphocytes [35]. The presence of tumor-infiltrating lymphocytes in the stroma is most often found in triple-negative, HER2-positive, and poorly differentiated breast carcinomas; also, its presence (and number of tumor-infiltrating lymphocytes) is associated with pathological complete response to neoadjuvant therapy, better disease-free survival, and better overall survival, being an independent prognostic factor [35–37]. The original method to evaluate this parameter was described by Denkert in 2010 [38]. The tumor-infiltrating lymphocytes should be reported for the stromal compartment as a percentage of the area of stromal tissue occupied by these cells over total intratumoral stromal area (as an average, not focusing on hot spots) (Fig. 18.11). As a consequence, tumor-infiltrating lymphocytes should only be evaluated within the borders of the invasive tumor component. The lymphocytes should be evaluated using a 20× or 40× objective on a Hematoxylin-eosin stained slide; immunohistochemical markers such as CD45, CD8, and CD3 can also be used (although there is no added value from these markers according to some studies) [35]. The international recommendations advise counting the stromal compartment (rather than the intratumor lymphocytes,

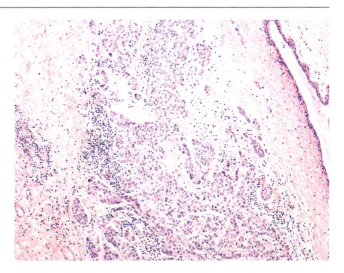

Fig. 18.11 The tumor-infiltrating lymphocytes should be reported for the stromal compartment as a percentage of the area of stromal tissue occupied by these cells over total intratumoral stromal area

that is, those cells in direct contact with nests of tumor cells) [35]. Also, it is advisable to avoid areas of necrosis, fibrosis (including biopsy-site) and crushing artifacts. Only mononuclear cells (lymphocytes and plasma cells) should be counted, while polymorphonuclear leukocytes, dendritic cells, and macrophages must be excluded. The counting should be done, if possible, on one full tumor section; core biopsies can be used only in the pre-treatment neoadjuvant setting. At this time there is no international clinical relevant tumor-infiltrating lymphocyte threshold (which vary between 50% and 60% stromal lymphocytes) [35].

18.2.7 An Extensive *In Situ* Component

The presence of an extensive *in situ* component is associated with a higher rate of local recurrence, especially in patients treated with conservative surgery associated with radiotherapy (the gold standard for patients with breast cancers) [39]. Those patients presenting an extensive DCIS component are more likely to have extensive DCIS in the remaining breast tissue after quadranectomy, and are the ones more likely to develop local recurrences, a fact that has been confirmed by numerous studies [40]. The presence of the extensive *in situ* component must be included in the final report, as well as the distance to the surgical margins (Fig. 18.12). Regarding the surgical margins, for pure DCIS, margins of at least 2 mm are associated with a reduced risk of local recurrence if the surgery is followed by radiotherapy [41], while for patients treated only with surgery, the optimal margin width is unknown, but should be at least 2 mm.

18.2.8 Status of Surgical Margins

Especially after conservative surgical treatment became the gold standard in breast cancer, evaluation of the surgical margins was considered a very important parameter, and the aspect of these margins is a prognostic factor when it is positively related to development of local recurrences [42]. The surgical margins are evaluated by the pathologist while grossing the surgical specimen, and on microscopic examination, but also by cytological examination, inking the specimen or separate examination of the cavity post-quadranectomy (Figs. 18.13 and 18.14). Defining a positive or negative surgical margin is very difficult, and the definition varies among pathologists, clinicians, and medical institutions. However, by establishing a good and evidence-based definition, one might avoid unnecessary surgery, morbidity, and high costs, and one can improve the cosmetic aspect of the remaining breast. Most data originate in retrospective studies and cutoffs of 1, 2, 5, and 10 mm have been used. According to the latest international guidelines, only the presence of ink

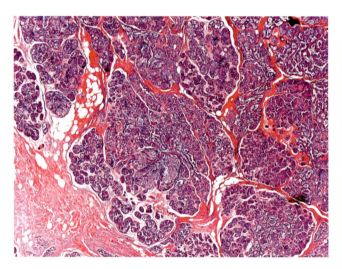

Fig. 18.12 Extensive lobular *in situ* carcinoma: the presence of this component should be reported in the final histopathological report

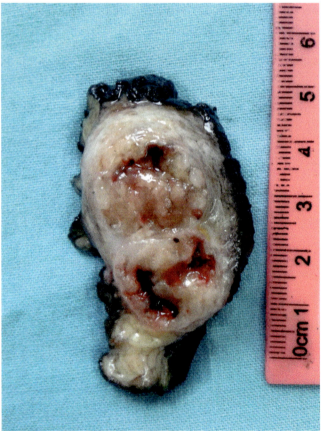

Fig. 18.13 Status of the surgical margins: the surgical margins are evaluated by the pathologist while grossing the surgical specimen; in this case, an infiltrating breast carcinoma of large size is infiltrating the surgical margin, marked with black ink

to the tumor cells is considered a positive margin, the goal not being to ensure that there is no residual tumor left after surgery, but to identify those patients more likely to have a large residual tumor burden and who would require further surgery (Figs. 18.15 and 18.16) [41, 43]. Requirements for optimal margin evaluation include: orientation of the surgical specimen, description of the gross and microscopic margin status, and reporting of the distance and orientation of any type of tumor (*in situ* or invasive) in relation to the closest margin [41].

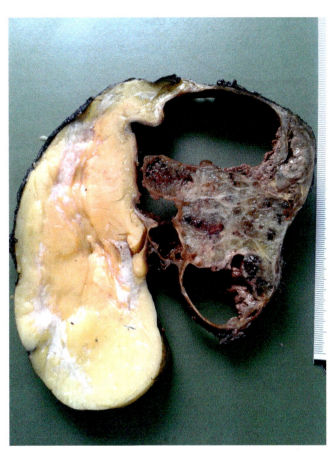

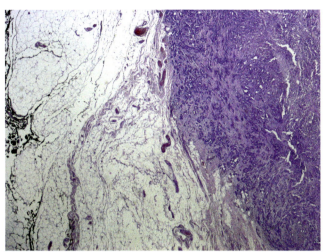

Fig. 18.15 Grade 1 infiltrating breast carcinoma: at the microscopic examination, the pathologist can appreciate that the tumor is located at distance from the surgical margin; however, the distance from the closest margin must be reported

Fig. 18.14 Status of surgical margins: at the macroscopic examination, the malignant tumor is infiltrating the surgical margin (inked with black color)

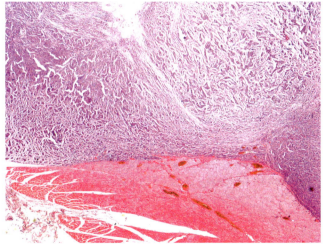

Fig. 18.16 Infiltrating breast carcinoma: the tumor is infiltrating the pectoral muscle, but is at a distance from the surgical margin

18.2.9 Lymph Node Metastases

Lymph node metastases are the most important prognostic factor for patients with breast carcinoma and can be assessed only via histopathological examination [24, 44, 45]. Patient survival depends on the presence or absence of lymph node metastases, the number of lymph nodes affected, the group of affected lymph nodes, the extent of metastasis, and the presence of tumor cells in peri-lymph node vessels and peri-lymph node fat tissue [46]. It is important to detect and sample as many axillary lymph nodes as possible. The number of normal lymph nodes present in one axilla varies from one patient to another. Also, the size of metastasis is important, but studies have shown that although small metastases (micrometastases) do have statistical significance, their impact on prognosis is less than 3% at 5 and 10 years when compared with node-negative patients, and they are not a discriminatory variable for predicting either recurrence or survival [47–50]. In micrometastasis, the metastasis is larger than 0.2 mm in diameter, but smaller than 2 mm in the largest dimension, and in macrometastasis, the metastasis is larger than 2 mm in diameter (Figs. 18.17, 18.18, 18.19, 18.20, and 18.21). There is also a third category of patients, in which only isolated tumor cells or small groups of tumor cells are present, called isolated tumor cells, with a diameter of less than 0.2 mm in the largest diameter (Fig. 18.22). According to the latest pTNM classification, these isolated tumor cells have no metastatic capacity and should therefore be classified as pN0 [24]. Macrometastases are easily detected even at low-power examination, while micrometastases and isolated tumor cells require more careful examination (especially examination of the subcapsular area), and in some situations also the use of ancillary stains (Figs. 18.23, 18.24, 18.25, and 18.26). All parameters to be specified in the status of axillary lymph nodes must be reported within the pTNM classification. If multiple foci of metastases are detected in an axillary lymph node, the size of the largest confluent focus is recorded (same as for multiple primary tumors) [18, 19]. When only clusters of tumor cells can be identified within afferent lymphatics of the node but not within the node parenchyma, the tumor should be classified according to the AJCC rules for metastases present, and this should not be confused with extranodal extension (extranodal extension should be reported separately). There are cases in which clinically or macroscopically one or more axillary lymph nodes have a size greater than 2 cm, but the microscopic examination does not reveal the presence of a metastasis. In these cases, only the changes observed during the microscopic examination are described, and they are classified in the pN0 category. Also, the presence of extracapsular extension (and its size) as well as the presence of tumor cells in the peri-lymph nodular vessels, must be recorded according to the pN classification (Fig. 18.27). If metastasis occurs in internal mammary lymph nodes, the survival of the patient is

even shorter. The presence of metastases in internal mammary lymph nodes is particularly associated with malignant tumors located in internal quadrants. Usually, patients with metastases in internal mammary lymph nodes also have axillary metastases.

Isolated tumor cells or foci of micrometastases can be recognized with ancillary studies like Cytokeratin stain; however, there are also other cells positive for cytokeratin, such as interstitial reticulum cells (usually positive for pan-Cytokeratin CAM 5.2 but not for pan-Cytokeratin AE1/AE3). Pan-Cytokeratin AE1/AE3 should be better used to identify isolated tumor cells.

Axillary lymph nodes are, in most cases (75%), filtration stations of tumor cells from a breast cancer. Research has shown that lymphatic drainage of the breast is done sequentially and, initially, a lymph node located in the lymph drainage path (called sentinel lymph node) is affected. Multiple studies have shown that sentinel lymph node biopsy, in addition to being minimally invasive, is a reliable method (accuracy close to 100%) for determining the status of regional lymph nodes in patients with breast cancer. The absence of metastases in the sentinel lymph node predicts the absence of metastasis in other lymph nodes in a proportion of 98%. In these cases, it is possible to apply a conservative surgical therapy [51].

There is no consensus on the technical processing and examination protocol of the sentinel lymph node in terms of pathology. Pathologists who have dealt with the detection of metastases in sentinel lymph nodes have developed different protocols for microscopic examination. The identification of the sentinel lymph node is made intraoperatively, and its microscopic examination is done on frozen sections, the sections being stained with hematoxylin-eosin. Subsequently, sentinel lymph node fragments cut at 2 mm apart from one another are embedded in paraffin blocks. The protocol of sectioning, examining, staging, and reporting the sentinel lymph node in breast pathology is presented in Chapter 23.

Lymph node metastases of breast cancer should not be confused with other pathological processes that affect a lymph node.

Of the reactive processes that may involve an axillary lymph node, one can encounter hyperplasia of lymphoid follicles and sinus histiocytosis (the presence of both lesions is associated by some reports with a better immune response to the presence of the breast carcinoma and a better survival) (Figs. 18.28 and 18.29). Also, an axillary lymph node can present fat tissue metaplasia, when normal lymphoid tissue is replaced by adipose tissue (this situation occurs more frequently in obese patients) (Fig. 18.30). The characteristic changes of toxoplasmosis type granuloma may also be encountered. Also, a sarcoid-like granulomatous lesion may sometimes occur, especially during chemotherapy or tumor necrosis factor blocker therapy, and sarcoidosis and tuberculosis must be ruled out [52] (Fig. 18.31). Very rarely, true sarcoidosis or tuberculosis affect the axillary lymph nodes (Fig. 18.32). Benign-appearing groups of nevus cells with a capsular location can sometimes occur in a lymph node. This is always an incidental finding (Fig. 18.33). The cells are oval, with pale cytoplasm, indistinct borders, sometimes contain melanin pigment within the cytoplasm, and present bland nuclei. Absence of mucin production, presence of melanin pigment, location within the capsule, and the immunohistochemical profile help to differentiate this lesion from metastatic process. Staining for HMB-45 and S-100 protein allows for identifying the melanocytic origin of these cells together with Cytokeratin, since some tumor cells may be positive for S-100 protein (Fig. 18.34). Of note, nevus cells can occur within the same node with metastases. Also, a lymph node may have benign glandular inclusions (also called endosalpingiosis), which are formed by epithelial cells without atypia, line the cystic spaces, and have varying

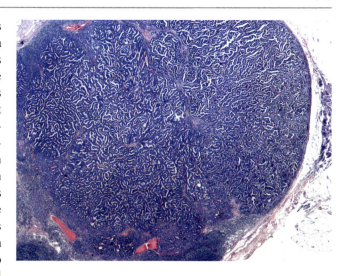

Fig. 18.17 Axillary lymph node macrometastasis from a grade 1 infiltrating breast carcinoma

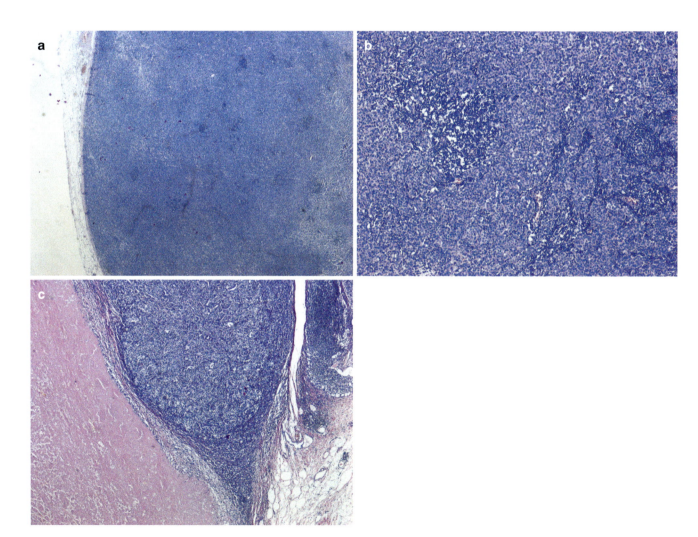

Fig. 18.18 Axillary lymph node macrometastasis from a grade 3 infiltrating breast carcinoma: (**a**) At low power, the lymph node architecture is replaced by tumor cells; (**b**) Higher power reveals that the tumor cells are of high grade and not forming tubular structures; (**c**) other areas contain also tumor necrosis

sizes (comparison with primary breast tumor morphology is of great help, as well as the positivity for WT-1, CA125, and estrogen receptors, and negativity for GCDFP-15 and GATA 3) (Fig. 18.35). This must be known by practicing pathologists and should not be confused with metastatic breast carcinoma, especially when the endosalpingiosis is of florid type [53]. Of interest, benign glandular inclusions represented by breast acini and ducts can also occur within axillary lymph nodes. This is important to know, since benign or malignant lesions similar to the ones in the breast can develop out of these inclusions. These acini and ducts are lined by epithelial, myoepithelial cells and have a basal membrane at the periphery. Silicone lymphadenopathy can occur, especially in the presence of silicone breast implants (empty or clear round spaces associated with inflammatory infiltrate, vacuolated histocytes, and multinucleate cells are present) (Fig. 18.36). Megakaryocytes can also be found in axillary lymph nodes, especially following neoadjuvant chemotherapy for local advanced breast cancer, being a potential source

of false-positive diagnosis of axillary metastases from breast cancer [54, 55]. Ancillary immunohistochemical studies, however, can rule out metastases. Lymph node metastases of breast cancer should not be confused with lymph node metastases of primary tumors from another location (especially from a thyroid carcinoma).

Displaced epithelium from benign breast tissue may occur, as might benign proliferative lesions or after the biopsy (Fig. 18.37) of breast lesions, especially after the biopsy of breast papillary lesions (of benign or malignant type) that are fragile. They are typically detected within the subcapsular sinus. Sometimes it is impossible to differentiate between benign or malignant cells (however, the presence of degenerative cells together with the presence of hemosiderin containing macrophages are in favor of displaced cells due to a biopsy). It is advisable that in patients with invasive carcinoma or DCIS, an explanatory note should be included at the end of the report mentioning that the possibility of metastasis cannot be excluded.

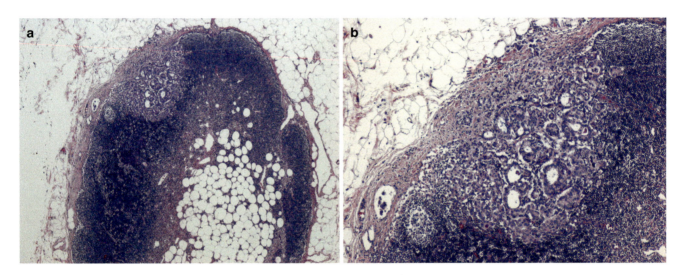

Fig. 18.19 (**a**) Micrometastasis in axillary lymph node; (**b**) High power reveals the presence of extracapsular extension and tumor emboli

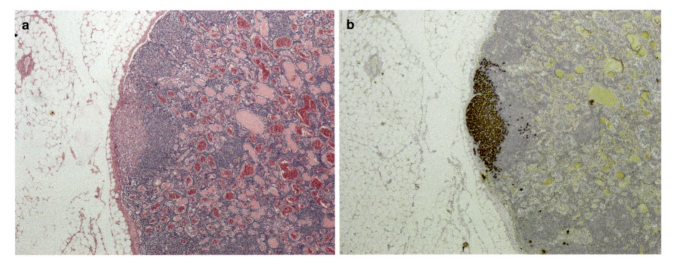

Fig. 18.20 Micrometastasis in axillary lymph node: (**a**) Especially in lobular carcinoma it is sometimes difficult to detect small size metastases on Haematoxylin-Eosin stain; (**b**) Ancillary stains can help, especially the use of Cytokeratin since the tumor cells are positive for this marker

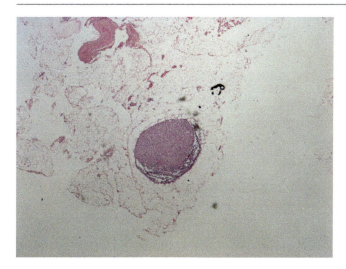

Fig. 18.21 Micrometastasis in a very small axillary lymph node demonstrating that all lymph nodes should be examined at the microscope for the detection of the metastases, despite their size

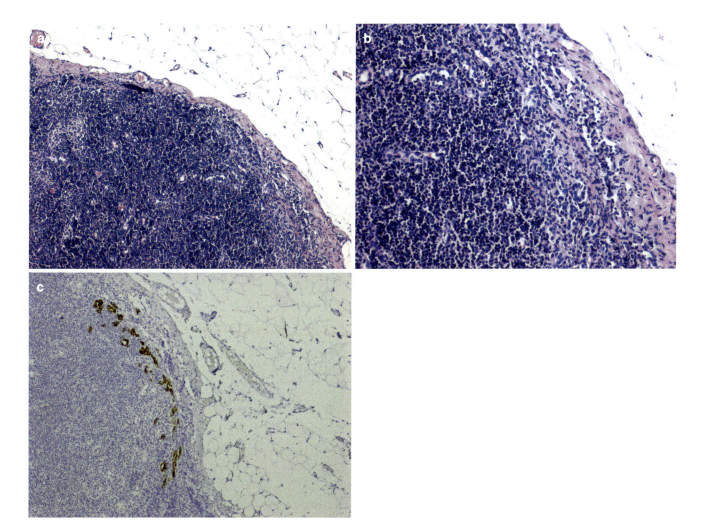

Fig. 18.22 Isolated tumor cells: (**a**) Small groups of tumor cells present in the subcapsular area; (**b**) Higher power examination reveals the presence of isolated small groups of atypical cells; (**c**) Cytokeratin stain can detect these cells better and the size of the lesion (less than 0.2 mm in the largest diameter) is better appreciated

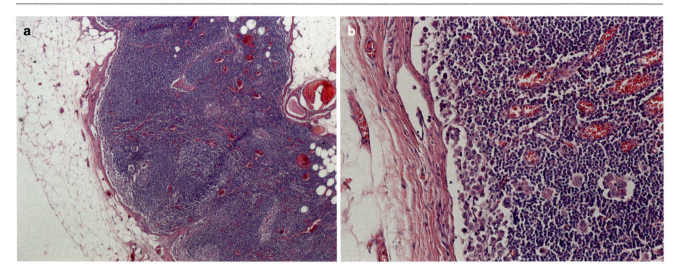

Fig. 18.23 (**a**) Small size metastases, especially when originating in lobular infiltrating breast carcinoma, are very difficult to detect while scanning at low-power examination; (**b**) Each suspected area has to be examined at high power as well

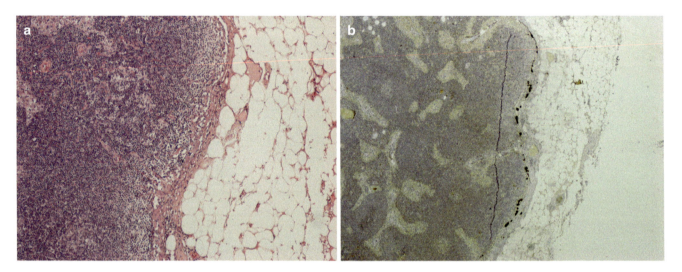

Fig. 18.24 (**a**) Isolated tumor cells requires more careful examination (especially examination of the subcapsular area) and (**b**) in some situations, also the use of ancillary stains such as Cytokeratin

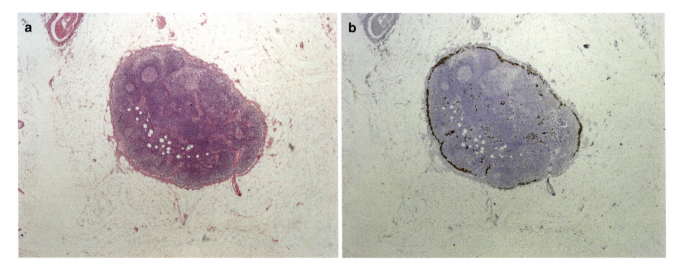

Fig. 18.25 (**a**) The presence and extent of small groups of cells within the subcapsular space (**b**) are better detected with ancillary stains such as Cytokeratin

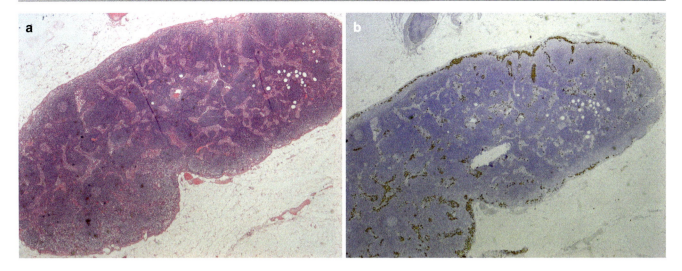

Fig. 18.26 Another case of axillary lymph node metastasis from breast carcinoma: (**a**) The presence and extent of small groups of cells within the subcapsular space are (**b**) better detected with ancillary stains such as Cytokeratin

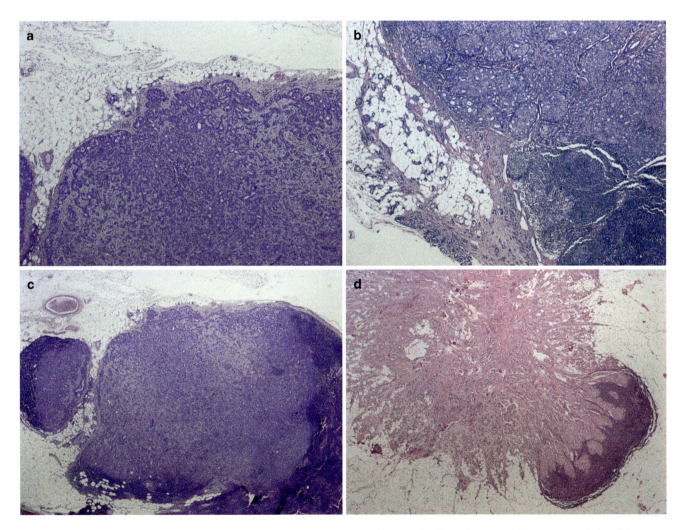

Fig. 18.27 (**a**) Extracapsular extension of lymph node metastasis from a grade 1 infiltrating breast carcinoma; (**b**) Different area with larger size; (**c**) Different case with extracapsular extension; (**d**) Massive extra-capsular extension in another case—the presence and size of the extra-capsular extension should be recorded in the final histopathological report

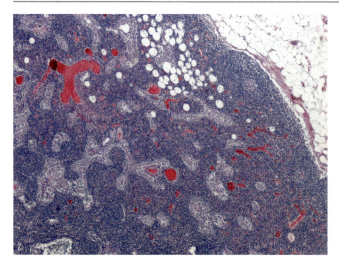

Fig. 18.28 Sinus histiocytosis involving axillary lymph node in a case of primary breast carcinoma

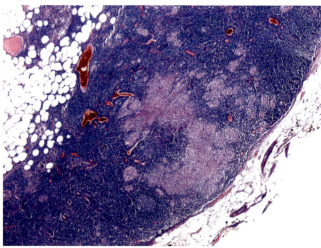

Fig. 18.31 Sarcoid-like granulomatous lesion involving axillary lymph node

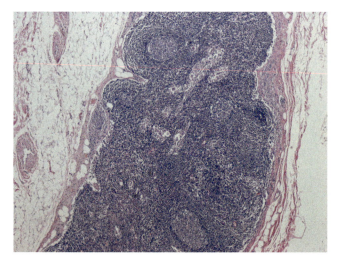

Fig. 18.29 Hyperplasia of lymphoid follicles involving axillary lymph node in a case of primary breast carcinoma

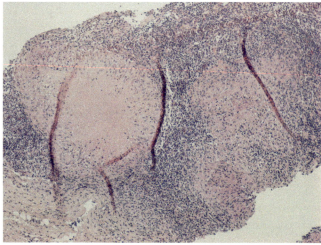

Fig. 18.32 Tuberculosis granulomatous lesions with central areas of necrosis involving axillary lymph node in a Tru-Cut biopsy

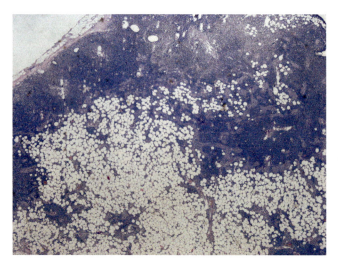

Fig. 18.30 Fat tissue metaplasia involving axillary lymph node: normal lymphoid tissue is replaced by adipose tissue with a variable extent

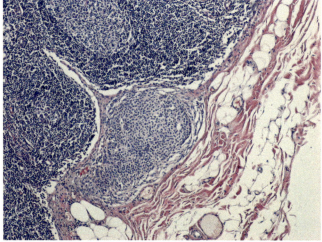

Fig. 18.33 Nevus cells with a capsular location in axillary lymph node: benign-looking cells, oval, with pale cytoplasm, bland nuclei, and indistinct borders; melanin pigment is not present in this case

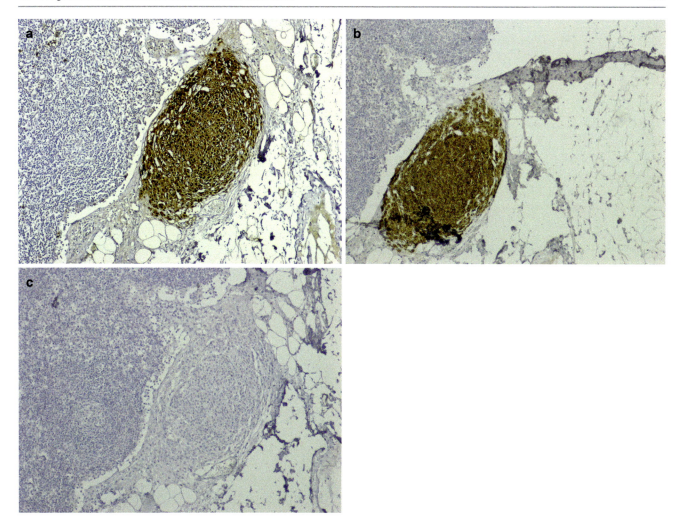

Fig. 18.34 Nevus cells with a capsular location are positive for (**a**) S-100 protein and (**b**) Melan A, and (**c**) negative for Cytokeratin

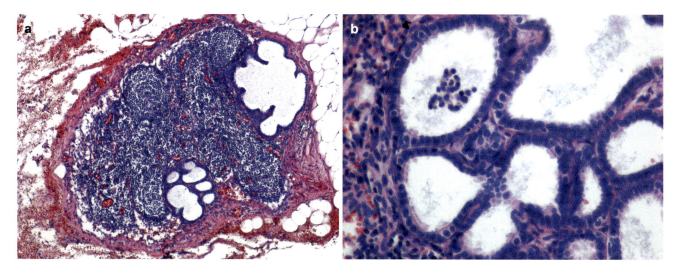

Fig. 18.35 Endosalpingiosis involving axillary lymph node: (**a**) Small glandular inclusions; (**b**) Lined by epithelial ciliated cells resembling the fallopian tube epithelium, without atypia

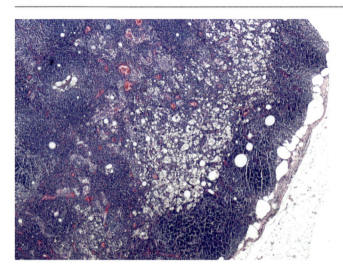

Fig. 18.36 Silicone lymphadenopathy: clear round spaces associated with inflammatory infiltrate, vacuolated histocytes, and multinucleate cells

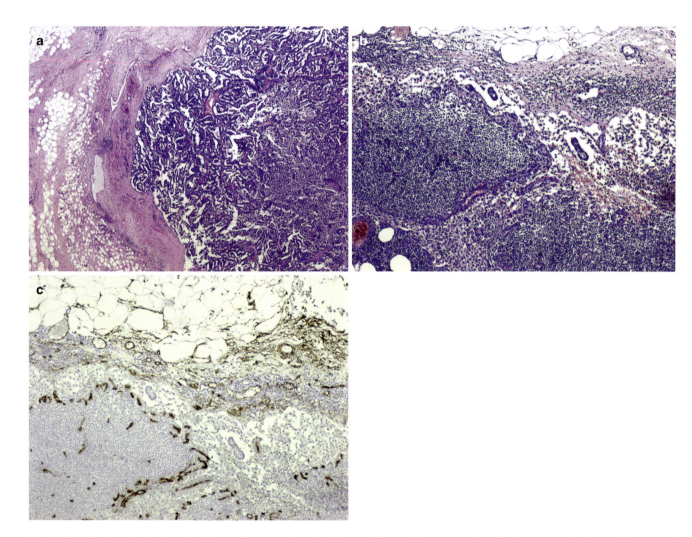

Fig. 18.37 Displaced epithelium involving axillary lymph node: (**a**) Primary breast tumor of encapsulated papillary breast carcinoma; (**b**) After Tru-Cut biopsy of the primary tumor, small groups of cells with papillary architecture are found in the subcapsular sinus of the removed sentinel lymph node; (**c**) CD34 is negative within the surrounding space

18.2.10 Nottingham Prognostic Index

A group of pathologists and oncologists in Nottingham formulated a prognostic indicator called the Nottingham prognostic index (NPI), the calculation of which takes into account the following parameters: tumor size, stage of axillary and internal mammary lymph nodes, and histological grade of the tumor in question [56]. Index calculation is made using the following formula:

$$NPI = 0.2 \times \text{tumor size} + \text{lymph node stage} + \text{histological grade}.$$

Tumor size is assessed in centimeters. The appearance of lymph nodes is estimated by 1, 2, or 3 points, depending on the presence of metastases in axillary or internal mammary lymph nodes.

Depending on the Nottingham prognostic index, patients can be classified into three categories: good prognosis (index below 3.4), moderate (index between 3.41 and 5.4), and poor prognosis (index higher than 5.41) [56]. The NPI has been validated by both retrospective and prospective studies. The NPI may assist the clinician in selecting which patients should receive systemic adjuvant therapy and what type of therapy.

18.3 Molecular and Genetic Prognostic Factors

Three molecular biomarkers are routinely used in the diagnosis and management of breast carcinoma: estrogen receptors, progesterone receptors, and HER2, all of which are indicators of effectiveness of therapies in breast carcinoma. Thus, correct assessment of these parameters is very important, and the pathologist dealing with these investigations has a very important role. Also, every laboratory performing these tests is responsible for providing accurate and reproducible results.

18.3.1 Hormonal Receptor

Determination of hormonal receptor status in breast carcinoma is a routine examination and is performed in all infiltrating breast carcinomas as well as in some *in situ* types. Estrogen receptor (ER) is a nuclear transcription factor involved in the breast developments as well as in tumorigenesis, and it regulates expression of genes such as progesterone receptor (PR). ER and PR levels are strongly and inversely correlated with other prognostic parameters. Also, ER and PR are prognostic and predictive factors, and their presence or absence is routinely assessed in all patients with breast cancer as a predictive factor for response to therapeutic and adjuvant hormonal therapy. This examination identifies patients who will respond to hormonal treatment. Approximately 55–65% of primary breast tumors and 45–55% of metastases present ER and PR. Studies have shown that 55–65% of patients with positive ER and PR respond to hormone therapy, compared to 8% of patients with negative ER responding to this treatment. Well-differentiated tumors usually have positive ER and a better prognosis. Approximately 45–60% of primary breast carcinomas and their metastases contain PR. If a breast tumor has both positive ER and PR, the response of these tumors to hormonal therapy increases from 55–60% to 75–80%. The presence of positive PR within a breast cancer is associated with a favorable prognosis. Approximately 46% of the ER-negative tumors, but positive PR, respond to hormonal therapy. Estrogen and progesterone receptors can be determined by immunohistochemical methods or molecular methods. Studies have shown that immunohistochemical determination correlates much better with assessing prognosis than conventional biochemical methods. Determination of hormone receptors by immunohistochemical methods can be done on fresh or paraffin-embedded tissue. The determination is made both on the *in situ* hormone receptor component, as well as the invasive one, and reporting of the results must indicate the percentage of tumor cells positive or negative for both receptor components; however, in invasive breast carcinomas, the positivity of the infiltrative component is taken into account when deciding the hormonal treatment. Also, for the cases of DCIS, the percentage of the tumor cells positive for ER will indicate the hormonal treatment. Assessment of positivity is only done on the nuclei of tumor cells, and cytoplasmic positivity is not taken into account (Figs. 18.38 and 18.39). For this purpose, the tumor must be properly fixed in formalin, immediately sectioned, and immersed in the suitable amount of fixation substance. Positive and negative control must be performed in every case. In most cases, normal breast tissue adjacent to the tumor represents a very good internal control because it normally contains ER and PR. A simpler method of assessment is to determine the hormone receptor positive tumor cell percentage. Different cutoffs have been used for the positivity of

ER and PR. Recent studies have shown, however, that a 1% cutoff is advisable since there are convincing data that patients with even a few cells positive will benefit from hormonal therapy [57].

Some laboratories use the H score to report immunohistochemical results. H score is calculated by taking into account both the percentage of positive nuclei and the intensity of the reaction. H score calculation is as follows: (1× % of weakly positive cells) + (2× % moderately positive cell) + (3× % of cells strongly positive). Percentage is calculated on 500–1000 tumor cells. By this calculation four grades are obtained:

Negative H Score: 0–50
Weakly positive H score: 51–100
Moderately positive H score: 101–200
Strongly positive H score: 201–300.

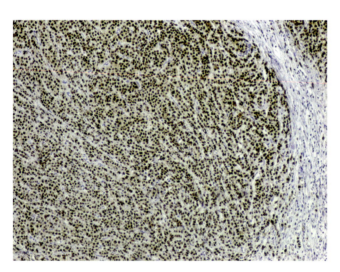

Fig. 18.38 Estrogen receptor is positive in more than 90% of the tumor cells in this case

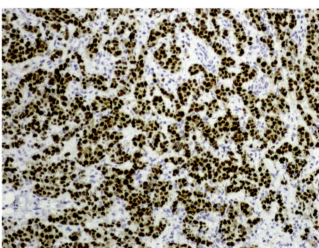

Fig. 18.39 Progesterone receptor is positive in more than 90% of the tumor cells in this case

18.3.2 Oncogene c-ErbB2

Oncogene c-ErbB2 or HER2/neu belongs to the ErbB oncogene family and is closely correlated with epidermal growth
factors. Studies have shown amplification of this oncoprotein
in about 15% of breast cancers. It is an independent factor
for assessing the prognosis of patients with axillary lymph
node metastases [57, 58]. The HER2 amplification is associated with poorly differentiated tumors with metastases in the
axillary lymph nodes, hormone receptor negativity, and a
poor prognosis [59]. HER2 testing should be performed in
all newly diagnosed invasive breast cancers and for first
recurrences of breast cancers. Amplification of c-ErbB-2
oncoprotein may be demonstrated by immunohistochemical
methods on the cell membrane or *in situ* hybridization (measuring the number of HER2 gene copies). Multiple studies
have shown, however, that the accuracy of HER2 assay used
in clinical practice is a major concern owing to false-positive
and false-negative results. This is why it is advised to perform the HER2 testing only in accredited laboratories.
Intracytoplasmic positivity is non-specific by diffusion from
the membrane, and it is not considered if it is not associated
with membranous positivity. The score performed using the
immunohistochemical method is calculated as follows:

Score 0 (negative): no staining is observed, or membrane
    staining is observed in less than 10% of the tumor cells.
Score 1+ (negative): a faint/barely perceptible membrane
    staining is detected in more than 10% of the tumor cells.
Score 2+ (weakly positive, equivocal): a weak-to-moderate
    complete membrane staining is observed in more than
    10% of the tumor cells.
Score 3+ (strongly positive): a strong, complete membrane
    staining is observed in more than 10% of the tumor cells
    (Fig. 18.40) [60].

Score 0 and 1 are considered as HER2 negative, Score 2 is
considered as equivocal; the recommendation is reflex
testing using the ISH method on the same specimen or
ordering a new test with immunohistochemistry or ISH if
a new specimen is available. Of interest, some invasive
carcinomas (like the micropapillary carcinoma) are HER2
1+ positive in 10–80% of cases, with intense but incomplete staining (basolateral or U-shaped) found to be HER2
amplified [60]. The pathologist should consider also
reporting these specimens equivocal and request reflex
testing using alternative test [60].

By using the ISH assay, ISH test is negative if average
HER2 copy number is less than 4 signals/cell, it is equivocal
if average HER2 copy number is between 4 and 6 signals/
cell and it is positive if average HER2 copy number is more
than 6 signals/cell. For the equivocal results, reflex test with
dual-probe ISH or with immunohistochemistry on the same
specimen must be ordered, or a new test with ISH or immunohistochemistry if a new specimen is available.

Evidence from trastuzumab adjuvant trials show that
HER2 testing by immunohistochemistry or ISH have similar
utility to predict clinical benefit from HER2-targeted
therapy.

Of recent drugs, Herceptin is used in patients with
c-ErbB-2 amplification and has proven effective in 20% of
these patients. Problems still exist with indeterminate IHC
cases, which need to be solved by FISH (an expensive
method), with a very well-trained pathologist experienced
with HER2 interpretation, as well as with rigorous quality
control programs.

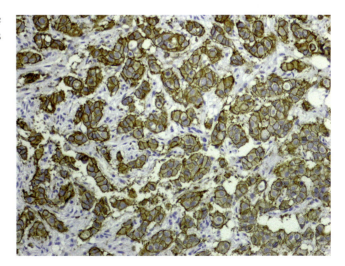

Fig. 18.40 Evaluation of HER2 positivity: score 3+ (strongly positive)
is diagnosed when a strong, complete membrane staining is observed in
more than 10% of the tumor cells

18.3.3 Proliferation Markers

Proliferation markers are represented by: the number of mitoses, Ki-67, and DNA content of tumor cells, and S-phase fraction (both determined by flow cytometry). Flow cytometry determines the DNA content of tumor cells and the histograms obtained indicate the euploidy or aneuploidy of these cells. Aneuploidy is associated with a poor prognosis. The S-phase fraction, which is proportional to the proliferation rate, can also be determined. The percentage of Ki-67 positive tumor cells allows patients to be grouped in those with good prognosis and those with poor prognosis. A high percentage of Ki-67 positive tumor cells advocates an unfavorable prognosis, but on the other hand it is a good indicator for better response to neoadjuvant chemotherapy [57]. Determination of Ki-67, however, reflects a more significant information about cell proliferation than DNA content, and the assessment of Ki-67 has become a major factor in treatment decisions of breast carcinoma patients, and is used in the routine work in some oncology centers as an additional factor for decision-making on adjuvant/neo-adjuvant treatment strategies. Also, in the 2015 St. Gallen Consensus Conference, the majority of panelists voted in favor of taking into account the Ki-67 index in the administration of adjuvant/neo-adjuvant chemotherapy in individual cases because Ki-67 score carries robust prognostic information and has a high value in predicting the benefit of addition of cytotoxic chemotherapy [61]. Ki-67 index is determined by immunohistochemical stains. Despite efforts within the last decade, however, an international cut-off for the low versus high index is still missing and different medical centers use different cutoffs (15%, 17%, 20%, 25%) (Fig. 18.41) [38, 61–66]. Also, breast intratumoral heterogeneity has been noted in breast carcinomas [66]. Since the Ki-67 index value could have an impact on clinical decisions, it is mandatory to evaluate the whole specimen and not only the core biopsy specimen, and to correlate it with the mitotic count.

18.3.4 Other Markers

Other markers such as overexpression of *p53* can be demonstrated by immunohistochemical methods in breast carcinoma, and its presence correlates with a poor prognosis. However, evaluation of p53 is not recommended for evaluation of breast carcinoma in routine practice. More recently, genomic, and expression microarray technology has been used to classify breast cancer patients into those with good versus worse prognosis. There are several commercial *multiparameter gene expression analysis tools* (like Oncotype DX, which is done on paraffin sections, or Mamma Print, which is done on fresh tissue) which are discussed in Chap. 19 of this book [67]. Also, several prospective clinical trials (like Tailorx, ONCOTYPE DX, MINDACT) have investigated the usefulness of these tests in the management of patients with breast cancer [66–73].

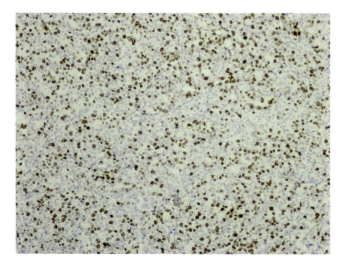

Fig. 18.41 High Ki67 index: more than 70% of the tumor cells are positive with variable intensity for Ki67 in this case

References

1. Wallack MK, Wolf JA Jr, Bedwinek J, Denes AE, Glasgow G, Kumar B, et al. Gestational carcinoma of the female breast. Curr Probl Cancer. 1983;7(9):1–58.
2. Petrek JA. Breast cancer during pregnancy. Cancer. 1994;74:518–27.
3. Petrek JA, Dukoff R, Rogatko A. Prognosis of pregnancy-associated breast cancer. Cancer. 1991;67:869–72.
4. Ruiz R, Herrero C, Strasser-Weippl K, Touya D, St Louis J, Bukowski A, et al. Epidemiology and pathophysiology of pregnancy-associated breast cancer. A review. Breast. 2017;35:136–41.
5. Fisher ER, Fisher B, Sass R, Wickerham L. Pathologic findings from the national surgical adjuvant breast project (protocol no 4). XI. Bilateral breast cancer. Cancer. 1984;54:3002–11.
6. Haagensen CD. Diseases of the breast. 2nd ed. Philadelphia, PA: WB Saunders; 1971. p. 449–58.
7. Leis HP Jr. Managing the remaining breast. Cancer. 1980;46:1026–30.
8. Robbins GF, Berg JW. Bilateral primary breast cancers; a prospective clinicopathological study. Cancer. 1964;17:1501–27.
9. Wanebo HJ, Senofsky GM, Fechner RE, Kaiser D, Lynn S, Paradies J. Bilateral breast cancer. Risk reduction by contralateral biopsy. Ann Surg. 1985;201:667–77.
10. Karakas Y, Kertemen N, Lacin S, Aslan A, Demir M, Ates O, et al. Comparison of prognosis and clinical features between synchronous bilateral and unilateral breast cases. JBUON. 2017;22(3):623–7.
11. Katz A, Strom EA, Buchholtz TA, Theriault R, Singletary SE, McNeese MD. The influence of pathologic tumor characteristics on locoregional recurrence rates following mastectomy. Int J Radiat Oncol Biol Phys. 2001;50(3):735–42.
12. Yerushalmi R, Kennecke H, Woods R, Olivotto IA, Speers C Gelmon KA. Does multicentric/multifocal breast cancer differ from unifocal breast cancer? An analysis of survival and contralateral breast cancer incidence. Breast Cancer Res Treat. 2009;117(2):365–70.
13. Tot T. The role of large-format histopathology in assessing subgross morphological prognostic parameters: a single institution report of 1000 consecutive breast cancer cases. Int J Breast Cancer. 2012;2012:395415.
14. Fish EB, Chapman JA, Link MA. Assessment of tumor size for multifocal primary breast cancer. Ann Surg Oncol. 1998;5:442–6.
15. Joergensen LE, Gunnarsdottir KA, Lanng C, Moeller S, Rasmussen BB. Multifocality as a prognostic factor in breast cancer patients registered in Danish Breast Cancer Cooperative Group (DBCG) 1996–2001. Breast. 2008;17:587–91.
16. Pedersen L, Gunnarsdottir KA, Rasmussen BB, Moeller S, Lanng C. The prognostic influence of multifocality in breast cancer patients. Breast. 2004;13:188–93.
17. Tot T. Clinical relevance of the distribution of the lesions in 500 consecutive breast cancer cases documented in large-format histologic sections. Cancer. 2007;110(11):2551–60.
18. Edge SB, Byrd DR, Compton CC, Fritz AG, Greene FL, Trotti AIII, et al. AJCC cancer staging manual, vol. 7. New York, NY: Springer; 2010.
19. Sobin LH, Gospodarowicz MK, Wittekind C, editors. TNM classification of malignant tumors 7. Oxford: Wiley-Blackwell; 2009.
20. Boros M, Marian C, Moldovan C, Stolnicu S. Morphological heterogeneity of the simultaneous ipsilateral invasive tumor foci in breast carcinoma: a retrospective study of 418 cases of carcinomas. Pathol Res Pract. 2012;208(10):604–9.
21. Boros M, Ilyes A, Nechifor Boila A, Moldovan C, Eniu A, Stolnicu S. Morphologic and molecular subtype status of individual tumor foci in multiple breast carcinoma. A study of 155 cases with analysis of 463 tumor foci. Hum Pathol. 2014;45(2):409–16.
22. Boros M, Voidazan S, Moldovan C, Georgescu R, Toganel C, Moncea D, et al. Clinical implications of multifocality as a prognostic factor in breast carcinoma: a multivariate analysis study comprising 460 cases. Int J Clin Exp Med. 2015;8(6):9839–46.
23. Tavassoli FA. Pathology of the breast. 2. Appleton and Lange: Stamford, CT; 1999.
24. Lakhani SR, Ellis IO, Schnitt S, Tan PH, van de Vijver MJ. World Health Organization classification of tumors of the breast. 4th ed. Lyon: IARC Press; 2012. p. 10–71.
25. Ellis IO, Galea M, Broughton N, Locker A, Blamey RW, Elston CW. Pathological prognosis factors in breast carcinoma. II. Histologic type. Relationship with survival in a large study with long-term follow-up. Histopathology. 1992;20:479–89.
26. Elston CW, Ellis IO. Pathological prognostic factors in breast cancer. I. The value of histological grade in breast cancer: experience from a large study with long-term follow-up. Histopathology. 1991;19:403–10.
27. Roylance R, Gorman P, Harris W, Liebmann R, Barnes D, Hanby A, et al. Comparative genomic hybridization of breast tumors stratified by histological grade reveals new insights into the biological progression of breast cancer. Cancer. 1999;59:1433–6.
28. Sotiriou C, Wirapati P, Loi S, Harris A, Fox S, Smeds J, et al. Gene expression profiling in breast cancer: understanding the molecular basis of histologic grade to improve prognosis. J Natl Cancer Inst. 2006;98:262–72.
29. Ellis IO, Elston CW. Histologic grade. In: O'Malley FP, Pinder SE, Mulligan AM, editors. Breast pathology. Philadelphia, PA: Elsevier; 2006.
30. Ro JY, Silva EG, Gallager HS. Adenoid cystic carcinoma of the breast. Hum Pathol. 1987;18(12):1276–81.
31. Rosen PP. Adenoid cystic carcinoma of the breast. A morphologically heterogeneous neoplasm. Pathol Annu. 1989;24Pt2:237–54.
32. Pinder SE, Ellis IO, Galea M, O'Rourke S, Blamey RW, Elston CW. Pathological prognostic factors in breast cancer. III. Vascular invasion: relationship with recurrence and survival in a large series with long-term follow-up. Histopathology. 1994;24:41–7.
33. Carlomagno C, Perrone F, Lauria R, de Laurentiis M, Gallo C, Morabito A, et al. Prognostic significance of necrosis, elastosis, fibrosis and inflammatory cell reaction in operable breast cancer. Oncology. 1995;52:272–7.
34. Ishihara A, Tsuda H, Kitagawa K, Yoneda M, Shiraishi T. Morphological characteristics of basal-like subtype of breast carcinoma with special reference to cytopathological features. Breast Cancer. 2009;16(3):179–85.
35. Salgado R, Denkert C, Demaria S, Sirtaine N, Klauschen F, Pruneri G, et al. The evaluation of tumor-infiltrating lymphocytes (TILs) in breast cancer: recommendations by an International TILs Working Group 2014. Ann Oncol. 2015;26:259–71.
36. Adams S, Gray RJ, Demaria S, Goldstein L, Perez EA, Lawrence N, et al. Prognostic value of tumor-infiltrating lymphocytes in triple-negative breast cancers from two phase III randomized adjuvant breast cancer trials. ECOG 2197 and ECOG 1199. J Clin Oncol. 2014;32(27):2959–66.
37. Loi S, Michiels S, Salgado R, Sirtaine N, Jose V, Fumagalli D, et al. Tumor infiltrating lymphocytes are prognostic in triple negative breast cancer and predictive for trastuzumab benefit in early breast cancer: results from the FinHER trial. Ann Onco. 2014;25:1544–50.
38. Denkert C, Loibl S, Noske A, Roller M, Müller BM, Komor M, et al. Tumor-associated lymphocytes as an independent predictor of response to neoadjuvant chemotherapy in breast cancer. J Clin Oncol. 2010;28:105–13.
39. Schnitt SJ, Connolly JL, Harris JR, Hellman S, Cohen RB. Pathologic predictors of early local recurrence in stage I and II breast cancer treated by primary radiation therapy. Cancer. 1984;53(5):1049–57.
40. Schnitt SJ, Connolly JL, Khettry U, Mazoujian G, Brenner M, Silver B, et al. Pathologic finding on re-excision of the primary site in breast cancer patients considered for treatment by primary radiation therapy. Cancer. 1987;59(4):675–81.
41. NCCN. NCCN clinical practice guideline in oncology (NCCN guidelines). NCCN.org: Breast Cancer; 2017.

42. Houssami N, Macaskill P, Marinovich ML, Dixon JM, Irwig L, Brennan ME, et al. Meta-analysis of the impact of surgical margins on local recurrence in women with early-stage invasive breast cancer treated with breast-conserving therapy. Eur J Cancer. 2010;46(18):3219–32.

43. Moran MS, Schnitt SJ, Giuliano AE, Harris JR, Khan SA, Horton J, et al. Society of Surgical Oncology-American Society for Radiation Oncology consensus guideline on margins for breast-conserving surgery with whole-breast irradiation in stages I and II invasive breast cancer. J Clin Oncol. 2014;32(14):1507–15.

44. Vinh-Hung V, Nguyen NP, Cserni G, Truong P, Woodward W, Verkooijen HM, et al. Prognostic value of nodal ratios in node-positive breast cancer: a compiled update. Future Oncol. 2009;5(10):1585–603.

45. Martin FT, O'Fearraigh C, Hanley C, Curran C, Sweeney KJ, Kerin MJ. The prognostic significance of nodal ratio on breast cancer recurrence and its potential for incorporation in a new prognostic index. Breast J. 2013;19(4):388–93.

46. Wilson RE, Donegan WL, Mettlin C, Natarajan N, Smart CR, Murphy GP. The 1982 national survey of carcinoma of the breast in the United States by the American College of Surgeons. Surg Gynecol Obstet. 1984;159:309–18.

47. Hurvos AG, Hutter RV, Berg JW. Significance of axillary macrometastases and micrometastases in mammary cancer. Ann Surg. 1971;173(1):44–6.

48. Chen SL, Hoehne FM, Giuliano AE. The prognostic significance of micrometastases in breast cancer: a SEER population-based analysis. Ann Surg Oncol. 2007;12:3378–84.

49. Weaver DL. Pathology evaluation of sentinel lymph nodes in breast cancer: protocol recommendations and rationale. Mod Pathol. 2010;23(Suppl 2):S26–32.

50. Weaver DL, Ashikaga T, Krag DN, Skelly JM, Anderson SJ, Harlow SP, et al. Effect of occult metastases on survival in node-negative breast cancer. N Engl J Med. 2011;364:412–21.

51. Weaver DL. Sentinel node biopsy and lymph node classification in the 6th edition staging manual. In: O'Malley FP, Pinder SE, Mulligan AM, editors. Breast pathology. Philadelphia, PA: Elsevier; 2006. p. 257.

52. Daien CI, Monnier A, Claudepierre P, Constantin A, Eschard JP, Houvenagel E, et al. Sarcoid-like granulomatosis in patients treated with tumor necrosis factor blockers: 10 cases. Rheumatology (Oxford). 2009;48(8):883–6.

53. Stolnicu S, Preda O, Kinga S, Marian C, Nicolau R, Andrei S, et al. Florid papillary endosalpingiosis of the axillary lymph nodes. Breast J. 2011;17(3):268–72.

54. Takhar AS, Ney A, Patel M, Sharma A. Extramedullary haematopoiesis in axillary lymph nodes following neoadjuvant chemotherapy for locally advanced breast cancer. BMJ Case Rep. 2013;pii:bcr2013008943. https://doi.org/10.1136/bcr-2013-008943.

55. Hoda SA, Resetkova E, Yusuf Y, Cahan A, Rosen PP. Megakaryocytes mimicking metastatic breast carcinoma. Arch Pathol Lab Med. 2002;126(5):618–20.

56. Galea MH, Blamey RW, Elston CE, Ellis IO. The Nottingham prognostic index in primary breast cancer. Breast Cancer Res Treat. 1992;22:207–19.

57. Mohsin SK. Molecular markers in invasive breast cancer. In: O'Malley FP, Pinder SE, Mulligan AM, editors. Breast pathology. Philadelphia, PA: Elsevier; 2006. p. 267.

58. Köninki K, Tanner M, Auvinen A, Isola J. HER2 positive breast cancer: decreasing proportion but stable incidence in Finnish population from 1982 to 2005. Breast Cancer Res. 2009;11:R37.

59. Ménard S, Fortis S, Castiglioni F, Agresti R, Balsari A. HER2 as a prognostic factor in breast cancer. Oncology. 2001;61(Suppl 2):67–72.

60. Wolff AC, Hammond EH, Hicks DG, Dowsett M, McShane LM, Allison KH, et al. Recommendations for human epidermal growth factor receptor 2 testing in breast cancer. American Society of Clinical Oncologu/College of American Pathologists clinical practice guideline update. J Clin Oncol. 2013;31:3997–4013.

61. Coates AS, Winer EP, Goldhirsch A, Gelber RD, Gnant M, Piccart-Gebhart M, et al. Tailoring therapies – improving the management of early breast cancer: St Gallen international expert consensus on the primary therapy of early breast cancer 2015. Ann Oncol. 2015;26(8):1533–46.

62. Dowsett M, Nielsen TO, A'Hern R, Bartlett J, Coombes RC, Cuzick J, et al. Assessment of Ki67 in breast cancer: recommendations from the international Ki67 in breast cancer working group. J Natl Cancer Inst. 2011;103:1656–64.

63. Denkert C, Liobl S, Müller BM, Eidtmann H, Schmitt WD, Eiermann W, et al. Ki67 levels as predictive and prognostic parameters in pretherapeutic breast cancer core biopsies: a translational investigation in the neoadjuvant GeparTrio trial. Ann Oncol. 2013;24:2786–93.

64. Denkert C, Budczies J, von Minckwitz G, Wienert S, Loibl S, Klauschen F. Developing Ki67 as a useful marker. Breast. 2015;24(Suppl 2):S67–72.

65. Polley MY, Leung SC, Gao D, Mastropasqua MG, Zabaglo LA, Bartlett JM, et al. An international study to increase concordance in Ki67 scoring. Mod Pathol. 2015;28(6):778–86.

66. Boros M, Moncea D, Moldovan C, Podoleanu C, Georgescu R, Stolnicu S. Intratumoral heterogeneity for Ki-67 index in invasive breast carcinomas: a study on 131 consecutive cases. Appl Immunohistochem Mol Morphol. 2017;25(5):338–40.

67. van de Vijver MJ, He YD, Van't Veer LJ, Dai H, Hart AA, Voskuil DW, et al. A gene-expression signature as a predictor of survival in breast cancer. N Engl J Med. 2002;347(25):1999–2009.

68. Zujewski JA, Kamin L. Trial assessing individualized options for treatment for breast cancer: the TAILORx trial. Future Oncol. 2008;4(5):603–10.

69. McVeigh TP, Hughes LM, Miller N, Sheehan M, Keane M, Sweeney KJ, et al. The impact of Oncotype DX testing on breast cancer management and chemotherapy prescribing patterns in a tertiary referral center. Eur J Cancer. 2014;50(16):2763–70.

70. Aalders KC, Kuijer A, Straver ME, Slaets L, Litiere S, Viale G, et al. Characterisation of multifocal breast cancer using the 70-gene signature in clinical low-risk patients enrolled in the EORTC 10041/BIG 03-04 MINDACT trial. Eur J Cancer. 2017;79:98–1.

71. Cardoso F, Piccart-Gebhart M, Van't Veer L, Rutgers E, TRANSBIG Consortium. The MINDACT trial: the first prospective clinical validation of a genomic tool. Mol Oncol. 2007;1(3):246–51.

72. Cardoso F, Van't Veer L, Rutgers E, Loi S, Mook S, Piccart-Gebhart MJ. Clinical application of the 70-gene profile: the MINDACT trial. J Clin Oncol. 2008;26(5):729–35.

73. Mook S, Van't Veer L, Rutgers EJ, Piccart-Gebhart MJ, Cardoso F. Individualization of therapy using mammaprint: from development to the MINDACT trial. Cancer Genomics Proteomics. 2007;4(3):147–55.

Basic Molecular Pathology in Breast Carcinoma

19

Maria Comanescu

Breast cancer is a multifactorial heterogeneous disease, reflected in a wide range of phenotypic subsets of tumors with varied degrees of aggressiveness and a significant global impact on women's health. In addition to defining the profiles of breast tumors, it is necessary to identify the individual gene and protein expression aberrations and their impact on the biology of the tumor. Molecular pathology changed the way we think about the classification of breast cancer, by no longer relying on just the histological alterations, but also on their biologic pathways. However, it should be noted that although the identification of breast cancer genes contributes to the detection of precursor lesions and prevention of invasive disease, a correlation between phenotype and genotype is necessary, as the sole assessment of gene alterations is insufficient for the identification of predictive and prognostic factors allowing the application of new and individualized cancer therapies. In conclusion, this chapter focuses on the basic molecular pathology knowledge needed in everyday routine practice.

19.1 Introduction

Diagnosis in breast cancer represents a multidisciplinary effort, combining clinical and imagistic features, histologic and immunohistochemical confirmation, and application of high-throughput technologies aiming to identify molecular targeted agents. The role of the pathologist is to apply in practice the new diagnostic tools to improve patient care (Fig. 19.1).

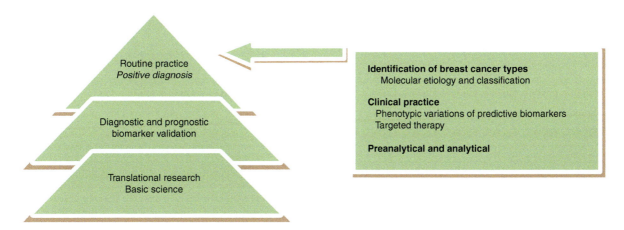

Fig. 19.1 How does molecular pathology fit into everyday practice? The ending point of all research is the development of assays that are robust and reproducible

M. Comanescu, MD, PhD
Department of Pathology, University of Medicine and Pharmacy
"Carol Davila", Bucharest, Romania

© Springer International Publishing AG, part of Springer Nature 2018
S. Stolnicu, I. Alvarado-Cabrero (eds.), *Practical Atlas of Breast Pathology*, https://doi.org/10.1007/978-3-319-93257-6_19

19.2 Identification of Breast Cancer Subtypes

Modern diagnosis is based on:

- Clinical and imagistic features
- Histological and immunohistochemical confirmation
- Identification of molecular targets for a personalized therapy (Fig. 19.2)

The molecular classification of breast carcinoma was first proposed by Perou et al. [1], who divided a set of 1753 genes into four categories based on their gene expression profile:

- Luminal-like
- Basal-like
- Her2/neu positive
- Normal-like

This classification, which first emphasized the division of all breast carcinomas into estrogen (ER)-positive and ER-negative, has been validated by multiple studies, and several subtypes have been added to the initial panel.

Immunohistochemical surrogate algorithms were created to bring this classification into practice.

Different phenotypes of breast cancer reflect different cell types. The neoplastic precursor lesions and breast carcinomas are formed by epithelial cells transformed as a result of genetic and epigenetic changes. The similarity between markers expressed by normal mammary gland cells and those identified in various tumors has resulted in the etymology used in the molecular classification of breast tumors.

As pictured in Fig. 19.3, the adult normal breast epithelium (disease-free) has alveoli lined by:

- Luminal cells (ductal and alveoli luminal cells)—basophile, ER+ and −.
- Basal cells—clear cytoplasm and oval nuclei with conspicuous nucleoli, ER-Cells that are HR receptor positive are different from the proliferating cells (ki67 positive)—the control mechanism of proliferation by ER is indirect [2].

Because cytokeratins (CK) have a constant expression during carcinogenesis, they indicate the cell of origin [3]:

- Luminal cells—low molecular weight CK - CK7, CK8, CK18, CK19
- Basal cells—high molecular weight CK - CK5/6 (Fig. 19.4), CK14, CK17 but also p63 (Fig. 19.5), SMA, CD10, S100

The present guidelines recommend the molecular classification based on several immunohistochemical markers (Fig. 19.6) [4]. Prognosis of patients with ER-positive breast carcinoma depends on the expression of proliferation-related genes [5].

"Immunohistochemistry-Based Molecular Subtyping" is used in practice due to its good correlation with gene expression assays [6], and it has clinical implications (Fig. 19.7).

The basal-like has received special attention due to its aggressive evolution and lack of targeted therapies. This subtype overlaps with the triple negative in ~80% overlap [10]. It has been characterized by the "core basal profile" [12]:

- ER negative, PR negative, HER2 negative
- CK5/6 and/or EGFR positive
- High-grade histologic features
- Pushing borders
- High-grade cytology
- Tumor-infiltrating lymphocytes

Many BRCA1 positive breast cancers are basal-like, but all basal-like cancers are not BRCA1 positive, and CK14 positivity improves the prediction of BRCA1 status [13].

This subgroup also includes several histologic subtypes that are low-grade adenoid cystic carcinoma, apocrine carcinoma, some metaplastic carcinoma variants.

Due to this heterogeneity, it has been divided in four subgroups [14]:

- Luminal androgen receptor subtype (AR positive)
- Mesenchymal subtype (stem-like and claudin low subtype)
- Basal-like immunosuppressed subtype (downregulation of immune regulating pathways)
- Basal-like immunostimulated subtype (upregulation of immune regulating pathways)

Several commercial multiparameter gene expression analysis tools have entered clinical care and are available to patients, such Oncotype DX or Mamma Print. Both of these include hormone receptor and Her2 evaluation:

- Mammaprint Fresh/ FFPE (Agendia, Irvine, CA www. agendia.com)
  - Separates tumors into two categories: high risk and low risk of recurrence
  - Identifies 70 genes by microarray (genes involved in cell cycle, invasion, metastasis, and angiogenesis) [15]
  - Requires fresh tissue as well as formalin-fixed paraffin embedded tissue
- Oncotype dx (Genomic Health, Redwood, CA, www. oncotypedx.com)
  - Separates tumors into three categories: high risk, low risk, and intermediate risk of recurrence
  - Has therapeutic implications
  - Identifies 21 genes by qRT-PCR
  - Requires formalin-fixed paraffin embedded tissue
- ADJUVANT! Online is an online algorithm to determine the benefit of chemotherapy based on clinical and pathologic data (www.adjuvantonline.com)

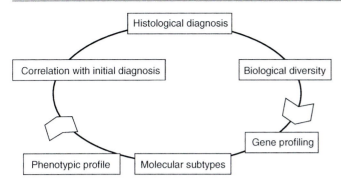

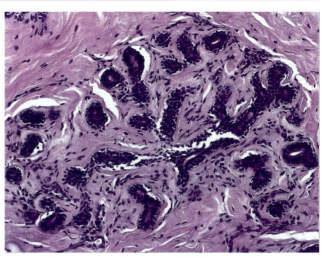

Fig. 19.2 Relationship between histological and molecular subtyping of breast carcinoma. Because all molecular information must be correlated with the clinical and histological findings, the first step is the identification of the morphologic variation of breast carcinoma. Histologically, most breast carcinomas will fall in the "invasive ductal carcinoma, not otherwise specified" type, disregarding the biological diversity. Although this initial "profiling," based on the Nottingham score, is important for therapy, there was a need for more information. The genetic study of breast cancers has brought new prognostic and predictive biomarkers into practice, as well as targeted therapies. On the other hand, molecular profiling is not available in a common pathology department

Fig. 19.3 Normal structure of the breast epithelium

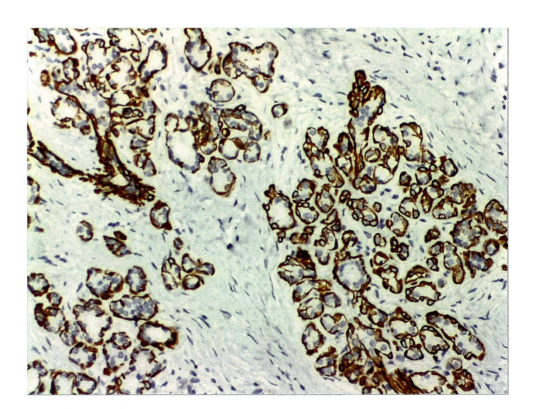

Fig. 19.4 CK5/6 positive in myoepithelial

Fig. 19.5 p63 positive in myoepithelial cells

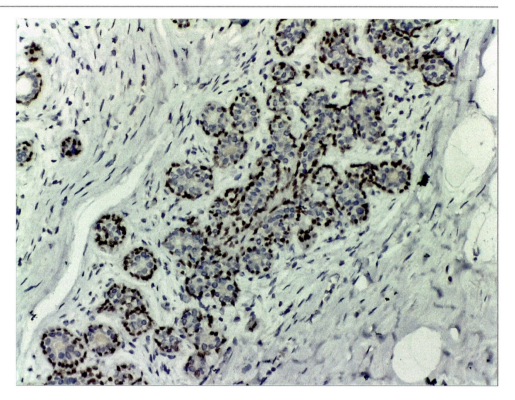

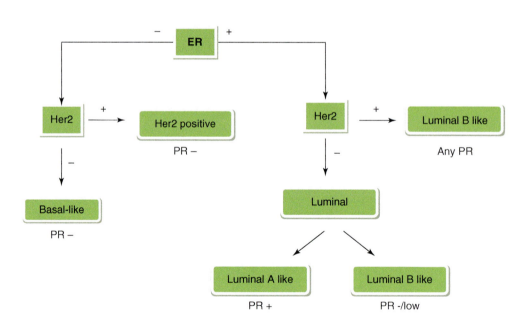

Fig. 19.6 Breast cancer "molecular" classification using immunohistochemical tests

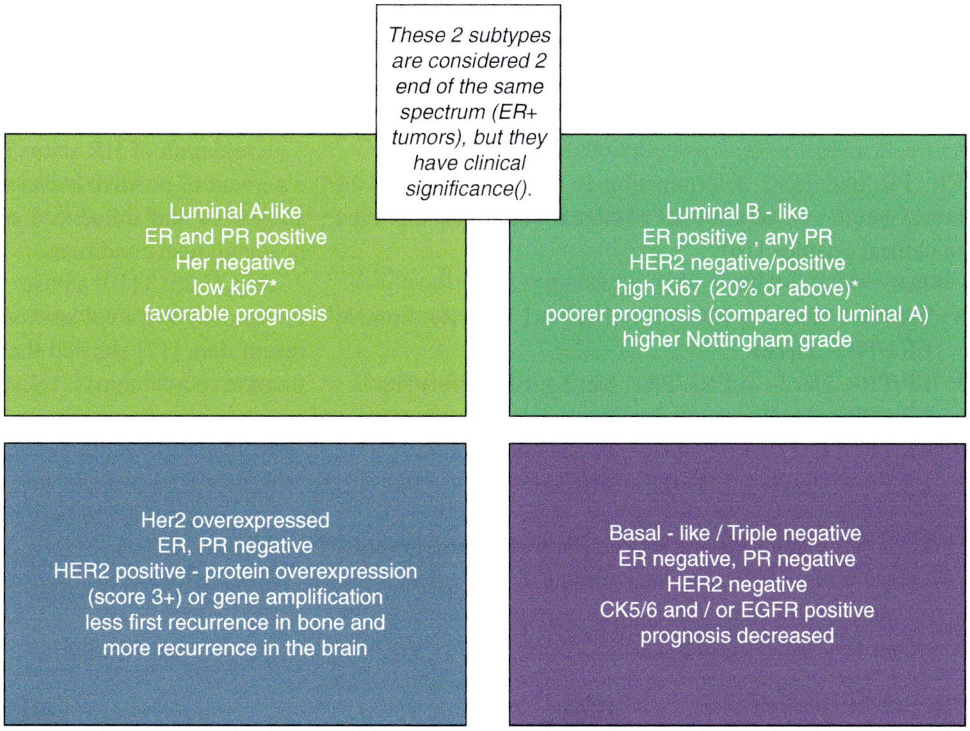

Fig. 19.7 Molecular subtypes of breast carcinomas. *ki 67—a 14% cutoff [9] and a cutoff of greater than 20% [10] per the 2013 St. Gallen Conference [7, 8, 11]

These 2 subtypes are considered 2 end of the same spectrum (ER+ tumors), but they have clinical significance().

Luminal A-like
ER and PR positive
Her negative
low ki67*
favorable prognosis

Luminal B - like
ER positive , any PR
HER2 negative/positive
high Ki67 (20% or above)*
poorer prognosis (compared to luminal A)
higher Nottingham grade

Her2 overexpressed
ER, PR negative
HER2 positive - protein overexpression
(score 3+) or gene amplification
less first recurrence in bone and
more recurrence in the brain

Basal - like / Triple negative
ER negative, PR negative
HER2 negative
CK5/6 and / or EGFR positive
prognosis decreased

Fig. 19.10 Schematic
representation of Her2 gene
and mechanism of Her2
activation [19]

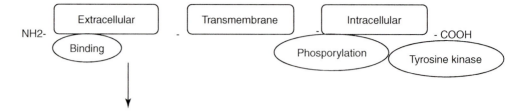

NH2-

Ligands bind to the ectodomain

Receptor dimerisation

Protein kinase activation

Autophosphorylation (self phosphorylation by the kinase)

PI3K/AKt and MAPK pathways - cell proliferation, cell survival, cell migration

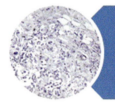

0 negative - no membrane staining or incomplete faint
staining <10% of the invasive tumor cells

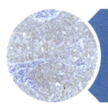

1+ negative incomplete faint/barely perceptible
membrane staining >10% of the invasive tumor cells

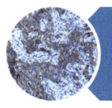

2+ equivocal incomplete and/or weak/moderate
circumferential membrane staining >10% of the invasive
tumor cells OR intense complete and circumferential
membrane staining ≤10% of the invasive tumor cells

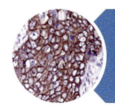

3+ positive - complete, intense circumferential membrane
staining of the invasive tumor cells

Fig. 19.11
Immunohistochemical
algorithm for the evaluation
of Her2 status [20]

Fig. 19.12 CISH
non-amplified

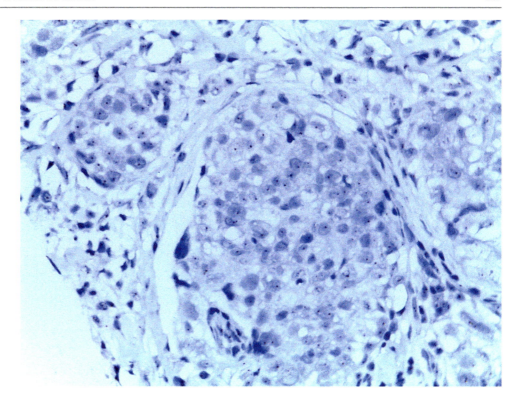

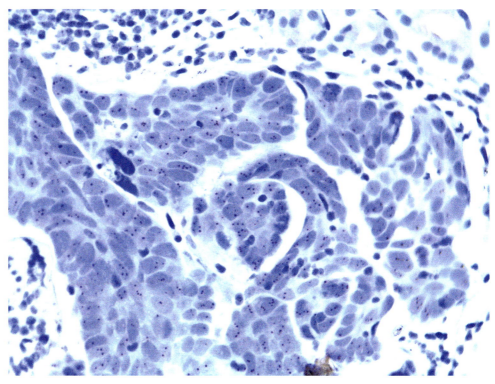

Fig. 19.13 CISH low level
amplification

Fig. 19.14 CISH high level amplification

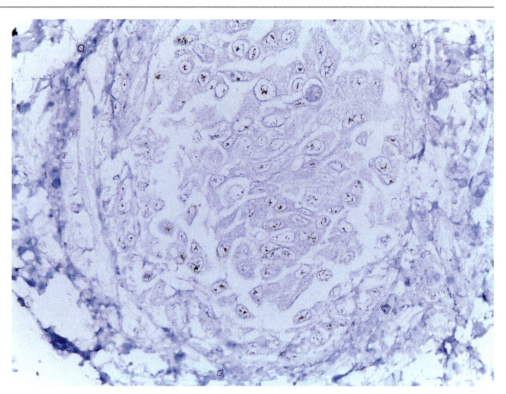

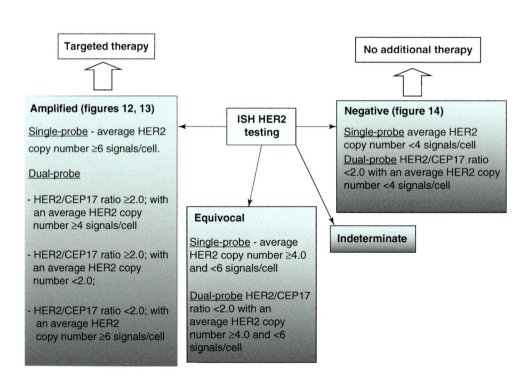

Fig. 19.15 ASCO–CAP HER2 test guideline recommendations (2013) [20]

Fig. 19.16 DISH amplified

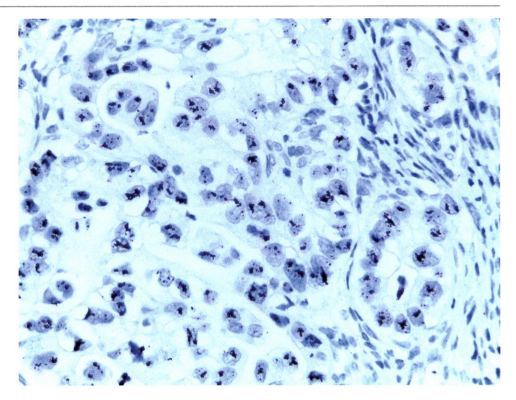

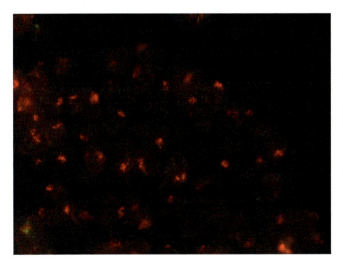

Fig. 19.17 Heterogenous breast cancer—background of Her2 amplified cells with high level amplification (red) together with isolated, intermingled nonamplified cells. Positive reaction

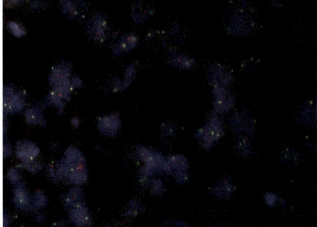

Fig. 19.18 Nonamplified tumor cells. Negative reaction

Fig. 19.19 Diagram showing polysomy and coamplification. (**a**) Polysomy. (**b**) Polysomy and Her2 amplification. (**c**) CEP 17 gain. (**d**) CEP17 gain and Her2 amplification

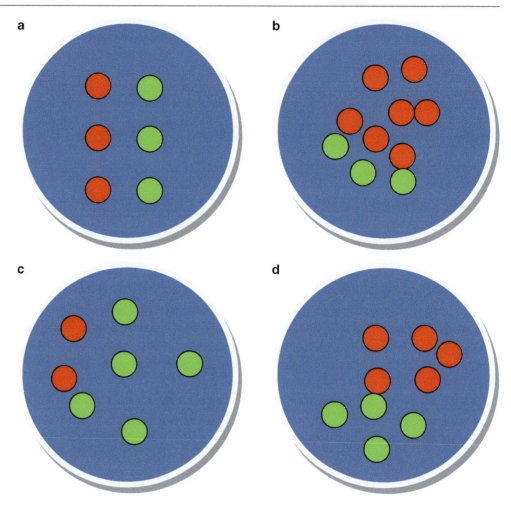

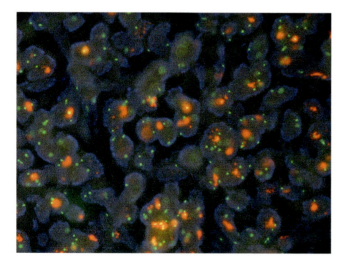

Fig. 19.20 Breast carcinoma. Her 2 amplified cells (red) and CEP 17 gain (green)

19.4 Cancer Predisposition

There are two types of genetic alterations that can initiate carcinogenesis [21]:

- Activation of protooncogenes
- Inactivation of suppressor genes

Around 10% of breast carcinomas are hereditary, tumors caused by mutations in a single high penetrance susceptibility gene, and they are histologically, phenotypically, and genotypically different from sporadic tumors.

The two-hit hypothesis explains the difference between hereditary and sporadic cancers and how mutations in suppressor genes occur [22] (Fig. 19.21).

Genetic/inherited breast cancers can be site-specific and are most commonly associated with BRCA1 or 2 mutations. They can be associated with other carcinomas, like the ones encountered in the Li-Fraumeni or Cowden syndrome.

BRCA1 and BRCA2 defects increase the lifetime risk of developing breast cancer (57% in BRCA1 mutation carriers and 49% in BRCA2 mutation carriers) [23].

The histopathological profile of hereditary tumors is different in the following ways:

- They appear in young women
- They have a higher histological grade

- They have abundant lymphocytic infiltrate
- They have pushing borders
- They are characterized by geographic necrosis
- They are usually triple negative, basal CK positive, high expression of p53
- They cluster with basal-like carcinomas

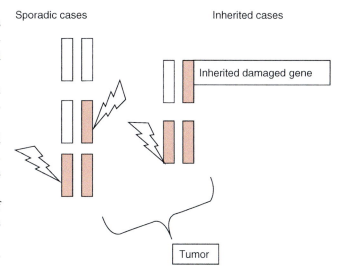

Fig. 19.21 The Knudson two-hit theory. Normally, there are two alleles of each tumor suppressor gene, and both must become inactivated in order to progress to cancer. In inherited cancers, there is already an inactivating mutation in one of the alleles

19.5   Circulating Tumor Cells

Circulating tumor cells (CTC) are migrating tumor cells that detach from the primary tumor and enter the blood stream, where they can suffer multiple transformations. Clinical detection of CTC has a prognostic relevance (Fig. 19.22).

Detection of CTC in the peripheral blood ("liquid biopsy") (Fig. 19.23) can be laborious owing to their very low concentrations, but detection has clinical importance because these cells have been demonstrated to have different genotypic profiles from the primary tumor [25].

CellSearch™ system (Veridex, LLC, Raritan, NJ, USA, www.cellsearchctc.com) is an FDA-approved method that works as an independent predictor of outcome, based on the number of CTC:

- <5 CTCs—more than 18 months survival
- ≥5 CTCs—less than 11 months survival

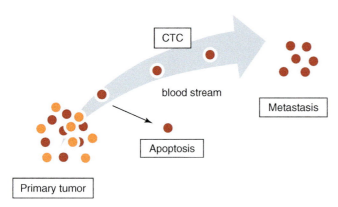

Fig. 19.22 CTC fate. CTC are released from the primary tumor in the blood flow, where they can undergo apoptosis or migrate to secondary sites (metastasis). Some CTC can become dormant [24]

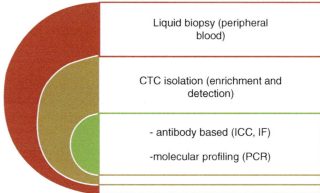

Fig. 19.23 Liquid biopsy is a noninvasive method of identifying CTC in the peripheral blood. Because of their low concentration and admixture with blood cells, special methods of isolation are needed, which generally involve labeling with cytokeratins and antibodies specific for leukocytes

19.6   Exosomes: Does the Future Lie There?

Exosomes (circulating miRNA) are small vesicles derived from cells which can cross the physiological barriers and are involved in breast cancer invasion and metastasis, drug resistance, angiogenesis and has dual effect on the immune system [26]

Conclusions

Although molecular high throughput techniques are not available in routine practice, the tissue needed for such procedures is. These tests require a proper preservation of tissues and special handling when being referred to specialized molecular laboratories (Fig. 19.24)

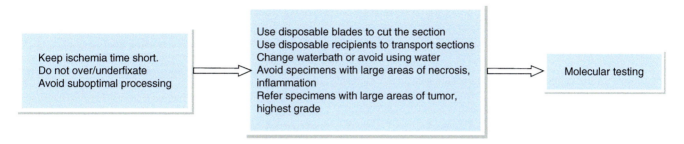

Fig. 19.24   Preparing tissue sections for molecular testing

References

1. Perou CM, Sørlie T, Eisen MB, van de Rijn M, Jeffrey SS, Rees CA, et al. Molecular portraits of human breast tumours. Nature. 2000;406:747–52.
2. Russo J, Yun-Fu H, Xiaoqi Y, Russo IH. Developmental, cellular, and molecular basis of human breast cancer. J Natl Cancer Inst Monogr. 2000;27:17–37.
3. Bannasch P. Cancer diagnosis: early detection. New York, NY: Springer; 1992. p. 170.
4. Coates AS, Winer EP, Goldhirsch A, Gelber RD, Gnant M, Piccart-Gebhart M, et al. Tailoring therapies—improving the management of early breast cancer: St Gallen International expert consensus on the primary therapy of early breast cancer 2015. Ann Oncol. 2015;26(8):1533–46.
5. Reis-Filho JS, Pusztai L. Gene expression profiling in breast cancer: classification, prognostication, and prediction. Lancet. 2011;378:1812–23.
6. Gomez-Wolff R, Garcia H, Ossa C. Impact of "immunohistochemistry-based molecular subtype" on chemo-sensitivity and survival in Hispanic breast cancer patients following neoadjuvant chemotherapy (NAC) [abstract]. In: Proceedings of the 2016 San Antonio breast cancer symposium; San Antonio, TX. Philadelphia (PA): AACR. Cancer Res. 2017;77(4 Suppl):Abstract no. P5-16-20.
7. Cheang MC, Chia SK, Voduc D, Gao D, Leung S, Snider J, et al. Ki67 index, HER2 status, and prognosis of patients with luminal B breast cancer. J Natl Cancer Inst. 2009;101:736–50.
8. Kimberly H, Allison MD. Molecular pathology of breast cancer: what a pathologist needs to know. Am J Clin Pathol. 2012;138(6):770–80.
9. Goldhirsch A, Wood WC, Coates AS, Gelber RD, Thürlimann B, Senn HJ, et al. Strategies for subtypes—dealing with the diversity of breast cancer–highlights of the St. Gallen international expert consensus on the primary therapy of early breast cancer 2011. Ann Oncol. 2011;22(8):1736–47.
10. Goldhirsch A, Winer EP, Coates AS, Gelber RD, Piccart-Gebhart M, Thürlimann B, et al. Personalizing the treatment of women with early breast cancer: highlights of the St. Gallen international expert consensus on the primary therapy of early breast cancer 2013. Ann Oncol. 2013;24(9):2206–23.
11. Vaz-Luis I, Ottesen RA, Hughes ME, Marcom PK, Moy B, Rugo HS, et al. Impact of hormone receptor status on patterns of recurrence and clinical outcomes among patients with human epidermal growth factor-2-positive breast cancer in the National Comprehensive Cancer Network: a prospective cohort study. Breast Cancer Res. 2012;14:R129.
12. Nielsen TO, Hsu FD, Jensen K, Cheang M, Karaca G, Hu Z, et al. Immunohistochemical and clinical characterization of the basal-like subtype of invasive breast carcinoma. Clin Cancer Res. 2004;10(16):5367–74.
13. Lakhani SR, Reis-Filho JS, Fulford L, Penault-Llorca F, van der Vijver M, Parry S, et al. Prediction of BRCA1 status in patients with breast cancer using estrogen receptor and basal phenotype. Clin Cancer Res. 2005;11:5175–80.
14. Burstein MD, Tsimelzon A, Poage GM, Covington KR, Contreras A, Fuqua SA, et al. Comprehensive genomic analysis identifies novel subtypes and targets of triple-negative breast cancer. Clin Cancer Res. 2015;21(7):1688–98.
15. Tian S, Roepman P, Van't Veer LJ, Bernards R, de Snoo F, Glas AM. Biological functions of the genes in the MammaPrint breast cancer profile reflect the hallmarks of cancer. Biomark Insights. 2010;5:129–38.
16. Onitilo AA, Engel JM, Greenlee RT, Mukesh BN. Breast cancer subtypes based on ER/PR and Her2 expression: comparison of clinicopathologic features and survival. Clin Med Res. 2009;7(1–2):4–13.
17. Halilovic A, Bulte J, Jacobs Y, Braam H, van Cleef P, Schlooz-Vries M, et al. Brief fixation enables same-day breast cancer diagnosis with reliable assessment of hormone receptors, E-cadherin and HER2/Neu. J Clin Pathol. 2017;70(9):781–6.
18. Lee EYHP, Muller WJ. Oncogenes and tumor suppressor genes. Cold Spring Harb Perspect Biol. 2010;2(10):a003236.
19. Dillon RL, White DE, Muller WJ. The phosphatidyl inositol 3-kinase signaling network: Implications for human breast cancer. Oncogene. 2007b;26:1338–45.
20. Wolff AC, Hammond ME, Hicks DG, Dowsett M, McShane LM, Allison KH, et al. Recommendations for human epidermal growth factor receptor 2 testing in breast cancer: American Society of Clinical Oncology/College of American Pathologists clinical practice guideline update. J Clin Oncol. 2013;31:3997–4013.
21. Van de Vijver MJ. Molecular genetic changes in breast cancer. In: Weinberg RA, editor. Oncogenes and the molecular origins of cancer. Cold Spring Harbor, NY: Cold Spring Harbor Laboratory Press; 1989. p. 25–60.
22. Chial H. Tumor suppressor (TS) genes and the two-hit hypothesis. Nat Educ. 2008;1(1):177.
23. Chen S, Parmigiani G. Meta-analysis of BRCA1 and BRCA2 penetrance. J Clin Oncol. 2007;25(11):1329–33.
24. Krawczyk N, Hartkopf A, Banys M, Meier-Stiegen F, Staebler A, Wallwiener M, et al. Prognostic relevance of induced and spontaneous apoptosis of disseminated tumor cells in primary breast cancer patients. BMC Cancer. 2014;14:394.
25. Aktas B, Kasimir-Bauer S, Müller V, Janni W, Fehm T, Wallwiener D, et al. Comparison of the HER2, estrogen and progesterone receptor expression profile of primary tumor, metastases and circulating tumor cells in metastatic breast cancer patients. BMC Cancer. 2016;16:522.
26. Wu CY, Du SL, Zhang J, Liang AL, Liu YJ. Exosomes and breast cancer: a comprehensive review of novel therapeutic strategies from diagnosis to treatment. Cancer Gene Ther. 2017;24:6–12.

Morphologic Changes Induced by the Oncologic Treatment for Breast Carcinoma (Chemotherapy, Radiotherapy, Hormonal Therapy)

20

Aziza Nassar

Neoadjuvant treatment has become a standard of care for selected high-risk breast cancers including tumors ≥2 cm and for locally advanced unresectable disease. Neoadjuvant chemotherapy (NAC) offers many advantages, including reducing the tumor size and potentially making patients candidates for breast conservation therapy (BCT), as well as allowing early assessment of response to chemotherapy treatment [1–3]. The main advantage of neoadjuvant chemotherapy is in shrinking tumors, which makes inoperable tumors amenable to surgery and allows better outcomes for patients [4–7]. NAC also provides information on tumor response to specific chemotherapeutic agents, and it provides data for investigating molecular determinants of chemotherapeutic response [8–10]. Pathologic complete response (pCR) provides an early surrogate marker of long-term survival, marking a benefit from chemotherapeutic treatment [4–7]. pCR is noted in only 10–20% of patients who were subjected to NAC [11]. There are several predictors of response to preoperative chemotherapy, including both clinical and pathologic variables such as estrogen-receptor negative (ER-) status, high-grade tumor, high proliferative activity, HER2 amplification, negative lymph node status, and smaller tumor size, among others [1, 4, 7, 12–16]. Histologic subtype also determines the response of the tumor to NAC; for example, lobular cancers do not respond well to NAC as compared to ductal cancers [2, 5, 8, 16, 17].

Studies have shown that the pathologic response rate varies from 15% to 30% depending on the tumor and type of chemotherapeutic agent used [5, 8, 18]. Therefore there is a recognized need for pre-treatment core biopsy to confirm the presence of cancer and to establish the hormonal receptors (ER and PR) and HER2 status of the primary cancer before treatment. It is also important to determine the pathologic features (grade, subtype, necrosis, lymphovascular invasion [LVI], etc.), since grade and receptor status can alter later treatment [3]. In addition, the degree of lymph node involvement following neoadjuvant chemotherapy is the strongest predictor of subsequent relapse. Therefore, axillary sentinel lymph node biopsy (fine-needle aspiration biopsy, core-needle biopsy, and excisional biopsy) is essential before neoadjuvant therapy, because 23–40% of patients with positive axillary node before NAC will become completely node-negative after induction chemotherapy [3, 8]. Clinical response to neoadjuvant therapy is preferably supported by mammographic assessment, ultrasound, and magnetic resonance imaging (MRI) [3]. The pathologic response in patients undergoing neoadjuvant chemotherapy usually represents eradication of the disease in both the breast and axillary lymph nodes (pCR; ypT0N0). However, in most instances, residual invasive and in situ disease may be identifiable following surgery. The assessment of residual disease burden is therefore of paramount importance.

A. Nassar, MD, MPH
Pathology and Laboratory Medicine, Mayo Clinic,
Jacksonville, FL, USA
e-mail: nassar.aziza@mayo.edu

© Springer International Publishing AG, part of Springer Nature 2018
S. Stolnicu, I. Alvarado-Cabrero (eds.), *Practical Atlas of Breast Pathology*, https://doi.org/10.1007/978-3-319-93257-6_20

20.1   Radiological and Macroscopic/ Gross Changes

20.1.1   Radiologic Changes

The establishment of residual tumor size is important in planning initial treatment and monitoring the treatment response. The published results of post-NAC clinical assessment and pathological findings are heterogeneous [9]. The accuracy of MRI in predicting post-NAC tumor size was lower for hormone receptor positive (HR+) breast cancers than for HER2+ or triple-negative breast cancers [19]. Both clinical physical examination (PE) and ultrasound (US) are associated significantly with the final histology. However, PE shows slightly better results than the US [16].

The limitation of PE is that tumors smaller than 2 cm are sometimes not detectable. In contrast, if a large tumor shows a considerable decrease in size by clinical examination, there could also be remaining small tumor foci with minimal residual disease on pathologic assessment [9]. These small foci, scattered over a relatively large area, could be defined as a residual tumor. This result implies that the clinical diagnosis of complete response (cCR) does not necessarily reflect the pathologic CR. Even if cCR is achieved, it is possible that viable tumor tissue is still present at the primary site in some cases. Magnetic resonance imaging, mammography, and ultrasound (US) cannot diagnose a pCR (ypT0) with sufficient accuracy to replace pathologic diagnosis of the surgical excision specimen (Figs. 20.1 and 20.2) [20]. The false negative rate was highest for the US (24%) followed by MRI (22%) and mammography (19%) [20]. Furthermore, MRI has a relatively high false positive rate of 11% for diagnosing pCR cases [20]. With respect to breast imaging, MRI was found to be the most accurate to evaluate tumor response to NAC [20].

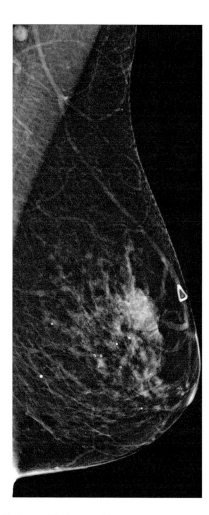

Fig. 20.1 Radiographic image of breast tumor pre-treatment

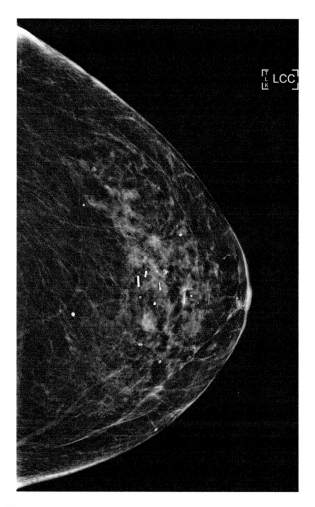

Fig. 20.2 Radiographic image of breast tumor post-treatment

20.1.2 Gross/Macroscopic Changes

Grossly the tumor bed may appear to be an irregular area of rubbery fibrous tissue (Fig. 20.3), and the residual tumor may be recognized as fleshy nodules within the tumor bed [10]. It is generally accepted that three types of information can be used to estimate the probability of pCR: the tumor response after two courses of treatment, molecular markers, and clinical phenotype including hormone receptor status, tumor subtype, grade, and age [1, 2]. Most studies have shown that patients with ER-negative and HER2-amplified breast cancer are more likely to achieve p CR [1, 2, 12, 16, 21]. Large clinical trials of neoadjuvant therapy have demonstrated that patients with pCR have better DFS and OS compared with those with residual tumors [2, 5–7, 12, 16, 21].

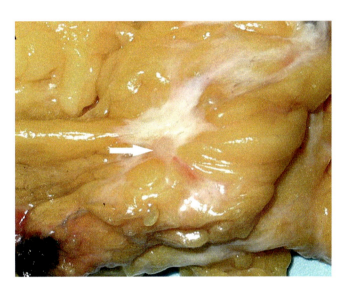

Fig. 20.3 Gross image of residual tumor. Post-treatment lumpectomy specimen with a grossly visible irregular area of fibrotic tumor bed with a small, tan nodule of residual invasive carcinoma

20.2 Histological Changes

The reported histopathologic response rates to preoperative chemotherapy range from 3–46% for complete responses and from 30% to 90% for partial responses [14]. Lee et al. reported that triple negative tumors frequently presented as a single mass in the pre-NAC MRI analyses and had a high overall (including in situ carcinoma) and invasive cancer cellularities in the pre-NAC biopsy specimens [19]. The different tumor subtypes retain their morphology after NAC [19], except for the loss of cellularity. Tumors with negative (HR−) hormonal receptors had higher nuclear and histological grade and denser lymphocytic infiltration than HR+ tumors. The tumor sizes were reduced significantly after NAC, and the HR− tumor will have higher homogenous invasive cancer composition and cancer cellularity than HR+ tumors. The in situ carcinoma and tumor emboli in vascular spaces are relatively resistant to treatment as compared to carcinoma invading the stroma [10].

20.2.1 Tumor Bed: Characteristics

Microscopically, the tumor bed is characterized by an area of hyalinized vascular stroma with stromal edema and fibro-elastosis, without glandular breast ducts and lobules. The stroma is infiltrated by foamy histiocytes, lymphocytes, and hemosiderin pigment (Fig. 20.4) [10, 22, 23]. The tumor bed of HR- tumors had more necrosis and less fibrosis compared to HR+ tumors, suggesting that HR- tumors will have more concentric shrinkage after chemotherapy [19]. Stromal changes, including fibrosis, elastosis, collagenization, hyalinization, micro-calcifications, and neovascularization are observed and reported in many studies (Fig. 20.5). These changes were observed by many authors, but they were not significantly related to response to chemotherapy [2, 8, 10, 22, 23]. Sethi et al. concluded that the changes which are significantly correlated with response are collagenization and giant cell reaction, and their presence was associated with better overall response to chemotherapy [24]. Necrosis was the most common event observed in neoadjuvant chemotherapy treated cases [24, 25].

Documentation of the tumor bed is essential in cases with pCR. The linear dimension of the largest contagious area of invasive carcinoma and the number of invasive foci or number of blocks with invasive carcinoma should be measured for evaluating the tumor size and extent [2, 8–10, 18, 22]. Lee et al. reported that triple-negative breast cancers have a higher correlation with MRI and pathological determined tumor size than other tumor subtypes. They also reported higher aggregation of macrophages in tumor bed after NAC in HR- tumors [19].

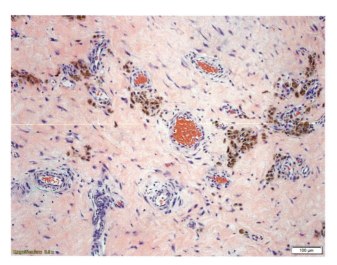

Fig. 20.4 Microscopic image of tumor bed with hemosiderin deposition

20.2.2 Tumor Cytopathic Changes at the Cellular and Stromal Level

When there is marked response, the residual invasive carcinoma is seen as multiple smaller nodules or scattered single tumor cells interspersed within a large, ill-defined tumor bed, which makes the determination of the tumor size difficult [10, 22, 26]. Some carcinomas [10] show cellular level treatment effect, which includes distortion of glandular architecture, cytomegaly, cytoplasmic vacuolization (Fig. 20.6) and occasional eosinophilic changes (Fig. 20.7), nuclear pleomorphism, nuclear enlargement and hyperchromasia (Fig. 20.8), and small nuclei with prominent nucleoli as well as bizarre nuclei (Fig. 20.9) and a decrease in mitotic activity [8, 10, 23]. Occasionally a tumor with relatively small cells may present with large epithelioid features after treatment [23, 26]. Paradoxical "squamoid differentiation," which is often due to prominent apocrine change and anaplastic giant cell formation with focal histiocytic change, can also be seen (Fig. 20.10) [23, 26]. Residual tumor cells are distributed either singly or in clusters (Fig. 20.11). Occasionally, residual tumor clusters may shrink away from the stroma, a feature that might be misinterpreted as lymphovascular invasion (LVI) (Fig. 20.12). In cases with complete response, there can be scattered degenerated single cells with multinucleation, hyperchromasia, and nuclear smudging [10, 22, 23, 26]. In general, the in situ component of the residual tumor shows pleomorphic cells with bizarre nuclei, and occasionally treated DCIS may show replacement of neoplastic cells by macrophages and might even mimic invasive carcinoma, necessitating the use of myoepithelial markers (Fig. 20.13) [8, 10, 22, 26]. In cases with scattered residual foci of invasive carcinoma or DCIS throughout the tumor bed, tumor bed changes at the margin may be predictive of residual tumor in the breast [8, 10, 26].

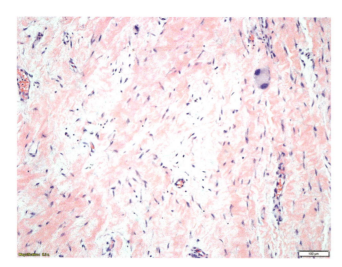

Fig. 20.5 Microscopic image of tumor bed with collagenization and hyalinization

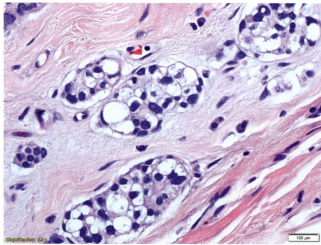

Fig. 20.6 Cytoplasmic vacuolization of residual tumor

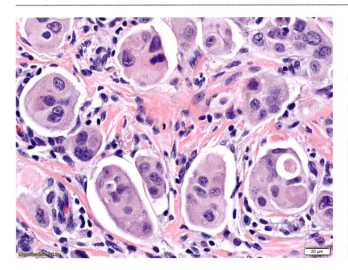

Fig. 20.7 Eosinophilic changes in residual tumor

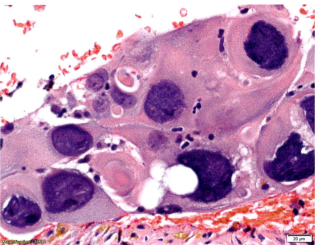

Fig. 20.10 Paradoxical squamoid change in residual tumor

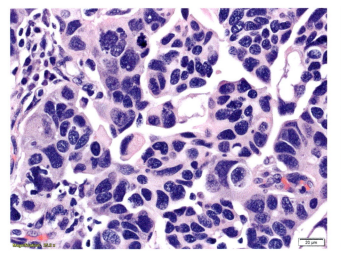

Fig. 20.8 Nuclear changes including nuclear pleomorphism, nuclear enlargement and hyperchromasia

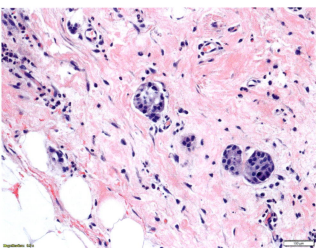

Fig. 20.11 Residual IDC tumor as single cells and clusters

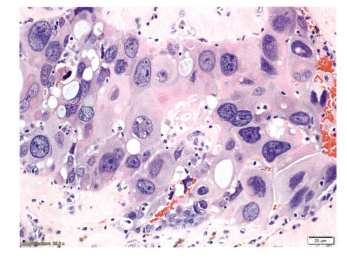

Fig. 20.9 Bizarre nuclei with prominent nucleoli

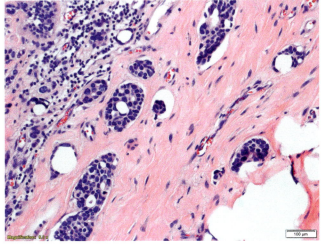

Fig. 20.12 Retraction artifact mimicking lymphovascular invasion

The tumor stromal response varies from elastosis and interstitial calcifications to a peculiar radial necrosis associated with mild lymphocytic infiltration almost mimicking a nodular-fasciitis-like scar [23, 24, 26].

Lymphocytic reaction, the presence of plasma cells and macrophages with the formation of histiocytic giant cell response, has been observed in many studies and may be indicative of host tissue response to the necrobiotic tumor [8, 11, 16, 23–27].

In general, the grade of the tumor may change to a higher or a lower grade as the result of the neoadjuvant chemotherapy (Fig. 20.14). The tumor grades according to the Modified Scarff-Bloom-Richardson Grade (MSBR grade 1–3) remain unchanged in 70% of the cases, but increased in 17% and decreased in 13%, due mainly to changes in mitotic rates [23]. On the other hand, neoadjuvant chemotherapy has no effect on the breast cancer subtype [9, 10, 18, 22].

The histologic type of breast carcinoma does not change after NAC. The cytological features of most carcinomas do not change after treatment except for the decrease in cellularity. Lobular carcinomas might be difficult to detect because these tumors are generally paucicellular with a minimal stromal response even before treatment, and after treatment, the tumor cells become sparse with abundant foamy cytoplasm resembling histiocytes (Fig. 20.15) [10, 22]. Residual invasive ductal carcinomas (or the so-called NST type) may be distributed singly in tumor bed mimicking lobular carcinoma (Fig. 20.16), and mucinous carcinoma may remain as mucinous pools after treatment (Fig. 20.17) [10, 22].

Mucinous patients have also been reported in 7.5% (3/40) of patients after chemotherapy [24]. In one case there was a transformation from ductal (NST type) to metaplastic carci-

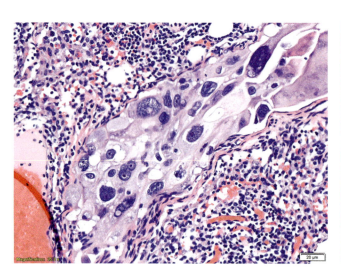

Fig. 20.13 Residual DCIS with bizarre nuclei, vacuolization and eosinophilic change

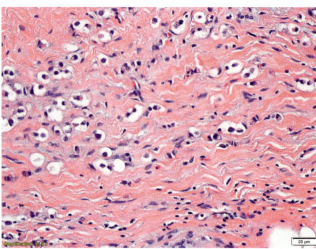

Fig. 20.15 Lobular carcinoma mimicking histiocytes

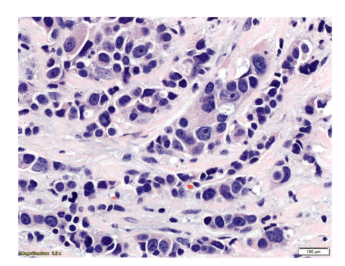

Fig. 20.14 Residual IDC with tumor grade change post-treatment

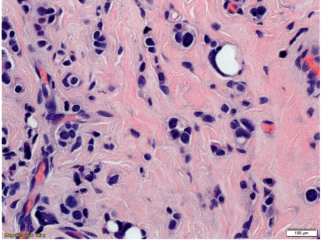

Fig. 20.16 Residual treated IDC mimicking lobular differentiation with single cell filing

noma, and in another case from papillary to ductal (NST type). Complete response was observed in apocrine carcinoma and disappearance of the apocrine component in mixed ductal with apocrine differentiation has also been reported [24]. Honkoop et al. noted a case with a mixed NST-mucinous carcinoma on initial pathologic assessment, and it was only the mucinous component that persisted after chemotherapy [27]. Lobular carcinoma was found to be less responsive to chemotherapy presumptively due to high stromal content [17]. Well-differentiated tubular carcinoma is found to be resistant to chemotherapy as well [28].

20.2.3 Normal/Native Epithelial Changes

The non-tumorous adjacent normal breast parenchyma shows moderate-to-marked sclerosis of basement membranes of both ductal and acinar components and lobular atrophy [8, 10, 26]. The native ductal epithelial cells may show cytological and nuclear enlargement and cytologic atypia (Fig. 20.18). Sometimes it may be impossible to distinguish residual DCIS with treatment changes from posttherapeutic alterations in the native benign breast epithelium and benign breast lesions [8, 10, 26].

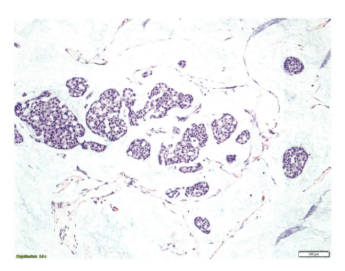

Fig. 20.17 Treated mucinous carcinoma with residual mucinous pools

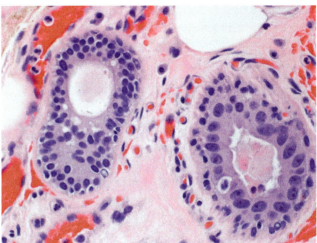

Fig. 20.18 Native ductal epithelium with treatment effect

20.2.4 Lymph Nodes' Treatment Changes

Lymph node status after NAC is a very significant prognostic factor for disease-free survival [5, 29, 30]. The detection rate of sentinel lymph node biopsy after NAC is limited by the effects of NAC, including anatomical alteration or disruption of lymphatics vessels by tumors, inflammation, or fibrosis, and blockage by necrotic and or apoptotic tumor cells. The specific patterns of pathologic findings within treated axillary lymph nodes include fibrosis, atrophy of the lymphoid tissue, the presence of mucin pools, and large aggregates of foamy histiocytes (Fig. 20.19) [8]. Some lymph nodes may show fibrous scarring, and pronounced lymphoid depletion with little or no residual carcinoma; whereas other nodes may have metastases with little evidence of treatment response [8]. Lymph nodes that show a complete response to therapy are often replaced with fibrosis, aggregates of macrophages, or mucin pools without viable tumor cells. Metastases in lymph nodes with partial response usually occur as single or small clusters of tumor cells (Fig. 20.20) sometimes surrounded by thin or thick hyaline fibrosis [8, 10]. Conversely, the metastatic tumor may completely respond to treatment without residual scarring or a small fibrous scar, making it difficult to ascertain prior metastatic involvement [10, 22]. Several studies have reported the association of axillary lymph node (ALN) status and the pathologic primary tumor response to NAC. Kim et al. reported that high histological grade and marked response of primary breast tumor (>80% decrease in primary tumor dimension) were associated with negative conversion of ALN after NAC [31].

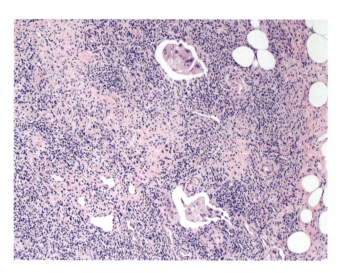

Fig. 20.19 Treated lymph node with stromal changes

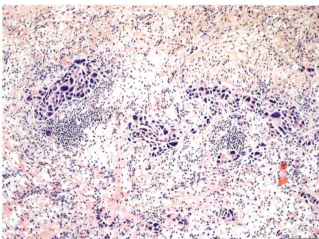

Fig. 20.20 Lymph node with residual tumor clusters with treatment effect, macrophages, and hemosiderin deposition

20.3 Biomarkers' Changes: Hormonal Receptors, HER2 and Ki-67

Changes in tumor markers like ER, PR, and Her2neu occur in a subset of cancers with residual disease after NAC. The discordance rate in untreated tumors between biopsy and the excisional specimen is low. With NAC, the reported discordance rate for hormonal receptors is higher (8–33%) and more frequent in tumors treated with targeted agents, particularly in studies where endocrine agents were used in the neoadjuvant setting. Discordance is likely due to heterogeneity in the tumor. A change from positive to a negative result is of uncertain significance. A change from negative to a positive result is most likely of clinical significance. Changes in HER2 status after non-targeted chemotherapy are uncommon. Loss of HER2 expression occurs in 0–17%, and gain of HER2 expression in 0–12% of treated cases [22].

When NAC includes HER2 targeted therapy, trastuzumab, loss of HER2 expression, is reported to be as high as 32–43% of the treated carcinomas. Loss of HER2 expression in post-treatment tumor is associated with reduced recurrence-free survival [22].

A significant change in proliferation index after treatment has been linked to a survival benefit. Also, post-treatment Ki-67 expression has been shown to be an independent predictor of recurrence-free and overall survival in both HR+ and HR- tumors [22].

20.4 Residual Cancer Burden

The residual cancer burden (RCB) represents the combination of the diameter of the residual primary cancer and the cellularity fraction of the invasive cancer with the diameter of the largest metastasis in the regional lymph nodes and number of positive lymph nodes in a formula termed the RCB index [3, 32].

Using measurements made on routine pathologic material, the RCB index identifies near pCR, especially in subgroups of resistant cancers, and has been validated as a predictor of distant relapse following anthracycline- or taxane-based neoadjuvant chemotherapy [3, 4, 32]. Higher pCR rates are seen more in ER-negative breast cancers than in ER-positive disease in some neoadjuvant trials [3, 5, 16]. Tumor biology has been demonstrated to predict pCR to some extent; e.g., triple-negative breast cancer (TNBC) shows pCR rates of up to 64%; whereas HER2 positive tumors (HER2+) have a response rate of up to 66% [20].

Conclusions

Neoadjuvant chemotherapy before breast cancer surgery is increasingly being used as a treatment modality. Since precise evaluation of histopathological changes is essential to assess the degree of response to therapy, pathologists play a significant role in evaluating tumor response. Therefore, detailed information about the gross findings, histopathological evaluation of the treated tumor, and lymph node changes that occur during neoadjuvant therapy is key to the assessment of neoadjuvant treatment response.

References

1. Tan MC, Al Mushawah F, Gao F, Aft RL, Gillanders WE, Eberlein TJ, et al. Predictors of complete pathological response after neoadjuvant systemic therapy for breast cancer. Am J Surg. 2009;198(4):520–5.
2. Pusztai L. Preoperative systemic chemotherapy and pathologic assessment of response. Pathol Oncol Res. 2008;14(2):169–71.
3. Thompson AM, Moulder-Thompson SL. Neoadjuvant treatment of breast cancer. Ann Oncol. 2012;23(Suppl 10):x231–6.
4. Rouzier R, Pusztai L, Delaloge S, Gonzalez-Angulo AM, Andre F, Hess KR, et al. Nomograms to predict pathologic complete response and metastasis-free survival after preoperative chemotherapy for breast cancer. J Clin Oncol. 2005;23(33):8331–9.
5. Kuerer HM, Newman LA, Smith TL, Ames FC, Hunt KK, Dhingra K, et al. Clinical course of breast cancer patients with complete pathologic primary tumor and axillary lymph node response to doxorubicin-based neoadjuvant chemotherapy. J Clin Oncol. 1999;17(2):460–9.
6. Jacquillat C, Weil M, Baillet F, Borel C, Auclerc G, de Maublanc MA, et al. Results of neoadjuvant chemotherapy and radiation therapy in the breast-conserving treatment of 250 patients with all stages of infiltrative breast cancer. Cancer. 1990;66(1):119–29.
7. Jiralerspong S, Palla SL, Giordano SH, Meric-Bernstam F, Liedtke C, Barnett CM, et al. Metformin and pathologic complete responses to neoadjuvant chemotherapy in diabetic patients with breast cancer. J Clin Oncol. 2009;27(20):3297–302.
8. Alvarado-Cabrero I, Alderete-Vázquez G, Quintal-Ramírez M, Patiño M, Ruíz E. Incidence of pathologic complete response in women treated with preoperative chemotherapy for locally advanced breast cancer: correlation of histology, hormone receptor status, Her2/Neu, and gross pathologic findings. Ann Diagn Pathol. 2009;13(3):151–7.
9. Marchiò C, Maletta F, Annaratone L, Sapino A. The perfect pathology report after neoadjuvant therapy. J Natl Cancer Inst Monogr. 2015;2015(51):47–50.
10. Sahoo S, Lester SC. Pathology of breast carcinomas after neoadjuvant chemotherapy: an overview with recommendations on specimen processing and reporting. Arch Pathol Lab Med. 2009;133(4):633–42.
11. Corben AD, Abi-Raad R, Popa I, Teo CH, Macklin EA, Koerner FC, et al. Pathologic response and long-term follow-up in breast cancer patients treated with neoadjuvant chemotherapy: a comparison between classifications and their practical application. Arch Pathol Lab Med. 2013;137(8):1074–82.

12. von Minckwitz G, Untch M, Blohmer JU, Costa SD, Eidtmann H, Fasching PA, et al. Definition and impact of pathologic complete response on prognosis after neoadjuvant chemotherapy in various intrinsic breast cancer subtypes. J Clin Oncol. 2012;30(15):1796–804.

13. Castaneda CA, Flores R, Rojas K, Flores C, Castillo M, Milla E. Association between mammographic features and response to neoadjuvant chemotherapy in locally advanced breast carcinoma. Hematol Oncol Stem Cell Ther. 2014;7(4):149–56.

14. Wang J, et al. Assessment of histologic features and expression of biomarkers in predicting pathologic response to anthracycline-based neoadjuvant chemotherapy in patients with breast carcinoma. Cancer. 2002;94(12):3107–14.

15. Mathew J, Asgeirsson KS, Cheung KL, Chan S, Dahda A, Robertson JF. Neoadjuvant chemotherapy for locally advanced breast cancer: a review of the literature and future directions. Eur J Surg Oncol. 2009;35(2):113–22.

16. Szentmartoni G, Tokes AM, Tokes T, Somlai K, Szasz AM, Torgyík L, et al. Morphological and pathological response in primary systemic therapy of patients with breast cancer and the prediction of disease free survival: a single center observational study. Croat Med J. 2016;57(2):131–9.

17. Tubiana-Hulin M, Stevens D, Lasry S, Guinebretière JM, Bouita L, Cohen-Solal C, et al. Response to neoadjuvant chemotherapy in lobular and ductal breast carcinomas: a retrospective study on 860 patients from one institution. Ann Oncol. 2006;17(8):1228–33.

18. Masood S. Neoadjuvant chemotherapy in breast cancers. Womens Health (Lond). 2016;12(5):480–91.

19. Lee HJ, Song IH, Seo AN, Lim B, Kim JY, Lee JJ, et al. Correlations between molecular subtypes and pathologic response patterns of breast cancers after neoadjuvant chemotherapy. Ann Surg Oncol. 2015;22(2):392–400.

20. Schaefgen B, Mati M, Sinn HP, Golatta M, Stieber A, Rauch G, et al. Can routine imaging after neoadjuvant chemotherapy in breast cancer predict pathologic complete response? Ann Surg Oncol. 2016;23(3):789–95.

21. Gianni L, Eiermann W, Semiglazov V, Manikhas A, Lluch A, Tjulandin S, et al. Neoadjuvant chemotherapy with trastuzumab followed by adjuvant trastuzumab versus neoadjuvant chemotherapy alone, in patients with HER2-positive locally advanced breast cancer (the NOAH trial): a randomised controlled superiority trial with a parallel HER2-negative cohort. Lancet. 2010;375(9712):377–84.

22. Sahoo S, Lester SC. Pathology considerations in patients treated with neoadjuvant chemotherapy. Surg Pathol Clin. 2012;5(3):749–74.

23. Moll UM, Chumas J. Morphologic effects of neoadjuvant chemotherapy in locally advanced breast cancer. Pathol Res Pract. 1997;193(3):187–96.

24. Sethi D, Sen R, Parshad S, Khetarpal S, Garg M, Sen J. Histopathologic changes following neoadjuvant chemotherapy in locally advanced breast cancer. Indian J Cancer. 2013;50(1):58–64.

25. Pu RT, Schott AF, Sturtz DE, Griffith KA, Kleer CG. Pathologic features of breast cancer associated with complete response to neoadjuvant chemotherapy: importance of tumor necrosis. Am J Surg Pathol. 2005;29(3):354–8.

26. Rajan R, Esteva FJ, Symmans WF. Pathologic changes in breast cancer following neoadjuvant chemotherapy: implications for the assessment of response. Clin Breast Cancer. 2004;5(3):235–8.

27. Honkoop AH, Pinedo HM, De Jong JS, Verheul HM, Linn SC, Hoekman K, et al. Effects of chemotherapy on pathologic and biologic characteristics of locally advanced breast cancer. Am J Clin Pathol. 1997;107(2):211–8.

28. Heil J, Schaefgen B, Sinn P, Richter H, Harcos A, Gomez C, et al. Can a pathological complete response of breast cancer after neoadjuvant chemotherapy be diagnosed by minimal invasive biopsy? Eur J Cancer. 2016;69:142–50.

29. von Minckwitz G. Neoadjuvant chemotherapy in breast cancer-insights from the German experience. Breast Cancer. 2012;19(4):282–8.

30. Rouzier R, Extra JM, Klijanienko J, Falcou MC, Asselain B, Vincent-Salomon A, et al. Incidence and prognostic significance of complete axillary downstaging after primary chemotherapy in breast cancer patients with T1 to T3 tumors and cytologically proven axillary metastatic lymph nodes. J Clin Oncol. 2002;20(5):1304–10.

31. Kim TH, Kang DK, Kim JY, Han S, Jung Y. Histologic grade and decrease in tumor dimensions affect axillary lymph node status after neoadjuvant chemotherapy in breast cancer patients. J Breast Cancer. 2015;18(4):394–9.

32. Symmans WF, Peintinger F, Hatzis C, Rajan R, Kuerer H, Valero V, et al. Measurement of residual breast cancer burden to predict survival after neoadjuvant chemotherapy. J Clin Oncol. 2007;25(28):4414–22.

Evaluation of Residual Tumor After Neoadjuvant Treatment

Aziza Nassar

The primary benefit of neoadjuvant chemotherapy (NAC) is reduction of breast tumor size and conversion of positive lymph nodes into negative ones. In 70–90% of cases, clinical tumor response is evident depending on the type of chemotherapy and number of courses [1]. Several randomized clinical trials have established that both long-term overall and, moreover, disease-free survivals are similar after adjuvant and neoadjuvant chemotherapies (NAC) [1]. The reported overall and disease-free survival for patients who achieved a complete pathological response (pCR) were 75% and 85% respectively, at a median follow-up of nine years, compared to 58% and 73% for patients with residual disease [2]. Regular monitoring of tumor response during neoadjuvant therapy is very critical to evaluate the patient's progress. When the patient's tumor is progressing despite treatment, neoadjuvant therapy has to be discontinued, and prompt referral to surgery or preoperative radiation therapy is necessary [1]. In clinical trials of patients subjected to neoadjuvant chemotherapy, pCR ranged from 6–26% [3]. In contrast, it appears that pCR infrequently occurs with patients treated with neoadjuvant endocrine therapy [3]. The reported rates of pCR for endocrine treatment (tamoxifen and letrozole) ranges from <1.0% to 6.5% [3]. Clinical response does not seem to be a good surrogate marker for pCR, as only 22% of patients with clinical response achieved pCR [4].

21.1 Assessment of Different Variables for Evaluating Pathologic Tumor Response

Complete clinical and pathologic response to therapy can make the pathologist's job more difficult for localizing the tumor bed, so it is necessary to place anatomical markings

(e.g., metallic clips, skin tattoo, etc.) [1]. Pathologic tumor size and nodal status have remained the most powerful predictors of long-term survival after preoperative chemotherapy treatment [1]. Therefore, complete pathologic response (pCR) has been adopted as the primary endpoint for NAC trials because of its consistent association with long-term survival [1, 5–7]. Complete pathologic response should include patients without residual invasive carcinoma in the breast and those with only residual ductal carcinoma in situ (DCIS) (ypT0) [1, 3]. Residual ductal carcinoma in situ after neoadjuvant chemotherapy has no adverse effect on any clinical outcome [1]. When there is no residual invasive cancer in the breast, the number of involved axillary lymph nodes (ALN) is inversely related to survival [1]. High histologic grade and more than 80% decrease in primary tumor dimension is associated with the negative conversion of ALN after NAC [8]. Similarly, Rouzier et al. have found that high histologic grade and more than 50% tumor response to chemotherapy were associated with the negative conversion of ALN after NAC [9].

Three types of information are necessary to estimate the probability of pCR to preoperative chemotherapy. These include (1) clinical tumor response after two courses of treatment; (2) clinical phenotype of the cancer including ER-status, tumor grade, and age; and (3) molecular markers [1, 3]. The discrepancy between pre- and post-treatment for hormonal receptors is reported to be 8–33%, and for HER2, 32% [10].

The tumor bed must be extensively sampled, with one block per centimeter for initial sampling [11]. If the residual tumor is present in the initial sections, additional sampling is not required. If the residual tumor bed is small, the entire area should be submitted. If the residual tumor is >5 cm, then at least five representative sections from the largest cross-sectional area should be submitted.

A. Nassar, MD, MPH
Pathology and Laboratory Medicine, Mayo Clinic,
Jacksonville, FL, USA
e-mail: nassar.aziza@mayo.edu

© Springer International Publishing AG, part of Springer Nature 2018
S. Stolnicu, I. Alvarado-Cabrero (eds.), *Practical Atlas of Breast Pathology*, https://doi.org/10.1007/978-3-319-93257-6_21

21.2 Predictors of Response to Neoadjuvant Chemotherapy

The pathologic response of tumors in the surgical excision specimens is usually divided into three parameters: (1) complete response (pCR) [no residual invasive tumor identified either in the breast or lymph nodes]; (2) partial response (pPR) [small foci of residual tumor and treatment effects identified]; and (3) no response (pNR) [no change in tumor size with no identifiable treatment effect] [12].

Some clinicopathologic features are associated with higher response rates to chemotherapy, and these include younger age, small tumor size, high histologic grade, tumor necrosis, the presence of tumor-associated lymphocytes, ER/PR-negative status, and negative lymph node status [1, 3–5, 9, 10, 13–18] Furthermore, HER2 amplification, triple-negative breast cancers, high Ki-67 percentage expression, as well as high OncotypeDX recurrence score, are associated with higher chemotherapy sensitivity [1, 3, 9, 10, 13, 15, 18]. The cut-off values of 9 for mitoses and 18% for the Ki-67 proliferative index was found to be a differentiating factor between non-responders versus partial and complete responders [10].

Several studies have shown that there is a strong association between pathologic response and nodal status, and patients with pCR are more frequently node-negative [3, 13]. Furthermore, changes in tumor size after NAC is also an independent and strong predictor of pathologic response [8, 19]. Patients with a smaller T-size tumor before chemotherapy have a higher rate of pCR [7, 13, 19]. Triple-negative breast cancers (TNBC) are more likely to achieve pCR than non-TNBC (23% versus 10% respectively) [3, 13]. Both TNBC and HER2 + breast tumors are characterized by a high proliferation index, which may account for the increased sensitivity to neoadjuvant chemotherapy [3, 13, 20]. Also, lobular carcinomas have a poor response to neoadjuvant chemotherapy [21, 22].

21.3 Procedures Required Before Starting Neoadjuvant Chemotherapy

It is critical to establish the diagnosis before starting neoadjuvant chemotherapy. A core biopsy should be performed and the following parameters documented: tumor type, tumor grade, presence or absence of necrosis, the presence of lymphocytic infiltrate, and lymphovascular invasion (LVI) [10, 21]. Additionally, a clip or a marker should be placed at the site of the tumor during initial tissue sampling or during the first few cycles of NAC [10, 21]. This clip/marker will make it easier to reliably locate the tumor bed following therapy [10, 21]. In addition, evaluation of biomarkers such as hormonal receptors, HER2, and Ki67 can also be performed on the initial biopsy. The status of the axillary lymph nodes can be evaluated both clinically and radiologically, and sampling of those lymph nodes can be performed using fine-needle aspiration biopsy and/or core-needle biopsy. An excisional biopsy can be performed in clinically negative axillary lymph nodes [10, 21].

21.4   Evaluation of Response to Neoadjuvant Chemotherapy

The response to neoadjuvant chemotherapy can be evaluated using different modalities: clinical physical examination (PE), breast imaging studies, and pathologic examination of post-treatment resected specimens. More recent advanced imaging devices are used to evaluate tumor response, and this includes magnetic resonance imaging (MRI), digital mammography, and positron emission tomography (PET) [10, 21]. Peintinger et al. have found that the overall agreement between predicted and pathologic responses was 53% for PE, 67% for mammography plus ultrasound (US), and 63% for PE plus mammography and US [23]. Szentmártoni et al. have found that both PE- and US-measured clinical remission associated significantly with pathological remission after NAC ($P < 0.001$ and $P = 0.004$, respectively) [18]. The accuracy of MRI in detecting residual disease is reported as high as 80% [19].

Neoadjuvant treatment induces several morphologic changes in the tumor. These changes are different depending on the degree of response, the distribution of the residual tumor, and the degree of treatment effect [10, 21].

The pathologist must have information regarding the pretreatment size and location and the presence of clips or radiologic calcifications marking the tumor. Furthermore, the pathologist must know about the presence or absence of multiple tumors and possible pretreatment involvement of the skin, nipple, and chest wall [10, 21, 24, 25].

The information about the primary tumor size and the location of the tumor prior to therapy is very critical. This information is usually obtained from the radiologic imaging studies, and a specimen radiograph at time of the post-surgical resection can also assist in locating the clip/markers. It is essential to obtain a specimen radiograph in wire-localized biopsies demonstrating the clip or density corresponding to the tumor. Mastectomies should undergo radiography before processing if there is no identifiable palpable mass. In the absence of radiographic images, the surgeon can place a suture at the site of interest, and the pathologist should have a detailed description of the pretreatment tumor location (i.e., quadrant and distance from nipple) [10, 21, 24]. For patients who underwent conservative breast surgery, the specimens should be differentially inked to assess margins in the event a residual tumor is detected during the microscopic examination [11, 24].

Sometimes, specifically after complete response to treatment, it is difficult to identify any grossly visible lesions. Therefore identification of the tumor bed and surrounding tissue is critical to selection of the correct area for tissue sampling and sectioning [10, 21, 24, 25]. The tumor bed may appear as a vague irregular rubbery area that is difficult to distinguish from the normal breast. Sometimes residual carcinoma is present as tan nodules within the tumor bed, and in many instances, the residual tumor is scattered as small foci that are difficult to visualize grossly. Both the tumor bed and any recognizable tumor should be documented, and the relationship to the margins noted. At least one section per centimeter of the pretreatment tumor size is suggested if the tumor bed is large (≥5 cm), or the entire bed could be sampled if it is ≤3 cm [11, 24, 25]. The MD Andrson web site that offers the residual cancer burden calculator (http://www.mdanderson.org/breastcancer_RCB) has some recommendations on tumor sampling [11, 24]. Tumor size is typically easy to measure if there is minimal or no tumor response; however, it becomes challenging when there are isolated tumor cells and clusters of residual tumor. In this scenario, the largest tumor focus or the entire dimension of the tumor should be measured and recorded [10, 21]. The size of the largest contiguous focus and the number of foci of invasive carcinoma are useful pieces of information [11, 24].

In general, smaller tumor sizes are a good prognostic feature, and residual tumors >2 cm are associated with higher rates of locoregional recurrence [10, 21].

Tumor cellularity can be used as a measure of response to therapy, and henceforth it is critical to evaluate the tumor cellularity prior to neoadjuvant therapy in the core-needle biopsy along with the type of stroma (sclerotic vs. edematous). The average tumor cellularity has to be documented after neoadjuvant chemotherapy, as loss of tumor cellularity correlates with better clinical outcome [10, 11, 24–26]. An estimation of the average cellularity over the tumor bed is used in some classification systems for pathologic response. The decrease in tumor cellularity is seen in both chemotherapy and hormonal therapy [11, 24, 25]. After neoadjuvant chemotherapy, tumor cellularity decreased from a median of 40% in core-needle biopsy to 10% in resection specimens ($P < 0.01$). The greatest reduction was observed in the cellularity of residual tumor that measured ≤1 cm (pathologic stage T1a [pT1a] and pT1b tumors) [26]. Similarly, both tumor grade and subtype should be evaluated before and after neoadjuvant chemotherapy, as the tumor grade tends to change following NAT [10, 21, 24].

It is important to find the previous biopsy site changes which are characterized by stromal fibrosis, macrophages, lymphocytes, and occasionally multinucleated giant cell reaction. Similarly, the recognition of the tumor bed is essential, and this is characterized by stromal fibrosis, histiocytic infiltrate, chronic inflammation, necrosis, and calcifications (Fig. 21.1). Sometimes it is hard to distinguish between inflammatory/reactive atypia and residual tumor cells. In these instances, it is helpful to use epithelial markers such as cytokeratin AE1/3 or CK7, and CD68 for histiocytes and myoepithelial markers (p63, smooth muscle myosin heavy chain, calponin, etc.), as deemed necessary. There are some histologic changes in the non-neoplastic breast tissue that can mimic residual tumors such as cytoplasmic and nuclear enlargement and sclerosis of basement membranes (Fig. 21.2) [10, 21].

It appears that DCIS and vascular tumor emboli are relatively resistant to neoadjuvant chemotherapy as compared to invasive carcinoma [10, 21]. Lymph nodes are hard to evaluate post-treatment because of atrophy and fibrosis. All lymph nodes should be thinly sectioned along the long axis and submitted completely for microscopic examination [11, 21, 24]. Assessment of post-treatment lymph nodes may require the use of cytokeratin immunostains to detect residual disease. Recognition of treatment response changes in lymph nodes includes pronounced lymphoid depletion, atrophy, and fibrosis (Fig. 21.3). The presence of tumor response without residual metastases in the lymph nodes is usually associated with a better prognosis [10, 21, 25]. Kuerer et al. showed that patients with incomplete tumor response were more likely to have metastases in ≥4 lymph nodes, compared with patients who had complete primary tumor response (*P* < 0.01) [7].

Studies have shown that there is an 8–33% discrepancy between pre- and post-treatment hormonal receptor status; and up to 32% discordance rate for HER2. Some of these discrepancies are attributed to preanalytical variables such as tissue fixation and processing, laboratory errors, tumor

heterogeneity, and change in tumor biology. The change in the rate of Ki-67 as a proliferation marker is regarded as a marker of response to NAC, particularly in patients with hormone receptor positive tumors who receive endocrine therapy [10, 24].

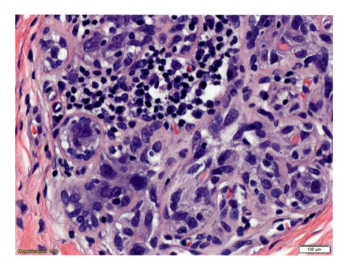

Fig. 21.2 Reactive atypia secondary to treatment in native ductal epithelium

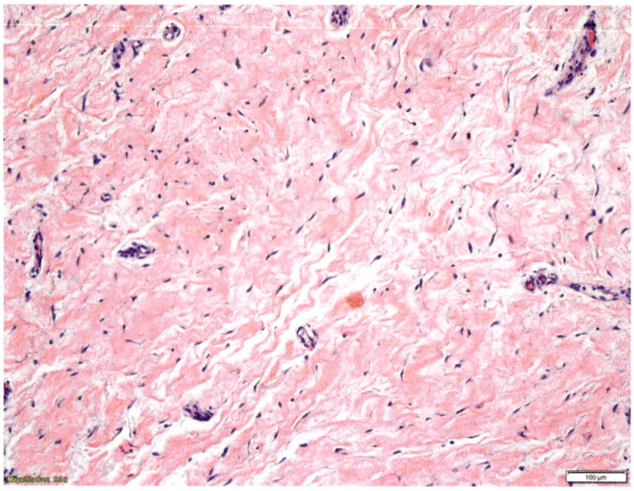

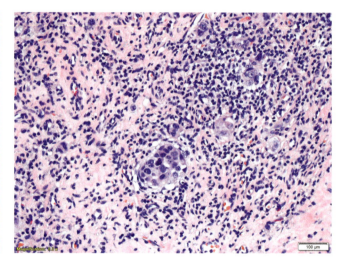

Fig. 21.3 Lymph node showing atrophy and fibrosis and residual tumor cell clusters with treatment response

Fig. 21.1 Tumor bed with dense collagenization and hyalinization

21.5 The Components of a Pathology Report

The pathology report should include the size of the tumor bed, tumor size, and extent of the residual tumor, assessment of tumor response to treatment, tumor grade, and tumor cellularity as compared to the primary tumor (Table 21.1). The final pathology report should also document the presence of mitoses, presence of necrosis, lymphovascular invasion, the presence of ductal carcinoma in situ, and the status of the margin with respect to the tumor bed. Ki-67 immunostaining of the tumor to evaluate the viability of the tumor cells can also be performed [10, 21].

The post-treatment tumor size is very critical for assessing residual disease (ypT) and should be estimated based on the combination of radiologic imaging, gross evaluation, and microscopic histologic findings [21]. Some radiologists will mark the area of the tumor before NAC with clips or tattoos, and this is particularly helpful when sampling surgical specimens with pCR [21]. The inclusion of the prefix "yp" for pathologic staging is also required in the pathology report. The final pathology report should also include the number of lymph nodes examined, the number of lymph nodes with metastasis and the size of the largest deposit, the status of tumor response, and the presence or absence of extranodal involvement [10, 21].

Table 21.1 Parameters that need to be documented in the clinical records and pathology reports for accurate evaluation of residual tumor

Variable	Different components that need to be documented	Optional information
Patient's information	• Patient's clinical information (age, distant metastasis) • Radiologic information before and after NAT (size, morphology, and location of the tumor, multifocality, ultrasound examination of the axilla) • NAT treatment details • Accurate histopathological features assessed on core biopsies before NAT	
Gross description	• Documentation of tumor bed—report size in 2 dimensions if possible • Description of macroscopic appearance and measurement of disease extension • If tumor is inconspicuous, it is best to proceed with macroblocks or multiple sampling with mapping	Photographic documentation can be helpful if tumor is inconspicuous
Non-pCR diagnosis	• Size and extent of residual invasive carcinoma: linear dimension of the largest contiguous area or number of invasive foci with the largest focus or number of blocks with invasive carcinoma • Tumor histological type, tumor grade, multifocality • Average tumor cellularity over the entire bed (compare with pretreatment carcinoma if available) • Presence of in situ component and percentage • Presence of lymphovascular invasion • Lymph node assessment (number of lymph nodes with metastasis, size of largest metastasis, presence of extranodal extension and number of metastases with evidence of treatment response and number of lymph nodes with treatment response but without viable tumor cells) • Staging (ypTNM) • Surgical margins with respect to tumor bed, DCIS and invasive carcinoma • Comment on overall response to treatment • Prognostic and predictive markers if sufficient residual carcinoma present	• Necrosis, fibrosis • Grading (modified Scarff-Bloom-Richardson grades 1–3)
pCR diagnosis	• Description of residual in situ lesion (if present) with margin evaluation • Comment on overall response to treatment	Description of changes induced by treatment (fibrosis, necrosis, calcifications) in both the breast and axillary lymph nodes
Categorization of tumor response according to published classification systems	• In the mammary gland • In the axillary lymph nodes	

21.6 Different Classification Systems and Nomograms for Estimating Residual Tumor Burden After Neoadjuvant Chemotherapy

The prognosis of breast cancer patients treated with NAC is influenced by the pretreatment clinical stage, the post-treatment pathologic stage, and lymph node status [11, 24]. Many histopathologic systems have been designed to sub-classify the larger group of patients with partial response (PR). The American Joint Committee on Cancer (AJCC) pretreatment stage is based on imaging findings and pre-treatment core biopsy. If the patient has a pretreatment stage IV disease (distant metastasis, M1), the post-treatment clas-sification does not change, regardless of the response to ther-apy. This staging system is based on the use of standard clinicopathologic parameters post-treatment. Although the criteria for classifying pathologic response have not been standardized, the degree of response to treatment correlates directly with survival. AJCC assigned a post-treatment carci-noma in both the T and N categories, indicated with the pre-fixes "y" and "p," which refer to the pathologic classification. The post-treatment stage relies mainly on tumor size and nodal status. The post-treatment pathologic tumor size (ypT) is based on the largest contagious focus of invasive carci-noma. If there are multiple microscopic foci scattered in the tumor bed, this is designated with a modifier "m." This sys-tem does not consider changes in cellularity and lymphovas-cular invasion [11]. The post-treatment ypN categories are the same as those for untreated tumor (pN). For example, isolated tumor cells (metastases no greater than 0.2 mm or fewer than 200 cells) are classified as ypNo(i+). The most common definitions for pCR includes the absence of both in situ and invasive cancer in the breast and axillary lymph nodes (ypT0 N0), irrespective of ductal carcinoma in situ (DCIS) (ypT0/is N0) and absence of invasive cancer in the breast irrespective of DCIS or lymph node involvement (ypT0/is) [9, 10].

The RCB index is one of the most utilized systems for evaluating residual breast cancer, and it was proposed by Symmans et al. as a good determinant of the extent of resid-ual disease in post-treatment surgical resection specimens of patients with NAC [27]. It provides an accurate surrogate endpoint for patient's survival. Residual cancer can be mea-sured as a continuous variable using the residual cancer bur-den (RCB) calculator, which utilizes several parameters including primary tumor dimensions, cellularity of tumor bed, and axillary nodal burden including the number of posi-tive axillary lymph nodes and diameter of the largest metas-tasis (www.mdanderson.org/breastcancer_RCB) [1, 28]. The RCB system uses residual invasive carcinoma cellularity over the tumor bed, the number of lymph nodes with metas-tasis, and size of largest metastasis combined mathemati-

cally into a continuous index to define four categories of RCB (RCB-0 through RCB-III) [11, 24].

The RCB index was found to be a continuous predictor of disease-free survival (DFS) and to predict relapse more strongly than the AJCC stage [4, 27]. RCB was noted to be an independent predictive variable for event-free survival (HR 1.59; 95% CI: 1.04–2.43), but pCR was not (HR 0.90; 95% CI: 0.52–1.57) [4]. Higher RCB scores correlated sig-nificantly with lower event-free survival and showed a trend toward a lower rate of overall survival [4, 27].

The original National Surgical Adjuvant Breast and Bowel Project (NSABP) B18 trial recognized two catego-ries: pCR, defined as no histologic evidence of residual inva-sive tumor cells in the breast, and pINV, indicating histologic evidence of residual invasive carcinoma cells. Miller-Payne grading provides a 5-step response scale based on tumor cel-lularity in the excision/mastectomy specimen as compared with the pre-treatment core biopsy. In this system, a grade 4 response (almost complete response) had a worse prognosis than a grade 5 (pCR), providing evidence that pCR should be kept as a separate group. However, this system does not account for response in lymph nodes for classification of pCR or the presence of lymphovascular invasion (LVI) or tumor size [11, 24, 29]. Sataloff et al. proposed a dual 4-tier system, separately assessing residual tumor and treatment in primary tumor site and lymph nodes, but this system does not include LVI [28, 30].

The Residual Disease in Breast and Nodes (RDBN) uses the formula RDBN = 0.2× tumor size (cm) + Modified Scarff – Bloom-Richardson Grade (MSBR grade 1–3) + lymph node stage (0–3), which takes into account tumor size, histologic grade and lymph node stage to deter-mine the levels of response. The modified Nottingham prog-nostic index developed for untreated carcinomas has been shown to have prognostic significance for post-treatment carcinomas. The prognostic index is divided into three groups based on total score [28].

Chevallier et al. devised a 4-step algorithm to grade response in both breast and lymph nodes (class I: no residual carcinoma in breast or lymph nodes; class II: only in situ car-cinoma remaining, nodes are negative; class III: invasive car-cinoma with stromal fibrosis; and class IV: no or few modifications in the tumor). Both classes I and II are consid-ered as pCR [28, 31]. Different nomograms were further developed to evaluate tumor response to neoadjuvant chemo-therapy. One is Rouzier's nomogram, which was developed to predict complete pathologic response (pCR) and metastasis-free survival after preoperative chemotherapy for breast can-cer [32]. The Rouzier nomogram estimates the probability of complete pathologic response (pCR) by integrating clinical TNM stage at diagnosis, ER status, modified SBR histologic grade, age, and the number of chemotherapy courses. The prediction of the model showed an AUC of 0.76 [32].

References

1. Pusztai L. Preoperative systemic chemotherapy and pathologic assessment of response. Pathol Oncol Res. 2008;14(2):169–71.
2. Wolmark N, Wang J, Mamounas E, Bryant J, Fisher B. Preoperative chemotherapy in patients with operable breast cancer: nine-year results from National Surgical Adjuvant Breast and Bowel Project B-18. J Natl Cancer Inst Monogr. 2001;30:96–102.
3. Tan MC, Al Mushawah F, Gao F, Aft RL, Gillanders WE, Eberlein TJ, et al. Predictors of complete pathological response after neoadjuvant systemic therapy for breast cancer. Am J Surg. 2009;198(4):520–5.
4. Nahleh Z, Sivasubramaniam D, Dhaliwal S, Sundarajan V, Komrokji R. Residual cancer burden in locally advanced breast cancer: a superior tool. Curr Oncol. 2008;15(6):271–8.
5. Jiralerspong S, Palla SL, Giordano SH, Meric-Bernstam F, Liedtke C, Barnett CM, et al. Metformin and pathologic complete responses to neoadjuvant chemotherapy in diabetic patients with breast cancer. J Clin Oncol. 2009;27(20):3297–302.
6. Jacquillat C, Weil M, Baillet F, Borel C, Auclerc G, de Maublanc MA, et al. Results of neoadjuvant chemotherapy and radiation therapy in the breast-conserving treatment of 250 patients with all stages of infiltrative breast cancer. Cancer. 1990;66(1):119–29.
7. Kuerer HM, Newman LA, Smith TL, Ames FC, Hunt KK, Dhingra K, et al. Clinical course of breast cancer patients with complete pathologic primary tumor and axillary lymph node response to doxorubicin-based neoadjuvant chemotherapy. J Clin Oncol. 1999;17(2):460–9.
8. Kim TH, Kang DK, Kim JY, Han S, Jung Y. Histologic grade and decrease in tumor dimensions affect axillary lymph node status after neoadjuvant chemotherapy in breast cancer patients. J Breast Cancer. 2015;18(4):394–9.
9. Rouzier R, Extra JM, Klijanienko J, Falcou MC, Asselain B, Vincent-Salomon A, et al. Incidence and prognostic significance of complete axillary downstaging after primary chemotherapy in breast cancer patients with T1 to T3 tumors and cytologically proven axillary metastatic lymph nodes. J Clin Oncol. 2002;20(5):1304–10.
10. Masood S. Neoadjuvant chemotherapy in breast cancers. Womens Health (Lond). 2016;12(5):480–91.
11. Sahoo S, Lester SC. Pathology of breast carcinomas after neoadjuvant chemotherapy: an overview with recommendations on specimen processing and reporting. Arch Pathol Lab Med. 2009;133(4):633–42.
12. Alvarado-Cabrero I, Alderete-Vázquez G, Quintal-Ramírez M, Patiño M, Ruíz E. Incidence of pathologic complete response in women treated with preoperative chemotherapy for locally advanced breast cancer: correlation of histology, hormone receptor status, Her2/Neu, and gross pathologic findings. Ann Diagn Pathol. 2009;13(3):151–7.
13. von Minckwitz G, Untch M, Blohmer JU, Costa SD, Eidtmann H, Fasching PA, et al. Definition and impact of pathologic complete response on prognosis after neoadjuvant chemotherapy in various intrinsic breast cancer subtypes. J Clin Oncol. 2012;30(15):1796–804.
14. Castaneda CA, Flores R, Rojas K, Flores C, Castillo M, Milla E. Association between mammographic features and response to neoadjuvant chemotherapy in locally advanced breast carcinoma. Hematol Oncol Stem Cell Ther. 2014;7(4):149–56.
15. Wang J, Buchholz TA, Middleton LP, Allred DC, Tucker SL, Kuerer HM, et al. Assessment of histologic features and expression of biomarkers in predicting pathologic response to anthracycline-based neoadjuvant chemotherapy in patients with breast carcinoma. Cancer. 2002;94(12):3107–14.
16. Mathew J, Asgeirsson KS, Cheung KL, Chan S, Dahda A, Robertson JF. Neoadjuvant chemotherapy for locally advanced breast cancer: a review of the literature and future directions. Eur J Surg Oncol. 2009;35(2):113–22.
17. Pu RT, Schott AF, Sturtz DE, Griffith KA, Kleer CG. Pathologic features of breast cancer associated with complete response to neoadjuvant chemotherapy: importance of tumor necrosis. Am J Surg Pathol. 2005;29(3):354–8.
18. Szentmartoni G, Tokes AM, Tokes T, Somlai K, Szasz AM, Torgyík L, et al. Morphological and pathological response in primary systemic therapy of patients with breast cancer and the prediction of disease free survival: a single center observational study. Croat Med J. 2016;57(2):131–9.
19. Fangberget A, Nilsen LB, Hole KH, Holmen MM, Engebraaten O, Naume B, et al. Neoadjuvant chemotherapy in breast cancer-response evaluation and prediction of response to treatment using dynamic contrast-enhanced and diffusion-weighted MR imaging. Eur Radiol. 2011;21(6):1188–99.
20. Gianni L, Eiermann W, Semiglazov V, Manikhas A, Lluch A, Tjulandin S, et al. Neoadjuvant chemotherapy with trastuzumab followed by adjuvant trastuzumab versus neoadjuvant chemotherapy alone, in patients with HER2-positive locally advanced breast cancer (the NOAH trial): a randomised controlled superiority trial with a parallel HER2-negative cohort. Lancet. 2010;375(9712): 377–84.
21. Marchio C, Maletta F, Annaratone L, Sapino A. The perfect pathology report after neoadjuvant therapy. J Natl Cancer Inst Monogr. 2015;2015(51):47–50.
22. Tubiana-Hulin M, Stevens D, Lasry S, Guinebretière JM, Bouita L, Cohen-Solal C, et al. Response to neoadjuvant chemotherapy in lobular and ductal breast carcinomas: a retrospective study on 860 patients from one institution. Ann Oncol. 2006;17(8):1228–33.
23. Peintinger F, Kuerer HM, Anderson K, Boughey JC, Meric-Bernstam F, Singletary SE, et al. Accuracy of the combination of mammography and sonography in predicting tumor response in breast cancer patients after neoadjuvant chemotherapy. Ann Surg Oncol. 2006;13(11):1443–9.
24. Sahoo S, Lester SC. Pathology considerations in patients treated with neoadjuvant chemotherapy. Surg Pathol Clin. 2012;5(3):749–74.
25. Rajan R, Esteva FJ, Symmans WF. Pathologic changes in breast cancer following neoadjuvant chemotherapy: implications for the assessment of response. Clin Breast Cancer. 2004;5(3):235–8.
26. Rajan R, Poniecka A, Smith TL, Yang Y, Frye D, Pusztai L, et al. Change in tumor cellularity of breast carcinoma after neoadjuvant chemotherapy as a variable in the pathologic assessment of response. Cancer. 2004;100(7):1365–73.
27. Symmans WF, Peintinger F, Hatzis C, Rajan R, Kuerer H, Valero V, et al. Measurement of residual breast cancer burden to predict survival after neoadjuvant chemotherapy. J Clin Oncol. 2007;25(28):4414–22.
28. Corben AD, Abi-Raad R, Popa I, Teo CH, Macklin EA, Koerner FC, et al. Pathologic response and long-term follow-up in breast cancer patients treated with neoadjuvant chemotherapy: a comparison between classifications and their practical application. Arch Pathol Lab Med. 2013;137(8):1074–82.
29. Ogston KN, Miller ID, Payne S, Hutcheon AW, Sarkar TK, Smith I, et al. A new histological grading system to assess response of breast cancers to primary chemotherapy: prognostic significance and survival. Breast. 2003;12(5):320–7.
30. Sataloff DM, Mason BA, Prestipino AJ, Seinige UL, Lieber CP, Baloch Z. Pathologic response to induction chemotherapy in locally advanced carcinoma of the breast: a determinant of outcome. J Am Coll Surg. 1995;180(3):297–306.
31. Chevallier B, Roche H, Olivier JP, Chollet P, Hurteloup P. Inflammatory breast cancer. Pilot study of intensive induction chemotherapy (FEC-HD) results in a high histologic response rate. Am J Clin Oncol. 1993;16(3):223–8.
32. Rouzier R, Pusztai L, Delaloge S, Gonzalez-Angulo AM, Andre F, Hess KR, et al. Nomograms to predict pathologic complete response and metastasis-free survival after preoperative chemotherapy for breast cancer. J Clin Oncol. 2005;23(33):8331–9.

Sentinel Lymph Node: Clinicopathologic Features

Isabel Alvarado-Cabrero and Sergio A. Rodríguez-Cuevas

The sentinel lymph node (SLN) is frequently the first node in the lymphatic basin that receives drainage from an anatomic region and is immunologically responsible for that region. Sentinel lymph node biopsy (SLNB) remains the standard of care for the assessment of clinically negative axillary lymph nodes in patients with invasive breast carcinomas. Accurate diagnosis of a SLNB can direct the surgeon with regard to the need for axillary dissection (AD), and it can affect post-operative treatment decisions, including decisions about radiation therapy. Furthermore, an accurate negative diagnosis on SLNB can spare the patient the increased risk of lymphedema that accompanies AD or post-operative treatments. Its relatively low false negative rate of 5–10% and high sensitive rate of 90–95% in the detection of cancer to the lymph node basin has made this minimally invasive operation a standard. The idea that the SLN serves as a limited target sample of the axillary lymph nodes aroused an interest and trend toward increased inspection of the sentinel lymph node for detection of metastatic carcinoma by the pathologist though serial sections and/or immunohistochemistry.

22.1 Introduction

Axillary lymph nodes status is an important prognostic factor and determinant of treatment for patients with breast carcinoma. For decades, axillary lymph node dissection (ALND) was the only procedure used for staging axillary lymph nodes in women with invasive breast carcinoma [1]. Axillary lymph node dissection, however, is associated with significant morbidity, including long-term complications such as limitation of shoulder movements, paresthesia and arm numbness, and lymphedema, which can have a significant impact on the patient's quality of life.

The feasibility of identifying a sentinel lymph node (SLN) intraoperatively in breast cancer was first investigated at the JWCI by Giulano et al. [2]. In October 1991, the group began to investigate the feasibility of lymphatic mapping and sentinel lymphadenectomy with isosulfan blue vital dye in breast cancer as a more accurate and less morbid approach to stage breast cancer. This prospective study demonstrated that sentinel node biopsy of the axilla is technically feasible, safe, and without added complications. With a defined technique and experience, 100% accuracy in predicting the status of axilla was subsequently achieved [2, 3].

The sentinel lymph node (SLN) is frequently the first node in the lymphatic basin that receives drainage from an anatomic region and is immunologically responsible for that region. The sentinel lymph node biopsy (SLNB) has become the standard of care in the assessment of metastatic spread to the lymph node basin. Its relative low false negative rate of 5–10% and high sensitivity rate of 90–95% in the detection of cancer to the lymph node basin has made this minimally invasive operation a standard [4].

Clinical trials have proven that SLN is equivalent to staging of the axilla in patients with clinically node-negative disease (cN0). In addition, recent trials show that ALND may be safely omitted in selected cN0 patients with metastatic carcinomas limited to one or two sentinel lymph nodes. No difference in regional control, disease-free survival, and overall survival have been found between sentinel lymph node biopsy and axillary lymph node dissection in patients with early breast cancer and clinically negative axillary lymph nodes [5, 6].

I. Alvarado-Cabrero, MD, PhD (✉)
Department of Pathology, Hospital de Oncologia, Centro Médico Nacional Siglo XXI, Instituto Mexicano del Seguro Social, Mexico City, Mexico

S. A. Rodríguez-Cuevas, MD
Breast Institute, FUCAM, Mexico City, Mexico

S. Stolnicu, I. Alvarado-Cabrero (eds.), *Practical Atlas of Breast Pathology*, https://doi.org/10.1007/978-3-319-93257-6_22

22.2 Patterns of Regional Nodal Drainage

The axilla is the primary site of drainage in about 95% of breast cancer cases, with isolated internal mammary drainage seen in less than 5% of cases. Primary drainage to other pathways, such as supraclavicular, cervical, or intercostal, and contralateral lymph nodes, is extremely uncommon [7].

22.3 Indications and Contraindications for Sentinel Lymph Node

Sentinel lymph node biopsy is indicated for staging patients with early T1-T2 invasive breast cancer and clinically negative axillary lymph nodes, irrespective of surgical therapy on the breast. Women with ductal carcinoma in situ undergoing mastectomy are SLNB candidates because the disruption of lymph channels during a mastectomy will prevent accurate subsequent SLNB if invasion is identified. SLNB is absolutely contraindicated in patients with inflammatory breast cancer and patients with clinically positive axillary lymph nodes. These patients require axillary lymph node dissection [8, 9].

22.4 Surgical Techniques

Sentinel lymph node biopsy typically begins with injection of one or two tracers (blue dye or radioactive colloid) into breast skin or parenchyma either in the vicinity of the tumor or under the areolar plexus. These tracers enter the lymphatic channels and passively flow to the draining lymph nodes. Sentinel lymph nodes are then identified as those first receiving drainage from the tumor by the presence of tracer, and are removed [10, 11].

The use of radiocolloids for SLN identification offer several advantages. The colloids are efficiently trapped in the SLN (whereas blue dyes typically pass into second echelon nodes). Radiocolloid enables pre-operative sentinel node imaging (Figs. 22.1 and 22.2). It also facilitates rapid and easy intraoperative detection by the surgeon using a gamma probe (Fig. 22.3). Several studies have shown better sentinel node identification rates, when compared with blue dye alone [12, 13].

Fig. 22.1 Breast imaging after radiocolloid injection. Two lymph nodes are seen: one infraclavicular and another in the axilla

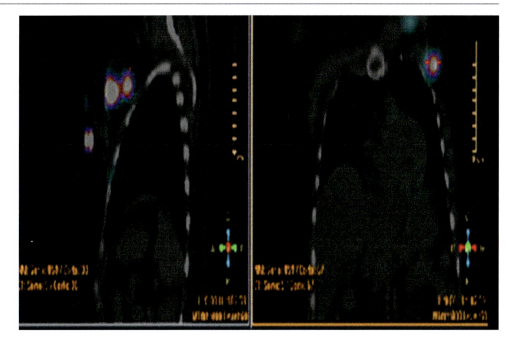

Fig. 22.2 Sentinel Lymph node imaging. Radiocolloid has been injected in the periareolar region. Two radioactive ("hot") nodules can be seen in the axilla. A ganglionar conglomerate and one lymph node

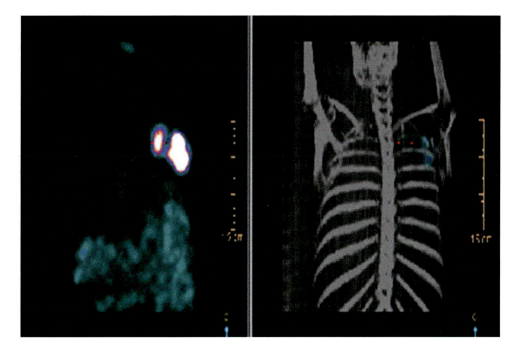

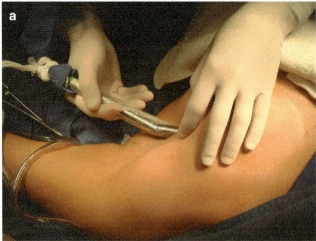

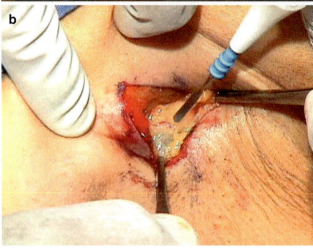

Fig. 22.3 Breast lymphatic mapping and sentinel lymph node. The two mapping agents, vital blue dye and radiocolloid, are injected into the subareolar plexus. (**a**) "Hot" Spots in the axilla can be identified before making the skin incision with the gamma probe. (**b**) Small incision in axilla, the sentinel lymph node is harvested

22.5 Pathological Axillary Lymph Node Staging

The pathological characterization of regional lymph nodes (pN) for breast carcinoma reflects the cumulative total regional lymph node burden of metastatic disease in the axillary, infraclavicular, supraclavicular, and ipsilateral internal mammary nodes. Pathologic classification (pN) is used only in conjunction with a pathological tumor assignment (surgical resection) (pT), and includes pathological evaluation of excised nodes from a sentinel lymph node biopsy and/ or lymph node dissection. Classification based solely on sentinel lymph node biopsy with fewer than six nodes evaluated and without subsequent axillary lymph node dissection is designated (sn) for "sentinel node" [2–6].

The American Joint Committee on Cancer (AJCC) and the Union for International Cancer Control TNM staging systems recognize three categories of lymph node involvement on the basis of size: isolated tumor cells (ITCs), micrometastasis, and macrometastasis (Table 22.1) [1]:

(a) Isolated Tumor Cells (pN0 [i+]): Isolated tumor cell clusters (ITCs) are defined as small clusters of cells not larger than 0.2 mm, or single tumor cells, or fewer than 200 cells in single histologic cross-section. ITCs may be detected by routine histology or by immunohistochemical methods (Figs. 22.4 and 22.5).

(b) Micrometastasis (pN1mi): Micrometastases are defined as tumor deposits larger than 0.2 mm but not larger than 2.0 mm in the largest dimension (Figs. 22.6, 22.7, 22.8, and 22.9).

(c) Macrometastasis (pN1): For patients who are pathologically node-positive with macrometastasis, at least one node must contain a tumor deposit >2 mm, and all remaining quantified nodes most contain tumor deposits larger than 0.2 mm (at least micrometastasis) (Figs. 22.10, 22.11, and 22.12).

A point that requires clarification pertains to measuring the size of the tumor deposit. When multiple tumor deposits are present in a lymph node with the isolated tumor cells or micrometastasis, the size of only the largest contiguous tumor is used to classify the node. This is regardless of whether the deposit is confined to the lymph node, extends outside the node, or is totally present outside the lymph node and invading adipose tissue. Some authors do not consider lesions purely outside the lymph node (e.g., in afferent lymphatic channels or perinodal fat) as evidence of nodal involvement (Fig. 22.13) [1, 3, 5].

Table 22.1 Definition of regional lymph nodes-pathological (pN)

pN category	pN criteria
pNX	Regional lymph nodes cannot be assessed (e.g., not removed for pathological study or previously removed)
pN0	No regional lymph node metastasis identified or ITCs only
pN0(i+)	ITCs only (malignant clusters no larger than 0.2 mm) in regional lymph node(s)
pN0(mol+)	Positive molecular findings by reverse transcriptase polymerase chain reaction (RT-PCR); no ITCs detected
pN1	Micrometastases; or metastases in 1–3 axillary lymph nodes; and/or clinically negative internal mammary nodes with micrometastases or macrometastases by sentinel lymph node biopsy
pN1mi	Micrometastases (approximately 200 cells, larger than 0.2 mm, but none larger than 2.0 mm)
pN1a	Metastases in 1–3 axillary lymph nodes, at least larger than 2.0 mm
pN1b	Metastases in ipsilateral internal mammary sentinel nodes, excluding ITCs
pN1c	PN1a and PN1b combined

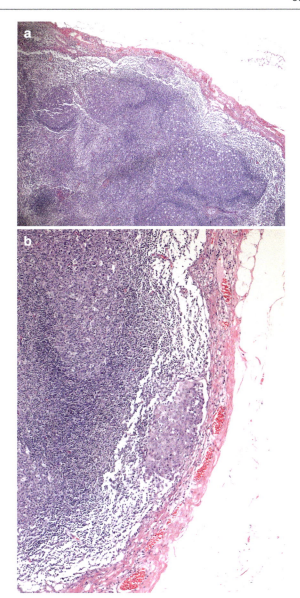

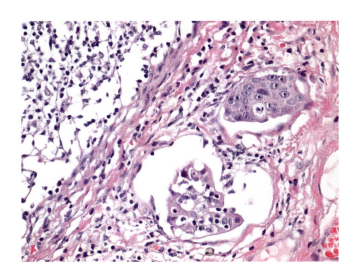

Fig. 22.4 Section of sentinel lymph node showing isolated tumor cells presenting as clusters

Fig. 22.6 Micrometastasis within a sentinel lymph node: (**a**) Low power and (**b**) High power

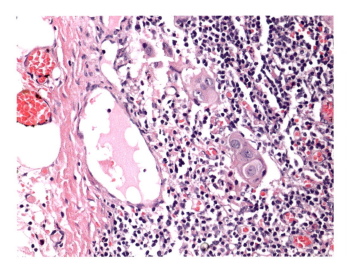

Fig. 22.5 Isolated tumor cell within a sentinel lymph node

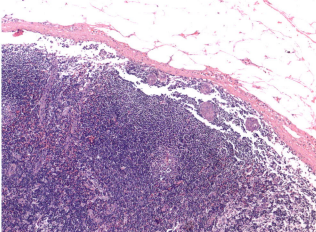

Fig. 22.7 Sentinel lymph node with multiple small clusters of metastatic cells dispersed in the subcapsular sinus. (**a**) Low power and (**b**) High power

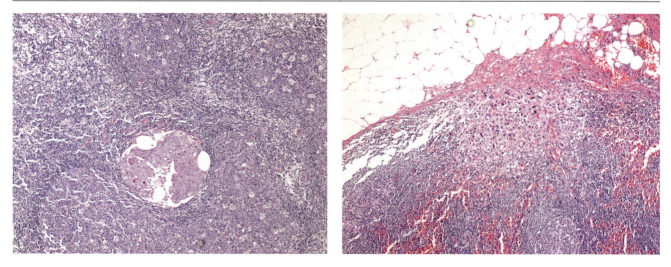

Fig. 22.8 Sentinel lymph node with small (<2 mm) deposit (micrometastasis) of invasive ductal carcinoma

Fig. 22.9 Micrometastasis within a sentinel lymph node

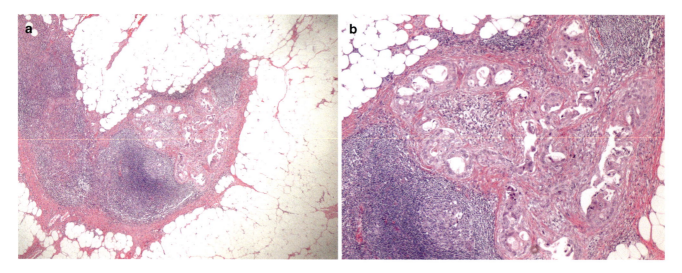

Fig. 22.10 Sentinel lymph node with metastatic deposits. (**a**) Section of lymph node showing macrometastatic (>2.0 mm) breast carcinoma. (**b**) Tumor deposits have induced a fibrous stromal reaction

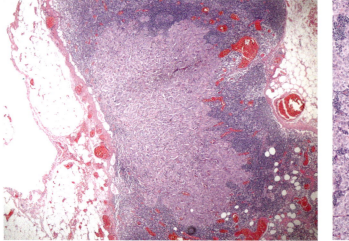

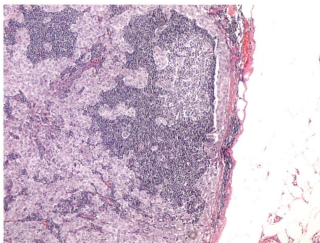

Fig. 22.11 Axillary lymph node macrometastases. The metastatic deposit in this case is >2 mm in size

Fig. 22.12 Sentinel lymph node with a large (>2 mm) macrometastases. Tumor involves the subcapsular sinus as well as the nodal parenchyma

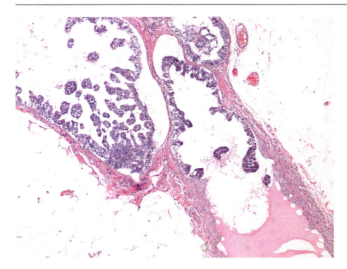

Fig. 22.13 Tumor deposits seen in afferent vessel

22.6 Occult Metastatic Disease

An occult metastasis is defined as any metastasis that is not identified on initial examination with a "standard" evaluation protocol. In one study, more intensive pathologic evaluation of the nodes by deeper sectioning and immunohistochemical staining increased the yield of occult metastases and led to an overall case conversion rate of 10.3% in patients who had an initial negative sentinel lymph node [14]. Occult metastases have no significance in terms of surgical management and patient outcomes. Routine immunohistochemical and reverse transcriptase polymerase chain reaction (PCR) are therefore not recommended for the evaluation of SLN [15].

22.7 Intraoperative Evaluation

Intraoperative detection of metastatic carcinoma in sentinel lymph nodes leads to immediate axillary lymph node dissection, avoiding the need for a delayed second surgical procedure. Intraoperative evaluation (IOE) of SLN at the time of primary breast surgery may be reserved for patients with clinically and radiologically negative axillae or suspicious intraoperative findings. The disadvantages of IOE of SLN include an increase in operation time and possible false-positive results. It is helpful for pathologists to be aware of the histologic type of carcinoma; metastatic invasive lobular carcinoma can be very difficult to diagnose in frozen sections [16, 17].

Frozen section (FS), imprint cytology (IC), or cytological smear (CS) can be used to evaluate sentinel lymph nodes intraoperatively. Cytological techniques are faster than FS, and do not cause significant loss of nodal tissue, but it may be difficult to confirm findings limited to the cytology material, and not present in H&E-stained sections (Fig. 22.14). FS is time-consuming (all slides should be frozen), freezing introduces artefactual tissue distortion, and sectioning of the frozen tissue block could potentially lead to the loss of critical tissue [17].

Recent studies have called the need for intraoperative sentinel lymph node assessment in situations where additional axillary dissection (AD) is unlikely to be performed even if metastasis is detected in the SLN. The ACOSOG Z0011 study showed no difference in local or regional recurrence between patients with 1–2 positive sentinel lymph nodes who were randomly treated with either SLNB-alone or SLNB plus axillary dissection. By applying the Z0011 criteria, it is estimated that approximately 75% of patients undergoing breast-conservation surgery could avoid additional AD [18]. Finally, intraoperative evaluations of SLN continue to be performed routinely at many hospitals for cN0 patients undergoing mastectomy, and pathologists should use the method (FS, IC, CS) that they are most comfortable with to avoid false-positive results [19].

22.7.1 Pathologic Evaluation

Despite specific recommendations from the College of American Pathologists (CAP) and ASCO, considerable heterogeneity remains among pathologists in the evaluation of sentinel lymph node pertaining to grossing, sectioning, cutting intervals, and use of immunohistochemistry or RT-PCR [20].

Fig. 22.14 Sentinel lymph node (SLN). Intraoperative evaluation. (**a**) Blue-stained SLN. (**b**) Imprint cytology in a blue stained node sectioned at 2–3 mm

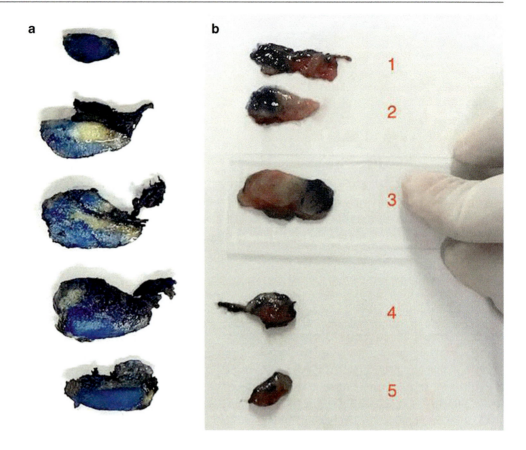

22.7.2 Gross Evaluation

First, we must inspect the node and any adherent fat. If any dimension is larger than 2.0 mm, the node must be sectioned. Most lymph nodes take the form of an asymmetric ellipsoid, or are bean shaped, with one long axis and two shorter axes. Most authors recommend cutting the node parallel to the long axis even though this is harder than sectioning perpendicular to this axis. Cutting parallel to the long axis produces fewer 2.0 mm slices to examine, and there is data that suggest afferent lymphatics are more likely to enter the node in this plane. The two opposing cut faces should be placed down in the cassette and full-face sections should be examined microscopically (Fig. 22.15) [20, 21].

22.7.3 Histologic Evaluation

Standard histopathologic evaluation of SLN has a sensitivity for the detection of both micrometastasis and macrometastasis at a rate of 83.4%. The assessment of levels in SLN is highly inconsistent among institutions, ranging from the performance of 1 H&E as advocated by CAP to 2–5–100 levels separated by intervals ranging from 2 to 500 µm, to a more labor-intensive and cost-intensive protocol with exhaustive sampling of the entire paraffin block at 50 µm. ASCO has endorsed limited step sections cut at 200–500 µm, to enhance detection of micrometastases [22].

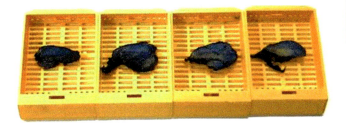

Fig. 22.15 Gross sectioning of sentinel lymph node. Node is serially sectioned; no slice is thicker than 2.0 mm

22.8 Extracapsular Extension

Metastatic carcinoma can invade through the lymph node (LN) capsule into the surrounding axillary fibroadipose tissue (Fig. 22.16). According to CAP, the presence of extracapsular extension (ECE) should be reported and the area of invasion outside of the LN capsule should be included when measuring the largest span of the LN metastasis.

The presence of tumor outside the lymph node is a prognostic parameter in breast cancer. It has also been shown to be associated with increased likelihood of non-sentinel lymph node involvement. Extranodal invasion is often further classified into minimal (if less than 1 mm beyond the capsule) or prominent (if greater than 1 mm) (Fig. 22.17).

Prominent extranodal invasion is often used by radiation oncologists to guide therapy, although there is no hard evidence that this makes a difference to the outcomes [22–24].

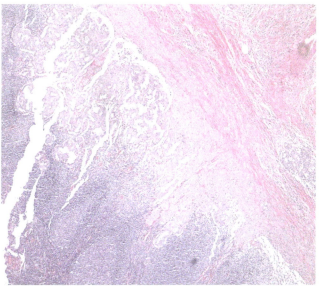

Fig. 22.16 View of pathologic findings, with extracapsular extension noted in the sentinel lymph node

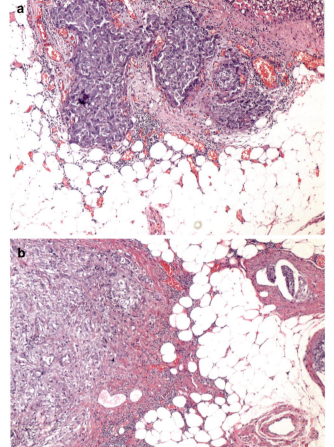

Fig. 22.17 Photomicrograph of metastatic tumor in axillary lymph nodes demonstrating extranodal extension. (**a**) The partial type with foci of extranodal extension. (**b**) Complete type with total destruction of the lymph node capsule

22.9 Sentinel Lymph Node Biopsy After Neoadjuvant Chemotherapy

Neoadjuvant chemotherapy (NAC) is a common treatment used for patients with locally advanced and lymph-positive breast cancer to reduce tumor size, increase the rate of breast-conserving surgery, and acquire information regarding chemotherapy sensitivity. The use of sentinel lymph node biopsy after NAC is controversial. A meta-analysis of studies in which SLNB was performed after NAC in patients with clinically node-negative cancer showed acceptable accuracy (Fig. 22.18) [25].

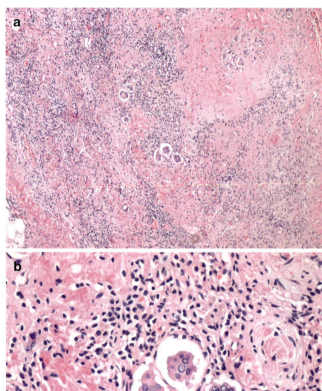

Fig. 22.18 Sentinel lymph node with residual metastatic carcinoma after neoadjuvant chemotherapy. (**a**) Low-power view showing residual metastatic carcinoma composed of small clusters of cells in desmoplastic stroma. (**b**) High-power view of the same lymph node

22.10 Immunohistochemistry

Immunohistochemical stains are commonly performed to increase the likelihood of detection of micrometastases. A number of different broad-spectrum or low-molecular-weight cytokeratin antibodies, including AE1/AE3, MNF 116, and CAM 5.2, have been used for this purpose. The results of two randomized trials (NSABP-B32 and ACOSOG Z0010) [15] have raised questions about the clinical significance of micrometastasis and isolated tumor cells. As a result, it has been suggested that routine evaluation of sentinel lymph node with cytokeratin immunostains should be abandoned. Immunohistochemistry is more commonly performed for evaluation of lymph nodes from a patient with lobular carcinoma (Fig. 22.19).

Immunostaining for cytokeratin does have a role in the evaluation of both sentinel and nonsentinel lymph nodes when there are cells identified on H&E-stained sections that are suspicious for, but not diagnostic of, tumor cells (Fig. 22.20). If cytokeratin staining is to be performed in this setting, it is important to recognize that other cell types in lymph nodes, particularly interstitial reticulum cells, demonstrate cytokeratin reactivity with some antibodies (especially antibody CAM 5.2); these cells much less frequently stain with cytokeratin AE1/AE3. Therefore, AE1/AE3 is preferable to CAM 5.2 for the confirmation of carcinoma cells in lymph nodes [26].

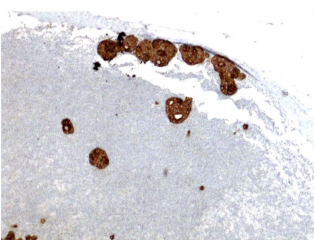

Fig. 22.20 Sentinel lymph node with micrometastases. Pancytokeratin immunostain highlights the tumor cell deposit(s)

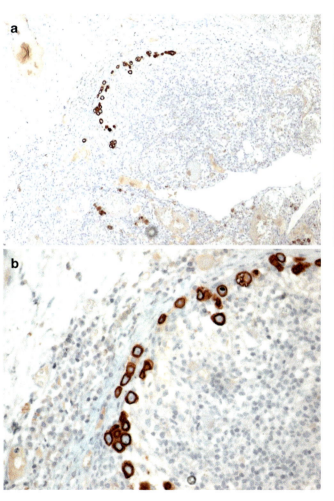

Fig. 22.19 Sentinel lymph node with metastatic lobular carcinoma. Pancytokeratin immunostain highlight the tumor cells which are dispersed within the nodal sinuses. (**a**) Low power and (**b**) High power

References

1. Amin M, Edge S, Greene F, Byrd DR, Brookland RK, Washington MK, et al., editors. The AJCC cancer staging manual. 8th ed. New York, NY: Springer International Publishing; 2017.
2. Giuliano AE, Kirgan DM, Guenther JM, Morton DL. Lymphatic mapping and sentinel lymphadenectomy for breast cancer. Ann Surg. 1994;220:391–8.
3. Lyman GH, Giulano AE, Somerfield MR, Benson AB 3rd, Bodurka DC, Burstein HJ, et al. American Society of Clinical Oncology guideline recommendations for sentinel lymph node biopsy in early-stage breast cancer. J Clin Oncol. 2005;23:7703–20.
4. McMaster KM, Tuttle TM, Carlson DJ, Brown CM, Noyes RD, Glaser RL, et al. Sentinel lymph node biopsy for breast cancer: a suitable alternative to routine axillary dissection in multi-institutional practice when optimal technique is used. J Clin Oncol. 2000;18:2560–6.
5. Veronesi U, Viale G, Paganelly G, Zurrida S, Luini A, Galimberti V, et al. Sentinel lymph node biopsy in breast cancer: ten-year results of a randomized controlled study. Ann Surg. 2010;25: 595–600.
6. Giuliano AE, Ballman K, Mc Call L, Beitsch P, Whitworth PW, Blumencranz P, et al. Locoregional recurrence after sentinel lymph node dissection with or without axillary dissection in patients with sentinel lymph node metastases: long-term follow-up from the American College of Surgeons oncology group (alliance) ACOSOG Z 011 randomized trial. Ann Surg. 2016;264:413–20.
7. Chatterjee A, Serniak N, Czerniecki BJ. Sentinel lymph node biopsy in breast cancer: a work in progress. Cancer J. 2015;21:7–10.
8. Apple SK. Sentinel lymph node in breast cancer: review article from a pathologist's point of view. J Pathol Transl Med. 2016;50: 83–95.
9. Hansen NM, Grube BJ, Giulano AE. The time has come to change the algorithm for the surgical management of early breast cancer. Arch Surg. 2002;137:1131–5.
10. Somasundaram SK, Chicken DW, Keshtgar M. Detection of the sentinel lymph node in breast cancer. Br Med Bull. 2007;84:117–31.
11. McMasters KM, Wong SL, Martin RC 2nd, Chao C, Tuttle TM, Noyes RD, et al. Dermal injection of radioactive colloid is superior to peritumoral injection for breast cancer sentinel lymph node biopsy: results of a multiinstitutional study. Ann Surg. 2001;233:676–87.
12. Maguire A, Brogi E. Sentinel lymph nodes for breast carcinoma. A paradigm shift. Arch Pathol Lab Med. 2016;140:791–8.
13. Weaver DL. Sentinel lymph nodes and breast carcinoma: which micrometastases are clinically significant? Am J Surg Pathol. 2003;27:842–7.
14. Weaver DL, Ashikaga T, Krag DN, Skelly JM, Anderson SJ, Harlow SP, et al. Effect of occult metastases on survival in node-negative breast cancer. N Engl J Med. 2011;364:412–21.
15. Weaver DL, Le UP, Harlow SP, Ashikaga T, Krag DN, Dupuis SL, et al. Metastasis detection in sentinel lymph nodes comparison of a limited widely spaced (NSABP protocol B-32) and a comprehensive narrowly spaced paraffin block sectioning strategy. Am J Surg Pathol. 2009;33:1583–9.
16. Van der Noordaa MEM, MTFD V-P, EJT R. The intraoperative assessment of sentinel nodes—standards and controversies. Breast. 2017;34:S64–9.
17. Barroso-Bravo S, Zarco-Espinoza G, Alvarado-Cabrero I, Valenzuela-Flores AG, Pichardo-Romero P, Rodríguez-Cuevas S. Lymphatic mapping and sentinel lymph node biopsies in order to avoid axillary dissection in early breast cancer. Cir Cir. 2005;73:437–41.
18. Cox C, Centeno B, Dickson D, Clark J, Nicosia S, Dupont E, et al. Accuracy of Intraoperative imprint cytology for sentinel lymph node evaluation in the treatment of breast carcinoma. Cancer. 2005;105:13–20.
19. Brogi E, Torres-Matundan E, Tan LK, Cody HS III. The results of frozen section, touch preparation, and cytological smear are comparable for intraoperative examination of sentinel lymph nodes: a study in 133 breast cancer patients. Ann Surg Oncol. 2005;12:173–80.
20. Weaver DL. Pathology evaluation on sentinel lymph nodes in breast cancer: protocol recommendations and rationale. Mod Pathol. 2010;23:S26–32.
21. Diaz LK, Hunt K, Ames F, Meric F, Kuerer H, Babiera G, et al. Histologic localization of sentinel lymph node metastases in breast cancer. Am J Surg Pathol. 2003;27:385–9.
22. Association of Directors of Anatomic and surgical Pathology. ADASP recommendations for processing and reporting lymph node specimens submitted for evaluation of metastatic disease. Am J Surg Pathol. 2001;25:961–3.
23. Aziz S, Wik E, Knutsuik G, Klingen TA, Chen Y, Davidsen B, et al. Extra-nodal extension is a significant prognostic factor in lymph node positive breast cancer. PLoS One. 2017;15:e0171853.
24. Cserni G. Axillary sentinel lymph node micrometastases with extracapsular extension: a distinct pattern of breast cancer metastasis? J Clin Pathol. 2008;61:115–8.
25. Xing Y, Foy M, Cox DD, Kuerer HM, Hunt KK, Cormier JN. Meta-analysis of sentinel lymph node biopsy after preoperative chemotherapy in patients with breast cancer. Br J Surg. 2006;93:539–46.
26. Lyman GH, Temin S, Edge SB, Newman LA, Turner RR, Weaver DL, et al. Sentinel lymph node biopsy for patients with early-breast cancer: American Society of Clinical Oncology. Clinical practice guideline update. J Clin Oncol. 2014;32:1365–83.

Mesenchymal Tumors of the Breast

Helenice Gobbi and Cristiana Buzelin Nunes

Mesenchymal breast lesions include a variety of benign and malignant neoplasms, as well as reactive and tumor-like lesions made up of mesenchymal cells. They frequently pose diagnostic challenges to surgical pathologists. This chapter provides a diagnostic approach to benign and malignant mesenchymal lesions of the breast, with emphasis on those that enter the differential diagnosis with spindle cell metaplastic carcinoma and malignant phyllodes tumor. Close clinicopathological correlation is recommended in the evaluation of both spindle cell/fibrous and vascular lesions of the breast.

23.1 Introduction

Mesenchymal breast lesions include a variety of benign and malignant neoplasms, as well as reactive and tumor-like lesions made up of mesenchymal cells. They frequently pose diagnostic challenges to surgical pathologists. To increase the difficulty, often the pathologist initially receives only a limited sample of material obtained by core needle biopsy from which to formulate a diagnosis [1–5].

Mesenchymal breast tumors and lesions are similar to those that occur in soft tissues at other anatomic sites. Virtually any type of benign mesenchymal tumor or sarcoma may occur in the breast as a primary lesion, including tumors with fibroblastic, adipocytic, histiocytoid, or vascular differentiation [6–9]. Primary sarcomas of the breast are extremely rare, however, most tumors with sarcomatous morphology in the breast are metaplastic carcinomas or malignant phyllodes tumors [10–12]. Extensive sampling and immunohistochemical stainings are recommended before concluding that a tumor is a primary breast sarcoma. Pathologists should also

consider the possibility of metastasis to the breast of a sarcoma from another anatomical site [1, 9].

It is important to separate out breast sarcomas as a distinct tumor group, to highlight their different clinical course and treatment response compared with breast carcinomas. Most benign spindle cell lesions of the breast are myofibroblastic tumors. Distinguishing mammary fibromatosis (which is locally aggressive) from nodular fasciitis or scar tissue can be difficult, especially in small biopsy samples. Tumors with histiocytoid differentiation are also a potential source of error because of their bland morphology and resemblance to reactive processes [2, 6, 8]. Angiosarcomas of the breast are more common than hemangiomas, and angiosarcomas may appear very bland; a dissecting growth pattern may be the diagnostic clue [7, 12].

This chapter provides a diagnostic approach to benign and malignant mesenchymal lesions of the breast, with emphasis on those that enter the differential diagnosis with spindle cell metaplastic carcinoma and malignant phyllodes tumor. Close clinicopathological correlation is recommended in the evaluation of both spindle cell/fibrous and vascular lesions of the breast.

23.2 Benign Mesenchymal Tumors and Reactive Lesions

Benign fibrous or myofibroblastic lesions of the breast are a challenge to pathologists because of the morphologic spectrum of these entities. There is also clinical, radiologic, and morphologic overlap between reactive and neoplastic fibrous lesions and also between fibrous and nonfibrous lesions [1]. Fibrous lesions of the breast include scars, reactive nodules, nodular fasciitis, pseudoangiomatous stromal hyperplasia, and benign tumors such as inflammatory myofibroblastic tumor, myofibroblastoma, and fibromatosis. Other benign mesenchymal tumors of the breast include lipoma, hamartoma, granular cell tumor, and vascular lesions [1–3, 8, 9, 13].

H. Gobbi, MD, PhD (✉)
Department of Surgery, Institute of Health Sciences, Federal University of Triangulo Mineiro, Uberaba, MG, Brazil

C. B. Nunes, PhD
Department of Anatomic Pathology, Faculty of Medicine, Federal University of Minas Gerais, Belo Horizonte, MG, Brazil

© Springer International Publishing AG, part of Springer Nature 2018
S. Stolnicu, I. Alvarado-Cabrero (eds.), *Practical Atlas of Breast Pathology*, https://doi.org/10.1007/978-3-319-93257-6_23

23.2.1 Reactive Spindle Cell Nodules

Reactive spindle cell nodules (RSCNs) of the breast arising after fine-needle aspiration or core biopsy of the breast are similar in appearance to the postoperative spindle cell nodules described in the genitourinary tract and thyroid. RSCNs are often associated with needle trauma to fibrosclerotic breast lesions such as papillary and complex sclerosing lesions [13]. The RSCNs are composed of intersecting fascicles of plump spindle cells with mild to moderate nuclear pleomorphism, intermixed with small blood vessels, plasma cells, macrophages, and lymphocytes (Fig. 23.1a). Normal epithelial elements may be seen entrapped with the prolifer-

ating spindle cells (Fig. 23.1b). Squamous metaplasia may be seen in ducts and lobules adjacent to the prior biopsy site (Fig. 23.1c). The spindle cells are positive for smooth and specific muscle actin, which is consistent with a myofibroblastic origin. The differential diagnosis includes other spindle cell proliferations such as nodular fasciitis, myofibroblastic inflammatory tumor, and low-grade metaplastic carcinomas. A history of previous needling procedure and the presence of other changes associated with biopsy sites, such as hemosiderin and foamy macrophages, favor a diagnosis of RSCN. Recognition of this reactive process will avoid overdiagnosis of mammary spindle cell benign or malignant neoplasms [3, 13].

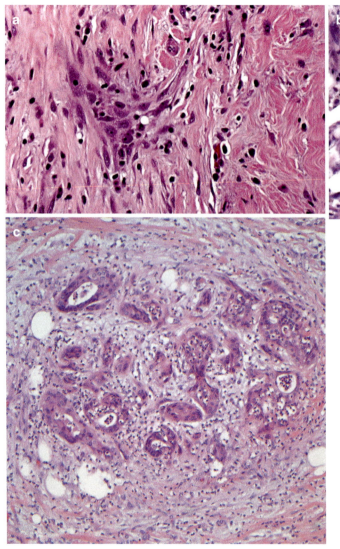

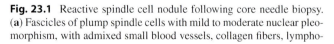

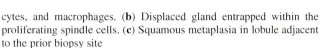

Fig. 23.1 Reactive spindle cell nodule following core needle biopsy. (**a**) Fascicles of plump spindle cells with mild to moderate nuclear pleomorphism, with admixed small blood vessels, collagen fibers, lympho-cytes, and macrophages. (**b**) Displaced gland entrapped within the proliferating spindle cells. (**c**) Squamous metaplasia in lobule adjacent to the prior biopsy site

23.2.2 Fat Necrosis and Histiocytic Reactions

Fat necrosis is common and often mimics malignancy clinically and mammographically, owing to its presentation as a firm mass, sometimes associated with microcalcifications. In approximately half the cases there is a history of injury to the breast, such as trauma, a needling procedure, surgery, or radiation [3], but often no previous history of injury can be elicited. The gross and histological appearances of fat necrosis depend on its age. Early fat necrosis consists of zones filled with lipid-laden histiocytes, hemorrhage, and various spaces surrounded by foreign body–type giant cells. An acute inflammatory cell infiltrate may be sometimes present (Fig. 23.2). Lipomembranous fat necrosis is a phenomenon in which delicate, eosinophilic membranes line the outlines of necrotic adipocytes. In older lesions, there is fibroblastic proliferation and deposition of collagen, forming a firm mass of dense, collagenous stroma or a scar-like appearance, often with dystrophic microcalcifications. Cavitation may occur as a result of liquefactive necrosis. Even in older lesions, foamy histiocytes and foreign body–type giant cells are usually seen [2, 3].

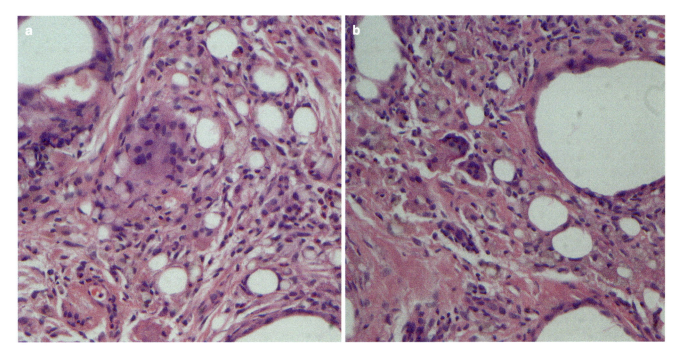

Fig. 23.2 Fat necrosis and histiocytic reaction. (**a**, **b**) Foamy histiocytes and foreign body-type giant cells

23.2.3 Pseudoangiomatous Stromal Hyperplasia

Pseudoangiomatous stromal hyperplasia (PASH) is a benign mammary lesion characterized by the proliferation of spindle-shaped myofibroblasts lining slit-like spaces simulating a vascular lesion. PASH may be an incidental finding in specimens with benign or malignant diseases, or it may form a slow-growing breast mass [14, 15]. Few cases with rapid growth, mimicking malignancy, have been described. PASH may be seen in males with gynaecomastia. On gross examination, PASH occurs as a sharply circumscribed, nonencapsulated nodule that on cut section is firm to rubbery and homogeneous; the nodules range in size from 1 to 12 cm (mean, 6 cm). Microscopic examination shows anastomosing, pseudovascular spaces intermixed with epithelial elements in a dense, collagenous, keloid-like stroma (Fig. 23.3).

Usually the spaces are empty, but they may contain a few erythrocytes. Some cases of PASH show a more fascicular pattern resembling myofibroblastoma. Rare cases of PASH show mild nuclear atypia and mitotic activity of the myofibroblasts. PASH is rarely observed in its pure form; more commonly, it is seen as scattered foci associated with proliferative breast disease, fibroadenoma, or malignancy. The myofibroblasts of PASH stain for CD34, vimentin, and progesterone receptor, and show a variable staining for smooth muscle actin and desmin; they are negative for CD31 and estrogen receptor [15]. The main differential diagnosis of PASH is a true vascular lesion, especially low-grade angiosarcoma. PASH is strongly positive for CD34, which is a potential pitfall when interpreted as evidence of endothelial differentiation. Immunostainings for CD31 and ERG are negative, which illustrates the importance of using multiple markers of endothelial lineage [3, 15].

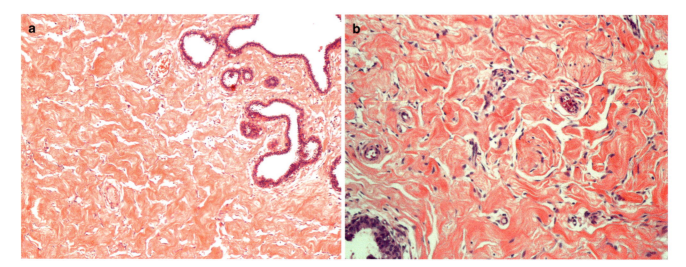

Fig. 23.3 Pseudoangiomatous stromal hyperplasia. (**a**) Slit-like interanastomosing spaces in a dense, collagenous, keloid-like stroma. (**b**) Spindle-shaped myofibroblasts lining spaces resembling endothelial cells

23.2.4 Nodular Fasciitis

Nodular fasciitis is a self-limited clonal proliferation of fibroblasts and myofibroblasts, very uncommon seen in the breast. The lesions grow rapidly and may be tender or painful; they arise in the subcutaneous tissue of the breast or less often, in mammary parenchyma. Nodular fasciitis is a relatively well-circumscribed but not encapsulated lesion composed of plump spindle cells (fibroblast and myofibroblasts) arranged in short fascicles and whorls. The nuclei are uniform, with prominent nucleoli. Mitoses are frequent and may be numerous. The stroma is loose, myxoid, and microcystic, with lymphocytes, erythrocytes, and thin-walled vessels. By immunohistochemistry, the tumor cells are consistently positive for actin, less often positive for desmin, and typically negative for keratins, S100, and CD34 [16, 17].

The differential diagnosis includes other reactive, benign, and malignant spindle cell lesions such as RSCN after biopsy, fibromatosis, and low-grade spindle cell metaplastic carcinomas, especially the fibromatosis-like type [18]. Numerous mitotic figures are frequent in nodular fasciitis and may be worrisome of malignancy, but the lack of nuclear atypia or hyperchromasia is a key distinguishing feature. Sarcomas and metaplastic carcinomas usually show greater nuclear atypia, and clusters of epithelioid cells may be seen in spindle cell metaplastic carcinomas. Nodular fasciitis does not have the infiltrative edge that enwraps adjacent normal structures and characterizes fibromatosis. Pathologists must be aware of an overlapping immunoprofile of nodular fasciitis and other myofibroblastic lesions [16, 17].

23.2.5 Inflammatory Myofibroblastic Tumor

Inflammatory myofibroblastic tumors are very rare benign neoplasms arising in the breast. They present as a painless, well-circumscribed mass that is firm, white to yellow or gray in color, and less than 5 cm in diameter. Histologic examination shows a low-grade neoplasm composed of bland, myofibroblastic spindle cells arrayed in interlacing fascicles admixed with plasma cells and occasionally lymphocytes and neutrophils (Fig. 23.4). Neoplastic cells are positive for smooth muscle actin and occasionally for desmin; they are usually negative for cytokeratins [19, 20]. The main differential diagnosis is with low-grade spindle cell metaplastic carcinoma, which shows positivity for cytokeratins and p63 [18].

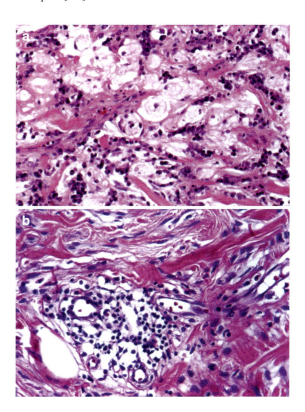

Fig. 23.4 Inflammatory myofibroblastic tumor. (**a–b**) Myofibroblasts admixed with collagen fibers, plasma cells, histiocytes, and lymphocytes

23.2.6 Myofibroblastoma

Myofibroblastomas are uncommon benign tumors of the breast that usually present as a well-circumscribed, firm, solitary, mobile nodule. Microscopically, there is a variety of histological variants: collagenized, cellular, infiltrative, myxoid, deciduoid, lipomatous, atypical, and epithelioid. Myofibroblastomas are composed of fibroblasts and myofibroblasts with bland nuclei, arranged in intersecting fascicles intermixed with bands of hyalinized, eosinophilic collagen (Fig. 23.5). Most cases present variable amounts of adipocytes, plasma cells, and lymphocytes, and the stroma may show smooth muscle differentiation and chondroid metaplasia. The neoplastic cells are positive for desmin, CD34, and vimentin, with variable positivity for smooth muscle actin, CD99, CD10, estrogen, progesterone and androgen receptors, and h-caldesmon by immunohistochemistry [21–23].

Because of the many microscopic patterns of myofibroblastomas, the differential diagnosis includes benign and malignant spindle cell lesions, including nodular fasciitis, fibromatosis, solitary fibrous tumor, spindle cell lipoma, leiomyoma, fascicular PASH, low-grade spindle cell sarcomas, and low-grade spindle cell metaplastic carcinoma. The epithelioid variant of myofibroblastoma should be differentiated from invasive lobular carcinoma, especially in tumors that express hormone receptors [18, 22, 23].

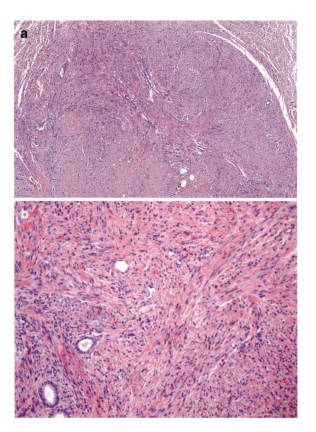

Fig. 23.5 Myofibroblastoma. (**a**) In this low-power view, the tumor border is well circumscribed. (**b**) In a high-power view, spindle cells are arranged in intersecting fascicles intermixed with bands of hyalinized, eosinophilic collagen, with a few entrapped normal ducts

23.2.7 Fibromatosis

Mammary fibromatosis, a locally infiltrative lesion without metastatic potential, is composed of fibroblasts or myofibroblasts occurring within the breast parenchyma or arising from the pectoral fascia extending into the breast [24, 25]. On gross examination, fibromatosis is a poorly circumscribed or stellate, white-gray mass, ranging from 0.3 to 15 cm in diameter (Fig. 23.6a). Microscopically, mammary fibromatosis is similar to desmoid-type fibromatosis of other sites. Tumors are characterized by an infiltrative growth pattern composed of long, sweeping and intersecting fascicles of bland spindle cells, with pale, eosinophilic cytoplasm and oval to elongated nuclei (Fig. 23.6b, c). Subtle undulations can be appreciated in the nuclear membrane. Atypia is an uncommon feature, and there are no or few mitoses. The cellularity may be variable, intermixed with collagen fibers and keloidal collagen, depending on the age of the tumor. Slit-like blood vessels are interspersed among the fascicles and have variable perivascular edema. Neoplastic cells infiltrate the adjacent breast stroma, surrounding and entrapping mammary ducts and lobules [24, 25].

By immunohistochemistry, fibromatosis shows weak and focal staining for smooth muscle actin; it less often stains for desmin and estrogen receptor, and it is usually negative for CD34. Aberrant nuclear staining for beta-catenin is present in 80% of breast fibromatosis lesions. However, other mammary spindle cell tumors, including solitary fibrous tumor, myofibroblastic sarcomas, metaplastic carcinomas, and phyllodes tumor, can also exhibit nuclear staining for beta-catenin [25, 26]. Expression of beta-catenin appears to be negative in scars and nodular fasciitis. Immunohistochemical stainings should be interpreted with caution, taking into consideration the other microscopic features of the tumors. The differential diagnosis of fibromatosis includes scar, fibromatosis-like metaplastic carcinoma, lipomatous myofibroblastoma, nodular fasciitis, and low-grade fibrosarcoma. The absence of immunoreactivity for epithelial and myoepithelial markers is critical in the distinction from spindle cell metaplastic carcinoma, fibromatosis-like. Fibromatosis shows long, sweeping fascicles of fibroblast with bland appearance and negative staining for cytokeratins. Myofibroblastomas are well-circumscribed tumors composed of short, parallel bundles of bland spindle cells intermixed with variable amounts of collagen and adipose tissue. Nodular fasciitis has a loose connective tissue containing bland myofibroblasts with frequent mitotic figures, erythrocytes, and cystic degeneration. There is no nuclear pleomorphism or hyperchromasia and no atypical mitoses [25].

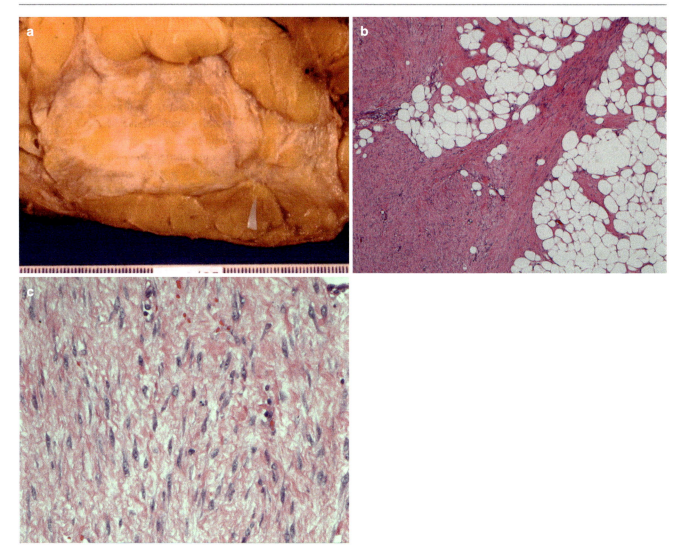

Fig. 23.6 Fibromatosis. (**a**) Poorly circumscribed, stellate, white-gray mass (*arrow*). (**a**) Fascicles of spindle fibroblasts extending into the adipose tissue. (**c**) High-power view shows bland spindle cells with elongated nuclei

23.2.10 Granular Cell Tumor

Granular cell tumors are composed of cells with eosinophilic, granular cytoplasm derived from Schwann cells of peripheral nerves; they are uncommonly found in the breast [32]. Mammary granular cell tumors represent less than 10% of all granular cell tumors. They are usually single, but may be multiple within the breast and in other sites. Clinically, patients usually present with a painless mass that may mimic malignancy because of its firm consistency, fixation to the pectoralis major muscle, and/or associated skin thickening, tethering, or dimpling [1]. Macroscopically, these tumors are firm, homogenous, white or tan, and usually well-defined or spiculated, mimicking invasive carcinoma on clinical examination, mammography, and gross examination. Granular cell tumors of the breast are identical to granular cell tumors of other sites. Histologically, granular cell tumors have an infiltrative growth pattern, forming sheets, cords, or clusters of round to polygonal cells with uniform round to oval nuclei (Fig. 23.9a, b). The cytoplasm shows prominent periodic acid-Schiff (PAS)/diastase-resistant granules, which correspond to secondary lysosomes upon electron microscopy [32]. Mitoses are generally scant. Perineural invasion may be seen and does indicate worse outcome in cases of malignancy [2]. Reactive pseudoepitheliomatous hyperplasia may occur when granular cell tumors are located close to the skin. Histologically, granular cell tumors must be distinguished from invasive mammary carcinomas and reactive and neoplastic processes because of the poorly circumscribed, infiltrative growth pattern. By immunohistochemistry, neoplastic cells of granular cell tumors show positivity for S100 protein (Fig. 23.9c), CD68, PGP 9.5, CD56, and NSE. They are negative for cytokeratin and for estrogen and progesterone receptors [1, 2, 32].

Most granular cell tumors are benign, but there are reports of malignant tumors arising in the breast [32, 33]. Tumors with three of the following microscopic criteria should be considered malignant:

- Necrosis
- Spindling
- Vesicular nuclei with large nucleoli
- Mitotic rate >2 per 10 HPF (200× magnification)
- High nuclear-to-cytoplasmic ratio
- Pleomorphism

Tumors with only one or two of these features are considered atypical and generally behave indolently [33].

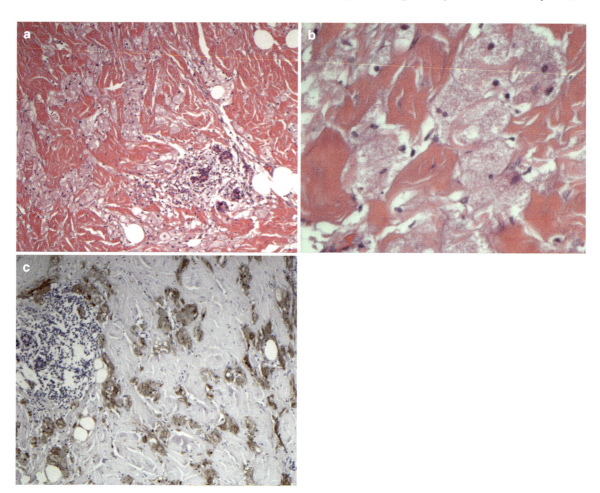

Fig. 23.9 Granular cell tumors. (**a**) The tumor has an infiltrative growth pattern and consists of groups of cells with pale, granular cytoplasm and uniform round to oval nuclei. (**b**) High-power view demonstrates the small nuclei and cytoplasmic granularity. (**c**) Immunohistochemistry shows reactivity for S100 protein

23.2.11 Benign Vascular Lesions

Vascular lesions of the breast comprise a range of benign and malignant lesions with significant overlap in histological features. Pathologists should be careful in their differential diagnosis, especially in small samples obtained by core needle biopsy, to avoid diagnostic pitfalls that can lead to over- or under-diagnosis of these lesions [34–36]. Pathologists should consider histological features and immunohistochemical studies along with clinical and imaging information. Any previous history of radiation therapy to the breast is also important.

23.2.11.1 Hemangioma

Hemangiomas are a benign proliferation of mature vessels; they may occur throughout the body but are rare in the breast. On gross examination, hemangiomas show a circumscribed, red or dark-brown spongy texture. Histologically, breast hemangiomas are classified as parenchymal or nonparenchymal in location, and cavernous (most common) or noncavernous. The noncavernous types include peri-lobular, capillary, complex, and venous hemangiomas [35, 37]. Cavernous hemangiomas consist of distended, congested vessels of various sizes, immersed in a fibrous stroma (Fig. 23.10a). The vessels are lined by endothelial cells showing neither nuclear atypia nor mitoses. Thrombosis is common, and organization may result in the formation of endothelial hyperplasia. Perilobular hemangiomas are microscopic lesions that are usually an incidental finding measuring <2 mm. They are composed of small, thin-walled, congested, capillary-sized blood vessels, involving the peri-lobular or extra-lobular breast stroma (Fig. 23.10b). They can be solitary or multiple. Most vessels are lined by flat, bland endothelial cells without atypia. Vascular anastomoses may be seen but are inconspicuous.

The differential diagnosis for hemangiomas includes benign lesions such as myofibroblastoma and angiolipoma, as well as malignant neoplasms including low-grade angiosarcoma. Perilobular hemangiomas are usually smaller than angiosarcomas, do not infiltrate the breast parenchyma, and do not demonstrate nuclear atypia or mitoses [35, 36].

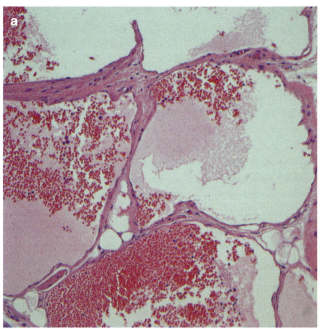

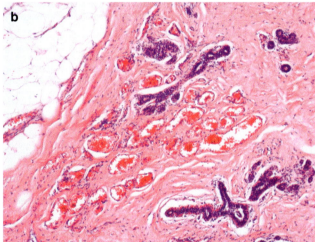

Fig. 23.10 Hemangioma. (**a**) Cavernous hemangioma with distended, congested vessels of various sizes, lined by bland endothelial cells without nuclear atypia or mitoses. (**b**) Perilobular hemangioma shows small blood vessels in association with a lobule

23.2.11.2 Angiomatosis

Angiomatosis is a very rare benign vascular lesion of the breast and may be locally aggressive [38]. Lesions present as a palpable mass, ranging from 9 to 17 cm, or as a typically painless swelling of the present breast. At macroscopy, the lesions are red, spongy, cystic, and may contain serosanguineous material. Histologically, there is a proliferation of anastomosing vascular channels infiltrating the breast interlobular stroma, displacing (but not disrupting) the lobular structures. The vascular channels are supported by scant, nonmuscular stroma, and are lined by thin walls and endothelial cells without hyperchromasia, nuclear atypia, or mitoses. The vessel lumina may be empty or filled with erythrocytes. The vessels surround but do not invade ducts and lobules—an important feature differentiating these lesions from low-grade angiosarcoma [35–38]. Hemangiomatous channels (containing red blood cells) and lymphangiomatous channels (lymph-containing or empty) with stromal lymphoid aggregates are present. The most important differential diagnosis is low-grade angiosarcoma; the distinction between these two entities is of great clinical importance because of the implications for prognosis and adequate therapy. In most core needle biopsies or small incisional specimens, this distinction cannot be made with certainty. Both lesions show an infiltrative growth pattern, with diffuse peri-lobular and extra-lobular invasion, but angiosarcoma also exhibits intra-lobular growth with destruction and distortion of lobules. Although angiomatosis is a benign lesion, often simple mastectomy is required because of the diffuse nature of the lesion. Local recurrences may occur when lesions are incompletely excised [35, 36].

23.2.11.3 Atypical Vascular Lesions

Atypical vascular lesions (AVLs) are benign cutaneous vascular proliferations that can develop in the skin after breast-conserving surgery and radiation therapy. A direct link has been made between adjuvant radiotherapy and the subsequent development of cutaneous angiosarcoma (AS) and AVLs in the radiation field [39, 40]. In 1994, Fineberg and Rosen [39] reported for the first time a series of cases of an unusual group of vascular lesions occurring in mammary skin after radiation therapy for breast carcinoma, which they called "atypical vascular lesions." AVLs are believed to arise because of lymphatic obstruction following surgery and/or radiotherapy, causing acquired dilatation of superficial vascular channels.

AVLs present as single or multiple papules on the breast and axillary skin, consisting of flesh-colored, brown, or erythematous small patches ranging from 1 to 60 mm in size, which occur following postoperative radiation therapy. The latency interval between radiation and presentation is most frequently between 3 and 6 years. Microscopically, AVLs are well-circumscribed, vascular proliferations involving the dermis, which rarely extend into the subcutaneous fat (Fig. 23.11a). The vessels are dilated and varied in size; they may anastomose, displaying branching contours. Dissection between bundles of dermal collagen may be present. The vascular spaces are lined by a single layer of plump or attenuated "hobnail" endothelial cells with prominent nuclei, but without nuclear atypia (Fig. 23.11b). The endothelial cells occasionally form thin papillary projections into the lumina (Fig. 23.11c). The vessels are ectatic and clustered in a "back to back" arrangement within the superficial dermis, but they eventually may show a more infiltrative growth pattern within the deep dermis [36, 39, 40].

Based on D2–40 positivity, AVLs are usually classified as one of two immunohistochemical patterns: the D2–40 positive lymphatic type (LT-AVL) (Fig. 23.11d) or the D2–40 negative vascular type (VT-AVL). Both types of AVL stain positive for CD31 (Fig. 23.11e) and are variably stained for CD34; most often the vascular type is positive for CD34. Occasionally, both types may be encountered simultaneously within the same lesion [35, 40]. Erythrocytes are rarely seen within the vascular spaces of both types, and extravasation of red blood cells into the surrounding dermis is not present. A chronic inflammatory cell infiltrate is often present, although it may be sparse in some cases (Fig. 23.11f). Most AVLs reported in the literature are LT-AVL, and the diagnosis of LT-AVL and VT-AVL seems to have different implications. VT-AVL seems to have worse prognosis than LT-AVL. After the first description, most data on outcomes favored a benign process, but some studies have questioned this concept, suggesting that AVL and post-radiation angiosarcoma represent a morphologic continuum, implying that AVL is a precursor to angiosarcoma. The risk of malignancy is still undefined, however, because of the small number of reported cases with follow-up information [35, 41].

Microscopically, the most important differential diagnosis of AVLs is low-grade secondary angiosarcoma. Both commonly arise in the skin with prior radiation or chronic lymphedema. AVLs are typically smaller (<1 cm) than secondary angiosarcomas, and they are typically limited to the dermis, whereas secondary angiosarcomas often invade the subcutis. Endothelial cells of secondary angiosarcoma show significant nuclear atypia, which is not seen in AVL. Ki67 is absent or low in AVL and is high (>20%) in angiosarcomas. The majority of secondary angiosarcomas show c-*MYC* amplification by FISH, or c-MYC protein expression by immunohistochemistry; AVLs do not demonstrate these molecular alterations [35, 41].

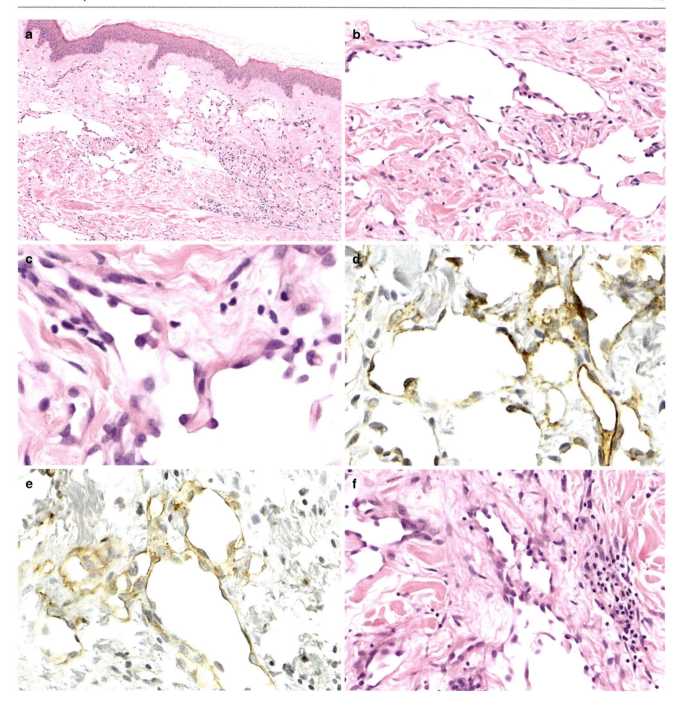

Fig. 23.11 Atypical vascular lesion (AVL). (**a**) Thin-walled vascular channels in the superficial dermis (H&E). (**b**) Irregular, branching vascular spaces within the dermal collagen (H&E). (**c**) Vascular space lined by a single layer of plump endothelial cells without atypia, forming a thin papillary projection into the lumina (H&E). (**d**) Lymphatic-type AVL immunostained for D2–40. (**e**) Vascular-type AVL immunostained for CD31. (**f**) Chronic inflammatory cell infiltrate adjacent to the vascular proliferation

23.3   Malignant Mesenchymal Breast Tumors

Breast sarcomas are a heterogeneous group of neoplasms arising from the nonepithelial components of the breast, including different histologic subtypes. They comprise less than 1% of breast malignancies and less than 5% of all sarcomas [4–7, 12].

23.3.1   Angiosarcomas

Angiosarcomas are the best known and most common vascular neoplasms arising in the breast. Angiosarcomas account for 0.05% of all malignant neoplasms of the breast and are the second most frequent sarcoma in the breast, after malignant phyllodes tumor, but they are still very uncommon [35, 42–44]. Angiosarcomas are divided into two categories: primary angiosarcoma (PAS) and secondary angiosarcoma (SAS), which follows conservative surgery and radiation therapy for breast cancer. Angiosarcomas may also arise in the upper limb and breast parenchyma secondary to chronic lymphedema following radical mastectomy (Stewart-Treves syndrome). The frequency of secondary angiosarcomas has been increasing since the late 1980s, reflecting the trend for breast-conserving surgery and the more frequent use of radiation therapy (0.9 per 1000 breast cancer patients). Patients with primary angiosarcomas have an average age of 35–40 years (range, 16–91 years) and are usually younger than those with secondary angiosarcomas, whose average age is 59–69 years (range, 36–96 years). The latency interval between radiation therapy and the diagnosis of secondary angiosarcoma ranges from 1 to 41 years, with a median of about 6–7 years, which is slightly longer than the interval for AVLs [35, 43].

Primary angiosarcomas are deeply located within the mammary parenchyma, and the majority present as a painless mass (Fig. 23.12a). About 10% of patients present with diffuse enlargement of the breast. When tumors involve the skin, areas of blue, violaceous, or bluish-red discoloration may be seen. Rare bilateral tumors more likely represent locoregional metastasis. Patients with secondary angiosarcoma characteristically present with cutaneous lesions, including skin thickening and red-purple, ecchymotic lesions (Fig. 23.12b) with or without ulceration, which may be associated or not with an underlying breast mass. Hemorrhagic tumors are friable, firm, or spongy, and areas of cystic necrosis may be evident.

Microscopically, angiosarcomas are characterized by vascular spaces dissecting the mammary stroma and invading lobules. The vascular spaces are lined by atypical endothelial cells that show nuclear hyperchromasia and mitosis. Extravasation of stromal erythrocytes is present to varying degrees (Fig. 23.12c, d). At the edge of many angiosarcomas, the vascular spaces are lined by bland endothelial cells with no or mild atypia; these may be difficult to differentiate from benign capillaries, angiolipomas, hemangiomas, or AVLs.

In 1981, Donnell et al. [34] proposed a grading criteria for angiosarcomas based on a combination of growth and other histological features indicative of the degree of differentiation. The features considered are endothelial tufting, papillary formations, solid and spindle cell foci, mitoses, blood lakes, and necrosis. It should be noted that the grade may vary within a given lesion. Low-grade angiosarcomas are characterised by anastomosing vascular channels with open lumina, which diffusely permeate mammary glandular elements. Endothelial cells show nuclear hyperchromasia, but mitoses are absent or scant. Papillary endothelial cell tufting and solid areas are absent. Intermediate-grade angiosarcomas show anastomosing vascular channels with hyperchromatic nuclei, as well as areas of increased cellularity, endothelial cell tufts, and papillary formations. Solid spindle cell foci with few or no vascular lumina may be present, and mitoses are present, particularly in areas of papillary growth [35, 37]. "Blood lakes" and necrosis are absent by definition [39]. High-grade angiosarcomas present malignant endothelial cells with nucleoli, frequent endothelial tufting, and papillary formations, occasionally with solid and spindled areas with inconspicuous vascular spaces. "Blood lakes" (areas of hemorrhage), necrosis, and high mitotic number are frequently found and characteristic of high-grade angiosarcomas. Some high-grade angiosarcomas are composed almost entirely of large, round, epithelioid cells, with vesicular nuclei and abundant cytoplasm (epithelioid angiosarcomas); these tend to be more aggressive. Epithelioid and poorly differentiated angiosarcomas may mimic spindle cell carcinomas, malignant phyllodes tumor, melanoma, and other sarcomas [34, 35]. A panel of immunohistochemical markers can aid in the differentiation between these lesions. Positivity for CD31, FLI1, ERG, factor VIII-related antigen (FVIII), and *Ulex euro-*

paeus lectin (UEL) can confirm the endothelial phenotype. Keratin may be expressed focally in some angiosarcomas, so this information should be interpreted in conjunction with information on other markers [42].

Secondary angiosarcomas are usually intermediate-grade or high-grade tumors, and the degree of atypia in these lesions is often out of proportion to the structural grade of the lesion [37]. Ginter et al. [35] suggest that angiosarcomas should be graded after complete excision, stating that "since the area of the highest grade is used to assign the overall tumor grade, it is important to recognize that low-grade areas may be present and even predominant within a higher-grade tumor. As such, pathologists should refrain from grading angiosarcomas in core biopsy samples, as higher-grade areas

may become evident when the entire lesion in the excisional biopsy specimen is evaluated."

Recent studies have shown *c-MYC* amplification in 54–100% of cases of secondary angiosarcomas (post-radiation and lymphedema-associated). The concordance between c-*MYC* amplification detected by FISH and c-MYC protein expression by immunohistochemistry ranges from 94% to 100% [35, 40]. Further studies have shown that a small subset of primary angiosarcomas also have c-*MYC* amplification, but much less often than in secondary angiosarcomas. c*MYC* amplification has not been found in post-radiation AVLs [41]. In cases with commingling AVLs and secondary angiosarcomas, *MYC* amplification is identified in the angiosarcomas, but not in the AVLs [41].

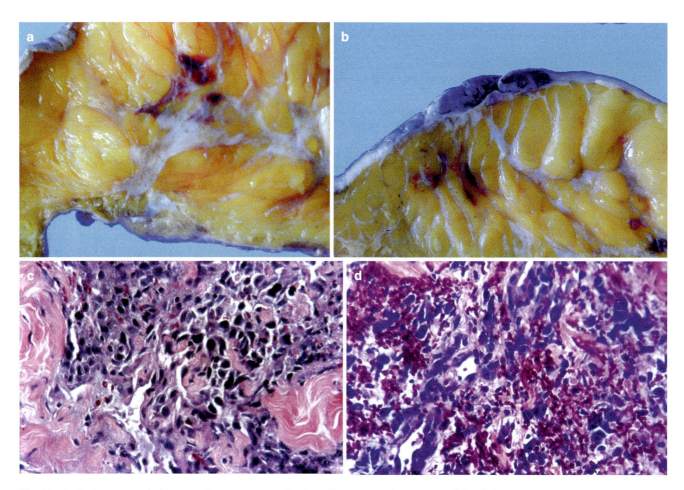

Fig. 23.12 Angiosarcoma. (**a**, **b**) cut surface at gross examination. (**a**) Primary angiosarcoma deeply located within the mammary parenchyma. (**b**) Secondary angiosarcoma presenting skin thickening with hemorrhagic lesions extending into the dermis. (**c**, **d**) High-grade angiosarcoma has a more solid, cellular growth pattern of atypical cells with areas of stromal hemorrhage. There is marked nuclear pleomorphism of the malignant endothelial cells

23.3.2 Other Primary Sarcomas of the Breast

Primary sarcomas of the breast other than angiosarcomas are extremely rare [4–8]. Some sarcomas arise in the chest wall and secondarily involve the breast, particularly those that develop after radiation therapy for breast cancer, such as liposarcoma. The majority of breast sarcomas are actually part of the heterologous component of a malignant phyllodes tumor (Fig. 23.13).

Virtually any histological type of sarcoma that occurs in other sites may occur in the breast as a primary tumor, including liposarcoma, leiomyosarcoma, rhabdomyosarcoma, fibrosarcoma, synovial sarcoma, malignant peripheral nerve sheath tumor, and osteosarcoma. Sarcomas of other

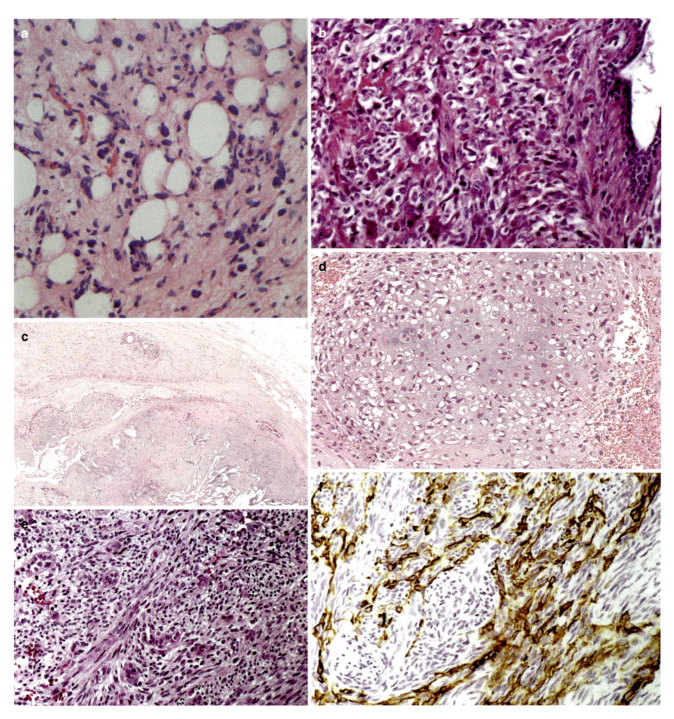

Fig. 23.13 Different types of heterologous differentiation within malignant phyllodes tumors of the breast, simulating primary breast sarcomas. (**a**) Myxoid liposarcoma composed of hyperchromatic lipoblasts within a myxomatous stroma. (**b**) Osteosarcoma showing pink osteoid formation among atypical spindle and ovoid cells. (**c, d**) Chondrosarcoma with multiple chondroblasts in single lacunae; some are multinucleated, with plump nuclei. (**e, f**) Synovial sarcoma showing proliferation of spindle and epithelioid cells immunostained positive for AE1/AE3 (**e, f**, cytokeratins AE1/AE3)

anatomical sites may metastasize to the breast. These sarcomatous lesions, whether primary or metastatic to the breast, are all histologically similar to those found in other sites [4–8]. Differentiating sarcoma subtypes based on molecular characteristics helps in differential treatment sensitivities and development of specifically targeted therapies in breast sarcomas [6].

23.3.2.1 Liposarcoma

Liposarcomas, which are tumors showing pure adipocytic differentiation, are the second most common type of primary mammary sarcoma, after angiosarcoma [45]. All types of soft-tissue liposarcomas (well-differentiated/atypical lipomatous tumor, myxoid, and pleomorphic) have been reported in the breast, more often as part of malignant phyllodes tumor. Atypical lipomatous tumor is most frequent in primary tumors, whereas in malignant phyllodes tumors, heterologous fatty components may be either pleomorphic or well-differentiated [11, 12].

Myxoid liposarcoma is the most commonly reported subtype of liposarcoma in the breast, but its presentation as a primary breast tumor is highly unusual and should prompt consideration that the breast mass may be a metastasis or part of a phyllodes tumor. Myxoid liposarcomas tend to metastasize to other soft tissue sites, so imaging studies of the extremities would be prudent. Myxoid liposarcomas are composed of hyperchromatic spindle cells within a myxomatous stroma with a delicate, plexiform capillary vasculature. There is variable lipoblastic differentiation, especially at the edge of the tumor nodules. Areas of high-grade transformation may be present, with increased cellularity of round, spindle, or pleomorphic cells and greater nuclear atypia and proliferative activity. The presence of more than 5% of round-cell components is considered an adverse prognostic factor. Thus, estimation of the percentage of round-cell components should be included in the pathological report.

Molecular findings show that myxoid liposarcomas have a t(12;16) translocation involving the *FUS* and *DDIT3* genes, resulting in *DDIT3-FUS* gene fusion. Pleomorphic liposarcoma has a nonspecific complex karyotype [45].

23.3.2.2 Osteosarcomas

Osteosarcomas are malignant soft-tissue tumors elaborating osteoid or bone in the absence of any other line of differentiation (e.g., epithelial, fibroepithelial, or nerve sheath). Before making a diagnosis of pure osteosarcoma of the breast, pathologists should distinguish it from heterologous osteosarcomatous differentiation in malignant phyllodes tumor or metaplastic carcinoma of the matrix-producing type. In some cases, osteosarcoma differentiation may represent >75% of the stroma of a phyllodes tumor, and extensive sampling is necessary to establish the correct diagnosis. Less frequently, the same situation is seen for metaplastic carcinoma, in which carcinomatous cells represent a minimal component of the whole tumor [4–7, 46]. Clinically, the tumor presents as a solitary mass associated with pain in 20% of cases. Tumors are sharply delineated and vary in size from 1.4 to 13 cm. At cut surface, the consistency varies from firm to stony hard, depending on the amount of osseous differentiation. Central cavitation and necrosis are seen in larger tumors. Histological features of osteosarcomas arising in the breast are similar to those of osteosarcomas at other sites. Tumors are composed of atypical spindle or ovoid cells associated with a variable amount of osteoid or osseous tissue. Cartilage is present in more than one third of cases. Fibroblastic, osteoclast-rich, and osteoblastic subtypes of osteosarcomas have been described in the breast.

Complex genetic alterations have been reported in osteosarcomas, including *VEGF*, *IGF*, *EGF*, *AKT*, *PDGF*, *MAPK*, and p70/s6 kinase, which may have an impact on prognosis and therapy [46].

References

1. Cheah AL, Billings SD, Rowe JJ. Mesenchymal tumours of the breast and their mimics: a review with approach to diagnosis. Pathology. 2016;48:406–24.
2. Torous VF, Schnitt SJ, Collins LC. Benign breast lesions that mimic malignancy. Pathology. 2017;49:181–96.
3. Schnitt SJ, Collins LC. Reactive, inflammatory, and nonproliferative lesions. In: Schnitt SJ, Collins LC, editors. Biopsy interpretation of the breast. 2nd ed. Philadelphia, PA: Lippincott Williams & Wilkins; 2013. p. 25–57.
4. Lim SZ, Ong KW, Tan BK, Selvarajan S, Tan PH. Sarcoma of the breast: an update on a rare entity. J Clin Pathol. 2016;69:373–81.
5. Adem C, Reynolds C, Ingle JN, Nascimento AG. Primary breast sarcoma: clinicopathologic series from the Mayo Clinic and review of the literature. Br J Cancer. 2004;91:237–41.
6. Voutsadakis IA, Zaman K, Leyvraz S. Breast sarcomas: current and future perspectives. Breast. 2011;20:199–204.
7. Pandey M, Mathew A, Abraham EK, Rajan B. Primary sarcoma of the breast. J Surg Oncol. 2004;87:121–5.
8. Schnitt SJ, Collins LC. Spindle cell lesions. In: Schnitt SJ, Collins LC, editors. Biopsy interpretation of the breast. 2nd ed. Philadelphia, PA: Lippincott Williams & Wilkins; 2013. p. 363–86.
9. Rakha EA, Aleskandarany MA, Lee AH, Ellis IO. An approach to the diagnosis of spindle cell lesions of the breast. Histopathology. 2016;68:33–44.
10. Reis-Filho JS, Lakhani SR, Gobbi H, Sneige N. Metaplastic carcinoma. In: Lakhani SR, Ellis IO, Schnitt SJ, Tan PH, van de Vijver MJ, editors. WHO classification of tumours of the breast. 4th ed. Lyon: IARC Press; 2012. p. 48–52.
11. Tan BY, Acs G, Apple SK, Badve S, Bleiweiss IJ, Brogi E, et al. Phyllodes tumours of the breast: a consensus review. Histopathology. 2016;68:5–21.
12. Thornton K. Sarcomas of the breast with a spotlight on angiosarcoma and cystosarcoma phyllodes. Surg Oncol Clin N Am. 2016;25:713–20.
13. Gobbi H, Tse G, Page DL, Olson SJ, Jensen RA, Simpson JF. Reactive spindle cell nodules of the breast after core biopsy or fine-needle aspiration. Am J Clin Pathol. 2000;113:288–94.
14. Powell CM, Cranor ML, Rosen PP. Pseudoangiomatous stromal hyperplasia (PASH). A mammary stromal tumor with myofibroblastic differentiation. Am J Surg Pathol. 1995;19:270–7.
15. Michal M, Badve S, Shin SJ. Pseudoangiomatous stromal hyperplasia. In: Lakhani SR, Ellis IO, Schnitt SJ, Tan PH, van de Vijver MJ, editors. WHO classification of tumours of the breast. 4th ed. Lyon: IARC Press; 2012. p. 129–30.
16. Gobbi H, Fletcher C. Nodular fasciitis. In: Lakhani SR, Ellis IO, Schnitt SJ, Tan PH, van de Vijver MJ, editors. WHO classification of tumours of the breast. 4th ed. Lyon: IARC Press; 2012. p. 126.
17. Montgomery EA, Meis JM. Nodular fasciitis. Its morphologic spectrum and immunohistochemical profile. Am J Surg Pathol. 1991;15:942–8.
18. Gobbi H, Simpson JF, Borowsky A, Jensen RA, Page DL. Metaplastic breast tumors with a dominant fibromatosis-like phenotype have a high risk of local recurrence. Cancer. 1999;85:2170–82.
19. Fletcher CDM. Inflammatory myofibroblastic tumour. In: Lakhani SR, Ellis IO, Schnitt SJ, Tan PH, van de Vijver MJ, editors. WHO classification of tumours of the breast. 4th ed. Lyon: IARC Press; 2012. p. 133.
20. Gobbi H, Atkinson JB, Kardos TF, Simpson JF, Page DL. Inflammatory myofibroblastic tumor of the breast: report of a case with giant vacuolated cells. Breast. 1999;8:135–8.
21. Wargotz ES, Weiss SW, Norris HJ. Myofibroblastoma of the breast. Sixteen cases of a distinctive benign mesenchymal tumor. Am J Surg Pathol. 1987;11:493–502.
22. Fukunaga M, Ushigome S. Myofibroblastoma of the breast with diverse differentiations. Arch Pathol Lab Med. 1997;121:599–603.
23. Magro G, Fletcher CDM, Eusebi V. Myofibroblastoma. In: Lakhani SR, Ellis IO, Schnitt SJ, Tan PH, van de Vijver MJ, editors. WHO classification of tumours of the breast. 4th ed. Lyon: IARC Press; 2012. p. 130–1.
24. Rosen PP, Ernsberger D. Mammary fibromatosis. A benign spindle-cell tumor with significant risk for local recurrence. Cancer. 1989;63:1363–9.
25. Lee A, Gobbi H. Desmoid-type fibromatosis. In: Lakhani SR, Ellis IO, Schnitt SJ, Tan PH, van de Vijver MJ, editors. WHO classification of tumours of the breast. 4th ed. Lyon: IARC Press; 2012. p. 131–2.
26. Abraham SC, Reynolds C, Lee JH, Montgomery EA, Baisden BL, Krasinskas AM, Wu TT. Fibromatosis of the breast and mutations involving the APC/beta-catenin pathway. Hum Pathol. 2002;33:39–46.
27. Gobbi H, Tan PH. Lipoma. In: Lakhani SR, Ellis IO, Schnitt SJ, Tan PH, van de Vijver MJ, editors. WHO classification of tumours of the breast. 4th ed. Lyon: IARC Press; 2012. p. 123–4.
28. Schnitt SJ, Collins LC. Other mesenchymal lesions. In: Schnitt SJ, Collins LC, editors. Biopsy interpretation of the breast. 2nd ed. Philadelphia, PA: Lippincott Williams & Wilkins; 2013. p. 408–18.
29. Tan PH, Tse G, Lee A, Simpson JF, Hanby AM. Fibroepithelial tumours. In: Lakhani SR, Ellis IO, Schnitt SJ, Tan PH, van de Vijver MJ, editors. WHO classification of tumours of the breast. 4th ed. Lyon: IARC Press; 2012. p. 142–7.
30. Daya D, Trus T, D'Souza TJ, Minuk T, Yemen B. Hamartoma of the breast, an underrecognized breast lesion. A clinicopathologic and radiographic study of 25 cases. Am J Clin Pathol. 1995;103:685–9.
31. Tse GM, Law BK, Ma TK, Chan AB, Pang LM, Chu WC, Cheung HS. Hamartoma of the breast: a clinicopathological review. J Clin Pathol. 2002;55:951–4.
32. Fox SB, Lee A. Granular cell tumor and benign peripheral nerve-sheath tumours. In: Lakhani SR, Ellis IO, Schnitt SJ, Tan PH, van de Vijver MJ, editors. WHO classification of tumours of the breast. 4th ed. Lyon: IARC Press; 2012. p. 134–5.
33. Fanburg-Smith JC, Meis-Kindblom JM, Fante R, Kindblom LG. Malignant granular cell tumor of soft tissue: diagnostic criteria and clinicopathologic correlation. Am J Surg Pathol. 1998;22:779–94.
34. Donnell RM, Rosen PP, Lieberman PH, Kaufman RJ, Kay S, Braun DW Jr, Kinne DW. Angiosarcoma and other vascular tumors of the breast. Am J Surg Pathol. 1981;5:629–42.
35. Ginter PS, McIntire PJ, Shin SJ. Vascular tumours of the breast: a comprehensive review with focus on diagnostic challenges encountered in the core biopsy setting. Pathology. 2017;49:197–214.
36. MacGrogan G, Skalova A, Shin SJ. Benign vascular lesions. In: Lakhani SR, Ellis IO, Schnitt SJ, Tan PH, van de Vijver MJ, editors. WHO classification of tumours of the breast. 4th ed. Lyon: IARC Press; 2012. p. 127–8.
37. Schnitt SJ, Collins LC. Vascular lesions. In: Schnitt SJ, Collins LC, editors. Biopsy interpretation of the breast. 2nd ed. Philadelphia, PA: Lippincott Williams & Wilkins; 2013. p. 387–407.
38. Rosen PP. Vascular tumors of the breast. III. Angiomatosis. Am J Surg Pathol. 1985;9:652–8.
39. Fineberg S, Rosen PP. Cutaneous angiosarcoma and atypical vascular lesions of the skin and breast after radiation therapy for breast carcinoma. Am J Clin Pathol. 1994;102:757–63.
40. Fraga-Guedes C, Gobbi H, Mastropasqua MG, Rocha RM, Botteri E, Toesca A, Viale G. Clinicopathological and immunohistochemical study of 30 cases of post-radiation atypical vascular lesion of the breast. Breast Cancer Res Treat. 2014;146:347–54.
41. Fraga-Guedes C, André S, Mastropasqua MG, Botteri E, Toesca A, Rocha RM, et al. Angiosarcoma and atypical vascular lesions of the

breast: diagnostic and prognostic role of *MYC* gene amplification and protein expression. Breast Cancer Res Treat. 2015;151:131–40.

42. Fletcher CDM, MacGrogan G, Fox SB. Angiosarcoma. In: Lakhani SR, Ellis IO, Schnitt SJ, Tan PH, van de Vijver MJ, editors. WHO classification of tumours of the breast. 4th ed. Lyon: IARC Press; 2012. p. 135–6.

43. Fraga-Guedes C, Gobbi H, Mastropasqua MG, Botteri E, Luini A, Viale G. Primary and secondary angiosarcomas of the breast: a single institution experience. Breast Cancer Res Treat. 2012;132:1081–8.

44. Scow JS, Reynolds CA, Degnim AC, Petersen IA, Jakub JW, Boughey JC. Primary and secondary angiosarcoma of the breast: the Mayo Clinic experience. J Surg Oncol. 2010;101:401–7.

45. Fletcher CDM, Eusebi V. Liposarcoma. In: Lakhani SR, Ellis IO, Schnitt SJ, Tan PH, van de Vijver MJ, editors. WHO classification of tumours of the breast. 4th ed. Lyon: IARC Press; 2012. p. 137.

46. Fletcher CDM, Eusebi V. Osteosarcoma. In: Lakhani SR, Ellis IO, Schnitt SJ, Tan PH, van de Vijver MJ, editors. WHO classification of tumours of the breast. 4th ed. Lyon: IARC Press; 2012. p. 138–9.

Because of the relative higher incidence of papillary carcinoma in men than in women [11], it may be prudent to assess the presence myoepithelial cells with the aid of immunostains such as p63, smooth muscle actin and calponin. If myoepithelial cells are present at the periphery of the lesion and inside (lining) the fibrovascular cores, we are dealing with a papilloma. If they are present only at the periphery, it is consistent with a papillary DCIS. Complete absence of myoepithelial cells is the hallmark of low-grade invasive papillary carcinoma [12].

Considering their benign behavior, both a conservative approach and surgical excision of papillary lesions are recommended [4].

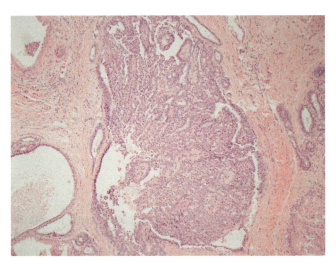

Fig. 24.1 Papilloma of male breast: low magnification shows multiple papillary fronds filling the duct, characterized by different sizes and shapes. Fibrovascular stalks are also evident

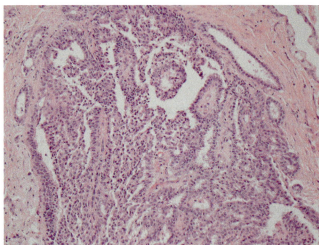

Fig. 24.2 Papilloma of male breast: papillary fronds in this benign intraductal papilloma show histological features overlapping with their female counterpart; fibrovascular stalks are lined by bland cuboidal or cylindrical ductal epithelial cells with underlying myoepithelial cells (not shown)

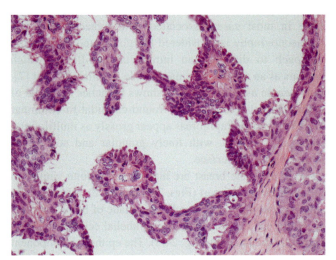

Fig. 24.3 Papillary frond in benign intraductal papilloma of male breast: papillae show variably sized fibrovascular stalks, typical of benign papillary lesions; epithelial lining shows frankly benign cytology, with cuboidal or columnar luminal cells with round/oval nuclei. Myoepithelial cells are also observed in fibrovascular stalk and ductal wall

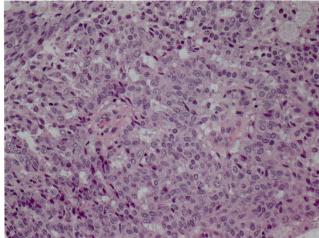

Fig. 24.4 Papilloma of male breast harboring usual ductal hyperplasia: this intraductal papilloma shows areas of epithelial proliferation, characterized by cohesive cells with variably sized and irregularly distributed nuclei; scattered irregular lumens are also noted. Such findings are all suggestive of usual ductal hyperplasia

24.1.3 Fibroepithelial Tumors

Fibroepithelial tumors are uncommon in men. Fibroadenomas (FA) most commonly arise in association to gynecomastia and underlying lobular differentiation [13–15]. Truth to be told, many case reports that described FA are mistaken and actually feature fibroadenomatoid nodules in gynecomastia [12]. FA can occur in patients who undergo hormonal therapy or male-to-female sexual transition [16–18]. There are also cases related to certain medications such as: spironolactone [13], digitalis [19], methyldopa, chlordiazepoxide, furosemide, and Lupron [15]. Age at diagnosis ranges from 15 to 71 years. FA up to 7 cm in size have been described [20]. Hamartomas can also occur in men [21]. Phyllodes tumors (PT) have been described in the literature, with most cases being benign [20, 22].

Patients with FA can present with breast swelling and palpable masses. The clinical presentation of PT is similar to FA, showing, however, palpable masses usually larger than fibroadenomas. FA and PT appear as solid and cystic masses sometimes harboring calcifications on mammography. Ultrasonography usually reveals well circumscribed hypoechoic masses, with solid and cystic features. FNA shows uniform epithelial cells arranged in sheets with a honeycomb pattern, on a background of stromal cells [23].

FA appears as firm, solid multilobulated nodules with a grey-whitish cut surface. Histologically, fibroepithelial lesions in men don't differ much from those described in women, with the remarkable frequent presence of gynecomastia in the background. FA are characterized by a uniformly distributed biphasic proliferation of glandular and stromal compartments with intracanalicular and pericanalicular patterns, exactly like their female counterparts. The glandular/stroma ratio is 1:1. The stromal component may show myxoid and/or hyaline features. Cytologic atypia is absent. Stromal overgrowth (including the characteristic "leaf-like" pattern) accompanied by cytologic atypia and increased mitotic count are rather features of PTs. FA are benign fibroepithelial lesions that are usually treated with surgical excision. PT require surgical excision with clear margins.

24.1.4 Duct Ectasia

Duct ectasia (DE) is a benign condition that rarely occurs in men. It clinically presents as a mastitis with nipple discharge, especially in children [24] and young adults [25]. Histologically, DE is fairly similar to that described in women and exhibits dilated ducts with variable periductal fibrosis and periductal inflammation (Figs. 24.5 and 24.6).

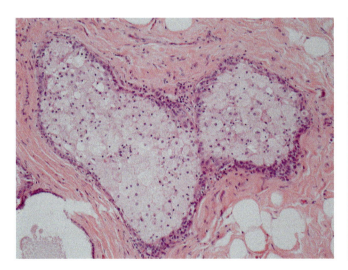

Fig. 24.5 Duct ectasia in male breast: cystically dilated duct containing intraductal foam cells; there is mild chronic inflammatory infiltrate in periductal stromal tissue

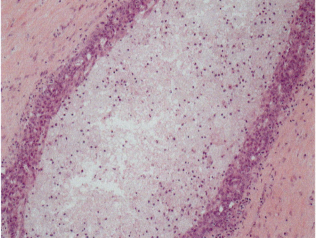

Fig. 24.6 Duct ectasia in male breast: acute and chronic inflammatory infiltrate composed by foamy macrophages, scattered neutrophils and lymphocytes are present inside the ectatic duct; ductal epithelial lining shows hyperplastic and regenerative changes

24.1.5 Fibrocystic Changes

Fibrocystic changes in the male breast are rare [26]. Usually this condition presents as abnormal swelling of the breast. Grossly the lesion appears white or gray, fibrotic and cystic. Histologically it looks identical to its female counterpart [27]: mammary ducts appear cystically dilated and crowded, apocrine metaplasia may be present. Usual ductal hyperplasia and papillary hyperplasia [26] can be also present. Bigotti et al. [28] reported a case of incidental sclerosing adenosis of the breast discovered at autopsy of a man with lung small cell carcinoma.

24.1.6 Myoepithelial Tumors

Myoepithelial neoplasms in male breasts are extremely uncommon. Adenomyoepitheliomas (AME) are benign neoplasms characterized by epithelial and myoepithelial differentiation. In men it is very rare, with only a handful of cases described in the literature [29–31]. Mammography usually reveals an opaque mass with focal indistinct margins and occasional microcalcifications. On gross examination they are described as nodular and well circumscribed lesions with solid or papillary features. Small, round, and bland glandular units with cuboidal or cylindrical epithelial layers are surrounded by a proliferation of polygonal myoepithelial cells with clearing of the cytoplasm; not infrequently, such myoepithelial cells may display spindle morphology (Figs. 24.7, 24.8, 24.9, and 24.10).

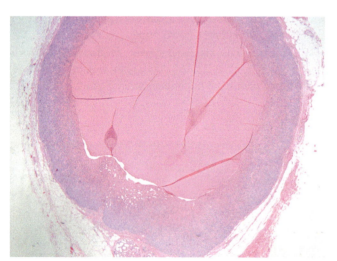

Fig. 24.7 Adenomyoepithelioma of male breast: low magnifications shows a well circumscribed, nodular lesion; the central part of this lesion is cystically dilated with intraluminal eosinophilic secretion

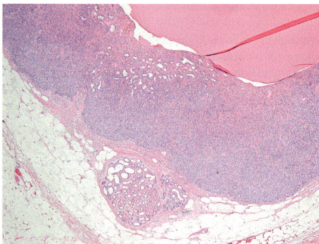

Fig. 24.8 Adenomyoepithelioma of male breast: such lesions could be mono or multinodular; even if they are well demarcated, there is a typical lack of a thick fibrous capsule

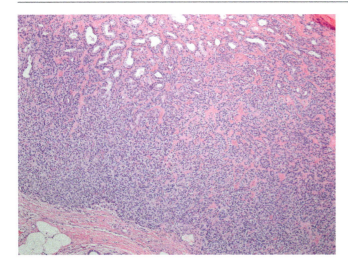

Fig. 24.9 Adenomyoepithelioma of male breast: this lesion shows solid and sometimes papillary structures with cords and cellular aggregates separated by fibrovascular collagenous stroma; they are sometimes organized in glandular units with bland appearance and mildly irregular lumens

24.1.7 Mesenchymal Neoplasms

Myofibroblastoma (MFB) is a mesenchymal neoplasm composed by myofibroblasts with smooth muscle differentiation. MFBs occur in both women and men, and breast parenchyma is a common location. They present as an asymptomatic mobile mass, usually monolateral, causing breast swelling. Radiographic findings are not specific: mammography and ultrasonography reveal round and well circumscribed benign-looking nodular lesions [32]. Grossly, MFB appear as a solid nodule, well circumscribed, with a white or yellow cutting surface. MFB consist of haphazardly arranged and variably sized fascicles of spindle cells, sometimes organized in storiform pattern, with eosinophilic cytoplasm and bland elongated nuclei. Atypical cytologic features, necrosis, and hemorrhage should not be present. Staghorn-like blood vessels may be present (Figs. 24.11, 24.12, 24.13, and 24.14).

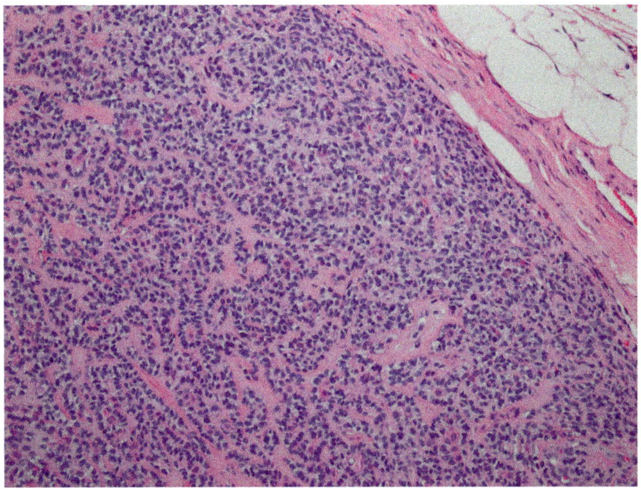

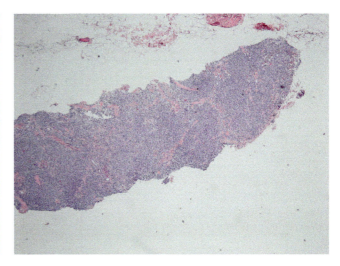

Fig. 24.10 Adenomyoepithelioma of male breast: cuboidal or columnar cells are surrounded by prominent myoepithelial cells with clear cytoplasm and polygonal shape. Sometimes such cells may show spindle shape

Fig. 24.11 Myofibroblastoma of male breast: this lesion is densely cellular and usually circumscribed, but an invasive rim may be observed

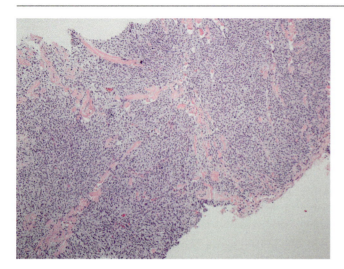

Fig. 24.12 Myofibroblastoma of male breast: the main histologic feature is the presence of spindle-shaped cells haphazardly arranged in fascicles with storiform pattern, with occasional interposed bands of dense collagen

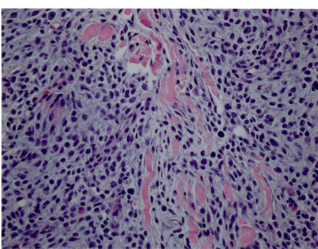

Fig. 24.14 Myofibroblastoma of male breast: bland cytology characterized by overall dark nuclei with inconspicuous nucleoli and occasional nuclear grooves. Mitotic figures are rare

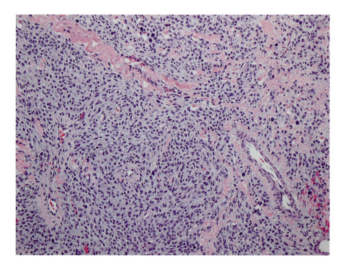

Fig. 24.13 Myofibroblastoma of male breast: spindle cells show eosinophilic cytoplasm with bland elongated nuclei. In this figure, inconspicuous "staghorn-like" blood vessels are also present

24.1.8 Gynecomastia

Gynecomastia is the most frequent benign lesion of the male breast. It is defined as an increase in size of the breast due to both epithelial and stromal proliferation. Gynecomastia has been observed mainly in neonatal and pubertal patients but can occur at all ages [33–35]. Bilateral synchronous involvement is seen in most patients. Although the main cause of gynecomastia seems to be a physiologic unbalance between estrogen and androgen hormones [33, 36], a conspicuous amount of literature describes cases of gynecomastia related to exogenous administration of estrogen [37], androgen, or other drugs such as Finasteride for the treatment of prostatic hyperplasia [38] and chemotherapeutic agents [39, 40]. Gynecomastia can be associated with multiple pathologic conditions such as cirrhosis, extramammary neoplasms causing paraneoplastic syndromes (lung cancer, germ cell tumors of the testis) [41, 42], and genetic diseases such as Klinefelter syndrome or other hypogonadism [41, 43].

Clinically, gynecomastia presents with bilateral or, less frequently, unilateral breast enlargement with the presence of a palpable mass associated with pain and/or tenderness. Nipple discharge or cutaneous involvement are rare.

Radiological findings associated with gynecomastia consist of three characteristic patterns: a nodular pattern, corresponding to the initial florid phase with a fan-shaped dense area with indistinct borders; a dendritic pattern that corresponds to the fibrotic phase of gynecomastia, with a flame-shaped mass that penetrates into the fat [7]; and the third pattern, so-called diffuse glandular pattern, that usually occurs in patients who received exogenous estrogen, and shows mixed radiological findings typical of dendritic and nodular patterns [44].

FNA displays large fragments of cohesive cells or flat monolayered sheets of epithelial cells, with oval nuclei in the background (Fig. 24.15). Minimal cytologic atypia and slight dyshesion may be occasionally observed. In the case of a fibrous lesion, scant material is commonly yielded.

Macroscopy reveals soft, somewhat rubbery or indurated white-gray tissue that may form a distinct mass. Regardless of the etiology, gynecomastia is classified in three phases: florid, intermediate, and fibrous, which reflect its physiological evolution. Florid gynecomastia is characterized by a proliferative ductal epithelium composed of clustering ducts embedded in a variably cellular stroma with fibroblasts and adipose tissue; periductal stroma may be edematous (Fig. 24.16). Epithelial proliferation consists of usual ductal hyperplasia, often with micropapillary architecture; ectatic ducts are infrequent (Figs. 24.17 and 24.18). The fibrous phase usually occurs after a prolonged proliferative gynecomastia (1 year or longer). Epithelial proliferation is decreased, and progressive ductal dilatation is observed. Acellular stromal fibrosis becomes prominent with decreased adipose tissue and vanishing periductal edema (Figs. 24.19 and 24.20). In some cases, pseudoangiomatous stromal hyperplasia may be seen (Fig. 24.21) [45]. Additional histologic findings include lobular formation, pseudolactational, squamous metaplasia, and apocrine metaplasia (Figs. 24.22, 24.23, 24.24, and 24.25). Micropapillary ductal hyperplasia sometimes shows mild cytologic atypia (Fig. 24.26), as reported by Zimmerman et al. [46] in a patient treated with Finasteride. The authors described cellular monotony and vacuolated cells resembling lobular carcinoma in cytologic smears. Intermediate gynecomastia shows histologic features of both florid and fibrotic phases. Male breast ducts in gynecomastia express estrogen and progesterone receptors. Of note, further studies revealed the presence of a three-layered epithelium [47] with complex immunophenotype. Such epithelium is composed of a basal myoepithelial cell layer (positive for myoepithelial cell markers) that surrounds two layers of epithelial cells, defined as intermediate (hormone receptors positive) and inner luminal (cytokeratin 5 positive).

Gynecomastia causes breast enlargement and variably palpable lesions; it must therefore be differentiated by breast volume increase due to adipose tissue (pseudogynecomastia). Male breast carcinoma, even if rare, should be considered in differential diagnosis considering its potential clinical presentation as a discrete palpable nodular lesion. Gynecomastia is a benign condition that is usually self-limiting, especially in the prepubertal setting. Medical treatment is based on correcting the underlying hormonal imbalance; drugs related to the onset of gynecomastia should be suspended. Surgery is the gold standard treatment in cases of cosmetic correction or removal of a persistent gynecomastic condition [48].

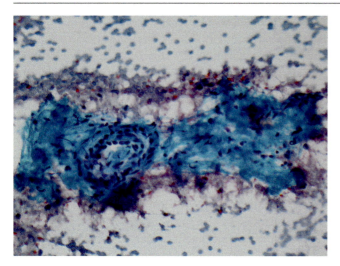 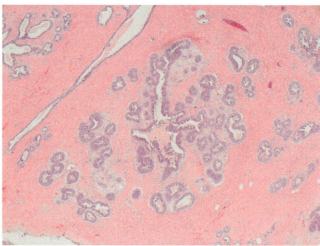

Fig. 24.15 Gynecomastia, cytology: this fine-needle aspiration shows a sheet of typical epithelial cells admixed with smaller and darker myo-epithelial cells; background is composed of fibrous and inconspicuous adipose tissue (Papanicolaou Stain)

Fig. 24.16 Gynecomastia, florid phase: clustering proliferating ducts within a fibrous stroma with periductal edema and condensation; note the lack of ectatic ducts

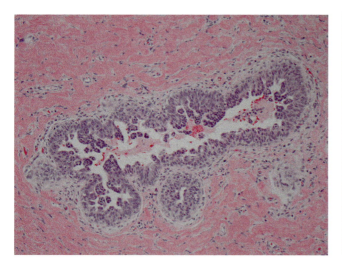 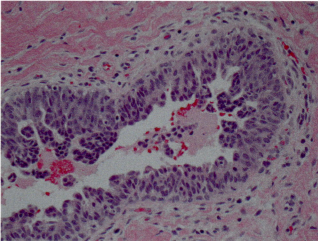

Fig. 24.17 Gynecomastia, usual ductal hyperplasia: ductal units in florid gynecomastia often show hyperplastic changes, mostly with micropapillary features

Fig. 24.18 Gynecomastia, usual ductal hyperplasia: micropapillary hyperplasia in gynecomastia with epithelium composed by cohesive bland proliferating cells, arranged in micropapillae and showing maturation as usually seen in usual ductal hyperplasia

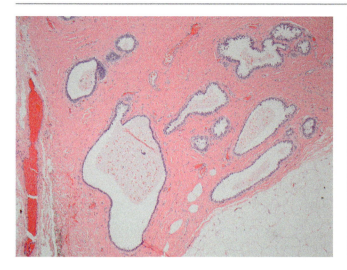

Fig. 24.19 Gynecomastia, fibrous phase: lack of epithelial proliferation, pronounced duct dilation and dense acellular fibrous stroma are typical of fibrous phase of gynecomastia

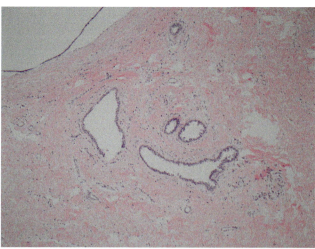

Fig. 24.20 Gynecomastia, fibrous phase: dense acellular stroma surrounds non-proliferating ductal units; note the decrease of periductal edema and stromal condensation

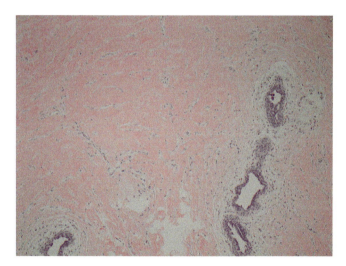

Fig. 24.21 Gynecomastia with pseudoangiomatous stromal hyperplasia: ductal units with mildly hyperplastic epithelium and decreased periductal edema are associated with fibrous stroma showing pseudoangiomatous stromal hyperplasia, with typical myofibroblasts with dark nuclei forming slit-like anastomosing channels

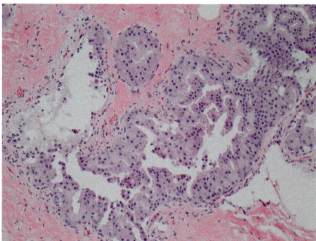

Fig. 24.22 Gynecomastia, apocrine change: this ductal unit is part of a nodule of gynecomastia; it shows apocrine metaplasia of epithelial cells, with evident eosinophilic cytoplasm and round dark nuclei

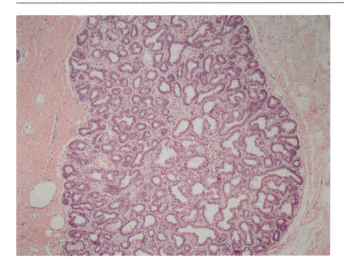

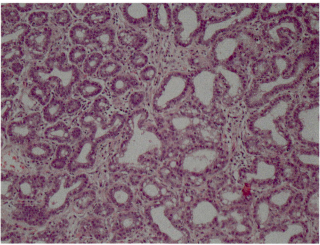

Fig. 24.23 Gynecomastia, pseudo-lactational changes: multiple ductal units showing a lobular configuration with pseudo-lactational changes

Fig. 24.24 Gynecomastia, pseudo-lactational changes: epithelial lining in these ducts is characterized by the presence of clear vacuoles, resembling lactational changes as seen in female breast

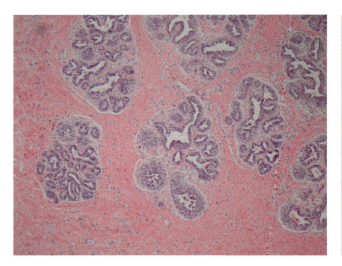

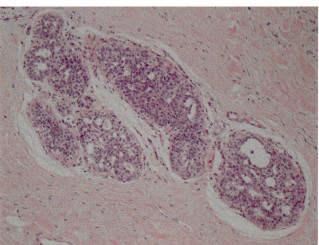

Fig. 24.25 Gynecomastia, lobule formation: in this gynecomastia nodule a lobular organization of ductal units can be appreciated. Common findings of gynecomastia are also present: micropapillary hyperplasia, periductal edema and pseudoangiomatous stromal hyperplasia of surrounding stroma

Fig. 24.26 Gynecomastia, atypical ductal hyperplasia: in this ductal unit, epithelial proliferation with mild cytologic atypia is present; nevertheless, the lack of architectural atypia favors atypical ductal hyperplasia

24.2   Malignant Lesions of the Male Breast

Male breast cancer has an incidence of 1.1 cases per 100,000 people a year in the USA [49] and accounts for 1% of cancers in males [50]. It occurs in an older age group than in women (mean age of 67 versus 61 years). Hormonal imbalance with an excess of estradiol seems to contribute to male breast cancer development, particularly in patients with testicular dysfunctions. Cryptorchidism, Klinefelter syndrome [51, 52], and obesity [53] are conditions associated with a high risk for developing male breast carcinoma because of their onset related to elevated levels of estradiol. Increased incidence of breast cancer has been observed in transgender patients who undergo hormonal therapy with prolonged administration of estrogen [54].

Medications that cause hormonal imbalance, utilized for the treatment of prostate cancer, may increase the risk; there is no convincing evidence of this, however, in part because of the lack of epidemiologic data and in part due to the fact that in some patients, breast cancer occurs prior to the onset prostate cancer, showing no cause-and-effect relationship between anti-androgen therapies for prostatic disease and breast carcinogenesis [55, 56]. A strong association between family history of breast or ovarian carcinoma and the incidence of breast neoplasia in males has been reported [57]. BRCA2 mutation and increased risk of male breast carcinoma has been well documented; other genetic alterations have also been related to male breast cancer, such as CHECK 2 [58]. There is no clear evidence of gynecomastia as a predisposing factor for breast cancer in males, and histopathologic transition between the two conditions is rare. Above all, common risk factors (for example, their coexistence in males with Klinefelter's syndrome and the presence of atypia in gynecomastic breast) for both the diseases suggest a mutual correlation [57]. Finally, occupational exposure to chemicals and similar industrial branches has been noted, correlating this phenomenon to increased incidence of breast neoplasm and gynecomastia [59].

The male breast presents with a unilateral and asymptomatic, or sometimes painful, swelling, with enlargement and palpable lump. Median age at diagnosis is 68 years in the United States [60]. Malignant neoplastic masses are commonly located centrally, behind the nipple, but peripheral nodules have been also described. Nipple discharge may be present, as well skin and nipple retraction; the latter two are more frequent in male than in female breasts.

Ultrasonography and mammography are the most useful radiological techniques for diagnostic approach [61]. At mammographic exam, invasive ductal carcinoma can be described as a dense, irregular, round or oval mass with spiculated margins; calcifications are uncommon. At ultrasonography, invasive ductal carcinoma is represented as an irregular, solid, or hypoechoic mass, with multilobular appearance and spiculated margins.

Cytologic findings are similar to those described in female breast carcinoma, in particular the ductal type.

As in most of the breast neoplasms, cytologic preparations obtained by invasive carcinomas of NST type are very rich in cellularity, with plenty of discohesive single epithelial cells, often monomorphic and atypical; sometimes they can be arranged in sheets, tridimensional clusters or glandular-like structures. Nuclei are eccentric and show prominent nucleoli. Myoepithelial cells are absent in invasive carcinomas, but their presence may be suggestive for ductal carcinoma in situ (Figs. 24.27 and 24.28). The background varies from a simple bloody component to the presence of necrosis and acute or chronic inflammatory cells. High-grade carcinomas are characterized by remarkable atypia, prominent mitoses, and necrotic background.

Such findings are commonly present also in atypical epithelial lesions—for example atypical ductal hyperplasia—but the lack of myoepithelial cells and the presence of morphologic criteria should drive the diagnosis toward invasive ductal carcinoma [62]. Papillary carcinomas are more frequent in males than in females; at fine-needle aspiration they are characterized by hypercellular smears with single atypical cells or branching cohesive tridimensional sheets. Papillary structures with fibrovascular cores may be present. Benign papillary lesions tend to show poorer smears and none or lesser atypia than the malignant counterpart [6].

Invasive carcinomas are grossly analogous to the neoplastic masses in the female breast: irregular and sometimes multinodular tumors with grey or whitish cut surface.

One of the main differentials to keep always in mind is metastatic prostatic adenocarcinoma [63]. Both breast and prostate carcinomas can be positive for estrogen receptor (ER) and androgen receptors, making a phenotypic distinction difficult. Also, rare positivity of male breast cancer for prostate specific antigen has been described [63], suggesting further caution with immunohistochemical interpretation in invasive neoplasms.

Surgical excision is the most effective therapeutic approach for male breast cancer, including mastectomy as the most common choice because of the central position of the cancer and the dimension of the breast [64]. Neoadjuvant therapy and radiotherapy for advanced stage cancer are also useful. As in female patients, ER positivity allows male patients to benefit of endocrine therapy with good response.

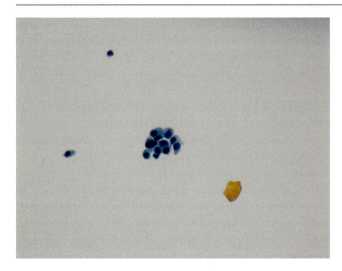

Fig. 24.27 Male breast carcinoma, cytology: fine-needle aspiration obtained from an invasive ductal carcinoma of male breast, neoplastic cells are single or arranged in sheets, showing marked eccentric atypical nuclei. Myoepithelial cells are absent (Papanicolaou)

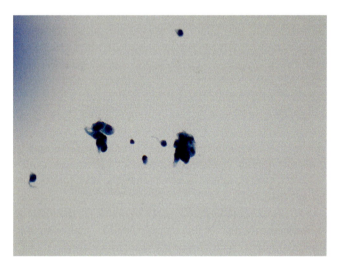

Fig. 24.28 Male breast carcinoma, cytology: invasive ductal carcinoma characterized by single atypical cells and tridimensional clusters; nuclear atypia and hyperchromasia are remarkable (Papanicolaou)

24.2.1 Ductal Carcinoma In Situ

Ductal carcinoma in situ (DCIS) represents 10% of all male breast carcinomas. Most of the malignant neoplasms (90%) in the male breast are invasive carcinomas not otherwise specified [65]. Men are usually affected by DCIS at an older age than females, with a remarkable difference in subtypes distribution: the most frequent variant in men is intraductal papillary carcinoma; the other subtypes such as cribriform, solid, and micropapillary are uncommon [66]. Comedonic DCIS is very rare (Figs. 24.29, 24.30, 24.31, 24.32, 24.33, 24.34, 24.35, and 24.36) [11].

Histopathologic features of intraductal papillary carcinoma in men are similar to those observed in women, the duct(s) are occupied by arborescent fibrovascular cores lined by epithelial cells with lack of myoepithelial cells. As in females, the distinction between pure papillary DCIS and preexisting papilloma involved by DCIS or atypical ductal hyperplasia must be made [67]. The diagnosis of DCIS within a preexisting papilloma must be considered when the atypical cell population is equal to or greater than 3 mm (or 90% of the entire lesion), or if nuclear grade is intermediate or higher grade, regardless of the extent of the lesion [68]. If these criteria are not met, such a lesion is best classified as atypical papilloma.

Papillary DCIS in men are for the most part intracystic. Fibrovascular stalks are thin and sometimes inconspicuous, surrounded by bland and uniform epithelial cells that may be round or columnar. Pleomorphism and high-grade atypia are rare. Myoepithelial cells are not present inside the papillary processes. Cribriform or micropapillary patterns may coexist within the same duct along with a papillary one (Figs. 24.37, 24.38, and 24.39).

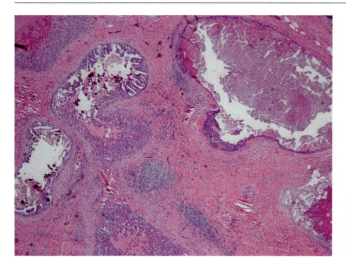

Fig. 24.29 Male breast ductal carcinoma in situ (DCIS): High-grade DCIS showing comedonic-type necrosis expanding the lumen. Histological features overlap with its female counterpart

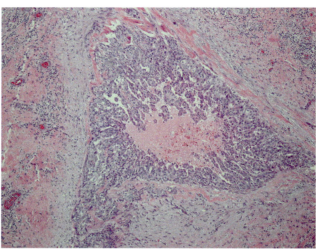

Fig. 24.30 Male breast DCIS: this focus of DCIS shows moderate-high-grade cytology and micropapillary architecture. Periductal stromal edema and condensation are also present, as seen in gynecomastia

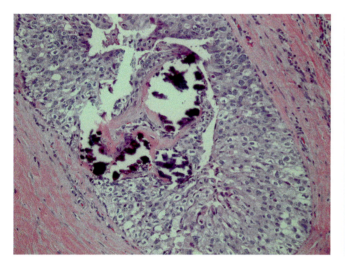

Fig. 24.31 Male breast DCIS: this high-grade DCIS harbors central calcifications. There are nuclear pleomorphism and prominent nucleoli; cells show solid proliferation with large cytoplasm and occasional vacuolization

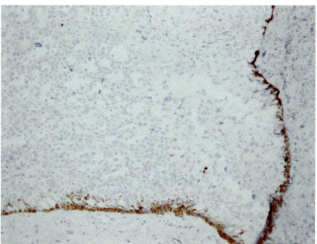

Fig. 24.32 Male breast DCIS, CK5/6 antibody: immunohistochemical marker for Cytokeratin 5/6 (CK5/6) is negative in luminal epithelial proliferating cells in this picture, corroborating the diagnosis of DCIS

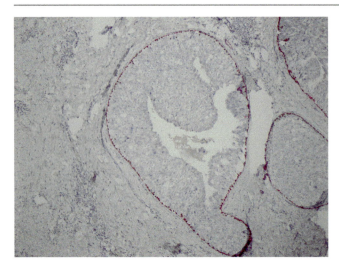

Fig. 24.33 Male breast DCIS, p63 antibody: DCIS shows positive staining of myoepithelial cells for antibody anti-p63

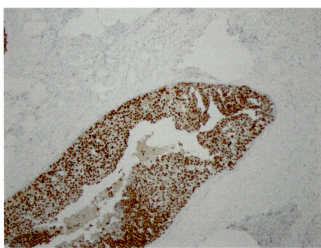

Fig. 24.34 Male breast DCIS, ER antibody: as in females, this DCIS of the male breast shows diffuse and strong positivity for Estrogen Receptor antibody

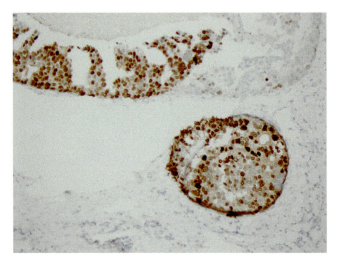

Fig. 24.35 Male breast DCIS, PR antibody: DCIS is strongly and diffusely immunoreactive for Progesterone Receptor antibody

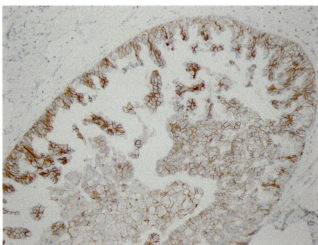

Fig. 24.36 Male breast DCIS, Cerb-B2(HER2) antibody: this micropapillary DCIS shows moderate-to-strong and complete membranous staining for HER2 antibody

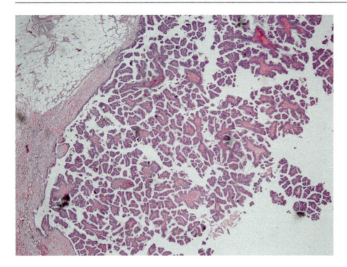

Fig. 24.37 Male breast, papillary DCIS: low-power view shows papillary DCIS, with variably thick or thin fibrovascular stalks surrounded by neoplastic epithelium

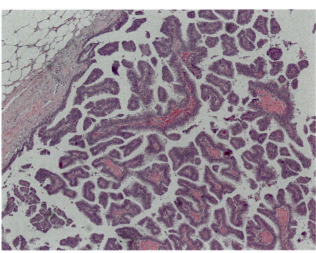

Fig. 24.38 Male breast, papillary DCIS: papillary projections fill the lumen creating classic papillae or luminal tufts; fibrovascular stalks may be inconspicuous, and sometimes only mildly ectatic blood vessels are evident

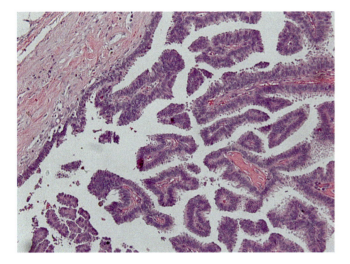

Fig. 24.39 Male breast, papillary DCIS: neoplastic cells are overall cuboidal and monomorphic, with elongated bland nuclei and apical snouts; peripheral duct wall shows some prominent myoepithelial cells

24.2.2 Paget Disease of the Nipple

Paget disease has a higher incidence in males than in females [66]; it presents as nipple erosion or erythema, sometimes with discharge. Underlying carcinoma may not be present [69]. The skin can be hyperkeratotic and hyperplastic, showing papillomatosis, and harboring large and atypical cells with clear cytoplasm and a dark nucleus that infiltrate epidermis (Figs. 24.40, 24.41, 24.42, and 24.43).

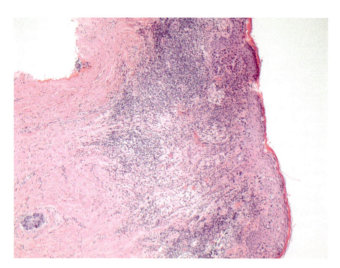

Fig. 24.40 Paget disease in male breast: low-power view shows skin with brisk dermal inflammatory infiltrate and some evident atypical epithelioid cell involving the epidermis

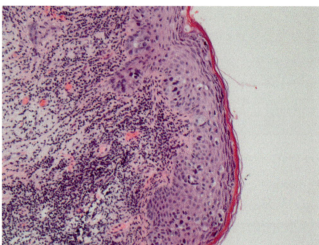

Fig. 24.41 Paget disease in male breast: the epidermis is involved by large atypical cells, with large cytoplasm and prominent nuclei. Note consensual epidermal hyperkeratosis

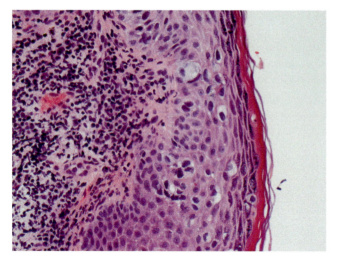

Fig. 24.42 Paget disease in male breast: high-power view shows atypical neoplastic cells scattered throughout the entire epidermal depth (Pagetoid spread)

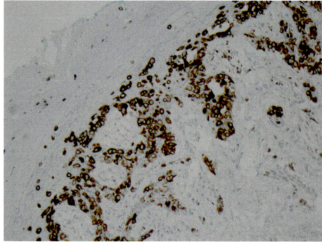

Fig. 24.43 Paget disease in male breast: Cytokeratin 7 positivity highlights neoplastic cells, confirming their origin from breast neoplastic tissue

24.2.3 Lobular Carcinoma

Lobular carcinoma is very uncommon in men, probably because of the lack of lobular units in the male breast. Rare cases of lobular carcinoma have been reported in patients affected by Klinefelter's syndrome [70, 71], suggesting a potential role of increased estrogen stimulation.

Most of the cases reported are invasive lobular carcinomas, described as small and discohesive cells with clear and granular cytoplasm, round vesicular nuclei, arranged in the classic Indian file. A pleomorphic variant with high nuclear/cytoplasmic ratio and focal signet ring cell formation have also been described [72]. As in women, lobular carcinomas of the male breast lack E-Cadherin expression.

24.2.4 Invasive Carcinoma

Invasive carcinoma of NST type [73–75] is by far the most common type of male breast cancer and is histologically identical to that of women (Figs. 24.44, 24.45, and 24.46) [11]. Invasive papillary carcinoma, on the other hand, is more frequent in men than in women. Special types of breast carcinoma, such as medullary, adenoid cystic, micropapillary, and secretory carcinoma, have been described in men,

although they are quite rare (Figs. 24.47, 24.48, 24.49, and 24.50) [74–76].

Histological grading is applied as in females. Of note, breast cancers in men tend to present with a higher grade than in women, with most of invasive carcinomas of NST type being grade II–III at the moment of diagnosis [77]. The prognosis depends on the same parameters considered in females: histologic grade, pathologic TNM staging system status and hormonal receptors status. Presentation with a higher stage, and at an older age, at the moment of diagnosis negatively influences the prognosis; this is partly due to the fact that breast screening exams are performed less frequent in men than in women [77].

Male breast cancers are frequently estrogen and progesterone receptor positive [78]; however, response to hormonal therapy is controversial. The role of Her2 status in male breast carcinoma is still unclear. Its amplification has been reported in a low percentage of cases (Figs. 24.51, 24.52, and 24.53). Prognostic relevance has also been observed in cytokeratin profile expression: the majority of male breast cancers exhibit luminal-like phenotype (CK18+, CK19+) while only a small fraction shows a basal-like pattern (CK5/6+, CK14+) with an incidence similar to the one diagnosed in women [79].

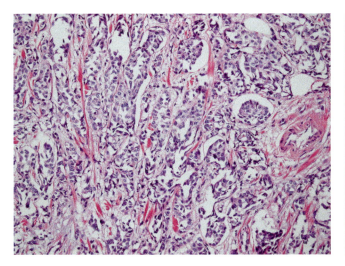

Fig. 24.44 Male breast, invasive carcinoma: invasive ductal carcinoma shows the same histological characteristics of its female counterpart

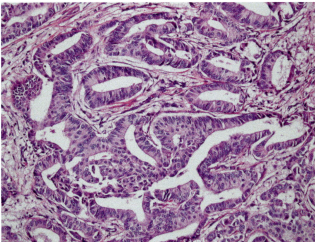

Fig. 24.45 Male breast, invasive carcinoma: this invasive ductal carcinoma shows irregular neoplastic ductal structures with high-grade atypical cytology, mitoses, prominent nucleoli, and pleomorphic nuclei

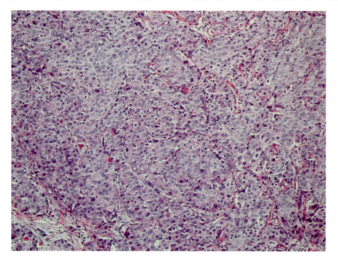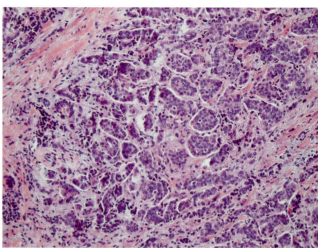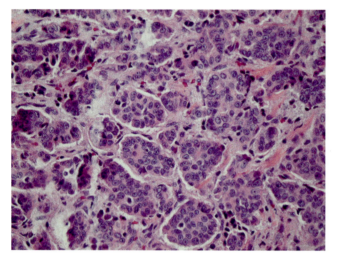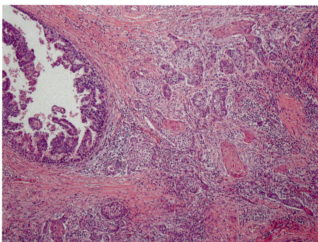

3

Fig. 24.46 Male breast, invasive carcinoma: invasive ductal carcinoma showing solid and cohesive sheets of neoplastic cells with inconspicuous blood vessels

Fig. 24.47 Male breast, invasive micropapillary carcinoma: this micropapillary invasive carcinoma is characterized by small clusters of cells (micropapillae) apparently suspended in clear spaces

Fig. 24.48 Male breast, invasive micropapillary carcinoma: apical surface of neoplastic cells shows "reverse" orientation toward the outside; this is a typical feature of micropapillary pattern of growth; moreover, micropapillae typically lack fibrovascular stalks

Fig. 24.49 Male breast, invasive carcinoma with squamous metaplasia: this invasive carcinoma shows large and irregular sheets of squamous keratinizing cells. In the same areas there is also a single focus of ductal carcinoma in situ with papillary and micropapillary features

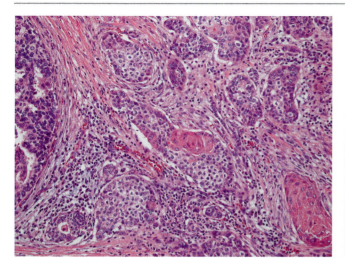

Fig. 24.50 Male breast, invasive carcinoma with squamous metaplasia: invasive carcinoma with squamous keratinizing metaplasia. There is a brisk inflammatory infiltrate around the invasive sheets of carcinoma

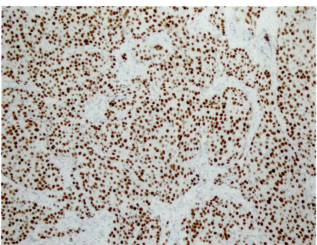

Fig. 24.51 Male breast, invasive carcinoma, ER: invasive ductal carcinoma showing strong and diffuse positivity for Estrogen Receptor immunohistochemical stain

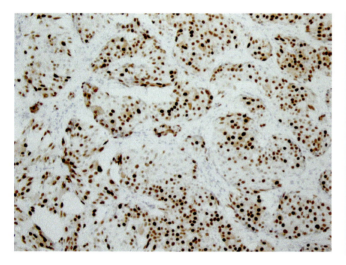

Fig. 24.52 Male breast, invasive carcinoma, PR: invasive ductal carcinoma showing, moderate-to-strong positivity for Progesterone Receptor immunohistochemical stain

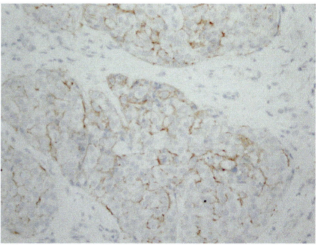

Fig. 24.53 Male breast, invasive carcinoma, HER2-neu: this invasive carcinoma of male breast shows incomplete circumferential membrane staining for HER2-neu, with weak-moderate intensity

References

1. Tavassoli FA. Male breast lesions. In: Tavassoli FA, editor. Pathology of the breast. 2nd ed. New York: McGraw-Hill; 1999.
2. González CC, Romero Manteola EJ. Intraductal metachronic papilloma: clinical case. Arch Argent Pediatr. 2015;113(6):e314–6.
3. Durkin ET, Warner TF, Nichol PF. Enlarging unilateral breast mass in an adolescent male: an unusual presentation of intraductal papilloma. J Pediatr Surg. 2011;46(5):e33–5.
4. De Vries FEE, Walter AW, Vrouenraets BC. Intraductal papilloma of the male breast. J Surg Case Rep. 2016;2016(2):rjw014.
5. Shim JH, Son EJ, Kim EK, Kwak JY, Jeong J, Hong SW. Benign intracystic papilloma of the male breast. J Ultrasound Med. 2008;27(9):1397–400.
6. Reid-Nicholson MD, Tong G, Cangiarella JF, Moreira AL. Cytomorphologic features of papillary lesions of the male breast: a study of 11 cases. Cancer. 2006;108(4):222–30.
7. Nguyen C, Kettler MD, Swirsky ME, Miller VI, Scott C, Krause R, et al. Male breast disease: pictorial review with radiologic-pathologic correlation. Radiographics. 2013;33:763–79.
8. Sara AS, Gottfried MR. Benign papilloma of the male breast following chronic phenothiazine therapy. Am J Clin Pathol. 1987;87:649–50.
9. Munitiz V, Illana J, Sola J, Piñero A, Rios A, Parrilla P. A case of breast cancer associated with juvenile papillomatosis of the male breast. Eur J Surg Oncol. 2000;26(7):715–6.
10. Pacilli M, Sebire NJ, Thambapillai E, Pierro A. Juvenile papillomatosis of the breast in a male infant with Noonan syndrome, café au lait spots, and family history of breast carcinoma. Pediatr Blood Cancer. 2005;45(7):991–3.
11. Burga AM, Fandare O, Lininger RA, Tavassoli FA. Invasive carcinomas of the male breast: a morphologic study of the distribution of histologic subtypes and metastatic patterns in 778 cases. Virchows Arch. 2006;449:507–12.
12. Murray MP, Brogi E. Benign proliferative lesions of the male breast. In: Hoda SA, Brogi E, Koerner FC, Rosen PP, editors. Rosen's breast pathology. 4th ed. Philadelphia: Lippincott Williams and Wilkins; 2014. p. 957.
13. Nielsen BB. Fibroadenomatoid hyperplasia of the male breast. Am J Surg Pathol. 1990;14(8):774–7.
14. Uchida T, Ishii M, Motomiya Y. Fibroadenoma associated with gynaecomastia in an adult man. Case report. Scand J Plast Reconstr Surg Hand Surg. 1993;27(4):327–9.
15. Shin SJ, Rosen PP. Bilateral presentation of fibroadenoma with digital fibroma-like inclusions in the male breast. Arch Pathol Lab Med. 2007;131(7):1126–9.
16. Adibelli ZH, Yildirim M, Ozan E, Oztekin O, Kucukzeybek B. Fibroadenoma of the breast in a man associated with adenocarcinoma of the rectum and polyposis coli. JBR-BTR. 2010;93(1):12–4.
17. Lemmo G, Garcea N, Corsello S, Tarquini E, Palladino T, Ardito G, et al. Breast fibroadenoma in a male-to-female transsexual patient after hormonal treatment. Eur J Surg Suppl. 2003;588:69–71.
18. Ansah-Boateng Y, Tavassoli FA. Fibroadenoma and cystosarcoma phyllodes of the male breast. Mod Pathol. 1992;5(2):114–6.
19. LeWinn EB. Gynecomastia during digitalis therapy; report of eight additional cases with liver-function studies. N Engl J Med. 1953;248(8):316–20.
20. Hilton DA, Jameson JS, Furness PN. A cellular fibroadenoma resembling a benign phyllodes tumour in a young male with gynaecomastia. Histopathology. 1991;18:476–7.
21. Amira RA, Sheikhb SS. Breast hamartoma: a report of 14 cases of an under-recognized and under-reported entity. Int J Surg Case Rep. 2016;22:1–4.
22. Karihtala P, Rissanen T, Touminen H. Male malignant phyllodes breast tumor after prophylactic breast radiotherapy and bicalutamide treatment: a case report. Anticancer Res. 2016;36(7):3433–6.
23. Ashutosh N, Virendra K, Attri PC, Arati S. Giant male fibroadenoma: a rare benign lesion. Indian J Surg. 2013;75(Suppl 1):353–5.
24. McHoney M, Munro F, Mackinlay G. Mammary duct ectasia in children: report of a short series and review of the literature. Early Hum Dev. 2011;87(8):527–30.
25. Aydin R, Baris Gul S, Polat AV. Detection of duct ectasia of mammary gland by ultrasonography in a neonate with bloody nipple discharge. Pediatr Neonatol. 2014;55(3):228–30.
26. Robertson KE, Kazmi SA, Jordan LB. Female-type fibrocystic disease with papillary hyperplasia in a male breast. J Clin Pathol. 2010;63(1):88–9.
27. McClure J, Banerjee SS, Sandilands DG. Female type cystic hyperplasia in a male breast. Postgrad Med J. 1985;61(715):441–3.
28. Bigotti G, Kasznica J. Sclerosing adenosis in the breast of a man with pulmonary oat cell carcinoma: report of a case. Hum Pathol. 1986;17(8):861–3.
29. Berna JD, Arcas I, Ballester A, Bas A. Adenomyoepithelioma of the breast in a male. AJR Am J Roentgenol. 1997;169(3):917–8.
30. Tamura G, Monma N, Suzuki Y, Satodate R, Abe H. Adenomyoepithelioma (myoepithelioma) of the breast in a male. Hum Pathol. 1993;24(6):678–81.
31. Wahab TA, Uwakwe H, Gillibrand R, Fafemi O. Male breast adenomyoepithelioma- a case report and literature review. Afr J Cell Pathol. 2017;8:43–4.
32. Omar LA, Rojanapremsuk T, Saluja K, Merchant KA, Sharma PB. Radiologic and histologic presentation of male mammary myofibroblastoma. Proc (Bayl Univ Med Cent). 2016;29(3):321–2.
33. Akgül S, Kanbur N, Güçer S, Safak T, Derman O. The histopathological effects of tamoxifen in the treatment of pubertal gynecomastia. J Pediatr Endocrinol Metab. 2012;25(7–8):753–5.
34. Haibach H, Rosenholtz MJ. Prepubertal gynecomastia with lobules and acini: a case report and review of the literature. Am J Clin Pathol. 1983;80(2):252–5.
35. Demirbilek H, Bacak G, Baran RT, Avcı Y, Baran A, Keleş A, et al. Prepubertal unilateral gynecomastia: report of 2 cases. J Clin Res Pediatr Endocrinol. 2014;6(4):250–3.
36. Bannayan GA, Hajdu SI. Gynecomastia: clinicopathologic study of 351 cases. Am J Clin Pathol. 1972;57:431–7.
37. De Pinho JC, Aghajanova L, Herndon CN. Prepubertal gynecomastia due to indirect exposure to nonformulary bioidentical hormonal replacement therapy: a case report. J Reprod Med. 2016;61(1–2):73–7.
38. Green L, Wysowski DK, Fourcroy JL. Gynecomastia and breast cancer during finasteride therapy. N Engl J Med. 1996;335:823.
39. Caocci G, Atzeni S, Orrù N, Azzena L, Martorana L, Littera A, et al. Gynecomastia in a male after dasatinib treatment for chronic myeloid leukemia. Leukemia. 2008;22:2127–8.
40. Tanriverdi O, Unubol M, Taskin F, Meydan N, Sargin G, Guney E, et al. Imatinib-associated bilateral gynecomastia and unilateral testicular hydrocele in male patient with metastatic gastrointestinal stromal tumor: a literature review. J Oncol Pharm Pract. 2012;18:303–10.
41. Dickson G. Gynecomastia. Am Fam Physician. 2012;85(7):716–22.
42. Williams MJ. Gynecomastia. Its incidence, recognition and host characterization in 447 autopsy cases. Am J Med. 1963;34:103–12.
43. Bojesen A, Gravholt CH. Klinefelter syndrome in clinical practice. Nat Clin Pract Urol. 2007;4(4):192–204.
44. Chen L, Chantra PK, Larsen LH, Barton P, Rohitopakarn M, Zhu EQ, et al. Imaging characteristics of malignant lesions of the male breast. Radiographics. 2006;26(4):993–1006.
45. Mizutou A, Nakashima K, Moriya T. Large pseudoangiomatous stromal hyperplasia complicated with gynecomastia and lobular differentiation in a male breast. Springerplus. 2015;4:282.

46. Zimmerman RL, Fogt F, Cronin D, Lynch R. Cytologic atypia in a 53-year-old man with finasteride-induced gynecomastia. Arch Pathol Lab Med. 2000;124(4):625–7.
47. Kornegoor R, Verschuur-Maes AH, Buerger H, van Diest PJ. The 3-layered ductal epithelium in gynecomastia. Am J Surg Pathol. 2012;36(5):762–8.
48. Johnson RE, Hassan Murad M. Gynecomastia: pathophysiology, evaluation, and management. Mayo Clin Proc. 2009;84(11):1010–5.
49. Age-adjusted SEER incidence rates by cancer site, all ages, all races, male 1975–2013. https://seer.cancer.gov/csr/1975_2014/browse_csr.php?sectionSEL=4&pageSEL=sect_04_table.05.html. Accessed 18 Feb 2018.
50. Jemal A, Siegel R, Xu J, Ward E. Cancer statistics, 2010. CA Cancer J Clin. 2010;60:277–300.
51. Bender PF, de Oliveira LL, Costa CR, de Aguiar SS, Bergmann A, Thuler LCS. Men and women show similar survival rates after breast cancer. J Cancer Res Clin Oncol. 2017;143(4):563–71.
52. Javidiparsijani S, Rosen LE, Gattuso P. Male breast carcinoma: a clinical and pathological review. Int J Surg Pathol. 2017;25(3):200–5.
53. Weiss JR, Moysich KB, Swede H. Epidemiology of male breast cancer. Cancer Epidemiol Biomark Prev. 2005;14(1):20–6.
54. Kanhai RC, Hage JJ, van Diest PJ, Bloemena E, Mulder JW. Short term and long term histologic effects of castration and estrogen treatment on breast tissue of 14 male-to-female transsexual in comparison with two chemically castrated men. Am J Surg Pathol. 2000;24:74–80.
55. Leibowitz SB, Gaber JE, Fox EA, Loda M, Kaufman DS, Kantoff PW, et al. Male patients with diagnoses of both breast cancer and prostate cancer. Breast J. 2003;9(3):208–12.
56. Lee UJ, Jones JS. Incidence of prostate cancer in male breast cancer patients: a risk factor for prostate cancer screening. Prostate Cancer Prostatic Dis. 2009;12(1):52–6.
57. Brinton LA, Richesson DA, Gierach GL, Lacey JV Jr, Park Y, Hollenbeck AR, et al. Prospective evaluation of risk factors for male breast cancer. J Natl Cancer Inst. 2008;100:1477–81.
58. Pritzlaff M, Summerour P, McFarland R, Li S, Reineke P, Dolinsky JS, Goldgar DE, et al. Male breast cancer in a multi-gene panel testing cohort: insights and unexpected results. Breast Cancer Res Treat. 2017;161(3):575–86.
59. McLaughlin JK, Malker HS, Blot WJ, Weiner JA, Ericsson JL, Fraumeni JF Jr. Occupational risks for male breast cancer in Sweden. Br J Ind Med. 1988;45(4):275–6.
60. Age-adjusted SEER incidence rates by age, male breast, all races, male, 1975–2013 (SEER 9). https://seer.cancer.gov/csr/1975_2014/results_single/sect_01_table.12_2pgs.pdfAge. Accessed 18 Feb 2018.
61. Chau A, Jafarian N, Rosa M. Male breast: clinical and imaging evaluations of benign and malignant entities with histologic correlation. Am J Med. 2016;129(8):776–91.
62. Schmitt F, Gerhard R, Stanley DE, Domanski HA. Breast. In: Domanski HA, editor. Atlas of fine needle aspiration cytology. London: Springer; 2014. p. 67–8.
63. Carder PJ, Speirs V, Ramsdale J, Lansdown MR. Expression of prostate specific antigen in male breast cancer. J Clin Pathol. 2005;58(1):69–71.
64. Fentiman IS, Fourquet A, Hortobagyi GN. Male breast cancer. Lancet. 2006;367:595–604.
65. Fentiman IS. Male breast cancer: a review. Ecancermedicalscience. 2009;3:140.
66. Hittmair AP, Lininger RA, Tavassoli FA. Ductal carcinoma in situ (DCIS) in the male breast: a morphologic study of 84 cases of pure DCIS and 30 cases of DCIS associated with invasive carcinoma--a preliminary report. Cancer. 1998;83(10):2139–49.
67. Pal SK, Lau SK, Kruper L, Nwoye U, Garberoglio C, Gupta RK, et al. Papillary carcinoma of the breast: an overview. Breast Cancer Res Treat. 2010;122(3):637–45.
68. O'Malley F, Visscher D, MacGrogan G, et al. Papilloma with ADH and DCIS. In: Lakhani S, Ellis I, Schnitt S, Tan P, van de Vijver M, editors. WHO classifications of tumors of the breast. 4th ed. Lyon: IARC Press; 2012. p. 101–2.
69. O'Sullivan ST, Mc Greal GT, Lyons A, Burke L, Geoghegan JG, Brady MP. Paget's disease of the breast in a man without underlying breast carcinoma. J Clin Pathol. 1994;47:851–2.
70. Sanchez AG, Villanueva AG, Redondo C. Lobular carcinoma of the breast in a patient with klinefelter's syndrome. A case with bilateral, synchronous, histologically different breast tumors. Cancer. 1986;57:1181–3.
71. Chandrasekharan S, Fasanya C, Macneill FA. Invasive lobular carcinoma of the male breast: do we need to think of Klinefelter's syndrome? Breast. 2001;10:176–8.
72. Rohini B, Singh PA, Vatsala M, Vishal D, Mitali S, Nishant S. Pleomorphic lobular carcinoma in a male breast: a rare occurrence. Pathol Res Int. 2010;2010:871369.
73. Flynn LV, Park J, Patil SM, Cody HS III, Port ER. Sentinel lymph node biopsy is successful and accurate in male breast carcinoma. J Am Coll Surg. 2008;206:616–21.
74. Donegan WL, Redlich PN, Lang PJ, Gall MT. Carcinoma of the breast in males. Cancer. 1998;83(3):498–509.
75. Sanguinetti A, Polistena A, Lucchini R, Monacelli M, Galasse S, Avenia S, et al. Male breast cancer, clinical presentation, diagnosis and treatment: twenty years of experience in our Breast Unit. Int J Surg Case Rep. 2016;20(Suppl):8–11.
76. Barr JG, Clayton ESJ, Sotheran W. A case of metaplastic breast cancer in a man. J Surg Case Rep. 2013. https://doi.org/10.1093/jscr/rjs047.
77. Giordano SH, Cohen DS, Buzdar AU, Perkins G, Hortobagyi GN. Breast carcinoma in men: a population-based study. Cancer. 2004;101(1):51–7.
78. Wang-Rodriguez J, Cross K, Gallagher S, Djahanban M, Armstrong JM, Wiedner N, et al. Male breast carcinoma: correlation of ER, PR, Ki-67, Her2-neu, and p53 with treatment and survival, a study of 65 cases. Mod Pathol. 2002;15(8):853–61.
79. Ciocca V, Bombonati A, Gatalica Z, Di Pasquale M, Milos A, Ruiz-Orrico A, et al. Cytokeratin profiles of male breast cancers. Histopathology. 2006;49:365–70.

Lesions of the Nipple

Simona Stolnicu

The nipple can present a variety of tumor or tumor-like lesions, involving the skin and skin appendages, but also, the subcutaneous tissue or lactiferous ducts. Most of these lesions are very rare, but when occurring, they sometimes can be mistaken for malignant lesions clinically and pathologically, although most of them are not malignant in nature.

25.1 Nipple Duct Adenoma

Adenoma of the nipple is a benign tumor, also called nipple duct adenoma, papillary adenoma, erosive adenomatosis, nipple florid papillomatosis, or subareolar duct papillomatosis. The lesion can occur in both females and males, it can be unilateral or bilateral; mean age of occurrence is 45 years. Clinically, it is associated with serous or hemorrhagic nipple discharge, nipple size enlargement, hardening, and erosion or ulceration of the overlying epithelium of the nipple (therefore, it may be clinically confused with Paget's disease of the nipple or other malignant lesion). It is associated with pain, itching, and burning sensation. Sometimes, however, the lesion is asymptomatic (especially when it has a small size). It originates in the lactiferous ducts and, by developing, it gradually replaces the nipple stroma. When a similar lesion occurs in the subareolar region without involving the substance of the nipple, the lesion is designated as "subareolar sclerosing duct hyperplasia" [1]. Macroscopically, it has well-defined edges, gray-white cut surface, and compression over the underlying lactiferous ducts can cause cystic cavities. Microscopically, however, the margins of the tumor are most often ill-defined. The lesion consists of a compact tubular (ductal) proliferation surrounded by a sclerotic stroma, which often causes compression and distortion of the lactiferous ducts located in the vicinity (similar in appearance to sclerosing adenosis) (Fig. 25.1). The tubules are round or oval and lined by the two characteristic layers (epithelial and myoepithelial cells). Some lesions may focally present apocrine or squamous metaplasia. Sometimes, florid ductal hyperplasia of solid or papillary appearance also can be observed (Fig. 25.2). At other times, this hyperplasia is associated with atypia or even necrosis, and these findings are especially likely to be misinterpreted as malignant features (Figs. 25.3 and 25.4). The atypical features are most likely of reactive type, and identifying a heterogeneous population of cells in the florid intraductal hyperplasia areas is essential to rule out the carcinoma [2]. In some of the lesions, however,

S. Stolnicu, MD, PhD
Department of Pathology, University of Medicine and Pharmacy, Tîrgu Mureș, Romania

© Springer International Publishing AG, part of Springer Nature 2018
S. Stolnicu, I. Alvarado-Cabrero (eds.), *Practical Atlas of Breast Pathology*, https://doi.org/10.1007/978-3-319-93257-6_25

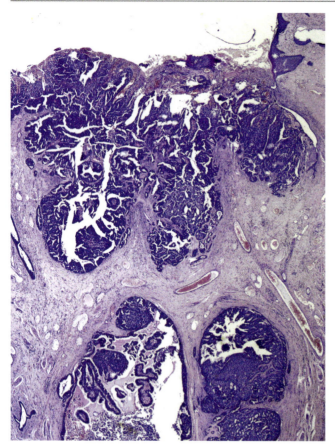

Fig. 25.1 Nipple duct adenoma: Compact tubular proliferation surrounded by a sclerotic stroma, producing the ulceration of the overlying skin; mixed adenosis, papillomatosis, and sclerosing papillomatosis patterns can be appreciated within the same lesion, lacking prognostic significance

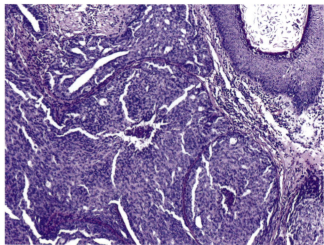

Fig. 25.3 Nipple duct adenoma: Areas of usual duct hyperplasia can present central necrosis, a feature not to be mistaken for a malignant lesion

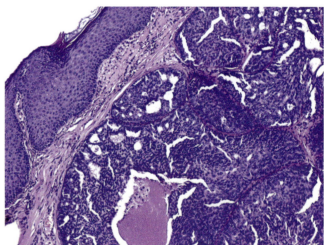

Fig. 25.4 Nipple duct adenoma: Areas of usual duct hyperplasia and central eosinophilic secretion within the tubular structures

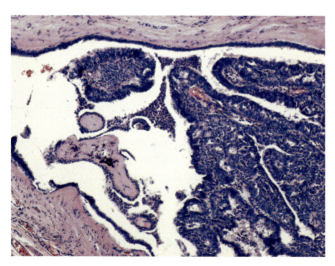

Fig. 25.2 Nipple duct adenoma: Papillomatosis areas are represented by fibrovascular cores lined by two cell layers, admixed with usual duct hyperplasia; areas of calcification can be appreciated within the fibrovascular cores

necrosis can occur even in the absence of atypia. The presence of necrosis and surface ulceration should not prompt a diagnosis of malignancy (Figs. 25.5 and 25.6). There was an attempt to classify the nipple duct adenoma into adenosis, but papillomatosis and sclerosing papillomatosis do not have any prognostic significance. Moreover, the three variants may be found mixed within the same lesion.

From a clinical point of view, differential diagnosis is made with Paget's disease (the microscopic appearance, however, allows differentiation between the two lesions). Microscopic differential diagnosis is made with an infiltrating breast carcinoma, and especially with a tubular infiltrating carcinoma; in this respect, immunohistochemical tests for myoepithelial cells (such as Actin, p63, CD10, Calponin)

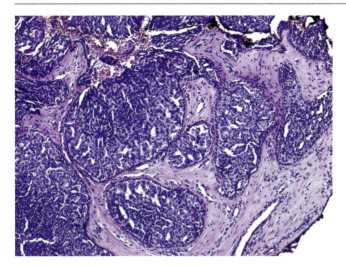

Fig. 25.5 Nipple duct adenoma: Areas of sclerosis can produce distortion of the tubular structures

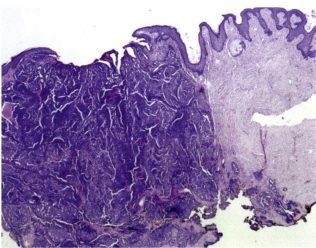

Fig. 25.7 Nipple duct adenoma: Another case with skin ulceration and pseudoinfiltrative pattern

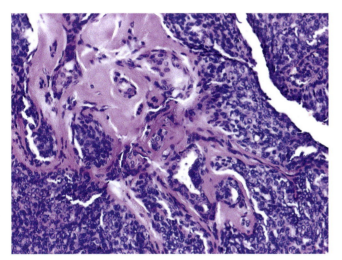

Fig. 25.6 Nipple duct adenoma: Areas of sclerosis can produce a pseudoinfiltrative pattern

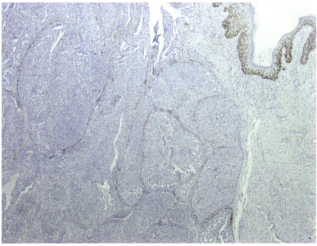

Fig. 25.8 Nipple duct adenoma: Immunohistochemical stain for p63 highlights the presence of the myoepithelial cells at the periphery of the papillary structures

confirm the presence of the myoepithelial cells around the tubules of the nipple adenoma, while tubular carcinoma lacks myoepithelial cells (Figs. 25.7 and 25.8). However, the differential diagnosis with infiltrating breast carcinoma is made especially in nipple duct adenoma with adenosis features. Of note, rare cases of nipple duct adenoma can harbor areas of intraductal or intralobular carcinoma. In this situation, the atypical cells are negative for CK 5/6. In contrast, the heterogeneity of the cells within the usual or florid ductal hyperplasia without atypia, which frequently accompanies nipple adenoma, can be demonstrated by using HMW-CK (like CK 5/6). Differential diagnosis should also be made with solitary central intraductal papilloma and sclerosing papilloma, both lesions developing from the lactiferous ducts, but with a papillary architecture, intraluminal location, not associated with a tubular proliferation in the nipple stroma, and usually not producing the ulceration of the nipple (Figs. 25.9 and 25.10). Nipple adenoma must also be differentiated from syringomatous adenoma (represented by tubular and trabecular structures associated with small keratin-containing cysts that infiltrate the nipple stroma between the muscle fibers and the perineal spaces, the cells lacking atypia and mitotic figures, and the stroma being usually sclerotic).

Nipple adenoma may undergo malignant transformation, and although the incidence of carcinoma developed on such a lesion varies from one author to another, it is nevertheless low. Typically, an *in situ* ductal or infiltrating carcinoma may develop. Since the tumor is imprecisely delimited, incomplete surgical excision of the nipple duct adenoma may lead to the development of local recurrences.

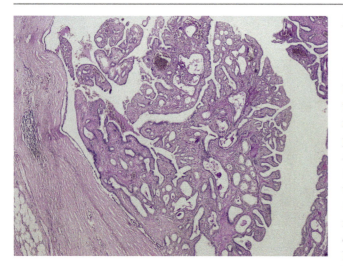

Fig. 25.9 Solitary central papilloma: A benign tumor developing from the lactiferous ducts, but with a papillary architecture represented by well-developed fibrovascular cores lined by epithelial and myoepithelial cells; tubular proliferation is not characteristic for a benign papilloma

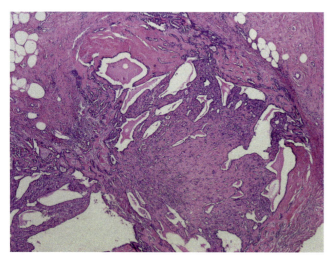

Fig. 25.10 Sclerosing papilloma: A benign tumor developed within a duct, but which underwent sclerotic central changes obscuring most of the papillary architecture; areas of entrapped glandular epithelium within collagen can be seen in the central area of the lesion; usually this lesion does not produce ulceration of the nipple

25.2 Syringomatous Adenoma of the Nipple

Syringomatous adenoma is a unilateral and non-metastasizing breast tumor, but it is locally infiltrative and has the potential for local recurrence. For this reason, it is also called infiltrating syringomatous adenoma. It is a rare lesion that occurs in patients with a mean age of 40 years. It appears to be skin adnexal in origin or differentiation, being microscopically similar to sweat gland ducts, and histogenetically similar to the microcystic adnexal carcinoma and sclerosing duct carcinoma [3]. Clinically, it develops as a nodular, firm, nipple mass that produces nipple region hardening, and can be associated with hyperkeratosis of the overlying epithelium. The lesion is very rarely associated with nipple discharge. Macroscopically, it is imprecisely defined, gray in color, with an average diameter of 1.5 cm, and may have small cystic cavities on the surface of the section. Microscopically, it consists of a tumor proliferation in the form of small angulated or compressed tubular (glandular) structures (with a characteristic comma-like shape or teardrop shape), arranged irregularly in a sclerotic stroma, or edematous, sometimes with mixoid or chondro-mixoid areas (Fig. 25.11). In some cases, the stroma can show reactive cellular areas (desmoplasia). Due to the sclerotic stroma, some of the tubular structures may look like cords or nests. Very rarely, these structures are connected to the overlying epithelium. This varied architecture alternates with small keratin-containing cysts (due to the squamous metaplasia of the internal epithelial layer, a very common finding) (Figs. 25.12 and 25.13). The tumor infiltrates the nipple stroma between smooth muscle fibers, and has infiltrating-appearing edges. Perineural invasion can also be detected. The epithelial tumor cells lin-

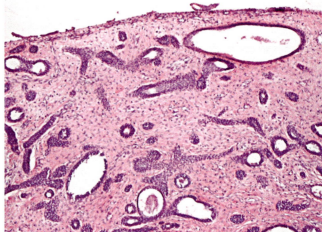

Fig. 25.11 Syringomatous adenoma of the nipple: Small angulated or compressed tubular structures, with a characteristic comma-like shape, arranged irregularly in a sclerotic stroma; due to the sclerotic stroma, some of the tubular structures may look like cords or nests

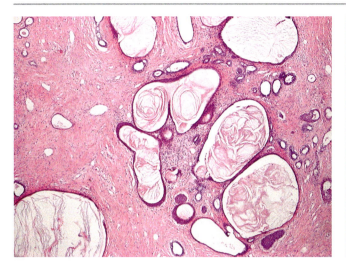

Fig. 25.12 Syringomatous adenoma of the nipple: The tubular structures alternate with small or large keratin-containing cysts

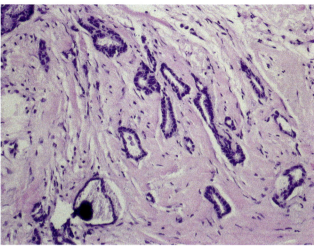

Fig. 25.14 Tubular carcinoma: Tubular structures with angulated shape, lined by only epithelial cells with low atypical nuclei; the myoepithelial cells are missing, as are the keratin-containing cysts; microcalcifications can be observed within the lumina of the tubular structures

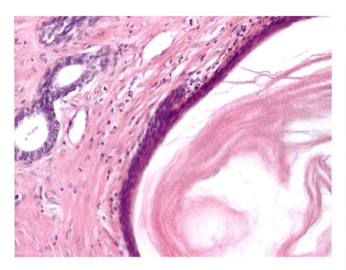

Fig. 25.13 Syringomatous adenoma of the nipple: Keratin-containing cysts, due to the squamous metaplasia of the internal epithelial layer

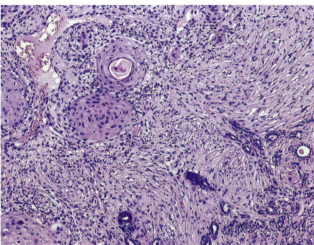

Fig. 25.15 Low-grade adenosquamous carcinoma: Well-developed tubular structures (right side of the picture), lined by only epithelial atypical cells intimately admixed with nests of squamous cells (myoepithelial cells are missing); the squamous cells form nests some of which contain central microcysts filled with keratin

ing the tubular structures are uniform in appearance, with eosinophilic cytoplasm and monomorphic round nuclei. These cells, of cuboid or flattened appearance, are peripherally surrounded by a layer of myoepithelial cells. The epithelial cells do not have atypical features, mitotic figures, and necrosis is absent. However, in some of the lesions, usual ductal hyperplasia may occur. Immunohistochemically, the internal epithelial cell layer is positive for CEA reaction, and the external one composed of myoepithelial cells is positive for Actin and p63 (but also for other myoepithelial markers). Sometimes, within the tumor proliferation, Langerhans cells may also appear and are positive for the S-100 Protein.

Differential diagnosis is made with nipple adenoma (localized in the nipple, with tubular architecture, associated with epithelial ductal hyperplasia, often with apocrine or squamous cells, with reduced stroma between the tubular

structures; of interest, syringomatous adenoma very rarely produces ulceration of the skin, while nipple adenoma is frequently associated with this feature) and tubular carcinoma (localized in deep breast tissue, made of tubular structures, arranged in a reactive abundant stroma, these structures not being associated with squamous metaplasia and not surrounded by myoepithelial cells) (Fig. 25.14). Differential diagnosis is also made with low-grade adenosquamous carcinoma (Fig. 25.15). Some authors believe that, despite morphological similarities, the two lesions are not variants of the same neoplastic process. Syringomatous adenoma originally develops in the nipple and infiltrates the underlying mammary parenchyma. Adenosquamous carcinoma develops in the terminal-acini duct and infiltrates the nipple. Also, the tubular structures of syringomatous adenoma are lined by two types of cells (epithelial and myoepithelial cells) while the structure of the low-grade adenosquamous carcinoma lacks myoepithelial cells. The tumor edge of adenosquamous carcinoma is also associated with aspects of intraductal carcinoma (Table 25.1).

Syringomatous adenoma is a benign tumor, and no metastases into axillary lymph nodes or distant metastases have so far been reported. Optimal treatment is surgical with free margins. No oncological treatment is needed [2, 3].

Table 25.1 Differential diagnosis of syringomatous adenoma

Lesion type	Localisation	Architecture	Tumor margins	Cell type
Syringomatous adenoma	Nipple	Tubular ± squamous metaplasia	Infiltrative	2 (epithelial and myoepithelial)
Nipple duct adenoma	Nipple	Tubular ± squamous metaplasia	Infiltrative	2 (epithelial and myoepithelial)
Tubular carcinoma	TDLU	Tubular ± squamous metaplasia	Infiltrative	1 cell type (epithelial)
Low-grade adenosquamous carcinoma	TDLU	Tubular ± squamous component	Infiltrative	2 cell type (epithelial and squamous)

TDLU terminal duct-lobular unit

25.3 Paget's Disease of the Nipple

Paget's disease is a rare lesion, represented by a proliferation of atypical cells located in the thickness of the squamous epithelium of the nipple. The lesion is almost always associated with an underlying breast carcinoma of *in situ* or infiltrating type (ductal or lobular), usually located in the central area of the breast. Therefore, Paget's disease should be regarded as a secondary sign of a breast carcinoma. Paget's disease of the nipple that is not associated with an underlying carcinoma is extremely rare. It can rarely be bilateral, but may develop in both sexes, sometimes even in a supernumerary nipple [4]. Studies have shown that tumor cells have a glandular-ductal origin (lesion development mechanisms are either by migration of tumor cells of an underlying ductal carcinoma to the epidermis, or by malignant transformation of an intraepidermal mammary duct, or by the epithelial differentiation of multipotential cells located at the basal level in the epidermis—this explains the rare cases of Paget's disease in which no underlying ductal carcinoma can be identified). Clinically, Paget's disease is characteristically localized in the nipple and appears either as a red lesion or, in more severe forms, as an eczematous lesion possibly associated with ulceration that can also spread to the areola region or, in more advanced cases, to the skin surrounding the areola (Figs. 25.16, 25.17, and 25.18). The skin lesion is accompanied by pruritus, and in half of the cases there is a painless tumor mass. In some cases, nipple retraction can be observed. Also, serous or bloody discharge often occurs in advanced cases. Of note, the presence of the clinical changes unaccompanied by microscopic characteristic is not sufficient for a diagnosis of Paget's disease. Microscopically, there is a proliferation of round-to-oval atypical cells (called Paget cells),

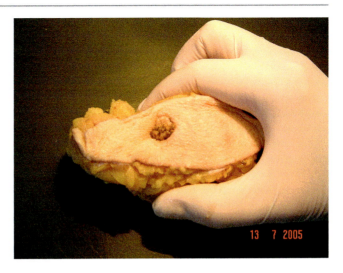

Fig. 25.17 Paget's disease: Eczematous brown-color lesion localized in the nipple and spread to the skin of the areolar region

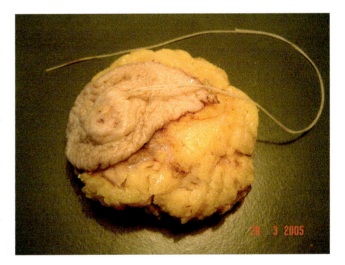

Fig. 25.18 Paget's disease: Tumor-like lesion involving the nipple with small areas of ulceration; microscopic examination revealed Paget atypical cells involving the skin and invasive breast carcinoma

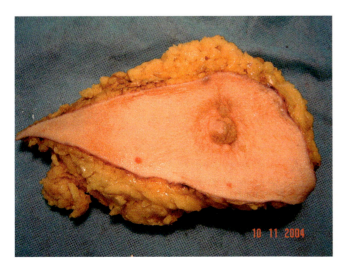

Fig. 25.16 Paget's disease: Eczematous lesion localized in the nipple; invasive carcinoma of NST subtype involved the breast parenchyma (not shown)

with abundant, clear, or eosinophilic cytoplasm, and large hyperchromatic nuclei with obvious nucleoli. These cells are located in nests, usually in the lower third of the epidermis, but can also appear as isolated cells in the upper part of the epidermis (Figs. 25.19, 25.20, 25.21, and 25.22). Also, on rare occasions, the cells may form acini (Figs. 25.23 and 25.24). Special stains usually reveal the intracytoplasmic presence of mucin (PAS- and Alcian-positive, Mucicarmin-negative), but in rare occasions when the Paget cells are anaplastic they may lack the mucin. They may sometimes also contain melanin pigment granules as a result of the phagocytosis process [5]. Hyperplasia and hyperkeratosis of the epidermis can occur while the underlying dermis can present an inflammatory infiltrate. The underlying lactiferous ducts usually present *in situ* ductal carcinoma and rarely *in situ* lobular carcinoma (Fig. 25.25).

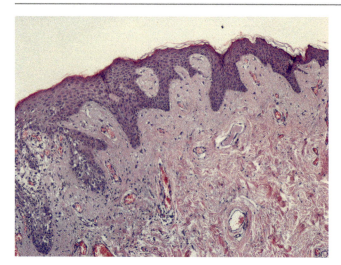

Fig. 25.19 Paget's disease: Normal epidermis (right) and thicker epidermis (left) due to the presence of Paget cells

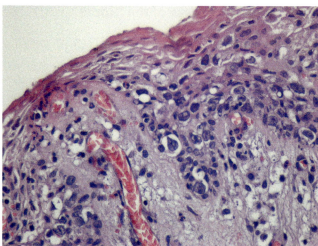

Fig. 25.22 Paget's disease: Nests of Paget cells involving two-thirds of the epidermis

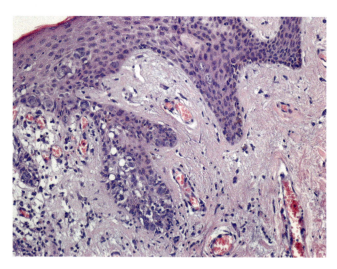

Fig. 25.20 Paget's disease: Proliferation of round-to-oval atypical cells (Paget cells) with eosinophilic cytoplasm, and large nuclei with obvious nucleoli; these cells are isolated, located in in the lower third of the epidermis; of note, few Toker cells are also located in the lower third of the epidermis

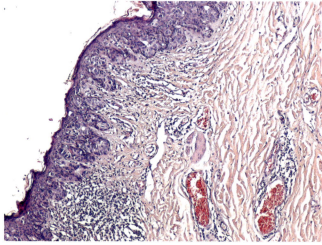

Fig. 25.23 Another case of Paget's disease: Paget cells in the full thickness of the epidermis

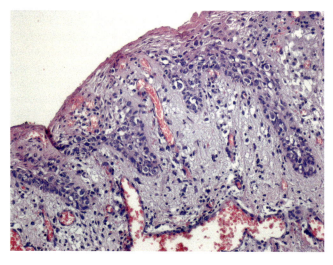

Fig. 25.21 Paget's disease: Multiple large Paget cells with abundant clear cytoplasm and atypical irregular nuclei

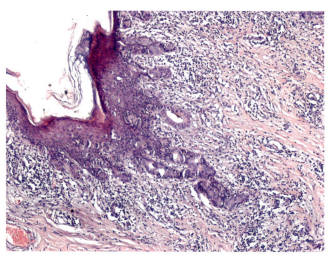

Fig. 25.24 Similar case to Fig. 25.23: Paget cells forming acinic structures; of note, an inflammatory infiltrate can be appreciated in the subjacent dermis

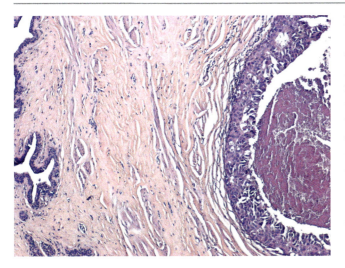

Fig. 25.25 Similar case to Fig. 25.23: Areas of ductal carcinoma *in situ* adjacent to a lactiferous duct; of note, the Paget cells within the epidermis are morphologically similar to the atypical cells within the duct with ductal carcinoma in situ

Immunohistochemically, tumor cells are positive for CEA (polyclonal), pan-Cytokeratin (like AE1/AE3 or CAM 5.2), Cytokeratin 7, EMA, MUC1, c-erbB-2, CK 8, 18, CK 5/6 and 34betaE12, GCDFP-15, and in some cases for estrogen receptor (ER), progesterone receptor (PR), androgen receptor (AR), HER2 (depending on the molecular profile of the underlying breast carcinoma), and are negative for Cytokeratin 20, HMB-45, and S-100 protein (Fig. 25.26). Occasionally, cells may be positive for S-100 Protein (important for differential diagnosis with malignant melanoma).

A variety of epithelial lesions may display a pagetoid appearance. Differential diagnostic problems occur especially when the tissue biopsy is poorly fixed, when the biopsy is collected from areas with degenerative lesions, when only a few atypical cells are present intraepithelially, or when these cells contain melanin pigment [3]. In all these difficult situations, repeating the biopsy is advisable. Also, from the pathologist's point of view, there is difficulty in establishing a correct diagnosis of borderline or difficult biopsy cases in

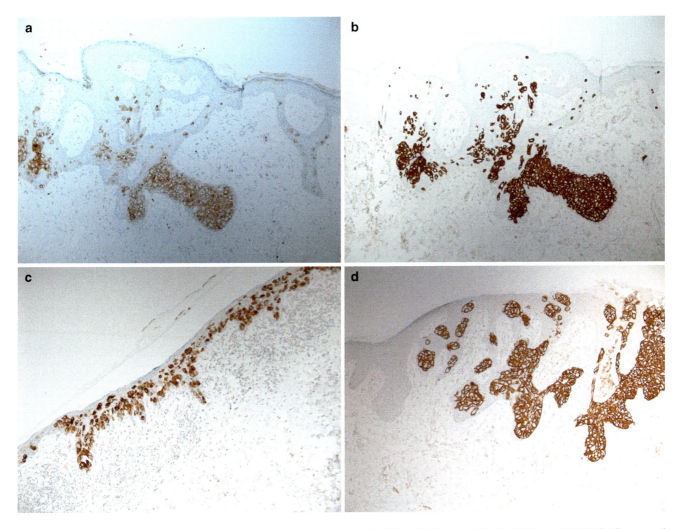

Fig. 25.26 Paget disease: Paget cells involving the epidermis are (**a**), positive for CEA; (**b**) Cytokeratin 7; (**c**), EMA; and (**d**) HER2. (Courtesy of Dr. Cristina Terinte)

the absence of clinical and/or radiological information about the patient.

Differential diagnosis is made with:

- *In situ* malignant melanoma (which may show pagetoid growth and melanin granules in tumor cells, but it is positive for HMB-45 and Protein S-100, and negative for CEA and Cytokeratin; of practical interest, some Paget cells may incorporate melanin from epidermal cells while some malignant melanomas are devoid of pigment);

- *In situ* squamous carcinoma (the presence of squamous dyskeratotic cells in the epidermal full thickness, positive for Cytokeratin (pan CK, CK 5/6, CK 34betaE12) and negative for CEA; of note, a variant of Paget's disease resembling Bowen's disease with full-thickness epidermal atypia, and severe nuclear atypia can occur) (Figs. 25.25, 25.26, and 25.27);

- Various inflammatory cutaneous lesions (also displaying chronic inflammatory infiltration in the dermis, but not associated with intraepidermic Paget cells or with an underlying breast carcinoma);

- Changes in epidermal keratinocytes, which can sometimes transform into cells with clear cytoplasm (also called Toker cells) or can undergo clear cell hyperplasia (keratinocytes do not show signs of atypia and have a different immunohistochemical profile; of interest, however, these clear cells may have a similar immunohistochemical profile with the Paget cells, some authors suggesting that there rare cases of Paget's disease without an identifiable underlying carcinoma that may derive from these clear cells) [6].

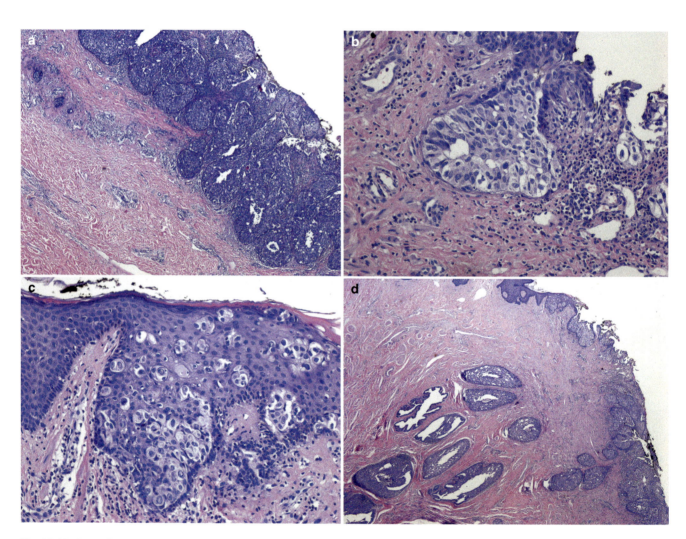

Fig. 25.27 Paget disease: (**a**) A variant of Paget's disease resembling Bowen's disease with full-thickness epidermal atypia and severe nuclear atypia; (**b**) Paget cells involve the full thickness of the epidermis and are arranged in acinic structures; (**c**) Paget cells have abundant cytoplasm and atypical nuclei; (**d**) the lesion is associated with ductal carcinoma *in situ*

From a practical point of view, however, most of these lesions are very rare in the nipple and when dealing with nipple changes, Paget disease should always be the first diagnosis ruled out. Simply by performing a mucin stain and few additional immunohistochemical stains, the diagnosis can be accurate.

The prognosis of Paget's disease depends on the presence, histological type, and molecular profile of the associated breast carcinoma, as well as on the size of the carcinoma and the condition of the axillary lymph nodes.

25.4 Other Nipple Lesions

Other nipple tumors or tumor-like lesion may develop very rarely. The nipple may develop Bowen disease (*in situ* squamous carcinoma), basal cell carcinoma, basal cell adenoma, malignant melanoma (distinct from infiltrating duct carcinoma with melanocytic features, a subtype of infiltrating breast carcinoma NST—no special type), leiomyoma, leiomyosarcoma, smooth muscle fiber hyperplasia, mucinosis (accumulation of mucinous and mixoid material in the mammary stroma without epithelial cells), hyperkeratosis (papillomatous elongation of the epidermis and underlying papillary connective tissue), extensive squamous metaplasia of lactiferous ducts (leading to the obstruction and rupture of these ducts with the consecutive development of a subareolar abscess) (Fig. 25.28) [3]. Also, the nipple, like the areola or breast parenchyma, can harbor metastases of malignant tumors, most frequently of malignant melanoma (Figs. 25.29, 25.30, and 25.31) [7].

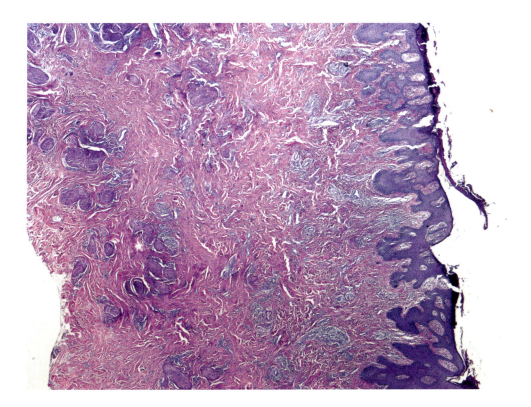

Fig. 25.28 Hyperkeratosis of the epidermis involving the nipple

Fig. 25.29 Multiple brown and round nodules involving the areolar area in a 42-year-old patient; the nodules represent metastases of a malignant melanoma originating in the interscapular skin

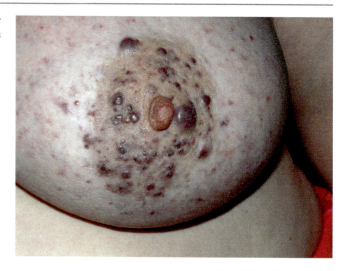

Fig. 25.30 Microscopic examination in the case of a 42-year-old patient with multiple metastases involving the nipple and areola: multiple nests of spindle atypical cells infiltrating the nipple (similar case to Fig. 25.29)

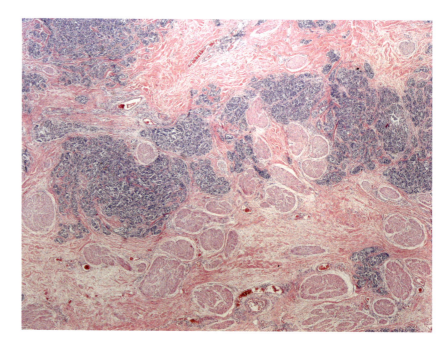

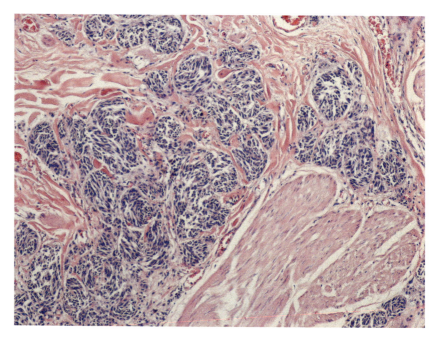

Fig. 25.31 Nests of atypical spindle cells infiltrating the muscle fibers of the nipple; of note, the melanin pigment is missing (similar case to Fig. 25.29)

References

1. Rosen PP. Subareolar sclerosing duct hyperplasia of the breast. Cancer. 1987;59:1927–30.
2. Moinfar F. Essentials of diagnostic breast pathology. Berlin: Springer; 2007. p. 355.
3. Tavassoli FA. Pathology of the breast. 2nd ed. New York: McGraw-Hill; 1999. p. 751–6.
4. Lopes S, Vide J, Moreira E, Pinheiro J, Azevedo F. Paget disease of the male breast. Dermatol Online J. 2017;23(4). pii: 13030/qt0t89d5dg.
5. Peison B, Benisch B. Paget's disease of the nipple simulating malignant melanoma in a black woman. Am J Dermatopathol. 1985;7:165–9.
6. Lundquist K, Kohler S, Rouse RV. Intraepidermal cytokeratin 7 expression is not restricted to Paget cells but is also seen in Toker cells and Merkel cells. Am J Surg Pathol. 1999;23:212–9.
7. Stolnicu S, Barsan I, Bauer O, Moldovan C, Chiriac A, Coros MF, et al. Areolar metastases of skin malignant melanoma- report of a unique case. Breast J. 2017;23(4):470–1.

Metastatic Tumors to the Breast

26

Isabel Alvarado-Cabrero

Metastases to the breast and axilla are rare and account for approximately 2% of all mammary malignancies. The first reported case of extra-mammary breast metastasis occurred in 1903, and case reports and reviews published in the English-language literature have reported fewer than 500 cases of metastasis to the breast. The most common metastatic lesion to involve the breast is a metastasis from a contralateral mammary cancer; however, reported primary tumors metastasizing to the breast include carcinoma from the lung, gastrointestinal, or genitourinary tract, and melanoma. The diagnosis of metastasis to the breast from extramammary malignancies is important for patient management. The prognosis is generally poor as most patients have widely disseminated disease.

26.1 Introduction

Metastases from non-mammary malignant neoplasms to the breast are rare and reportedly account for approximately 2% of all malignant mammary tumors. Metastases to the male breast are encounter even less frequently [1]. The most common metastatic lesion to involve the breast is a metastasis from a contralateral mammary cancer. If hematologic malignancies are also excluded, the number of non-mammary metastasis drop to well below 1% [2].

The first reported case of an extra-mammary organ metastasizing to the breast was published in 1903 [3]. In a 90-year study of tumor registry from Royal London Hospital, only 60 out of nearly 14,000 patients with breast cancer were identified to have a metastatic deposit in the breast from hematologic and non-hematological malignances. Out of these 60 patients, approximately 30% were identified postmortem [4].

More than 500 cases of breast metastases from extramammary sites have been reported in the literature, mainly as small series or case reports. Excluding contralateral mammary tumors, the most common sources of primary tumor metastases to the breast are, in decreasing order of frequency, melanoma, lung, and ovarian cancer [5, 6].

The diagnosis of metastases to the breast from extramammary malignancies, and distinction from primary mammary malignancy, is important for patient management. The prognosis is generally poor, as most patients have widely disseminated disease [4–6].

26.2 Clinical Presentation

Among metastatic carcinomas to the breast, the male to female ratio is 1 to 6; the average age is 48 years in women and 61 in men [2, 4–6]. Patients typically present with a rapidly growing painless firm palpable breast mass. Some reports emphasize that the masses are often superficial, but usually they are not bound to the skin. Diffuse skin involvement is rare [7].

Rarely, pain and nipple discharge are reported. Metastatic carcinomas to the breast are relatively well-circumscribed, and freely mobile mass is often misinterpreted as a benign breast lesion, such as a fibroadenoma. In about 30% of cases, the breast is the first sign of malignancy [8].

In those patients with a history of malignancy, the interval between initial diagnosis and mammary metastasis varies between 1 month and 15 years [9].

I. Alvarado-Cabrero, MD
Department of Pathology, Hospital de Oncologia, Centro Medico
Nacional Siglo XXI, Instituto Mexicano del Seguro Social,
Mexico City, Mexico

© Springer International Publishing AG, part of Springer Nature 2018
S. Stolnicu, I. Alvarado-Cabrero (eds.), *Practical Atlas of Breast Pathology*, https://doi.org/10.1007/978-3-319-93257-6_26

26.3 Imaging

On mammography, most metastases present as circumscribed or ill-defined masses; few cases present as irregular masses, and multiple masses are present in a minority. Calcifications usually are absent, but may occur in metastatic müllerian carcinomas (tubal, ovarian, or peritoneal). Extensive calcifications outside of tumor favor breast carcinoma associated with ductal carcinoma in situ [10].

Ultrasonography typically shows the lesion to be hypoechoic without spiculations.

Magnetic Resonance Imaging (MRI) has been used to evaluate breast metastases, and may be useful in young patients with breast parenchyma and in cases of metastatic melanoma where high signal with T-1 weighting and T-2 weighting tumor [10, 11].

26.4 Histopathology

Recognizing a breast tumor as being metastatic is crucial for appropriate treatment and prognosis. About two-thirds of cases will have histological features raising the possibility of metastases. For the other third, the history is vital for diagnosis [7, 12].

The diagnosis of metastases should be suspected when the histologic pattern is unusual for breast carcinoma. Unusual histologic patterns include: clear cells (Fig. 26.1), well-formed papillae, tall columnar cells, psammoma body calcifications, and discohesive cells with high grade nuclei [7, 12, 13].

Among the metastatic carcinomas in the breast that are more likely to be mistaken for a breast primary are those arising in the lung, ovary, müllerian system, and bowel [6, 8]. Some types of breast tumors such as small cell, adenoid cystic, and mucoepidermoid carcinomas can occur in other organs, and appropriate clinical workup is prudent in these cases. Metastatic neuroendocrine carcinomas of various organs generally share histologic features with primary mammary carcinoma [2, 5, 6, 8].

Rhabdomyosarcomas have a predilection for spreading to the breast, and it has been estimated that up to 10% of alveolar rhabdomyosarcomas metastasize to the breast during clinical course. Of 22 cases of rhabdomyosarcoma involving the breast at Armed Forces Institute of Pathology, 18 were metastatic and occurred in children or women under 40 years of age [13].

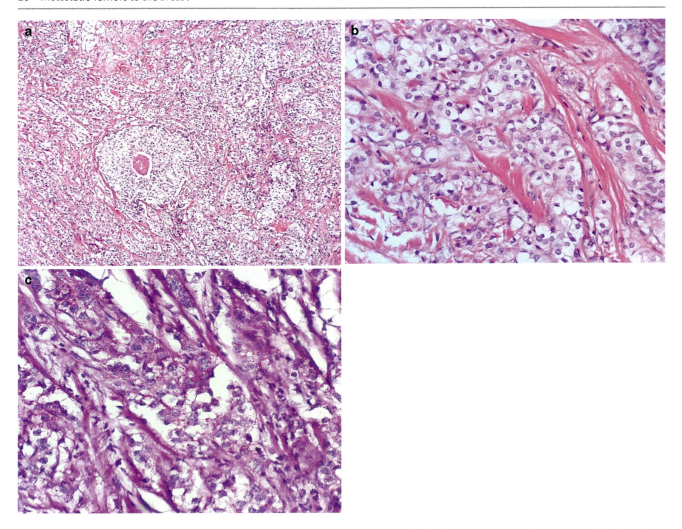

Fig. 26.1 Glycogen-rich carcinoma. (**a**) The invasive component usually exhibits the histologic growth pattern of a conventional invasive ductal carcinoma. (**b**) Invasive component form cords and solid nests. (**c**) PAS-positive, diastase resistant, intracytoplasmic hyaline droplets

26.5 Malignant Melanoma

Hematic or lymphatic metastases from malignant melanoma occur in 20% of cases. Liver, lung, and brain represent the common sites of hematic metastases, although any organ could be involved. Metastases to the breast from malignant melanoma or other extra-mammary tumors are rare and represent 1.3–2.7% of all malignant breast tumors (Fig. 26.2).

The microscopic diagnosis of metastatic melanoma can be challenging for several reasons, such as: it has a broad spectrum of clinical presentation; it has a remarkable histologic ability to mimic a variety of cellular (Fig. 26.3) and architec-

ture phenotypes; the results of immunohistochemical stains are sometimes equivocal; and it has the potential to occur as a metastatic lesion in practically any anatomic site [14].

Melanoma in the breast could be primary in the breast skin, primary in the breast tissue, metastatic in the breast (Fig. 26.4), or in transit metastasis to breast tissue and breast skin. Metastasis is more common in the outer half of the breast because of good vascularity and the presence or more glandular tissue.

Secondary breast lesion could be the first manifestation of melanoma, with metastasis to the breast in 40% of the affected patients [15].

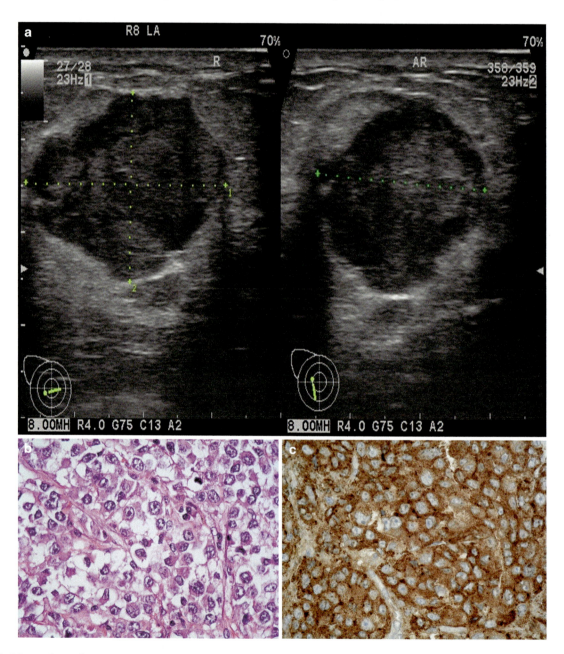

Fig. 26.2 Metastatic malignant melanoma (MM). A 30-year-old woman presented with bilateral palpable breast masses. (**a**) Breast ultrasound shows multiple bilateral predominantly hypoechoic lesions with irregular outlines. (**b**) Histological section of malignant melanoma metastatic to the breast. (**c**) The tumor is stained with immunoperoxidase reaction for HMB-45

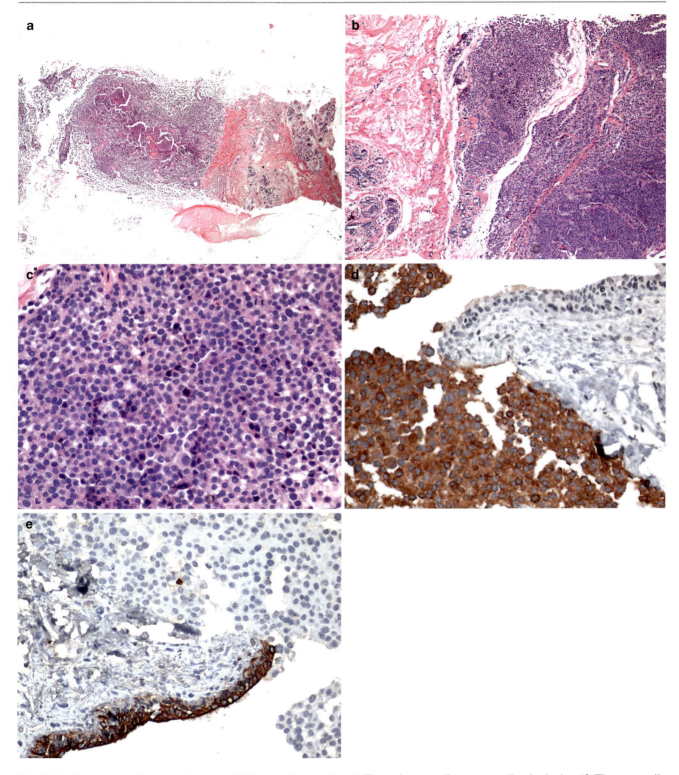

Fig. 26.3 Metastatic malignant melanoma (MM). A 68-year-old woman presented with a left palpable mass. (**a** and **b**) This needle core biopsy of the breast shows diffusely infiltrating malignant melanoma. (**c**) The melanoma cells appear small and cohesive. (**d**) The tumor cells are immunoreactive for Melan-A. (**e**) The tumor cells are negative for cytokeratin

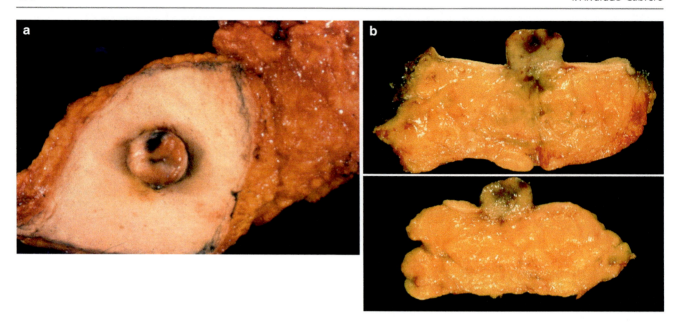

Fig. 26.4 Metastatic malignant melanoma to the breast. A 72-year-old woman presented with a left metastatic breast nodule. The patient had a history of primary malignant melanoma (MM) removed from the left ankle 2 years before her presentation with the breast nodule. (**a**) Left radical mastectomy shows a well define 3 × 3 cm mass. (**b**) The cut surface of the tumor is nodular with a white pigmented cut surface

26.6   Primary Lung Cancer

Breast masses presenting as metastatic spread from primary lung cancer can be difficult to diagnose in the absence of new and concerning respiratory symptoms (e.g., cough, hemoptysis). Patients with breast metastases from pulmonary adenocarcinoma usually present a rapidly growing, painless, firm, well-circumscribed, and palpable mass with predilection to the upper quadrant (Fig. 26.5) [16].

Histopathology can provide the diagnosis; in most instances, however, immunohistochemical staining is required. TTF-1 is a useful marker of pulmonary adenocarci-

noma with a reported frequency of 68–80%; however, no stains are positively detected in breast carcinoma. Napsin A can be confirmatory of lung primary. The mammary origin is supported by the expression of ER, GCDFP-15, and mammoglobin [6, 8].

Small cell carcinoma can be primary or metastatic in the breast. The diagnosis of primary small cell carcinoma of the breast is supported by the concurrent presence of a conventional ductal type of invasive and/or in situ carcinoma. Metastatic small cell carcinoma is more often multifocal and multicentric (Fig. 26.6). Squamous cell carcinoma of the lung has rarely been reported to metastasize to breast.

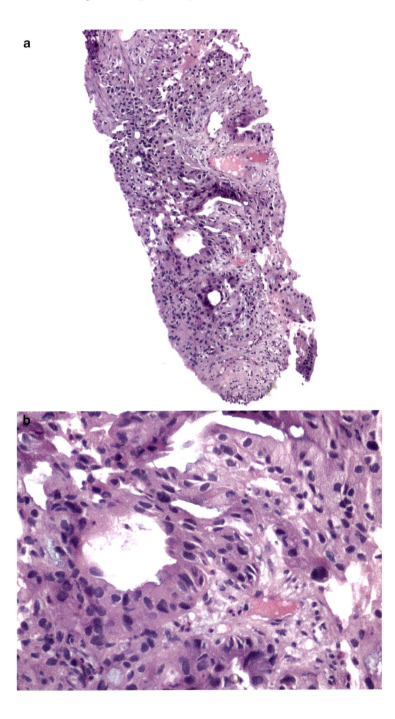

Fig. 26.5 Lung metastasis from pulmonary carcinoma. (**a** and **b**) Adenocarcinoma in a needle biopsy of the breast. The growth pattern is unusual for a mammary primary

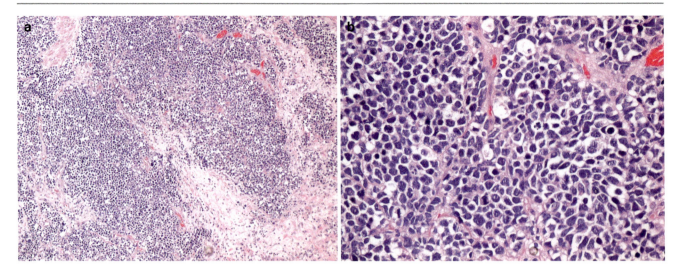

Fig. 26.6 Metastatic lung carcinoma. An 82-year-old woman presented with a mass in the right breast. The patient had a history of a lung cancer diagnosed at age 80. (**a** and **b**) Metastatic small cell neuroendocrine carcinoma of the lung

26.7 Gastrointestinal Tumors

Adenocarcinomas originating in the gastrointestinal tract, especially in the colon and rectum, are rarely the source of metastatic carcinoma in the breast, despite their relatively higher prevalence. The colon cancer metastasized to the breast can be synchronous or metachronous (Fig. 26.7). Only a few cases have been reported in the literature. Immunohistochemistry can be very valuable to confirm the primary site being in the colon [17]. According to a study by Bayrak et al. [18], the CK7−/CK 20+ phenotype was found in 65.8% of the patients with colorectal cancer.

The intestinal type of gastric carcinoma may resemble invasive ductal carcinoma of the breast, and diffuse gastric carcinoma may resemble invasive lobular carcinoma of the breast (Fig. 26.8). ER and GCDFP-15 are rarely expressed by gastric carcinoma, whereas CK20 and CDX2 are occasionally positive in gastric carcinoma.

Guanghui et al. [19] reported one case of hilar cholangiocarcinoma with synchronous metastases to breast and skeletal muscle (Fig. 26.9). About three cases of hepatocellular carcinomas metastatic to the breast have been reported [4, 7, 10].

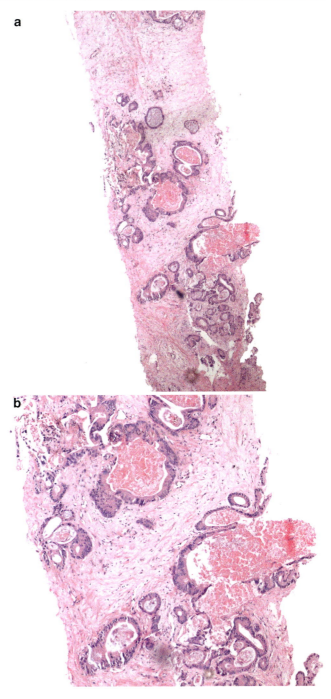

Fig. 26.7 Metastasis from colorectal carcinoma. (**a** and **b**) Sections show adenocarcinoma with intraluminal necrosis and high-grade nuclear atypia

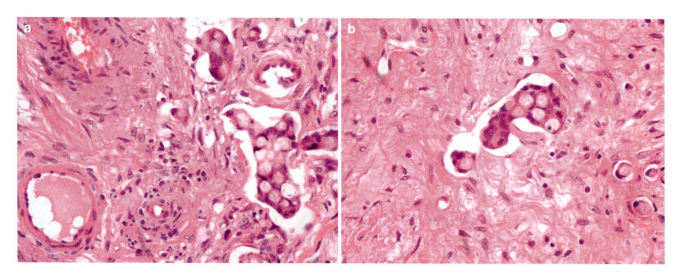

Fig. 26.8 Metastatic gastric carcinoma, diffuse type in breast. (**a** and **b**) sections show poorly differentiated adenocarcinoma with signet-ring cells

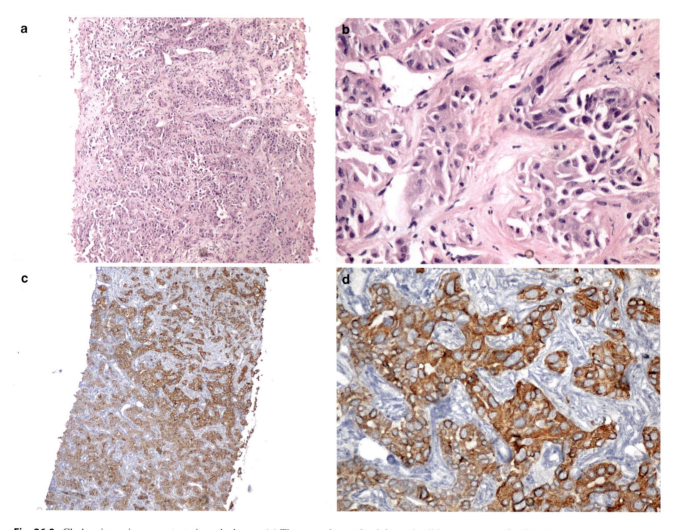

Fig. 26.9 Cholangiocarcinoma metastatic to the breast. (**a**) The tumor has a glandular and solid arrangement. (**b**) Glandular structures with high-grade nuclei. (**c** and **d**) Cholangiocarcinoma with extensive expression of cytokeratin 19

26.8   Neoplasias of Gynecological Organs

The first case report of ovarian cancer with metastases to the breast was in 1907 by Sitzenfrey. To date, a total of only 40 cases have been reported in the English-language literature [20]. Ovarian metastases to the breast carcinoma is even more infrequent, with only seven cases reported. Breast metastases from a serous carcinoma of müllerian origin usually display a papillary appearance with abundant psammoma bodies (Fig. 26.10).

Primary ovarian tumor is generally diagnosed an average of 2 years after the initial diagnosis of ovarian cancer.

The typically immunoprofile of these neoplasias is CK7 +, CK 20 −, CA-125 +, WT1 +, and PAX 8 +. By combining the tumor markers OC125 and OV 632, Yamasaki et al. [21] found a sensitivity of 86% and specificity of 89% for the diagnosis of metastatic ovarian cancer. Secondary breast involvement from an ovarian tumor suggests widespread dissemination and is associated with a poor prognosis.

Choriocarcinoma metastatic to the breast, originating in gynecological organs, have been reported (Fig. 26.11) [22].

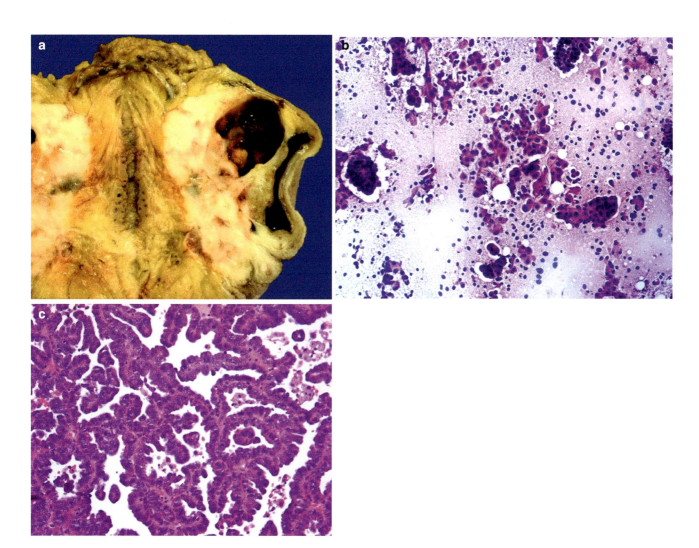

Fig. 26.10 Breast metastasis from serous carcinoma of the ovary. (**a**) Total mastectomy shows a 3 × 2 cm solid and multiloculated cystic mass. (**b**) Fine-needle aspiration of breast mass shows papillary aggre- gates with increased cellularity, including single cells with cytologic atypia. (**c**) Typical papillary architecture and high-grade nuclear atypia

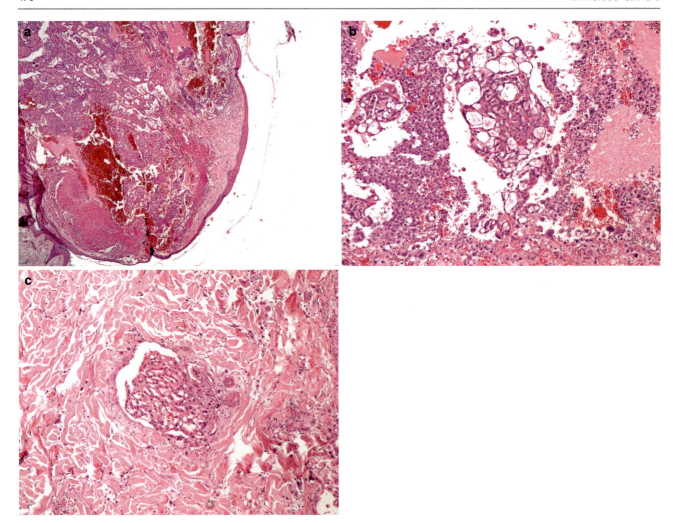

Fig. 26.11 Metastatic choriocarcinoma to the breast. A 29-year-old woman with a nodule in the left breast. The patient had a history of choriocarcinoma that had developed after a molar pregnancy. (**a**) Metastatic choriocarcinoma to the nipple. (**b**) Section shows a trimor- phic proliferation of syncytiotrophoblast, cytotrophoblast and interme- diate trophoblast. (**c**) Vascular invasion by cells with abundant eosinophilic cytoplasm and multinucleated cells

26.9 Genitourinary Tract Tumors

Metastases from renal cell carcinoma to the breast is very rare. It has been suggested that, as a metastatic route to the breast, tumor cells transit into the right ventricle from the inferior vena cava and spread to the breast after passing through the lungs in the arterial circulation (Fig. 26.12). In addition, the paravertebral venous plexus route has been suggested [23].

About 24 cases of breast metastases from renal cell carcinoma (RCC) have been described in the literature. The average age at onset is 67.4 years (47–82 years), and all patients have been female. Metastatic RCC in the breast may precede the diagnosis of the occult RCC, or metastases may occur decades later (≤18 years), after initial resection [24].

Conventional renal clear cell carcinoma is the most common renal malignancy that metastasizes to the breast. The abundant clear or granular cytoplasm with a relatively low nuclear-to-cytoplasmic ratio and prominent fine vessels are useful clues to correct diagnosis.

While the morphotype of renal cell carcinomas is usually discernible on examination of the H&E-stained section, markers are often useful for confirming diagnosis in difficult cases. PAX 2 is positive in more than 75% of clear cell renal carcinomas. PAX 8 shows similar labeling as PAX 2 [25].

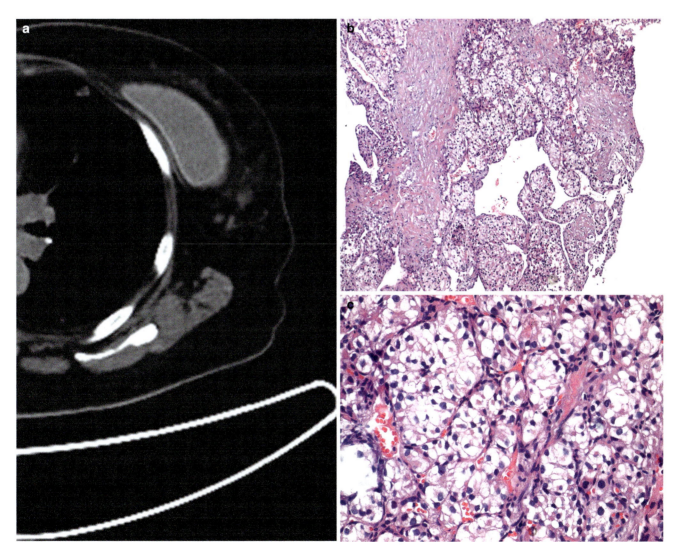

Fig. 26.12 Metastasis of renal cell carcinoma to breast. (**a**) Contrasted-enhanced axial CT of the chest shows two metastatic masses located nearby the breast implant. (**b**) Section shows a tumor with compact alveolar (nested) and acinar growth pattern. (**c**) Malignant epithelial cells with clear cytoplasm interspersed with intricate, arborizing vaculature

26.10 Sarcomas

Sarcomas are an extremely rare tumor source of breast metastases, and those that do present are mainly seen as a component of metaplastic carcinoma or phyllodes tumor.

Metastatic sarcomas to the breast includes rhabdomyosarcomas, liposarcomas, synovial sarcomas (Fig. 26.13), and Ewing sarcomas, among others [1, 2, 4–7].

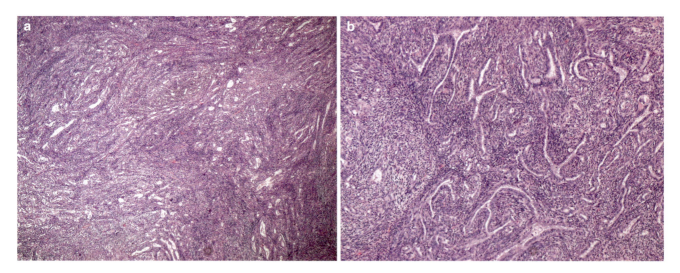

Fig. 26.13 Synovial Sarcoma. (**a** and **b**) Biphasic pattern of synovial sarcoma shows an admixture of glandular structures lined by columnar epithelium set in a sarcomatous stroma

References

1. Alvarado-Cabrero I, Carrera-Álvarez M, Pérez-Montiel D, Tavassoli FA. Metastases to the breast. Eur J Surg Oncol. 2003;29:854–5.
2. Williams SA, Ehlers RA, Hunt KK, Ehlers RA II, Hunt KK, Yi M, Kuerer HM, Singletary SE, et al. Metastases to the breast from non-breast solid neoplasms: presentations and determinants of survival. Cancer. 2007;110:731–7.
3. Trevithick E. A case of chloroma, with clinical history and account of post-mortem appearances. Lancet. 1903;2:158–60.
4. Georgiannos SN, Chin J, Goode AW, Sheaff MM. Secondary neoplasms of the breast. A survey of the 20th century. Cancer. 2001;92:2259–66.
5. Akçay MN. Metastatic disease in the breast. Breast. 2002;11:526–8.
6. Hoda SA, Rosen PP, Brogi E, Koerner FC. Rosen's diagnosis of breast pathology by needle core biopsy. 4th ed. Philadelphia: Wolters Kluwer; 2017.
7. DeLair DF, Corben AD, Catalano JP, Vallejo CE, Brogi E, Tan LK. Non-mammary metastases to the breast and axilla: a study of 85 cases. Mod Pathol. 2013;26:343–9.
8. Dabbs DJ. Breast pathology. 2nd ed. Philadelphia: Elsevier; 2017.
9. Lakhani SR, Ellis IO, Schnitt SJ, Hoon Tan P, van de Vijver MJ. WHO classification of tumours of the breast. Lyon: IARC; 2012.
10. Bartella L, Kaye J, Perry NM, Malhotra A, Evans D, Ryan D, et al. Metastases to the breast revisited: radiological-histopathological correlation. Clin Radiol. 2003;58:524–31.
11. McCrea ES, Johnston C, Haney PJ. Metastases to the breast. AJR Am J Roentgenol. 1983;141:685–90.
12. Lee AHS. The histological diagnosis of metastases to the breast from extramammary malignancies. J Clin Pathol. 2007;60:1333–41.
13. Tavassoli FA, Eusebi V. Tumors of the mammary gland. AFIP atlas of tumor pathology. Washington, DC: Amer Registry of Pathology; 2009.
14. Bacchi CE, Wludarski SC, Ambaye AB, Lamovec J, Salviato T, Falconieri G. Metastatic melanoma presenting as an isolated breast tumor. Arch Pathol Lab Med. 2013;137:41–9.
15. Moschetta M, Telegrafo M, Lucarelli NM, Martino G, Rella L, Stabile Ianora AA, et al. Metastatic breast disease from cutaneous malignant melanoma. Int J Surg Case Rep. 2014;5:34–6.
16. Babu KS, Roberts F, Bryden F, McCafferty A, Downer P, Hansell DT, et al. Metastases to the breast from primary lung. J Thorac Oncol. 2009;4:540–2.
17. Alvarado-Cabrero I, Sánchez-Vivar AE, Mohs-Alfaro M. Breast metastases from a colonic adenocarcinoma: a case report and literature review. Gac Med Mex. 2011;147:361–4.
18. Bayrak R, Yenidünya S, Haltas H. Cytokeratin 7 and Cytokeratin 20 expression in colorectal adenocarcinomas. Pathol Res Pract. 2011;207:156–60.
19. Ding G, Yang J, Cheng S, Gong H, Liu K, Dai B, et al. Hilar cholangiocarcinoma with synchronous metastases to breast and skeletal muscle: a case report and literature review. Chinese-German J Clin Oncol. 2006;5:216–8.
20. Klein RL, Brown AR, Gomez-Castro CM, Chambers SK, Cragun JM, Grasso-Lebeau L, et al. Ovarian cancer metastatic to the breast presenting as inflammatory breast cancer: a case report and literature review. J Cancer. 2010;1:27–31.
21. Yamasaki H, Saw D, Zdanowitz J, Faltz LL. Ovarian Carcinoma metastatic to the breast: a case report and review of the literature. Am J Surg Pathol. 1993;17:193–7.
22. Kalra N, Ojili V, Gulati M, Prasad GR, Vaiphei K, Suri S. Metastatic choriocarcinoma to the breast appeareance on mammography and Doppler sonography. Am J Roentgenol. 2005;184:S53–5.
23. Takayuyi I, Kinoshita S, Shimada N, Miyake R, Suzuki M, Takeyama H. Breast metastases nine years after nephrectomy for renal cell carcinoma: a case report. Int J Surg Case Rep. 2017;39:145–9.
24. Vassalli L, Ferrari VD, Simoncini E, Rangoni G, Montini E, Marpicati P, et al. Solitary breast metastases from a renal cell carcinoma. Breast Cancer Res Treat. 2001;68:29–31.
25. Truong LD, Shed SS. Immunohistochemical diagnosis of renal neoplasms. Arch Pathol Lab Med. 2011;135:92–109.

Sampling and Evaluation of the Breast Surgical Specimens

27

Raquel Valencia-Cedillo

Breast biopsies are common surgical specimens to search for possible cancer via evaluation of palpable masses, radiologic lesions, or nipple discharge. It is crucial for the pathologist to have the knowledge of all the breast specimens that could be received, and the best manner to process them, in order to provide accurate information about the diagnosis, prognostic factors (e.g., tumor staging, histologic type, precursor lesions, etc.) and assessment of treatment response. Appropriate grossing of breast specimens is indeed a cornerstone for achieving a quality diagnosis. We also must consider that grossing of breast specimens has been evolving over the past few decades. As image-guided core-needle biopsy has gradually replaced surgical biopsy in the initial assessment of breast lesions, most patients have a definitive diagnosis at the time of excision.

27.1 Grossing Breast Specimens

In the process of grossing breast specimens, as with all specimens that pathologist study, we first must consider that we are in the preanalytical phase of quality control in pathology. It is not just the responsibility of the pathologist, but of all hospital personnel involved, to ensure that each patient's specimen is appropriately and safely handled and processed in order to achieve maximum benefit for the patient and the physicians caring for her or him [1].

When a pathologic study is requested, it must come with the following information:

- Patient identification (name, date birth/age, ID number)
- Identification of the medical doctors requesting the examination
- Procedure date (to calculate the fixation time)
- Summary of clinical history
- Specimen identification (kind of specimen: Tru-Cut, incisional or excisional biopsy, lumpectomy, mastectomy. Laterality of the specimen, referred margins)

Breast biopsies are common surgical specimens for the evaluation of palpable masses, radiologic lesions, or nipple discharge, to search for possible cancer [1]. Breast-conserving therapy is now well accepted as a definitive treatment procedure. Neoadjuvant therapy is also selected by many patients. To provide accurate information for tumor staging and assessment of treatment response, breast grossing has never been more dependent on clinicopathologic correlation [2].

There are different types of biopsies or resection specimens with which to diagnose and/or assess treatment of breast diseases (Fig. 27.1): core-needle biopsy, incisional biopsy, excisional biopsies (mastectomy specimen, breast-conserving surgery, re-excisions, and duct dissections). These are discussed in the remainder of this chapter.

R. Valencia-Cedillo, MD
Department of Pathology, Hospital de Oncologia, Centro
Medico Nacional Siglo XXI, Instituto Mexicano del Seguro Social,
Mexico City, Mexico

© Springer International Publishing AG, part of Springer Nature 2018
S. Stolnicu, I. Alvarado-Cabrero (eds.), *Practical Atlas of Breast Pathology*, https://doi.org/10.1007/978-3-319-93257-6_27

Fig. 27.1 Different biopsies or resection specimens to diagnose and/or treat breast diseases

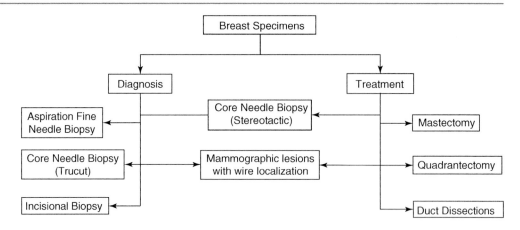

27.2 Core-Needle Biopsies

Large core-needle biopsies may be performed for palpable masses (Tru-Cut) (Fig. 27.2) without radiologic guidance; or under ultrasound guidance to sample non-palpable masses; or mammographically directed ("stereotactic") for either calcifications or mammographic densities; or using MRI to detect enhancing lesions (Fig. 27.3) [1].

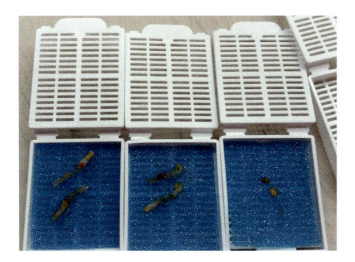

Fig. 27.2 Core-needle biopsy (Tru-Cut; these are usually taken with a 14-G needle) of a mucinous carcinoma

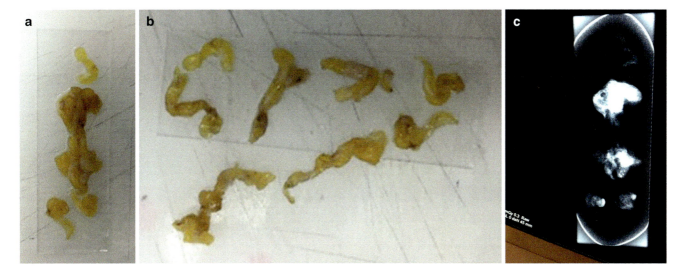

Fig. 27.3 (**a**) Core-needle biopsy (stereotactic; these are usually thicker cores taken with a 9–11 G needle). (**b**) Carefully separate the cores to submit them. (**c**) Radiographic image from the stereotactic biopsy showing the microcalcifications within the cores

27.2.1 Specimen Processing

1. Describe the number of cores, color, and size.
2. Submit 1–3 cores in each cassette. They must be wrapped in paper or held on with a sponge to provide them a flat surface, which results in the most possible uniform histologic slide (Fig. 27.4).

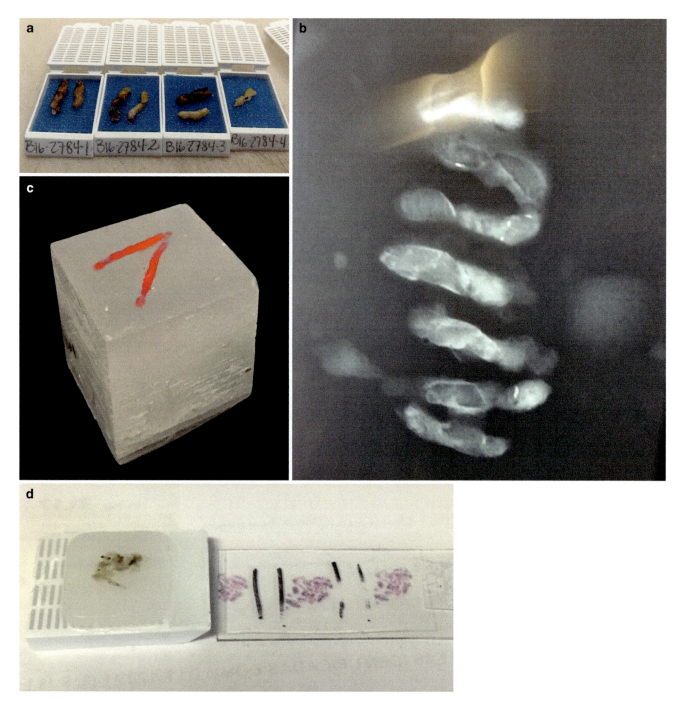

Fig. 27.4 (**a**) Core-needle biopsies submitted two cores by cassette, with a sponge in order to provide them a flat surface. (**a–c**) A paraffin block with two core-needle biopsies. (**d**) Avoid the overlapping of the cores, as the tissue can be lost in the slides and become insufficient to obtain the estrogen receptors, progesterone receptors, and HER2 status

27.3   Incisional Biopsy

Incisional biopsies are less frequently used and are almost always performed to evaluate unresectable invasive carcinomas. Often the purpose of the biopsy is to confirm the clinical diagnosis and to obtain hormone receptors and HER2 status (Fig. 27.5) [1].

27.3.1   Specimen Processing

The specimen can consist of a single fragment or of multiple small fragments of tissue.

1. Describe the number of fragments and global size, color, consistency.
2. There is no need to ink the specimen, because it is an incisional biopsy.
3. Submit all the fragments.

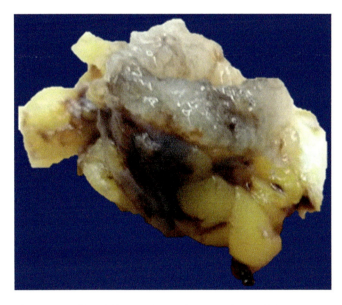

Fig. 27.5 Incisional biopsy of a mucinous carcinoma. It is not necessary to ink this kind of specimen. Just submit it completely

27.4   Excisional Biopsies

Excisional biopsies are defined as procedures intended for the primary evaluation of a breast lesion with complete removal of the lesion. If there has been a prior diagnosis of malignancy (e.g., by core biopsy), the intent of the procedure is to obtain adequate margins. The processing of an excisional biopsy will vary depending on the type of lesion resected [1].

27.4.1   Mastectomy Specimen

- *Radical mastectomy*: This is currently a rare procedure. It consists of en bloc removal of the entire breast, underlying and adjacent adipose tissue, pectoralis major and minor muscles, and axillary contents.
- *Supraradical mastectomy*: This procedure is no longer performed. It consisted of radical mastectomy, chest wall, various ribs, sternum, internal mammary vessels and nodes, and variable pleura.
- *Modified radical mastectomy*: This is a very common procedure. It preserves the pectoralis muscles, some skin (but nipple, areola, and surrounding areas are excised), and some lymph nodes containing fat from ipsilateral axilla (Fig. 27.6).
- *Simple mastectomy*: This procedure excises most or all mammary tissue, nipple, and variable adjacent skin, without lymph nodes of the axilla; it may sometimes include 1–4 axillary lymph nodes (Fig. 27.7). Simple mastectomy can be performed as a prophylactic surgery to reduce the risk of developing breast cancer.

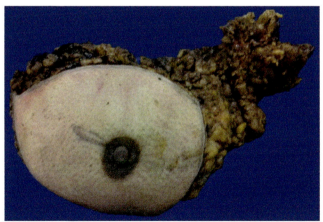

Fig. 27.6 A modified radical mastectomy includes skin, areola and nipple, and axillary lymph node dissection

- **Subcutaneous mastectomy**: This procedure excises most of the mammary tissue, without skin or nipple and variable axillary tail (Fig. 27.8).
- **Reduction mammoplasty**: The tissue excised consists of fragments of breast tissue with attached skin. The nipples are not present. It is almost always a bilateral procedure. This procedure is considered therapeutic if the specimen weighs over 300 g (e.g., to relive back pain), but cosmetic if the specimen weighs less than this [1].

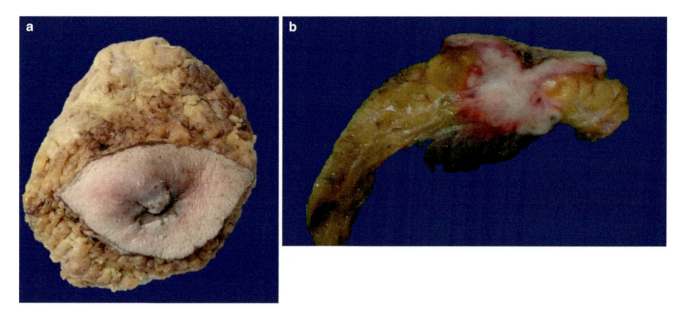

Fig. 27.7 (**a**) A simple mastectomy of a male patient with skin changes like redness, and nipple retraction. (**b**) The cut surface of the simple mastectomy shows a big tumor with spiculated and lobulated borders, infiltrating in the upside the skin, and downside the pectoralis muscle

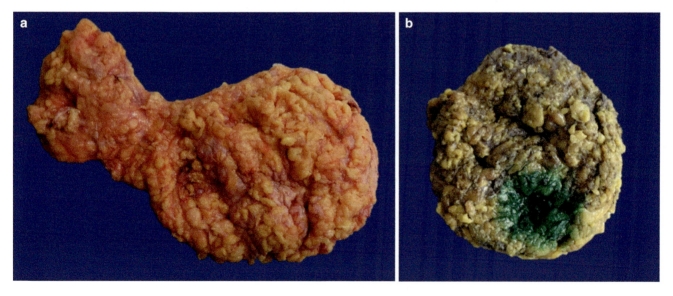

Fig. 27.8 (**a**) Subcutaneous mastectomy with axillary lymph node dissection. The anterior surface is irregular. (**b**) Subcutaneous mastectomy without axillary lymph node dissection. The retroareolar zone is green inked

27.4.1.1 Specimen Processing

Prior to gross examination of the specimen it is usually necessary to review the medical record to determine the number and type of lesions present, as well as whether any preoperative therapy has been given [1].

1. Measure (total size of breast and size of axillary dissection) and weigh specimen, including skin and nipple, and describe if any macroscopic lesion is seen (e.g., ulceration, nipple retraction, scars, pigmented lesions, etc.) (Fig. 27.9).
2. Ink deep margin (usually consists of a smooth fascial plane overlying the pectoralis muscle; in radical specimens, because the breast is a pendulous organ, we just need this margin). Palpate the specimen for masses and correlate with radiograph (if present) (Fig. 27.10).
3. Orient by using axillary fat as upper-external, and divide breast into quadrants (with marker or mentally).
4. Serial section entire breast into 1 cm thick slices, but do not cut through the skin; examine for tumor or suspicious areas (Fig. 27.11). Describe the number of tumors. If there are multiple lesions, describe the distance between lesions when they are close to each other [2], size, location, shape (pushing borders, spiculated), consistency (indurated, solid, cystic), with or without macroscopic necrosis, and distance from the deep margin (Fig. 27.12). The deep margin is always taken as the perpendicular margin because this is a true tissue plane and even a tiny rim of tissue (e.g., less than 0.1 cm) would be considered a negative margin. Any skeletal muscle present is sampled to look for muscle invasion (Fig. 27.13) [1].
5. The specimen must be fixated in buffer formalin (10%) for at least 24 hours before submission.
6. If possible, separate axillary nodes into level I (low: inferior to lower border of pectoralis minor muscle in radical mastectomy specimens); level II (middle: between upper and lower borders of pectoralis minor muscle); and level III (high: superior to upper border of pectoralis minor muscle). If pectoralis minor muscle is not present, separate lymph nodes into upper and lower half; one must find between 13 and 20 lymph nodes in a typical radical mastectomy [1].
7. Record the number and size of the lymph nodes. Try to leave a small amount of extranodal soft tissue (a few millimeters) for the evaluation of extranodal extension [2].
8. In a specimen after neoadjuvant therapy, if residual carcinoma is difficult to evaluate grossly, a specimen radiograph may be helpful to identify tissue distortion/density, residual calcifications that may be associated with the tumor bed, or biopsy marker clips, all of which may guide tissue sampling. Sections can be taken to map out the tumor bed based on the gross and/or radiographic findings and the original location and size of the tumor [2].

Sections: Nipple (perpendicular cuts to maximize cross-sectional area) (Fig. 27.14), deep margin, scar, tumor (at least three sections or 1 per cm of diameter, whichever is greater; include center and periphery of tumor and adjacent tissue), other gross lesions, areas of mammographic abnormality, representative sections of non-adipose tissue from each quadrant (upper-outer, lower-outer, upper-inner, lower-inner) and all lymph nodes (separate into upper and lower half or levels, for radical mastectomy) [3, 4]. If the lymph nodes are small, submit them entirely, but if they are big, submit just the half of each node, in order to not overestimate the number of lymph nodes.

In a specimen after neoadjuvant therapy, submit the entire tumoral bed and adjacent tissue.

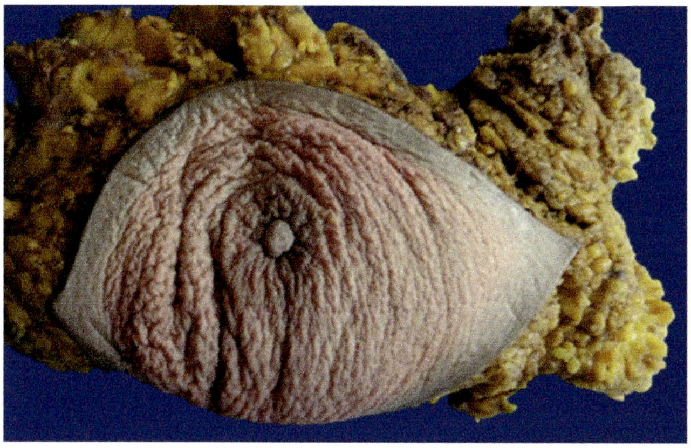

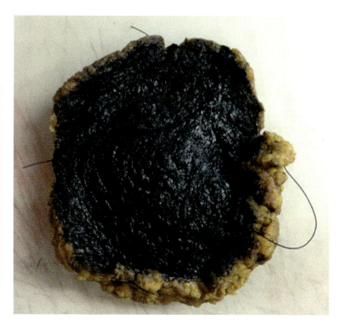

Fig. 27.9 A modified radical left mastectomy with redness of the skin. Describe and measure the skin and nipple, and notice if there are any scars or other abnormalities

Fig. 27.10 The inked deep margin of a simple mastectomy

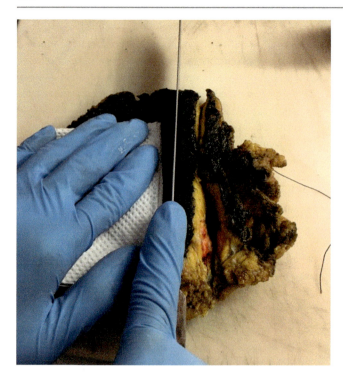

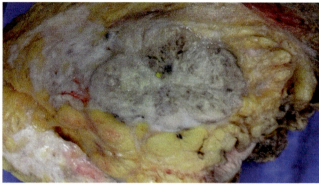

Fig. 27.12 A modified radical mastectomy, with a large tumor, gray-tan, solid, with pushing borders and macroscopic necrosis

Fig. 27.11 Section entire breast into 1 cm thick slices. Do not separate from the skin

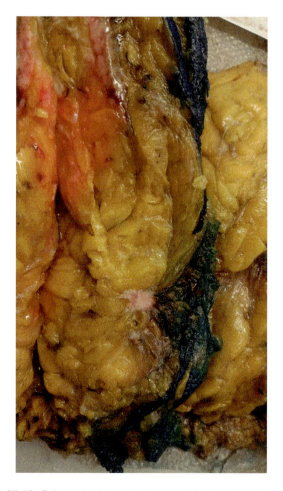

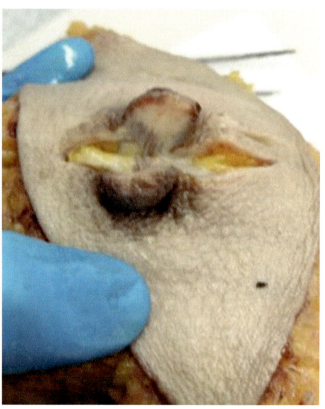

Fig. 27.14 Slice the nipple perpendicular, to see the relation between the skin and lactiferous ducts

Fig. 27.13 Submit the deep margin perpendicular to the tumor, to measure the distance between the tumor and the margin in the histologic section

27.4.2 Breast-Conserving Surgery

These specimens are more difficult and time-consuming to gross than mastectomy specimens, and more sections are often required. The pathologist should always consider that margin assessment is crucial.

Partial mastectomy includes excisional biopsy and segmental mastectomy, or lumpectomy. These can be performed with or without needle localization. Most partial mastectomy specimens are oriented by the surgeon. This is usually done by placing sutures on the specimen (e.g., short suture—superior, long suture—lateral) (Fig. 27.15a). If there is any question regarding the orientation, the surgeon should be contacted for clarification before the specimen is further processed [2].

Excisional biopsies for mammographic lesions with wire localization: Mammographic (non-palpable) lesions are biopsied by placing a wire in the breast at the site of the mammographic abnormality. After excision, the biopsy is sent to mammography for a specimen radiograph as well as the interpretation by the radiologist (Fig. 27.15b) [1].

Margin evaluation is an exercise in probabilities (not absolutes). Patients with positive margins are more likely to have residual disease at or near the primary site than those with negative margins.

A positive margin does not guarantee residual disease, and a negative margin does not preclude extensive residual disease.

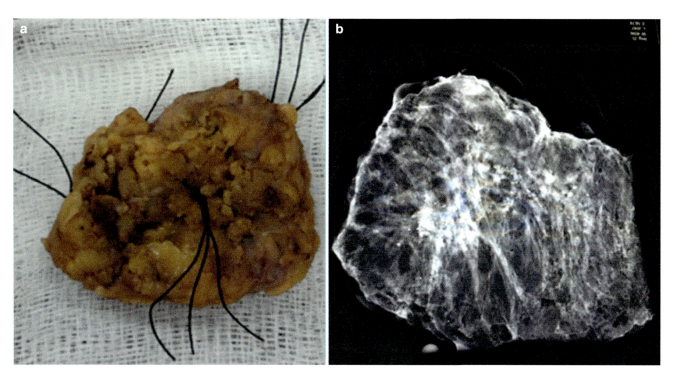

Fig. 27.15 (**a**) An excisional biopsy must come with referred margins by the surgeon; this could be done with sutures or with a written indication about each margin. (**b**) An x-ray image must accompany an excisional biopsy when it is performed for a nonpalpable lesion. See the architectural distortion and microcalcifications

27.4.2.1 Specimen Processing

1. Measure the specimen in three dimensions. Measure the attached skin if present [2].
2. The specimen can be inked one color if not oriented or multiple colors if oriented (e.g., anterior, yellow; posterior (deep), black; superior, blue; inferior, green; medial and lateral, red) (Fig. 27.16).
3. Blot excess ink.
4. If localization wires are present, it is the best to remove them before slicing the specimen, using the specimen radiograph as reference.
5. Slice the entire specimen (Fig. 27.17).
6. Identify gross lesions and record the location (which slices are involved), size, and distance from each margin for each lesion. If there are multiple lesions, describe the distance between lesions (Fig. 27.18) [2].
7. If there is no gross lesion, and the site of the calcifications cannot be identified (e.g., because the wire had fallen out the specimen), then the sliced tissue should be re-radiographed. Small specimens may be submitted in their entirety without additional radiography [1].
8. At least one section from each of the six margins should be submitted. Always submit perpendicular margin sections. Multiple sections of a close margin(s) can be submitted. It is better to include a portion of the lesion when submitting a margin section if the lesion is close enough to be included so that the distance can be measured microscopically (Fig. 27.19).

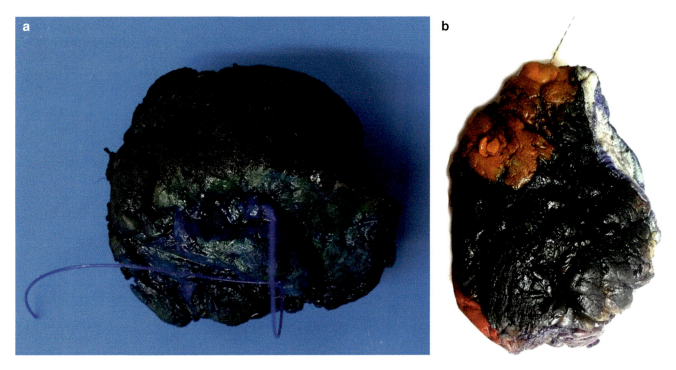

Fig. 27.16 (**a**) When an excisional biopsy comes without margin reference, you may ink it in just one color. (**b**) An excisional biopsy with referred margins could be inked in different colors to facilitate the measure of the lesion to each margin

Fig. 27.17 (**a**) Examine all the slices of an excisional biopsy; most of the time, if it is a non-palpable mass, you will not see an specific alteration of the breast parenchyma. (**b**) This is an example of a simple mastectomy with an extensive ductal in situ carcinoma. Note the yellow chinning; the slide will show a comedocarcinoma

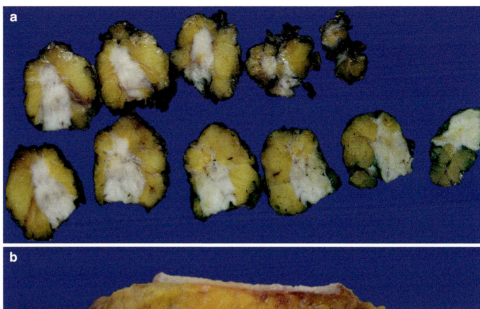

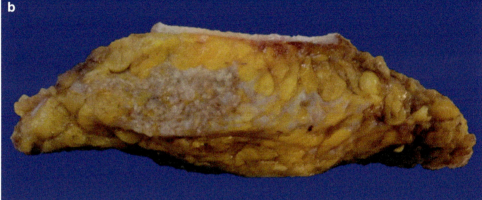

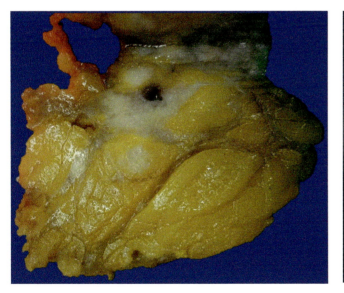

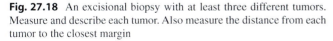

Fig. 27.18 An excisional biopsy with at least three different tumors. Measure and describe each tumor. Also measure the distance from each tumor to the closest margin

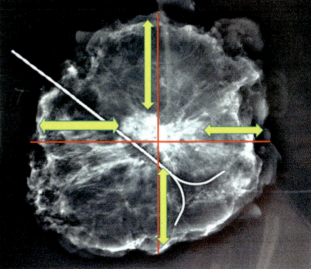

Fig. 27.19 A radiograph of a wire excision may help identify a tumor and see the relation of it with the margins

27.4.3 Re-excisions

Breast re-excision is a general term for larger excisions of an excisional biopsy site when malignancy has been found.

- Lumpectomy: The term is used loosely because a "lump" is usually no longer present at the time this procedure is performed.

- Quadrantectomy: This term refers to a larger resection of an entire breast quadrant.
- Sometimes even mastectomy can be done.

Re-excisions often have a small ellipse of skin, which may be oriented with sutures of different lengths (Fig. 27.20).

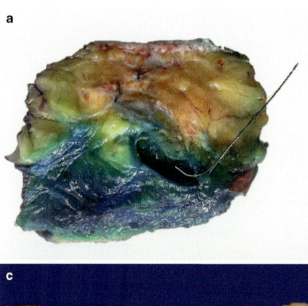

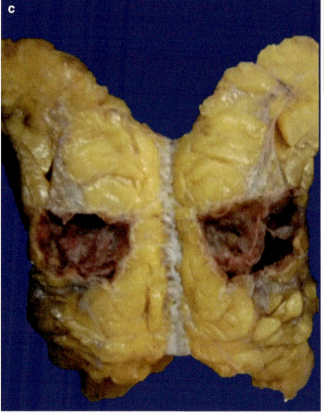

Fig. 27.20 (**a**), A wire-guided quadrantectomy. The tip of the wire is located in the previous excision cavity. It is stained with blue because a sentinel lymph node excision was also performed. (**b**) Mastectomy specimen with a residual tumor; note the hemorrhagic areas caused by a previous core-needle biopsy. (**c**) Mastectomy with excision cavity, from a previous wire resection with positive margins

27.4.3.1 Specimen Processing

1. Record the total dimensions, size, and color of skin ellipse (if present), and size and condition of scar (well-healed, recent) [1].
2. Orient the specimen through information provided by the surgeon.
3. Ink the entire specimen. Use different colors of ink if this will help in identifying margins, or one color if no orientation is provided.
4. Section the specimen sequentially from one end to the other.
5. Examine the tissue around the previous excision cavity for firm areas that may represent residual tumor [2].
6. Submit the entire specimen if it is small. Or, submit up to four sections of the biopsy cavity, selecting areas that are most suspicious for residual carcinoma close to the margins.
7. Sample the margins. Twelve cassettes (corresponding to two sections of each six margins) are usually adequate unless there are multiple suspicious areas [1].
8. Sample the skin to evaluate possible dermal lymphatic involvement or direct skin invasion [1].

27.4.4 Duct Dissections

Duct dissections are usually performed to evaluate nipple discharge, and the most common lesion found is a large papilloma (Fig. 27.21). A duct dissection specimen is usually small, and large ducts may be grossly visible (Fig. 27.22).

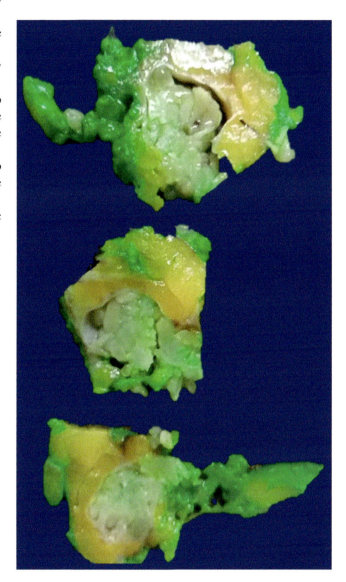

Fig. 27.21 A large papilloma resection

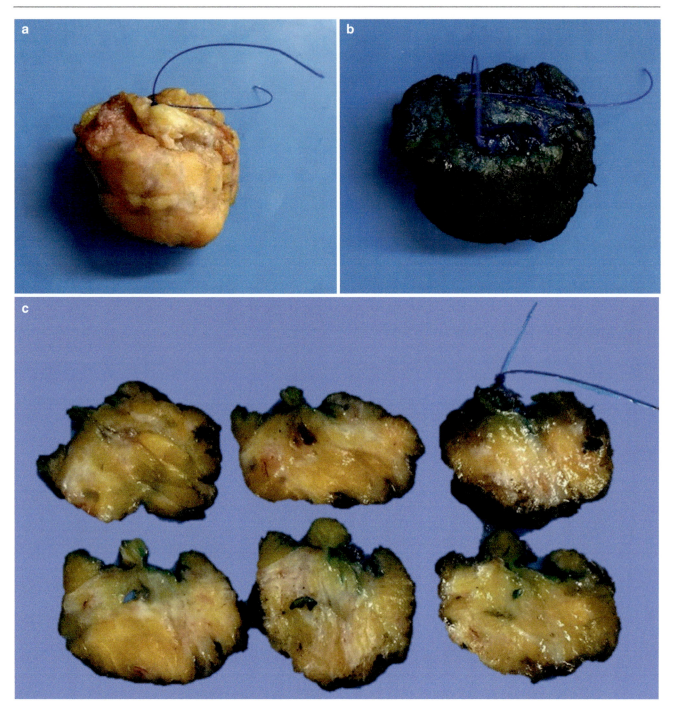

Fig. 27.22 A duct dissection specimen, with a suture indicating the nipple side (**a**); measure and ink the specimen (**b**), then slice all the specimens perpendicularly and look for dilated ducts and lesions inside them (**c**)

27.4.4.1 Specimen Processing

1. Record the total dimensions.
2. Orient the specimen through information provided by the surgeon; they frequently use a suture to signal the retroareolar tissue.
3. Ink the entire specimen.
4. Section the specimen sequentially from one end to the other, parallel to the duct direction.
5. Examine the tissue and describe if any nodule or papilloma is seen, size, color, texture.
6. Submit the entire specimen.

References

1. Lester SC. Manual of surgical pathology. 3rd ed. Philadelphia, PA: Elsevier; 2010. p. 262–88.
2. Huo L. A practical approach to grossing breast specimens. Ann Diagn Pathol. 2011;15:291–301.
3. Roychowdhury M. Grossing (histologic sampling) of breast lesions. PathologyOutlinescom. http://www.pathologyoutlines.com/topic/breastmalignantgrossing.html. Accessed 20 Nov 2017.
4. Gupta D, Nath M, Layfield LJ. Utility of four-quadrant random sections in mastectomy specimens. Breast J. 2003;9:307–11.

Dermatologic Diseases of the Breast and Nipple

Anca Chiriac

28.1 Dermatitis

Eczema and dermatitis are synonyms, describing the same disease. It is characterized clinically by erythema, oozing, edema, papules or vesicles, scaling, lichenification, and is associated with pruritus and scratch. It is histopathologically characterized by by intercellular edema.

28.1.1 Nipple Dermatitis (Nipple Eczema)

Nipple atopic eczema is the hallmark of atopic dermatitis of the breast and a minor criterion in Hanifin and Rajka's diagnostic criteria for atopic dermatitis [1, 2]. Clinical image is suggestive by showing erythema and exudation in acute phase; erosions, crusts, fissures, excoriations ("dry eczema") in sub-acute phase and even lichenification in chronic phase, associated mostly with pruritus or burning sensation (Fig. 28.1). In atopic patients, nipple dermatitis has flares and remissions and is related to other signs of atopy.

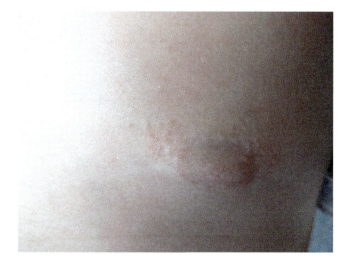

Fig. 28.1 Nipple and periareolar atopic eczema ("dry eczema")—discrete erythema and desquamation, small papules

A. Chiriac, MD, PhD
Department of Dermatology, Nicolina Medical Center, Iaşi, Romania

Department of Dermato-Physiology, Apollonia University, Iaşi, Romania

P. Poni Institute of Macromolecular Chemistry, Iaşi, Romania

© Springer International Publishing AG, part of Springer Nature 2018
S. Stolnicu, I. Alvarado-Cabrero (eds.), *Practical Atlas of Breast Pathology*, https://doi.org/10.1007/978-3-319-93257-6_28

28.1.2 Allergic Contact Dermatitis

Allergic contact dermatitis can cause nipple eczema by contact sensitization to specific allergens. Specific sensitivity can occur after years of chronic low-grade exposure, but allergic contact dermatitis, in a sensitized person, can develop within hours or days of recent exposure (Fig. 28.2).

Several reports have been published arguing in favor of allergic contact dermatitis of the breast area caused by: Cl + Me-isothiazolinone, cobalt chloride, thimerosal, nickel sulfate, and 4-tert-butylphenol-formaldehyde resin, which are found in preservatives, detergents, and fabric softeners [3]; p-tert-butylphenol formaldehyde resin bra associated [4]; and beeswax nipple-protective [5].

When lesions are bilateral and extend to the periareolar skin, allergic contact dermatitis should be suspected, and patch tests performed.

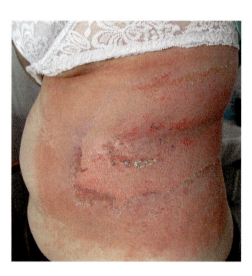

Fig. 28.2 Allergic contact dermatitis on the left part of the thorax and inframammary area caused by adhesive in hepatic transplanted recipient

28.1.3 Irritant Contact Dermatitis

Irritant contact dermatitis is a localized inflammatory skin lesion induced by direct contact with chemical or physical agents, including friction (mechanical trauma). The clinical manifestations are similar to other causes of nipple eczema (Fig. 28.3).

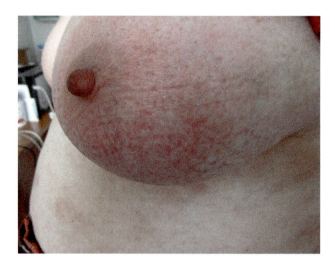

Fig. 28.3 Irritant contact dermatitis induced by mechanical trauma

28.2 Psoriasis

28.2.1 Inframammary Psoriasis (Inverse Psoriasis)

Inframammary psoriasis (inverse psoriasis) is a common form of psoriasis, mostly in women, clinically characterized by bilateral well-demarcated plaques, with no scales, discrete erythema or pink-moist appearance; it is symptom-free or associated with burning sensation or itch. Differential diagnosis should be done with seborrheic dermatitis, bacterial or fungal intertrigo. Similar lesions can be observed in the axillary regions or can be associated with typical plaque-psoriasis (Fig. 28.4).

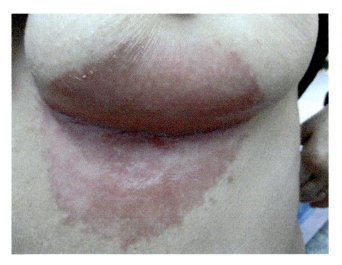

Fig. 28.4 Inframammary psoriasis (inverse psoriasis)—pink-moist appearance plaque, well demarcated, with no satellite papules and no scales

28.2.2 Plaque-Psoriasis (Psoriasis Vulgaris)

Plaque-psoriasis (psoriasis vulgaris) can be localized on other areas of the breast. It is diagnosed by the presence of unique or multiple rose pink papules or erythematous plaques covered by thick silvery-white scales (Figs. 28.5 and 28.6).

Psoriasis is diagnosed by the characteristic clinical findings; however, skin biopsy can be performed for certifying the diagnosis. The hallmarks of pathological findings in psoriasis are thickening of the epidermis, hyperkeratosis, parakeratosis, and neutrophilic infiltration under the horny cell layer (Munro's microabscess).

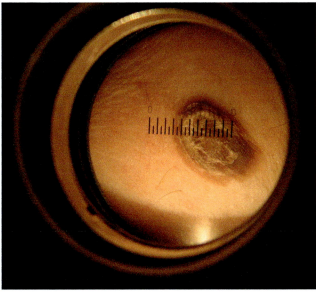

Fig. 28.5 Nipple psoriasis (through a lens): thick silvery-white scales covering the nipple

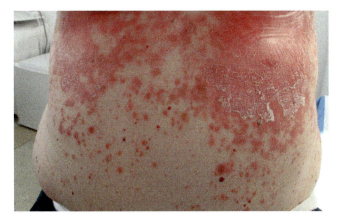

Fig. 28.6 Plaque-psoriasis: multiple and of variable size erythematous scaly plaques

28.3   Vitiligo

Vitiligo is an autoimmune depigmentation of the skin of unknown etiology, characterized by the presence of sharply circumscribed depigmented skin areas (leukoderma) as a result of destruction of epidermal melanocytes. Its prevalence is estimated to 0.5% of the general population [6]. Vitiligo has been recently classified into generalized vitiligo, segmental vitiligo, and unclassified/undetermined vitiligo or focal vitiligo (Fig. 28.7) [6].

White macules or patches can be spread around the nipple or any area of the breast. The lesions are irregular in shape and size, and they often coalesce in large plaques. It is asymptomatic.

Vitiligo should be differentiated from:

- Nevus depigmentosus (hypopigmented patches seen at birth or shortly thereafter, unique or several, with irregular shape and flu edges, localized mostly on the trunk, sometimes band-like).
- Vogt-Koyanagi-Harada disease (irregular-shaped diffuse cutaneous leukoderma associated with uveitis, leukotrichia and alopecia).
- Pityriasis versicolor (light brown or hypopigmented macules and patches, with discrete scales, localized on the trunk, caused by *Malassezia furfur*, a fungal yeast infection).

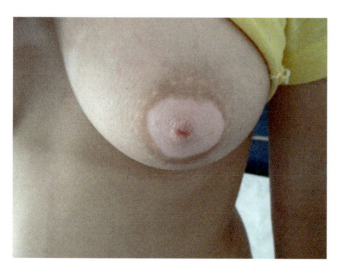

Fig. 28.7 Vitiligo: bilateral circumscribed depigmented area around the nipple

28.4   Hyperkeratosis of the Nipple

Hyperkeratosis of the nipple was described in 1938 by Levy-Franckel and classified in three types [7]:

(a) Type 1 or "nevoid hyperkeratosis of the nipple and areola" as a part of a unilateral verrucous (epidermal) nevus.
(b) Type 2 or "hyperkeratosis of the nipple associated with other disorders": ichthyosis, acanthosis nigricans, Darier disease, and lymphoma; mostly bilateral in distribution.
(c) Type 3 or "idiopathic hyperkeratosis of the nipple and/or areola," predominantly reported in women (at puberty, in adulthood, or during pregnancy), but also in men (treated with diethylstilbestrol for prostate cancer) [8–11].

During recent decades, although few cases have been reported in the literature, a new classification of hyperkeratosis of the nipple and/or areola has been released [12]:

(a) Primary hyperkeratosis of the nipple and areola accompanying other disorders of keratinization: ichthyosis, acanthosis nigricans, and Darier disease;
(b) Secondary hyperkeratosis of the nipple and areola associated with hormonal changes, lymphoma, neoplastic diseases;
(c) Idiopathic hyperkeratosis of the nipple and areola (Fig. 28.8).

Sparse cases of hyperkeratosis of the nipple and areola have been communicated during recent years by its association with *Malassezia furfur* infection [13, 14], or as a cutaneous side effect of Vemurafenib (for treating metastatic melanoma) [15].

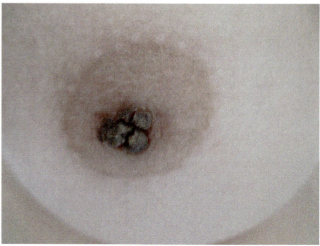

Fig. 28.8 Idiopathic hyperkeratosis of the nipple

28.5 Bacterial, Fungal and Viral Infections of the Breast

28.5.1 Bacterial Infections

28.5.1.1 Folliculitis

Folliculitis represents a localized bacterial infection of the hair follicles, caused by *Staphylococcus aureus* or group-A b-hemolytic *Streptococcus,* clinically presented as small pustules and erythema around the hairs (Fig. 28.9). When a pustular plug is present in the center of folliculitis and affects only one hair follicle, the disease is named *furuncle*; when the infection spreads to multiple hair follicles it is a *carbuncule*; multiple furuncles evolving over a long period of time is called *furunculosis* (Fig. 28.10).

Folliculitis can progress, in immune compromised hosts, to deep dermal layer and subcutaneous inflammation disorder named *cellulitis.*

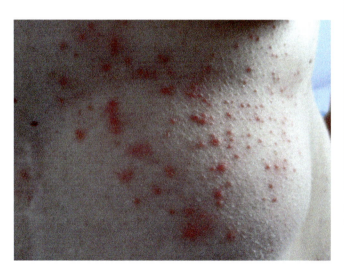

Fig. 28.9 Folliculitis: widespread small papules and pustules accompanied by erythema

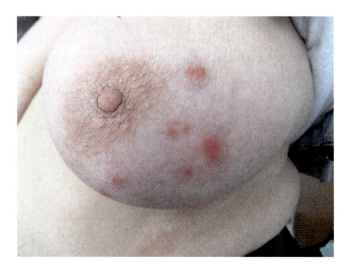

Fig. 28.10 Furunculosis: red, swollen, and tender nodules (deep infection of the hair follicle associated with accumulation of pus and necrotic tissue)

28.5.1.2 Impetigo

Impetigo is a superficial bacterial infection (localized at the horny layer), not related to hair follicles, caused by toxins released by *Staphylococcus aureus* (impetigo bullous type) or by group-A b-hemolytic *Streptococcus (Streptococcus pyogenes)* (non-bullous type). Impetigo bullous is characterized by the presence of vesicles, flaccid bullae, and erosive erythematous patches, accompanied by pruritus and scratching (which contributes to spreading the infection) (Fig. 28.11). Although it is highly contagious, it heals without scars. The hallmark of non-bullous impetigo is the yellowish-brown crust (honey-like) adherent to small erythematous macules.

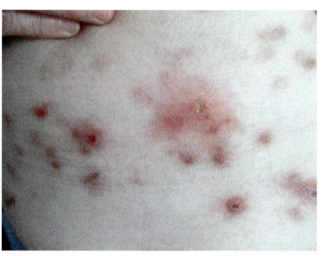

Fig. 28.11 Impetigo: yellowish-brown crusts ("honey-like") adherent to small erythematous macules, erosions on the inframammary area

28.5.2 Fungal Diseases

28.5.2.1 Superficial Dermatophytic Infections

Dermatophytes feed on keratin from the epidermal horny cell layer and hair follicles, causing tinea superficialis (tinea corporis) (Fig. 28.12). Initially small erythematous papules appear, they spread centrifugally forming a ring-shape lesion, with skin that appears normal in the middle and papules and vesicles distributed at the periphery; pruritus can be present.

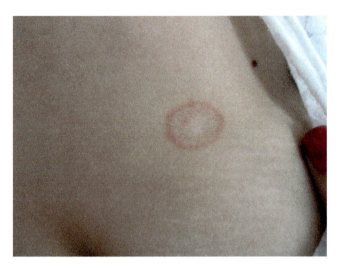

Fig. 28.12 Tinea corporis: scaly plaque, with central normal appearing skin, annular in shape, with scales, papules, vesicles at the advancing border

28.5.2.2 Candidiasis

Nipple Candidiasis

Nipple candidiasis is diagnosed mostly in breastfeeding mothers who complain of pain, burning sensation and erythematous nipple and areola, mild edema, and, sometimes, fissures around the areola [16].

Candida Intertrigo

Candida intertrigo is diagnosed clinically by the presence in the inframammary area of unilateral or bilateral moist, erythematous plaques ("beefy erythema") with no clear margins; fissures are sometimes present; with a whitish ring; papules and pustules spread to the adjacent healthy skin (Figs. 28.13 and 28.14).

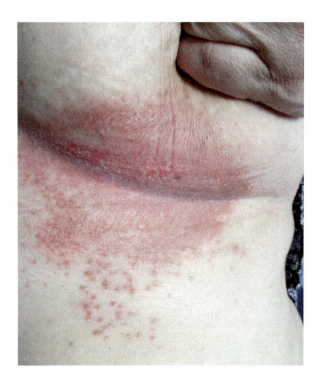

Fig. 28.13 Localized Candida intertrigo: under breast bright red ("beefy erythema") and moist plaques associated with satellite papules

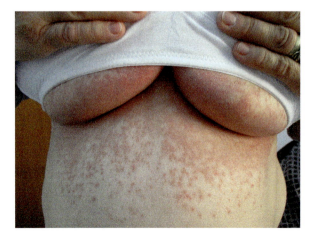

Fig. 28.14 Extended Candida intertrigo: under breast bright red ("beefy erythema") and moist plaques associated with satellite papules

28.5.3 Viral Infections

28.5.3.1 Herpes Simplex Infection

Herpes simplex is caused by herpes simplex virus type 1 (HSV-1) or type 2 (HSV-2). It may occur on any part of the body and is seen extremely rarely on the breast area. Clinically it is characterized by localized aggregation of grouped small vesicles that form, in the following days, pustules, erosions, and crusts on an erythematous base. Itching can be present. Healing is in one week (Fig. 28.15).

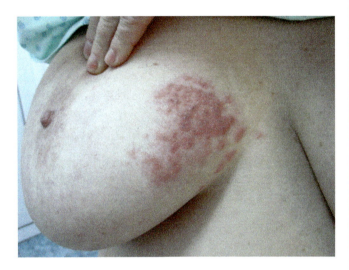

Fig. 28.15 Herpes simplex: localized aggregation of grouped small vesicles

28.5.3.2 Herpes Zoster

Herpes zoster is caused by the reactivation of latent varicella zoster virus (VZV). Herpetic vesicles are spread over certain innervated regions in a band-like pattern. Blisters rupture and form erosions covered by crusts, and in severe cases can be associated with intense, necrotic lesions. Neuralgic pain can precede or can be continuously present after crust formation (post herpetic neuralgia) (Figs. 28.16 and 28.17).

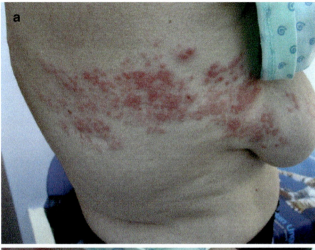

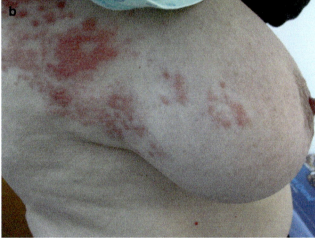

Fig. 28.16 (**a**, **b**) Herpes zoster: unilateral dermatomal grouped herpetiform vesicles

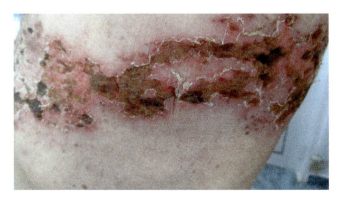

Fig. 28.17 Necrotic herpes zoster: necrotic lesions and scarring can occur if deeper epidermal and dermal layers have been affected

28.5.3.3 Pityriasis Rosea

Pityriasis rosea (originally described by Gibert) is an erythemato-squamous dermatosis that affects young people. It has a presumed viral etiology of human herpes virus 6 and 7, and lesions typically spread on the trunk and roots of limbs.

The initial lesion is named "herald patch" or "mother patch," and it is a solitary, salmon-colored round or oval macule, with size varying from 1 to 10 cm, and with a characteristic small fine scale in the center of the lesion (Fig. 28.18). Within hours and days of its appearance many thin papules with similar aspect—oval or round, pink or slight erythematous, small—spread on the trunk and extremities in a "Christmas tree" pattern (Fig. 28.19). Diagnosis is made by putting in evidence the "collarette" of scale around the border and free edges seen in each lesion (like in herald patch). In most cases it resolves spontaneously in a few weeks [17].

In daily practice the most important differential diagnosis should be made with secondary syphilis by serological test and by keeping in mind that syphilitic lesions do not have scales.

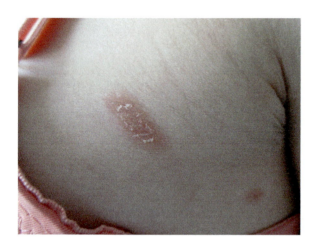

Fig. 28.18 Pityriasis rosea: "herald patch" or "mother patch": oval pink or red plaque of a few cm in diameter, with a "collaret" scale inside the edge of the lesion

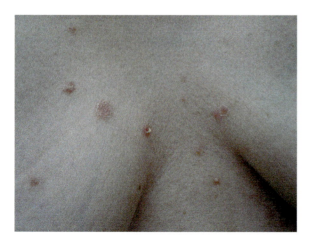

Fig. 28.19 Pityriasis rosea: secondary lesions, smaller than the herald patch, also oval, with an inner "collaret" of scale, distributed "in a Christmas tree" pattern on the trunk, thighs and arms

28.6 Morphea and Lichen Sclerosus et Atrophicus

28.6.1 Morphea

Morphea (localized scleroderma) should be distinguished from systemic scleroderma by the lack of lack of sclerodactyly, Raynaud's disease, microvascular lesions (visible on capillaroscopy), and internal organ involvement [18]. Etiology is still unknown; it is a localized sclerosis of the skin caused by fibrosis of the dermis and of the underlying tissues.

Plaque morphea is characterized clinically by well circumscribed ivory plaques surrounded by a typical lilac ring. Lesions can be unique or disseminated. Morphea can be divided into superficial localized scleroderma (fibrosis limited to the epidermis and superficial dermis) and deep scleroderma (fibrosis affecting deep dermis, hypodermis, subcutis, and fascia). Diagnosis is made by clinical examination; confirmation is done by skin biopsy showing thickening and horizontalization of collagen bundles associated with close atrophy; lymphocytic infiltrate is put in evidence in the lilac ring area (Figs. 28.20 and 28.21).

Although very typical in its appearance, localized scleroderma on the breast area should be differentiated from carcinoma "en cuirasse," chronic radiation dermatitis, lichen sclerosus et atrophicus, and other types of localized sclerosis (post-traumatic, drug induced).

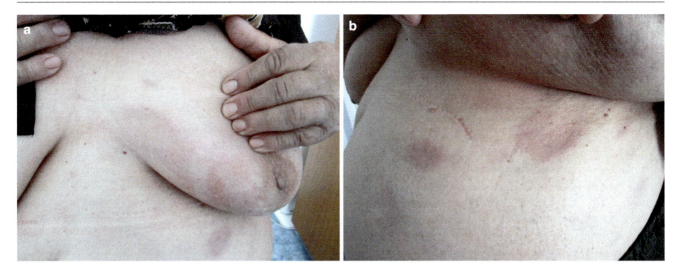

Fig. 28.20 (**a**, **b**) Morphea: well circumscribed ivory plaques surrounded by a typical lilac ring

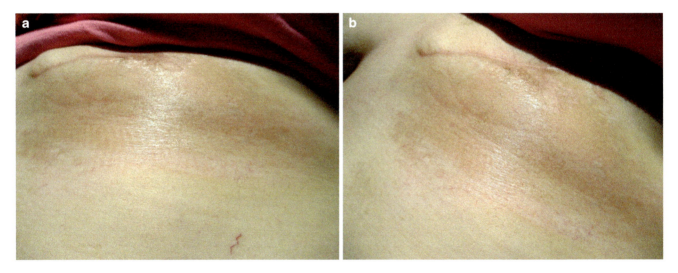

Fig. 28.21 (**a**, **b**) Morphea localized around the surgical scar

28.6.2 Lichen Sclerosus et Atrophicus

Lichen sclerosus et atrophicus is a chronic disease of post-menopausal women, clinically described as white firm plaques of different size, with a characteristic "crepe-like appearance" or "porcelain-white" atrophic plaques, associated with severe pruritus (Figs. 28.22 and 28.23). It is mostly localized in the ano-genital region, although extragenital form has been reported in 2.5% of cases. It is rarely seen on the breast or inframammary area [19].

Etiology is unknown, and various hypotheses have been postulated, such as hormonal disturbances, predisposition (HLA II DQ7), infection (*Borrelia burgdorferi*), traumatic events, and immunological mechanism (the presence of autoantibodies against extracellular matrix 1).

Pathology confirms epidermal atrophy, homogeneous collagen fibers in the dermis, and band-like lymphocytic infiltrate in the dermis.

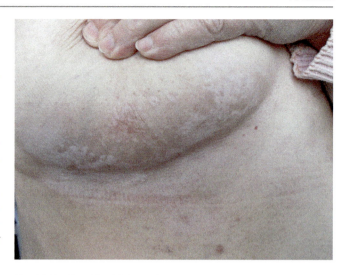

Fig. 28.23 Localized lichen sclerosus et atrophicus: "porcelain-white" atrophic plaques

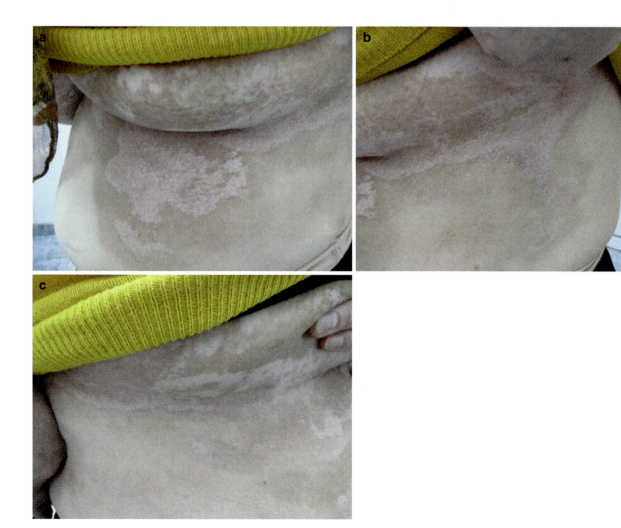

Fig. 28.22 (**a–c**) Extended lichen sclerosus et atrophicus: "porcelain-white" atrophic plaques

28.7 Factitial Disease (Dermatitis Artefacta, Patomimia)

Factitial disease it is a self-inflicted (auto-induced) skin disease, part of psychocutaneous disorders (Fig. 28.24).

"Neurotic excoriations," "psychologic excoriations," and "scratch marks" are commonly seen in patients diagnosed with depression, anxiety, or other psychiatric diseases [20].

Diagnosis of dermatitis artefacta is a challenge and is based on the following criteria:

- A multitude of clinical signs that cannot sustain any other known skin disease.
- Patients deny the cause of the skin lesions and do not accept aid from psychiatrist, psychotherapist, or psychologists.
- Lesions are always located in the areas easily accessible to auto-induced trauma; breast area is frequently involved, especially in young women (Fig. 28.25).
- Skin lesions vary from simple erythema to bizarre injuries, and are geometric and angular.
- Skin lesions heal under occlusive dressings and with psychiatric treatment.

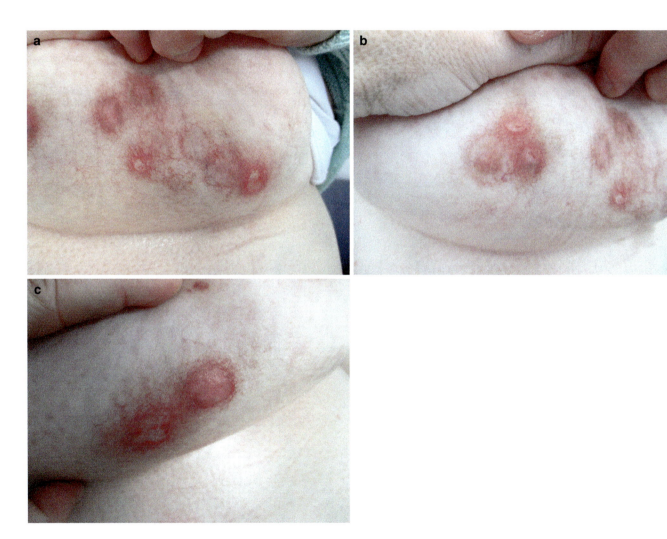

Fig. 28.24 (a–c) Factitial disease: self-inflicted lesions by cigarette

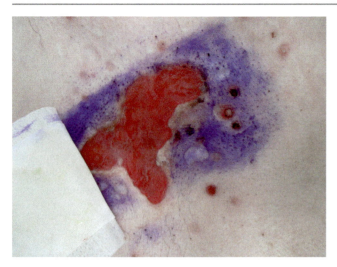

Fig. 28.25 Dermatitis artefacta: auto-induced skin lesion by chronic trauma with a sharp knife

28.8 Lyme Disease (Cutaneous Borreliosis)

Cutaneous borreliosis is a tick-borne disease. The main vector, a tick of the genus Ixodes (Fig. 28.26), transmits bacteria belonging to the *Borrelia burgdorferi* family during a blood meal. After 36 h Borrelia is inoculated in the skin of the affected person [21, 22]. Peak incidence of the disease is early spring to mid-summer.

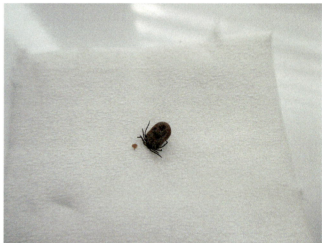

Fig. 28.26 Tick (Ixodes genus)

28.8.1 Erythema Migrans

Erythema migrans is the hallmark of the first stage of Lyme disease. It is an erythematous macule that appears at the site of inoculation after 7–14 days after tick bite; it expands centrifugally, with central clearing and well-delineated borders. Healing is without scars and can occur even in the absence of any treatment (Figs. 28.27 and 28.28) [23].

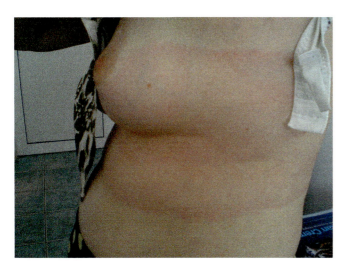

Fig. 28.27 Erythema migrans (stage I Lyme disease): gyrate erythema with clear center caused by the tick bite

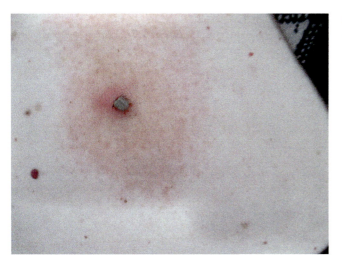

Fig. 28.28 Tick bite with early erythema

28.8.2 Borrelia Lymphocytoma

A rare manifestation of Lyme disease, Borrelia lymphocytoma manifests as a bluish-red nodule observed weeks–months after a tick bite, not at the site of inoculation, but commonly on the earlobe, nipple, genitalia, or face (Fig. 28.29) [24]. Diagnosis is based on anamnesis, clinical image, serology (PCR and culture) and skin biopsy (polyclonal B cell lymphocytic infiltrate mimicking a lymph node or a lymphoma) [25]. Spontaneous resolution occurs in years, in the majority of cases.

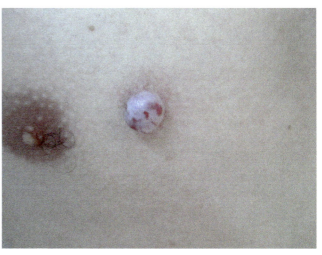

Fig. 28.29 Borrelia lymphocytoma: bluish-red nodule weeks-months after tick bite

28.9 Vascular Malformations and Steroid Purpura

28.9.1 Vascular Malformations

Hemangiomas and vascular malformations belong to the category of *vascular anomalies*. Vascular malformations have the following diagnostic criteria [26]:

- They are present at birth.
- Sex ratio: equal.
- They continue to grow proportionally with the growth rate of the body.
- They do not present any sign of involution.
- They are histologically "self-perpetuating" embryologic tissues with malformed vessels caused by defects of embryogenesis (vasculogenesis/angiogenesis).
- Duplex sonography and MRI attest the malformations.

Vascular malformations are classified in: capillary, venous, arterio-venous, and lymphatic malformations (Fig. 28.30).

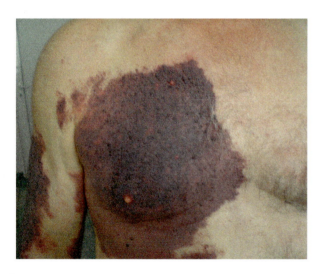

Fig. 28.30 Vascular malformation (malformed vessels)

28.9.2 Steroid Purpura

Steroid purpura occurs in the elderly as a consequence of prolonged used of systemic and/or topical steroids that alter the capillary walls, causing purpura to appear even after minimal trauma (Fig. 28.31). On the breast area, steroid purpura is described in patients who have been diagnosed with psoriasis and were treated for years with potent topical steroids.

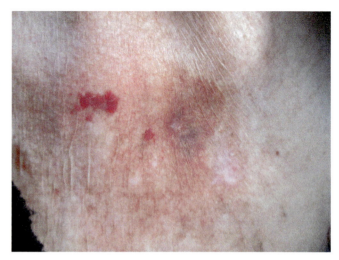

Fig. 28.31 Steroid purpura (purple skin lesions produced by bleeding in the dermis or subcutaneous tissues)

28.10 Cutaneous Erythematous Lupus

Sub-acute cutaneous lupus erythematosus (SCLE) is characterized by the presence of annular lesions with scaly borders arranged in a polycyclic pattern (Fig. 28.32) [27].

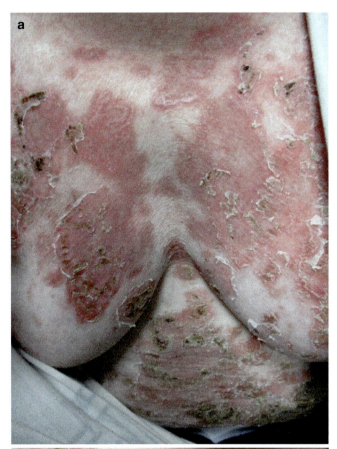

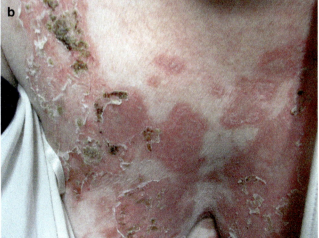

Fig. 28.32 (**a**, **b**) Sub-acute cutaneous lupus erythematosus: papulosquamous annular polycyclic lesions

28.11 Autoimmune Blistering Disorders

28.11.1 Intra-Epidermal Blistering (Pemphigus Group)

Diseases with intra-epidermal blistering (pemphigus group) are characterized by erosions in the oral cavity and blisters, erosions, ulcerations, and crusts spread on the skin (Fig. 28.33). Diagnosis is made by pathology (showing acantholysis and intra-epidermal blistering), direct immunofluorescence (identifying intercellular in IgG deposition), and ELISA (by detecting anti-desmoglein 3 and 1 antibodies).

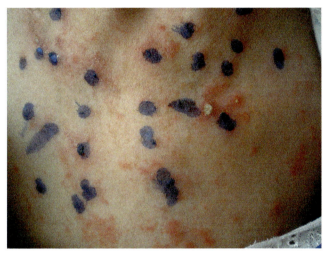

Fig. 28.33 Pemphigus: blisters, erosions, ulcerations and crusts spread on the skin (painted with ethyl blue)

28.11.2 Subepidermal Blistering (Pemphigoid Group)

Diseases with subepidermal blistering (pemphigoid group) are diagnosed mainly in elderly patients and are characterized by tense blisters that do not rupture easily owing to subepidermal cleavage caused by antibodies against epidermal basement membrane (Fig. 28.34). Linear IgG and C3 deposition in the basement membranes is detected by direct immunofluorescence and ELISA identify autoantibodies against Type XVII collagen in bullous pemphigoid.

Conclusion

The breast is a skin area that holds medical interest not only for surgeons specialized in breast pathology or gynecologists but for dermatologists as well. An interdisciplinary approach can prevent incorrect or misdiagnosed disorders.

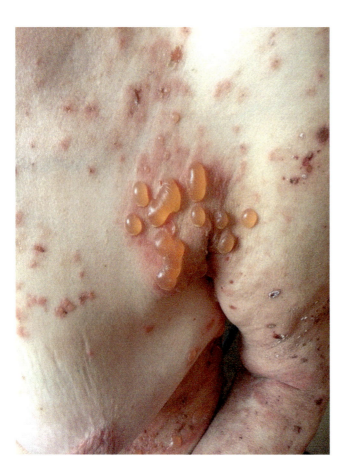

Fig. 28.34 Bullous pemphigoid: characteristic tense blisters

References

1. Whitaker-Worth DL, Carlone V, Susser WS, Phelan N, Grant-Kels JM. Dermatologic diseases of the breast and nipple. J Am Acad Dermatol. 2000;43:733–51. quiz 752–4
2. Hanifin JM, Rajka G. Diagnostic features of atopic dermatitis. Acta Dermatovenerol. 1980;60:44–7.
3. Kim SK, Won YH, Kim SJ. Nipple eczema: a diagnostic challenge of allergic contact dermatitis. Ann Dermatol. 2014;26:413–4.
4. Herro EM, Friedlander SF, Jacob SE. Bra-associated allergic contact dermatitis: p-tert-butylphenol formaldehyde resin as the culprit. Pediatr Dermatol. 2012;29:540–1.
5. Garcia M, del Pozo MD, Díez J, Muñoz D, de Corrès LF. Allergic contact dermatitis from a beeswax nipple-protective. Contact Dermatitis. 1995;33:440–1.
6. Boniface K, Taïeb A, Seneschal J. New insights into immune mechanisms of vitiligo. G Ital Dermatol Venereol. 2016;151:44–54.
7. Levy-Franckel A. Les hyperkeratoses de l'areole et du mamelon. Paris Med. 1938;28:63–6.
8. Ortonne J, el Baze P, Juhlin L. Nevoid hyperkeratosis of the nipple and areola mammae: ineffectiveness of etretinate therapy. Acta Derm Venereol. 1986;66:175–7.
9. Mehregan AH, Rahbari H. Hyperkeratosis of the nipple and areola. Arch Dermatol. 1977;113:1691–2.
10. Rodallec J, Moral P, Guilaine G, Civatte J. Hyperkeratose de l'areole mammaire unilateral recidivante chez une femme enceinte. Ann Dermatol Venereol. 1978;105:527–8.
11. Schwartz RA. Hyperkeratosis of the nipple and areola. Arch Dermatol. 1978;114:1844–5.
12. Mehanna A, Malak JA, Kibbi AG. Hyperkeratosis of the nipple and areola: report of 3 cases. Arch Dermatol. 2001;137:1327–8.
13. Li C, Ran Y, Sugita T, Zhang E, Xie Z, Cao L. Malassezia associated hyperkeratosis of the nipple in young females: report of three cases. Indian J Dermatol Venereol Leprol. 2014;80:78–80.
14. Parimalam K, Chandrakala C, Ananthi M, Karpagam B. Nipple hyperkeratosis due to malassezia furfur showing excellent response to itraconazole. Indian J Dermatol. 2015;60:324.
15. Vanneste L, Wolter P, Van den Oord JJ, Stas M, Garmyn M. Cutaneous adverse effects of BRAF inhibitors in metastatic malignant melanoma, a prospective study in 20 patients. J Eur Acad Dermatol Venereol. 2015;29:61–8.
16. Tanguay KE, McBean MR, Jain E. Nipple candidiasis among breastfeeding mothers. Case-control study of predisposing factors. Can Fam Physician. 1994;40:1407–13.
17. Drago F, Broccolo F, Rebora A. Pityriasis rosea: an update with a critical appraisal of its possible herpesviral etiology. J Am Acad Dermatol. 2009;61:303–18.
18. Fett N, Werth VP. Update on morphea: part I. Epidemiology, clinical presentation and pathogenesis. J Am Acad Dermatol. 2011;64:217–28.
19. Ballester I, Bañuls J, Pérez-Crespo M, Lucas A. Extragenital bullous lichen sclerosus atrophicus. Dermatol Online J. 2009;15:6.
20. Koblenzer CS. Dermatitis artefacta: clinical features and approaches to treatment. Am J Clin Dermatol. 2000;1:47–55.
21. Stanek G, Wormser GP, Gray J, Strle F. Lyme borreliosis. Lancet. 2012;379:461–73.
22. Sood SK, Salzman MB, Johnson BJ, Happ CM, Feig K, Carmody L, et al. Duration of tick attachment as a predictor of the risk of Lyme disease in an area in which Lyme disease is endemic. J Infect Dis. 1997;175:996–9.
23. Asbrink E, Hovmark A. Early and late cutaneous manifestations in Ixodes-borne borreliosis (erythema migrans borreliosis, Lyme borreliosis). Ann N Y Acad Sci. 1988;539:4–15.
24. Lipsker D. Dermatological aspects of Lyme borreliosis. Med Mal Infect. 2007;37:540–7.
25. Colli C, Leinweber B, Müllegger R, Chott A, Kerl H, Cerroni L. Borrelia burgdorferi-associated lymphocytoma cutis: clinicopathologic, immunophenotypic, and molecular study of 106 cases. J Cutan Pathol. 2004;31:232–40.
26. Lee BB, Laredo J. Hemangioma and venous/vascular malformations are different as an apple and an orange! Acta Phlebol. 2012;13:1–3.
27. Francès C, Barète S, Piette JC. Manifestations dermatologiques du lupus. Rev Med Interne. 2008;29:701–9.

Index

A

Adenoma(s), 4, 18, 69, 147, 165–170, 177, 178, 187, 189, 191–193, 209, 210, 445–450

Adenomyoepithelioma, 110, 156, 166, 170, 171, 173, 177–180, 193, 276, 423, 426, 427

Adenosis, 45, 77, 126, 127, 135, 136, 140, 143, 146–157, 161, 165, 166, 173, 175, 176, 185–187, 190, 192, 193, 240, 252, 267, 305, 314, 316, 426, 446

Angiosarcoma(s), 78, 403, 406, 413, 414, 416–419

Atypical ductal hyperplasia (ADH), 71, 109, 110, 115, 116, 133, 136, 142–144, 188, 205, 207–209, 213–224, 423, 432, 434

Atypical lobular hyperplasia (ALH), 175, 176, 243, 244

Atypical vascular lesion (AVLs), 414–417

Axillary lymph node (ALN), 4, 5, 94, 97–100, 106, 125, 261, 293, 332, 337, 342–344, 348, 353, 373, 380, 383, 384, 388, 391, 392, 394, 396, 397, 450, 455, 479, 480

B

Biopsy, 37, 39, 40, 43, 48–50, 52, 55, 56, 59, 66, 67, 69, 70, 76, 82, 91, 95, 99, 107, 109, 112, 118, 121, 122, 125, 126, 138–140, 144, 159, 161, 163, 173, 175, 176, 193, 196, 197, 199, 201, 240, 287, 321, 344, 348, 370, 381, 384, 385, 391, 392, 400, 403, 404, 407, 417, 453, 475, 477, 479, 481, 483, 484, 486, 487, 493, 498, 503

Breast, 1–6, 10, 15, 19–25, 27–29, 31–38, 41, 43–45, 47–49, 59, 60, 63, 64, 69–72, 74–80, 82–89, 91–101, 103–107, 109–111, 117–121, 125–128, 133–136, 141, 146, 150, 156, 159, 161–163, 165, 166, 169, 173, 174, 177–180, 183–187, 189, 190, 192–194, 200, 201, 205, 210, 211, 213, 217, 221, 224, 227, 239, 240, 243, 251, 252, 261–264, 266–268, 270, 272–277, 282, 284–287, 293–325, 327–354, 357–371, 373–381, 383–385, 388, 391, 392, 394, 403–419, 423–442, 446, 451, 454, 455, 459–473, 475–489, 491–506

Breast cancer(s), 1, 2, 4, 5, 21, 27, 44, 47, 84, 88, 111, 174, 175, 180, 211, 227, 236, 240, 263, 270, 272–274, 284, 287, 294, 327, 328, 330, 332, 339, 340, 342, 351, 353, 354, 357–359, 363, 367, 369, 371, 373–375, 378, 381, 384, 388, 391, 392, 400, 433, 439, 459, 460, 465, 479

Breast imaging reporting and data system (BI-RADS), 27, 33–35, 40, 41

Breast fibroepithelial lesions, 183–202, 210, 425

Breast infarct, 106

Breast lesion(s), 1–4, 22, 43, 44, 63, 71, 98, 100, 106, 107, 127, 136, 155, 246, 344, 379, 403, 404, 423–442, 459, 462, 475, 479

Breast mass, 63, 67, 69, 70, 75, 88, 95, 107, 163, 296, 406, 416, 419, 459, 462, 465

Breast specimens, 43, 61, 475

C

Cancer, 35, 47, 64, 72, 125, 127, 189, 205, 217, 287, 330, 358, 369, 373, 381, 383, 385, 391, 394, 400, 429, 433, 459, 465–467, 469, 475

Carcinoma(s), 4, 48, 49, 52, 54–57, 60, 63, 67, 70, 72, 74–80, 82–85, 87–89, 91, 92, 94–98, 100–103, 106, 107, 109–111, 115–122, 125–127, 136, 143–148, 150, 153, 155–157, 159, 161–166, 169, 175–177, 179, 180, 186, 187, 190, 193, 194, 199–202, 205, 208–210, 213–215, 217–220, 223, 224, 227–229, 231–233, 239–241, 243, 246–248, 251–287, 293, 298, 305, 308, 311, 314–316, 319, 321–325, 327–354, 357–371, 373–381, 384–386, 388, 391, 394, 396, 397, 399, 401, 403, 407, 408, 412, 419, 423, 426, 429, 433, 434, 438–441, 447–451, 454, 455, 459–461, 465, 467, 469, 471, 472, 477, 479, 481, 487, 498

Central papilloma, 110, 111, 448

Chemoprevention, 217

Classification, 109, 110, 118, 120, 180, 195, 200, 217, 220, 222, 227, 231, 251, 260, 263, 268, 325, 330, 332, 342, 357, 358, 385, 388

Collagenous spherulosis, 159, 161, 173, 176, 218, 246, 282, 309

Core biopsy, 43, 74, 109, 121, 148, 186, 189, 192–194, 197, 200–202, 211, 217, 223, 224, 243, 247, 354, 373, 384, 388, 404, 417, 479

Core-needle biopsy (CNB), 43, 44, 47, 49, 59, 60, 109, 110, 121, 122, 268, 384, 385, 475, 477

D

Definition, 40, 109, 111, 180, 239, 240, 251, 328, 340, 395

Dermatitis, 491–493, 498, 501

Diagnosis, 27, 43, 44, 55, 67, 71, 72, 79, 80, 84, 88, 91, 93, 106, 107, 109, 116, 121, 122, 125, 126, 133, 136, 142, 143, 146–148, 153, 155, 161, 163, 165, 166, 177, 179, 189, 192, 193, 199, 201, 202, 205, 209, 211, 216–221, 223, 224, 227, 239, 240, 245, 251, 252, 262, 264, 267, 268, 270, 274–276, 284, 293, 299, 307, 308, 311, 315, 330, 337, 351, 357, 358, 362, 374, 384, 391, 403, 404, 414, 419, 425, 433, 434, 446, 451, 455, 459, 460, 462, 465, 469, 471, 475, 479, 493, 498, 501, 503, 505

Differential diagnosis, 4, 27, 75, 78, 79, 82, 87, 89, 91, 93–98, 101, 104, 106, 107, 109, 110, 116, 120, 127, 143, 146, 147, 155–157, 159, 165, 166, 183, 190, 199, 201, 202, 217, 240, 252, 261, 262, 264, 276, 282, 284, 285, 287, 301, 307, 308, 315, 319, 323, 403, 404, 406–408, 413, 414, 429, 446, 447, 449, 450, 453, 454, 493

Ductal carcinoma in situ (DCIS), 40, 47–49, 63, 73, 103, 104, 109,
        110, 115–117, 121, 127, 143, 161, 175, 205, 208–210,
        213–215, 217–224, 227–236, 239, 276, 307–309, 314, 337,
        383, 387, 423, 433–435, 451, 453, 454
Ductal differentiation, 252, 309, 310
Ductal in situ carcinoma, 485

E
Encapsulated papillary carcinoma (EPC), 48, 55, 109, 117–120, 122, 313

F
Fat necrosis, 70, 91, 100–103, 106, 122, 134, 405
Fibroadenoma (FA), 35–37, 40, 63, 64, 67, 71, 72, 79, 126, 132, 159,
        161, 163–167, 183–197, 199, 202, 406, 425, 459
Fibrocystic changes, 66, 125–134, 136, 146, 159, 161, 162, 175, 205,
        210, 426
Fibroepithelial lesions, 183, 187, 190, 192, 197, 199, 202, 210, 425
Fibromatosis, 199, 200, 275, 276, 279, 280, 319, 403, 407–409
Fine needle aspiration (FNA), 43, 63, 67, 69, 72, 75, 76, 79, 82, 88,
        110, 121, 122, 126, 127, 264, 266–270, 273–276, 281, 283,
        373, 384, 404, 423, 433, 434, 469
Fine-needle aspiration cytology (FNAC), 121
Folliculitis, 495

G
Gene(s), 78, 87, 248, 270, 274, 282, 284, 285, 325, 351, 353, 354,
        357, 358, 363, 364, 369, 419
Granuloma, 94, 96–101, 105, 107, 342
Gynecomastia, 209, 423, 425, 429–432

H
Hamartoma(s), 173, 183, 190, 192, 210, 212, 403, 410–412
High-grade, 40, 47, 48, 73, 76, 78, 116, 117, 200, 201, 224, 231, 232,
        234, 236, 239, 240, 243, 256, 261, 263, 273, 275, 279, 282,
        284, 307, 319, 324, 332, 336, 358, 373, 416, 417, 419,
        433–435, 460, 467
Histology, 1–5, 44, 66, 69, 76, 77, 89, 190, 272, 374, 394, 423
Histopathological changes, 381
Hyperkeratosis, 448, 451, 455, 493, 494

I
Imaging, 27, 32, 34, 35, 41, 43, 44, 48, 49, 56, 59, 61, 67, 106, 109,
        110, 177, 189, 193, 194, 205, 263, 268, 275, 284, 373, 374,
        385, 387, 388, 392, 419, 460
Imaging-pathology correlation, 43
Immunohistochemical stain, 84, 106, 116, 143, 147, 157, 166, 175,
        177, 178, 200, 252, 264, 266, 270, 317, 354, 397, 401, 403,
        441, 447, 455, 462, 465
Immunohistochemistry (IHC), 78, 79, 84, 88, 109, 110, 117, 187, 201,
        202, 236, 270, 305–325, 353, 363, 391, 397, 401, 407, 408,
        412, 414
Inflammation(s), 91–96, 98, 99, 103, 105, 122, 127, 159, 231, 232,
        240, 385, 425, 495
Intermediate-grade, 47, 117, 119, 202, 217–219, 224, 233, 314, 416
Intraductal, 35, 38, 48, 82, 106, 109–114, 116, 117, 119, 121, 122,
        147, 148, 159, 161, 166, 176, 177, 193, 205, 214, 217, 220,
        224, 227, 233, 239–241, 261, 309, 311, 312, 331, 423, 424,
        434, 445, 447, 450
Invasive ductal carcinoma (NOS), 36, 37, 49–51, 64, 73, 308–309,
        359, 378, 396, 433, 441, 461, 467
Invasive papillary carcinoma, 109, 120, 311, 424

L
Lexicon, 27, 33, 40, 41
Lobular carcinoma in situ (LCIS), 49, 58, 175, 176, 243–249, 263,
        305, 308–310
Low-grade, 63, 67, 73, 110, 117, 118, 120, 143, 144, 153, 155, 156,
        159, 176, 200, 208, 213, 214, 217–224, 228–230, 236, 267,
        275, 276, 279, 280, 284, 285, 305, 307, 316, 319, 324, 336,
        358, 404, 407, 408, 413, 414, 416, 424, 449, 450, 492
Lymph node (LN), 3, 5, 14, 79, 106, 143, 196, 240, 268, 270, 293,
        303, 322, 330, 337, 342–351, 373, 380, 381, 384, 386, 388,
        391–402, 479, 481, 503
Lymphoma(s), 79, 95, 264, 293, 294, 296–302, 323,
        494, 503

M
Malignant myoepithelioma, 173
Management, 43, 71, 88, 120, 125, 187, 190, 196, 202, 205, 217, 308,
        325, 327, 329, 330, 332, 351, 354, 397, 459
Mesenchymal tumor, 403–419
Metastasis, 4, 5, 75, 84, 87, 88, 196, 251, 262, 264, 267, 270, 272,
        276, 282, 285, 337, 342, 344, 358, 363, 370, 371, 381, 388,
        397, 399, 403, 416, 419, 459, 462
Metastatic breast carcinoma, 84, 88
Microinvasion, 135, 239, 240
Molecular diagnosis, 357, 358
Molecular profile, 240, 328, 329, 332, 453, 455
Morphologic changes, 373–381, 385
Morphological features, 449
Morphology, 1, 40, 64, 65, 67, 141, 143, 180, 183, 193, 200, 210, 214,
        263, 264, 267, 268, 270, 272–279, 285, 328, 344, 363, 375,
        403, 423, 426
Myoepithelial carcinoma, 173, 174, 180, 181
Myofibroblastoma (MFB), 319, 320, 403, 406, 408, 413, 423, 427, 428

N
Needle core biopsy (NCB), 63, 72, 74, 75, 79, 82, 88, 463
Neoadjuvant therapy, 339, 373, 378, 381, 383, 385, 433, 475
Nipple, 445–457, 459, 470, 475, 479–481, 487, 491–506
Nipple discharge, 82, 97, 100, 110, 116, 117, 119, 125, 166, 227, 425,
        433, 445, 448, 459, 475, 487
Nipple eczema, 491, 492
Nodular fasciitis, 403, 407, 408
Normal anatomy, 27, 28, 32

P
Paget lesion, 445, 451
Papillary ductal carcinoma in situ, 116, 117
Papillary tumors, 82, 120
Papilloma, 38, 82, 111–116, 136, 143, 159–161, 166, 177, 193, 205,
        211, 311, 314, 423–424, 434, 447, 487, 489
Pathologic response, 332, 373, 383–385
Pathology report, 59, 240, 327, 328, 331, 387
Peripheral papillomas, 109–111, 113, 114
Phyllodes, 183, 185, 190, 191, 194–196, 198–202, 276, 319, 416, 418,
        419, 425, 472
Phyllodes tumor, 165, 319, 403, 408, 416, 418, 419, 425, 472
Prognosis, 79, 116, 118, 127, 252, 262, 263, 273, 277, 327–330, 332,
        337, 338, 342, 351, 353, 358, 386, 388, 414, 419, 439, 455,
        459, 460, 469
Protein, 4, 95, 96, 146, 155–157, 159, 161, 236, 248, 262, 270, 305,
        319, 322, 323, 363, 412, 414, 417, 449, 453, 454
Pseudoangiomatous stromal hyperplasia (PASH), 192, 319, 406, 408
Psoriasis, 493

R

Radiologic changes, 374–375
Residual tumor, 337, 341, 374–376, 383–388, 487

S

Sampling, 63, 71, 72, 75, 76, 136, 192, 201, 220, 223, 328, 383–385, 387, 399, 403, 419, 475–489
Sarcoma(s), 78, 106, 261, 319, 403, 407, 408, 416, 418, 419
Sentinel lymph node (SLN), 5, 156, 196, 322–323, 342, 350, 373, 391–402
Solid papillary carcinoma, 109, 119, 120, 285, 286, 311
Special type, 63, 72, 118, 120, 143, 145, 239, 439, 455
Spindle cell metaplastic carcinomas, 180, 319, 403, 407, 408
Stage, 2, 5, 70, 91, 92, 103, 105, 143, 147, 152, 221, 227, 254, 270, 274, 330, 351, 388, 433

Staging, 4, 44, 120, 330, 331, 391, 392, 394–397, 439, 475
Syringomatous adenoma, 143, 447–450

T

Taxonomic, 263

U

Usual ductal hyperplasia, 110, 113, 114, 119, 132, 133, 138, 139, 141–143, 147, 148, 175, 176, 187, 189, 205–215, 217–219, 224, 308, 424, 426, 429, 430, 449

V

Vitiligo, 494

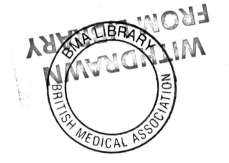

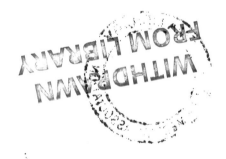